POSTOPERATIVE PAIN MANAGEMENT

POSTOPERATIVE PAIN MANAGEMENT:
An Evidence-Based Guide to Practice

GEORGE SHORTEN, MD, PhD, FRCA, FFARCSI
Department of Anesthesia and Intensive Care Medicine
Cork University Hospital and University College Cork
Cork, Ireland

DANIEL B. CARR, MD, FABPM, FFPMANZCA(Hon)
Professor of Anesthesiology and Medicine (Adjunct)
Tufts University School of Medicine
Saltonstall Professor of Pain Research
Tufts–New England Medical Center
Boston, Massachusetts
Chief Executive Officer and Chief Medical Officer
Javelin Pharmaceuticals, Inc.
Cambridge, Massachusetts

DOMINIC HARMON, MD, FRCA, FFARCSI
Consultant Anaesthesia/Pain Medicine
Mid-Western Regional Hospital
Dooradoyle
Limerick, Ireland

MARGARITA M. PUIG, MD, PhD
Professor of Anaesthesiology and Pain Management
Universitat Autónoma of Barcelona
Vice-Chair of Anaesthesiology
Hospital del Mar
Barcelona, Spain

JOHN BROWNE, FFARCSI
Director of Pain Management Services
Cork University Hospital
Cork, Ireland

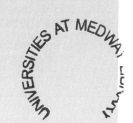

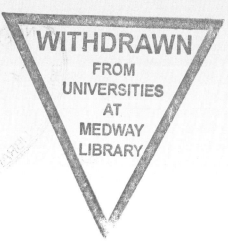

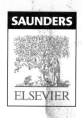

SAUNDERS

ELSEVIER

SAUNDERS
ELSEVIER

1600 John F. Kennedy Blvd.
Ste 1800
Philadelphia, PA 19103-2899

POSTOPERATIVE PAIN MANAGEMENT: ISBN-13: 978-1-4160-2454-9
AN EVIDENCE-BASED GUIDE TO PRACTICE   ISBN-10:   1-4160-2454-9

Copyright © 2006 by Saunders, an imprint of Elsevier Inc.

Library of Congress Cataloging-in-Publication Data
Postoperative pain management: an evidence-based guide to practice/[edited by] George Shorten...[et al.].
   p. ; cm.
   ISBN 1-4160-2454-9
   1. Postoperative pain–Treatment. 2. Postoperative care. 3. Evidence-based medicine. I. Shorten, George.
   [DNLM: 1. Pain, Postoperative–therapy. 2. Evidence-Based Medicine. WO 184 P8578 2006]
   RB127.P672 2006
   617′.9195–dc22   2005056313

Executive Publisher: Natasha Andjelkovic
Developmental Editor: Jean Nevius
Publishing Services Manager: Tina Rebane
Project Manager: Amy Norwitz
Design Direction: Steven Stave
Cover Designer: Steven Stave
Marketing Manager: Dana Butler

Printed in the United States of America

Last digit is the print number: 9   8   7   6   5   4   3   2   1

CONTRIBUTORS

SALAHADIN ABDI, MD, PhD
Associate Professor of Anesthesiology
Harvard Medical School
Director, Massachusetts General Hospital Pain Center
Boston, Massachusetts
The Principles of Evidence-Based Practice

DONAL BUGGY, MD, MSc, DME, FRCPI, FFARCSI, FRCA
Senior Lecturer in Anaesthesia and Intensive Care
  Medicine
University College Dublin
Consultant in Anaesthesia and Intensive Care Medicine
Mater Misericordiae University Hospital
Dublin, Ireland
Nonconventional and Adjunctive Analgesia

DANIEL B. CARR, MD, FABPM, FFPMANZCA(Hon)
Professor of Anesthesiology and Medicine (Adjunct)
Tufts University School of Medicine
Saltonstall Professor of Pain Research
Tufts–New England Medical Center
Boston, Massachusetts
Chief Executive Officer and Chief Medical Officer
Javelin Pharmaceuticals, Inc.
Cambridge, Massachusetts
Accessing and Assessing Medical Evidence

JEREMY N. CASHMAN, BSc, MB,BS, MD, FRCA
Honorary Senior Lecturer
St. George's Hospital Medical School
Consultant Anaesthetist
St. George's Hospital
Department of Anaesthetics
London, England
Patient-Controlled Analgesia

RACHEL A. FARRAGHER, MB, FCARCSI
Lecturer in Anaesthesia
University College Hospital Galway
Galway, Ireland
Postoperative Pain Management after Cesarean Section

KATE FITZGERALD, MSc, FCARCSI, SpR in Anaesthesia
Specialist Registrar in Anaesthesia
University College Dublin
Mater Misericordiae University Hospital
Dublin, Ireland
Nonconventional and Adjunctive Analgesia

HENRY FRIZELLE, MD, FFARCSI
Consultant Anaesthetist
Mater Misericordiae University Hospital
Dublin, Ireland
Mechanisms of Postoperative Pain—Nociceptive

DOMINIC HARMON, MD, FRCA, FFARCSI
Consultant Anaesthesia/Pain Medicine
Mid-Western Regional Hospital
Dooradoyle
Limerick, Ireland
**Regional and Peripheral Techniques;
  Postoperative Pain Management in the Elderly;
  Postoperative Pain Management in the Ambulatory
  Setting**

JAMES HELSTROM, MD

Instructor
Harvard Medical School
Assistant in Anesthesia
Massachusetts General Hospital
Boston, Massachusetts
**Nonsteroidal Anti-inflammatory Drugs in Postoperative
  Pain**

ROBERT W. HURLEY, MD, PhD

Fellow in Pain Medicine
Johns Hopkins Medical Institutions
Baltimore, Maryland
Postoperative Pain Management and Patient Outcome

GABRIELLA IOHOM, MD, PhD

Senior Lecturer
National University of Ireland
University College Cork
Consultant Anaesthetist
Cork University Hospital
Cork, Ireland
Clinical Assessment of Postoperative Pain

SHYAMALA KARUVANNUR, MD

Assistant Professor
State University of New York at Stony Brook
Stony Brook School of Medicine
Stony Brook, New York
Medical Director of Women's Health
Department of Veterans Affairs
Northport, New York
**Postoperative Pain Management in the Ambulatory
  Setting**

JOEL KATZ, PhD

Professor and Canada Research Chair in Health Psychology
Department of Psychology
York University
Director, Acute Pain Research Unit
Department of Anesthesia and Pain Management
Toronto General Hospital and Mount Sinai Hospital
Toronto, Ontario
Canada
**Prediction and Prevention of Acute Postoperative Pain:
  Moving Beyond Preemptive Analgesia**

BRIAN KINIRONS, MB, FFARCSI

Consultant Anaesthetist
Department of Anaesthesia and Intensive Care
University College Hospital Galway
Consultant Anaesthesiologist
Galway Regional Hospitals
Galway, Ireland
Regional and Peripheral Techniques

JOHN G. LAFFEY, MD, MA, BSc, FFARCSI

Clinical Lecturer
Department of Anaesthesia
National University of Ireland
Consultant Anaesthetist
University College Hospital Galway
Galway, Ireland
**Postoperative Pain Management after Cesarean
  Section**

YUAN-CHI LIN, MD, MPH

Associate Professor of Anaesthesia and Pediatrics
Harvard Medical School
Senior Associate in Anesthesia and Pain Medicine
Department of Anesthesiology, Perioperative and Pain
  Medicine
Children's Hospital Boston
Boston, Massachusetts
**Postoperative Pain Management in Infants and
  Children**

WILLIAM A. MACRAE, MB,ChB, FRCA

Honorary Senior Lecturer
University of Dundee
University of St. Andrews
Consultant Anaesthetist and Pain Specialist
Ninewells Hospital
Dundee, Scotland
Can We Prevent Chronic Pain after Surgery?

LAXMAIAH MANCHIKANTI, MD

Department of Anesthesiology
University of Louisville School of Medicine
Louisville, Kentucky
Medical Director, Pain Management Center of Paducah
Paducah, Kentucky
The Principles of Evidence-Based Practice

COLIN J. L. McCARTNEY, MB,ChB, FCARCSI, FRCA, FRCPC

Assistant Professor of Anesthesia
University of Toronto Faculty of Medicine
Staff Anesthesiologist
Toronto Western Hospital
Toronto, Ontario
Canada
Use of Opioid Analgesics in the Perioperative Period

DIARMUID McCOY, FFARCSI, FFPMANZCA, DPM(CARCSI)

Consultant in Anaesthesia and Pain Medicine
Department of Anaesthesia, Perioperative Care and Pain
     Medicine
The Geelong Hospital
Barworth Health
Geelong, Victoria
Australia
Postoperative Pain Management in the Elderly

CONNAIL R. McCRORY, LRCP&SI, FFARCSI, FIPP, MD

Clinical Lecturer
Department of Surgery
Trinity College
Consultant Anaesthetist and Pain Specialist
Lead Clinician Pain Medicine
Department of Anaesthesia, Intensive Care and Pain
     Medicine
St. James's Hospital
Dublin, Ireland
Mechanisms of Postoperative Pain—Neuropathic

PETER G. MOORE, MD, PhD

Professor and Chair
Department of Anesthesiology and Pain Medicine
University of California, Davis, School of Medicine
Sacramento, California
Defining Pain Management Objectives

MARCUS MÜLLNER, MD, MSc(Epidemiol)

Associate Professor
Department of Emergency Medicine
Medizinuniversität Wien/Allgemeines Krankenhaus Wien
Vienna, Austria
Accessing and Assessing Medical Evidence

DAMIAN MURPHY, FFARCSI, MD

Consultant Anaesthetist
Department of Anaesthesia, Intensive Care, and Pain
     Relief Service
Cork University Hospital
Wilton, Cork
Ireland
Applied Clinical Pharmacology of Opioids

SRDJAN S. NEDELJKOVIĆ, MD

Assistant Professor of Anaesthesia
Harvard Medical School
Director, Fellowship Education
Pan Management Center
Department of Anesthesiology
Perioperative and Pain Medicine
Brigham and Women's Hospital
Boston, Massachusetts
**Postoperative Pain Management for Patients with Drug
     Dependence**

AHTSHAM NIAZI, FCARCSI

Consultant Anaesthetist
Our Lady's Hospital
Navan, County Meath
Ireland
Use of Opioid Analgesics in the Perioperative Period

JOSEPH PERGOLIZZI, MD

Adjunct Assistant Professor
Department of Medicine
Johns Hopkins University School of Medicine
Baltimore, Maryland
Board of Directors, Coalition for Pain Education
New York, New York
Senior Partner, Naples Anesthesia and Pain Associates
Naples, Florida
Multimodal Analgesic Therapy

NARINDER RAWAL, MD, PhD

Professor of Anesthesiology and Intensive Care
University Hospital
Örebro, Sweden
Acute Pain Services

H. PAUL REDMOND, BSc, MCh, FRCSI

Professor and Head, Department of Surgery
National University of Ireland (Cork)
Professor of Surgery
Cork University Hospital
Wilton, Cork
Ireland
**The Neurohumoral, Inflammatory, and Coagulation
     Responses to Surgery**

CARL E. ROSOW, MD, PhD

Professor of Anaesthesia
Harvard Medical School
Anesthetist
Department of Anesthesia and Critical Care
Massachusetts General Hospital
Boston, Massachusetts
**Nonsteroidal Anti-inflammatory Drugs in Postoperative
     Pain**

NAVPARKASH SANDHU, MS(Surg), MD

Assistant Professor of Anesthesiology
New York University School of Medicine
Associate Attending
Bellevue Hospital Center
Assistant Attending
New York University Medical Center
New York, New York
Postoperative Pain Management in the Ambulatory Setting

CONOR J. SHIELDS, MD, AFRCSI

Senior Specialist Registrar in Surgery
Cork University Hospital and National University of Ireland (Cork)
Wilton, Cork
Ireland
The Neurohumoral, Inflammatory, and Coagulation Responses to Surgery

ULRIKE M. STAMER, MD

Associate Professor of Anesthesiology and Pain Medicine
Department of Anesthesiology and Intensive Care Medicine
University of Bonn
University Hospital Bonn
Bonn, Germany
Postoperative Pain—Genetics and Genomics

FRANK STÜBER, MD

Professor of Anesthesiology and Intensive Care Medicine
Department of Anesthesiology and Intensive Care Medicine
University of Bonn
Bonn, Germany
Postoperative Pain—Genetics and Genomics

RICHARD M. TALBOT, FCARCSI

Clinical Research Fellow
School of Biomolecular and Biomedical Science
The Conway Institute of Biomolecular and Biomedical Research
University College Dublin
Specialist Registrar
Department of Anaesthesia, Intensive Care and Pain Medicine
St. James's Hospital
Dublin, Ireland
Mechanisms of Postoperative Pain—Neuropathic

JEFFREY UPPINGTON, MB,BS, FRCA

Professor of Anesthesiology and Pain Medicine
University of California, Davis, School of Medicine
Vice Chairman, Department of Anesthesiology and Pain Medicine
University of California, Davis, Medical Center
Sacramento, California
Guidelines, Recommendations, Protocols, and Practice

AJAY D. WASAN, MD, MSc

Instructor, Departments of Anesthesiology and Psychiatry
Harvard Medical School
Instructor, Department of Psychiatry
Brigham and Women's Hospital
Boston, Massachusetts
Postoperative Pain Management for Patients with Drug Dependence

OLIVER H. G. WILDER-SMITH, MD, PhD

Associate Professor for Nociception and Pain
Radboud University
Consultant in Anesthesiology and Pain Medicine
Nijmegen Medical Centre
Nijmegen, The Netherlands
Opioids: Excitatory Effects—Hyperalgesia, Tolerance, and the Postoperative Period

LEONARD M. WILLS, BSc

Remedica Medical Education and Publishing
London, England
Multimodal Analgesic Therapy

CHRISTOPHER L. WU, MD

Associate Professor of Anesthesiology and Critical Care Medicine
Johns Hopkins University School of Medicine
Baltimore, Maryland
Postoperative Pain Management and Patient Outcome

FOREWORD

The subject of this book, acute pain management, has come of age only relatively recently. As long ago as 1971, I published one of the first papers to examine the impact of effective acute pain management on an objective parameter linked to outcome.[1] However, very little momentum existed at that time to pursue improvements in acute pain management and to evaluate efficacy, side effects, and outcomes in a rigorous manner. Thus, when I was asked to assemble a monograph on acute pain management in critical care in 1984, I found only small improvements in the situation[2]; surprisingly, although there have now been major improvements in postoperative pain management, there is a substantial lack of high-quality studies on pain management in critical care units even today.

The major international body responsible for fostering research in the field of pain, the International Association for the Study of Pain (IASP), had focused predominantly on the treatment of chronic noncancer pain since its inception in 1974. When I became president of IASP in 1987, I identified acute pain management as a new major target for IASP, resulting in the production of a key IASP policy document that set a clinical framework for improved acute pain management.[3] This document, however, did not provide a critical analysis of the research literature underpinning acute pain management that was rapidly accumulating. In 1992, a milestone was achieved by one of the editors of this textbook, Professor Dan Carr, who chaired the committee producing the first evidence-based medicine clinical practice guideline on acute pain management.[4] The Agency for Health Care Policy and Research (AHCPR) publication from the United States was the first in a broad-ranging program to develop guidelines for clinical care, and thus the choice of acute pain was particularly significant.

In 1995, I was recruited to chair a Working Party of the Australian National Health and Medical Research Council (NHMRC), which produced a very broad-ranging clinical practice guideline on all aspects of acute pain management across medical and surgical disciplines in 1998.[5] This NHMRC document was revised and published by the Australian & New Zealand College of Anaesthetists in mid-2005.[6] Thus, the current era represents a major change with respect to the availability of higher quality studies and a rigorous process for accessing and assessing medical evidence, to provide a basis for improved treatment of acute pain. Also, the milieu for changing attitudes to and practices regarding acute pain

has been set by editorials calling for acute pain management to be a basic human right.[7,8]

It is in this milieu that *Postoperative Pain Management: An Evidence-Based Guide to Practice* has been produced. The editors, George Shorten, Daniel Carr, Dominic Harmon, Margarita Puig, and John Browne, have surpassed themselves in making a major contribution to the improved management of postoperative pain. Their book draws on all of the important materials referred to and places evidence-based acute pain management in the broader context of evidence-based medicine.

The text is assembled such that it is accessible to the reader and is more like a textbook than the practice guidelines that have been published to date. There is also an emphasis on providing the clinician with the means to bridge the gap between current knowledge and practice. The first three chapters provide a readable introduction to evidence-based practice, accessing and assessing medical evidence, and the differences between guidelines, standards, protocols, and policies. An important distinction is made in Chapter 1 between the loose term "evidence-based medicine" and the term "evidence-based practice," which integrates the best available evidence with all aspects of individual patient decision-making to determine the best clinical care of the patient. This distinction highlights the fact that this text is clearly pitched at the clinician. Thus, readers will find important insights into accessing and assessing medical evidence and how such material is integrated into guidelines, recommendations, protocols, and practice.

All healthcare professionals will benefit from the precise and up-to-date coverage of the scientific basis of postoperative pain and analgesia in Section II of the text. Although such material is available elsewhere, there are particularly clear presentations of the injury response to surgery and the mechanisms of nociceptive and neuropathic postoperative pain. The chapter on genetics and genomics provides some up-to-the-minute insights into how genetics is likely to influence the management of postoperative pain at the present time and to a much greater degree in the future. This is certainly an exciting prospect. Another important topic highlighted in the text is the influence of effective postoperative pain management on patient outcome.

Section III, on the various options for management of postoperative pain, is very comprehensive and has drawn appropriately on clinical practice guidelines and other material.

The "levels of evidence" approach is used in some of the chapters (such as Chapter 16, Patient-Controlled Analgesia), but in other chapters a more descriptive approach is used to indicate the strength of the evidence for various treatments. In either case, the reader obtains a clear picture of the strength of evidence for all of the treatment options.

An important chapter deals with the more contemporary concept of "prediction and prevention" of acute postoperative pain, rather than the earlier concept of "preemptive analgesia." Also, a key chapter on multimodal analgesia gives a very lucid rationale for what has clearly become a major new framework for improved postoperative pain management. As has been the case in recent clinical practice guidelines, appropriate attention is given to the management of postoperative pain in specific clinical settings, such as in children and the elderly, in those with drug dependence, and in the settings of cesarean section and ambulatory surgery. Finally, an issue of major humanitarian and economic importance is considered—namely, prevention of chronic pain after surgery. New insights into mechanisms and improved management options presented in this text give new hope that the goal of prevention of persistent pain after surgery might be realized. This is recognized as an increasingly important subject in view of mounting evidence that persistent pain after surgery is much more prevalent than was previously recognized and thus contributes a substantial segment of the massive problem of persistent or chronic pain.

In my assessment, this text makes a major contribution to the field of acute pain management, and I congratulate the editors and authors.

REFERENCES

1. Cousins MJ, Wright CJ: Graft, muscle and skin blood flow changes after epidural block in vascular surgery. Surg Obstet Gynecol 1971;133:59–65.
2. Cousins MJ, Phillips GD: Acute Pain Management. Clinics in Critical Care Medicine. London, Churchill Livingstone, 1986.
3. Ready LB, Edwards WT: Management of Acute Pain: A Practical Guide. Seattle, Wash, IASP Publications, 1992.
4. Carr DB, Jacox AK, Chapman CR, et al: Acute Pain Management: Operative or Medical Procedures and Trauma. Clinical Practice Guideline No.1; AHCPR Publication No. 92-0032. Rockville, Md, AHCPR, 1992.
5. Acute Pain Management: Scientific Evidence (1st ed). Canberra, Australia, NHMRC, 1998, http://www.nhmrc.gov.au/publications/synopses/cp104syn.htm.
6. Acute Pain Management: Scientific Evidence (2nd ed). Melbourne, Australia, ANZCA, 2005, http://www.nhmrc.gov.au/publications/synopses/cp104syn.htm..
7. Cousins MJ: Relief of acute pain: A basic human right? Med J Aust 2000;172:3–4.
8. Cousins MJ, Brennan F, Carr DB: Pain relief: A universal human right. Pain 2004;112:1–4.

Professor Michael J. Cousins, AM, MD
Professor and Director
Pain Management Research Institute
University of Sydney at Royal North Shore Hospital
St. Leonards, New South Wales
Australia

PREFACE

In 1906, George Bernard Shaw wrote in *The Doctor's Dilemma,* "When doctors write or speak to the public about operations, they imply that chloroform has made surgery painless. People who have been operated upon know better." Surprisingly little progress was made in controlling postoperative pain in the ensuing century, until a confluence of factors directed attention to the generally poor state of postoperative pain control. First was progress in understanding both the neurobiology of pain and the association between poor pain control and the risks of postoperative complications such as respiratory insufficiency and myocardial infarction. Second was the rise of consumerism, culminating in the recognition of pain control as a human right and healthcare standard. Third was the increasing economic pressure on healthcare systems worldwide, which led to incentives for earlier postoperative discharge. Recognition that inadequate pain control can delay discharge or increase the likelihood of readmission added a strong motive to control pain effectively during elective surgery.

The growth in medical interest in acute pain control led to the development of acute pain services by departments of anesthesia and fostered intellectual interest in the previously overlooked topic of postoperative pain control. Hundreds of studies of one or another technique appeared, and clinicians found themselves challenged by the amount and variable quality of this new information. Evidence-based guidelines on acute pain control began to appear in the early 1990s, and since then professional and governmental organizations have prepared practice guidelines and evidence reviews to increasingly higher standards. Still, current quality assessments point to a continuing gap between what could be achieved in clinical practice by following best practices, and what is actually achieved.

Although important scientific and technical advances in postoperative pain management have taken place during the past decade, their effect on clinical practice has been limited by several factors: (1) the rapid rate at which new information has become available (information inflation); (2) inadequate or inconsistent training and education to understand new techniques or drugs; (3) uncertainty among clinicians as to which advances justify a change in practice (i.e., are supported by credible evidence); and (4) practical or logistical issues such as costs, local factors (availability of equipment or expertise), patient expectations, and insufficient support staff.

Our textbook addresses the first three of these factors in the following ways:
- By providing a framework within which readers can decide if practices are justified (or not) by the best evidence currently available.
- By presenting this information in a way that is accessible to all healthcare workers responsible for the management of postoperative pain. These practitioners include anesthesiologists, nurse anesthetists, surgeons, clinical nurse specialists, recovery room (PACU) nurses, and those working on surgical wards.
- By being suitable to both trainees and practitioners who wish to adopt current best practices.
- By providing a companion self-assessment interactive CD-ROM to maximize the educational impact of the information presented.

Since the first use of the term "evidence-based medicine" in 1992 by Guyatt and his colleagues and its adoption in the first governmental clinical practice guideline on acute postoperative pain management that same year, this approach has been adopted enthusiastically in principle (but more slowly in practice) around the world. As clinicians, the editors of this textbook have, in our combined experience, managed many thousands of patients with postoperative pain. We are strong supporters of an evidence-based approach to the prevention and treatment of postoperative pain, although we cannot recommend or advise methods that are not feasible and practical. We believe that the "knowledge to practice" gap must be kept narrow so that no patients fall through it. Postoperative pain is unforgiving of delayed or suboptimal treatment. The interval during which we can effectively intervene is short, and the implications of failing to do so can last a patient's lifetime.

The evidence base available to us is incomplete but improving in amount and quality. Still, the proportion of investigations that lack validity is great. The "recipe" approach to postoperative pain management is still widespread. Also, many important clinical questions will not be formulated until the problems have been recognized.

Integration of best evidence with an individual patient's preferences, circumstances, and suffering is more important and more difficult in pain management than in almost any other clinical problem. The difficulties range from opioid tolerance or dependence in the preoperative state, to the presence of anticoagulants that contraindicate certain regional anesthetic techniques, to patient distress and anxiety caused by sleeplessness or ominous surgical findings. Sadly, the responsibility for postoperative pain management may rest with someone who regards it as incidental, unimportant, or peripheral to his or her "main" duties. In other cases, management may be suboptimal not because of lack of awareness but because of lack of technical expertise (e.g., for peripheral nerve blockade) or because of economic or administrative factors (e.g., inability to support an acute pain management team).

The editors and authors of this textbook firmly believe that the principles of evidence-based practice can be applied to postoperative pain management in the "real world."

Convincing others of this view is an ambitious aspiration but is supported by leaders in the pain community worldwide. We hope that you, the reader, will find that the investment of your time in reading the text and using the CD-ROM is well rewarded.

George Shorten
Daniel B. Carr
Dominic Harmon
Margarita M. Puig
John Browne

ACKNOWLEDGMENTS

Dr. Shorten offers thanks to Bronagh, Geraldine, and Jack for their unfailing support, and to that most expert solver of problems, Mrs. Renee Mooney.

Dr. Carr gratefully acknowledges the administrative assistance of Evelyn Hall at Tufts–New England Medical Center; the ongoing support for scholarly activities provided by the Saltonstall Fund for Pain Research of Tufts–New England Medical Center; and the encouragement and understanding for the time commitment required for this volume on the part of his family and his colleagues at Javelin Pharmaceuticals, Inc.

Drs. Shorten and Carr, like so many before them, are grateful for the support and encouragement of Dr. Richard J. Kitz in their early academic pursuits.

CONTENTS

1 The Principles of Evidence-Based Practice

SALAHADIN ABDI • LAXMAIAH MANCHIKANTI

Evidence-based medicine is defined as the conscientious, explicit, and judicious use of the current best evidence in making decisions about the care of individual patients.[1] The past decade has been marked by unprecedented interest in evidence-based medicine and the development of various resources that can provide valid and reliable information about healthcare, including clinical practice guidelines. Thus, clinical decisions are increasingly being made on the basis of research-based evidence rather than expert opinion or clinical experience alone.

The need for careful scientific evaluation of clinical practice became a prominent focus during the second half of the 20th century. Tunis et al,[2] affiliated with Centers for Medicare and Medicaid Services and the Agency for Health Care Research and Quality, described that the demonstration of pervasive and persistent unexplained variations in clinical practice[3] and high rates of inappropriate care,[4] combined with increased expenditures, has fueled a steadily rising demand for evidence of clinical effectiveness. It is believed that the limited amount of high-quality evidence is partly responsible for geographical differences in practice, inappropriate care, and also the limited success of quality improvement efforts.[5,6] As a result, spurred by the growing ease of access to and retrieval of large amounts of biomedical information over the Internet, policymakers, clinicians, and patients and their families have become interested in applying valid and reliable information in their everyday healthcare choices.

The practice of evidence-based medicine requires the integration of individual clinical expertise with the best available external evidence from systematic research. Decisions that affect the care of patients should be made with due weight being accorded to *all* valid, relevant information. This information includes valid and relevant clinical evidence derived from randomized controlled trials, and *all* types of evidence, patient preferences, and resources. *All* implies that an active search should be made for all information that is valid and relevant and that an assessment should be made of the accuracy of the information and the applicability of the evidence to the decision in question. On the other hand, evidence-based practice assigns more weight to evidence that is unbiased than to evidence that is likely to be biased.

The following four basic tenets originally defined evidence-based practice[7]:

1. Recognition of the patient's problem and construction of a structured clinical question.
2. The ability to efficiently and effectively search the medical literature to retrieve the best available evidence to answer the clinical question.
3. Critical appraisal of the evidence.
4. Integration of the evidence with all aspects of individual patient decision-making to determine the best clinical care of the patient.

Thus, *evidence-based medicine* is a loose term that has been used at different times not only to present a particular view but also to advance personal philosophy, bias, and conjecture. This distortion of motives and methods has led to a multitude of questions as to whether evidence-based medicine is truly based on evidence.

Searching for the Evidence

To achieve balance in evidence-based pain management and also to include all types of evidence, one must literally include all types of evidence—not only systematic reviews and randomized clinical trials but also all published reports of observational studies and diagnostic test studies. Thus, a search strategy should include all sources easily available to obtain the literature. On the other hand, because of differences in the strength and consistency of published literature about many pain treatments, many authorities have advocated including separate dimensions to describe the nature of the evidence compared with its strength and consistency. For example, two weakly powered, low-quality, randomized controlled trials that reach opposite conclusions may, in aggregate, be less persuasive than one large, carefully conducted observational trial.

It has been shown that if one uses only MEDLINE to search the literature, roughly half of all known published randomized controlled trials can be identified, depending on the area and specific question.[1] Systematic reviews of analgesic trials and other studies have described under-representation of non–English language references in MEDLINE and the inclusion of only published articles.[1] Thus, there is the potential for publication bias and language bias. Further, these reviews showed that depending on the country of origin, there is also potential for geographical bias. For example, publications from China were more likely to find acupuncture efficacious than publications from outside China.

Another problem with using only databases for a literature search is that even though many of the studies may be included in a database such as MEDLINE, it may not be easy to identify all those that are relevant. Possible reasons for poor retrieval are (1) the search used was too narrow, (2) the indexing of studies in MEDLINE is inadequate, and (3) the original reports may have been too vague. The same issues are applicable to EMBASE. In general, MEDLINE provides wide coverage of many English language journals. In contrast, EMBASE can be used to increase coverage of articles in the European languages. The overlap between MEDLINE and EMBASE is approximately 34%, even though it can vary between 10% and 75% for specific topics. Thus, one cannot rely on searching a single database if one wishes to prepare a comprehensive review of the literature. Further, dependence on databases may miss many non-indexed journals, proceedings of scientific meetings, and peer-reviewed articles from scientific newsletters. Search of the reference lists of articles found through databases may also identify further studies for consideration. In fact, the Cochrane Collaboration (www.cochrane.org) advises that reviewers should check the references of all relevant articles that are obtained through a database search. Thus, additional potentially relevant articles that are identified should be retrieved and assessed for possible inclusion in the review. When doing this type of search, however, one should keep in mind the potential for reference bias and for a tendency to cite only studies supporting one's own views. One can guard against this bias by using a multitude of search strategies.

Assessing an Original Report

The acme of clinical research is the randomized, double-blind, controlled trial. Randomized controlled trials were introduced into clinical medicine in the 1940s, when streptomycin was evaluated in the treatment of tuberculosis.[8] Since then, randomized controlled trials have become the "gold standard" for assessing the effectiveness of therapeutic agents.[9–11] In 1982, Sacks et al[12] compared published randomized controlled studies with those that used observational designs. In this landmark evaluation, they showed that the agent being tested was considered effective in 44 of 56 trials (79%) in observational studies using historical controls but in only 10 of 50 randomized controlled trials (20%). Thus, these researchers concluded that bias in patient selection may irreversibly weigh the outcome of historically controlled trials in favor of new therapies in observational studies.

However, a 2002 evaluation by Kjaergard and Als-Nielsen[13] of randomized clinical trials published in the *British Medical Journal* explored the association between competing interests and authors' conclusions. This epidemiological study concluded that authors' interpretations of results in randomized clinical trials significantly favored the experimental interventions whenever financial competing interests (i.e., funding of trials by for-profit organizations) were declared. These conclusions were based on review of 159 trials from 12 medical specialties. These investigators also concluded that presence of other competing interests (personal, academic, or political) were not significantly associated with authors' conclusions. Similar conclusions were drawn in a study of trials of multiple myeloma by Djulbegovic et al.[14] These researchers found that authors' interpretations of their trial results favored the experimental interventions over the standard interventions more in trials that were funded by the pharmaceutical industry than in trials that were funded by nonprofit organizations.[14]

The random assignment of subjects to either experimental or controlled status is considered to be scientifically impeccable. However, random assignment does not confer an absolute protection against bias. It simply reduces the likelihood that such bias occurs. Because randomized controlled trials are often complicated and difficult to conduct, they are usually restricted to very homogeneous groups of patients. Often, the investigators are not actively concerned about how subjects are obtained and rely on random allocation to distribute any differences equally between the two groups. As a result, randomized trials often trade internal validity (similar demographics in experimental and control groups, and tightness of comparisons) for external validity (generalizability).[15] Hence, randomization does not provide the protective shield that some believe it does. Further, many patients refuse to participate in the process with the belief that randomization always puts them in the control groups. Thus, it does not seem feasible to rely exclusively on randomized controlled trials for all, or even most, of the needed empirical data linking outcome to the process of care.[16]

In such circumstances, particularly when randomized controlled trials are unavailable, one must rely on outcomes research. Generally, a difference in outcome between a treatment and a control group can be caused by chance, by confounding, or by bias due to differences between the groups, differences in handling the groups, and the true effect of intervention. Confounding and bias are avoided in the design of a trial by randomization, single blinding, or double blinding. Thus, randomization is considered to be a cornerstone of trial design to avoid bias and maintain similarity between treatment and control groups. Randomization by the tossing of a coin (or any equivalent method) ensures that the physician running the trial is not consciously or unconsciously allocating certain patients to a particular group. Without randomization, trials of surgical versus medical techniques are susceptible to selection bias. It is assumed that low-risk patients are much more likely to be assigned to the surgical group, leaving high-risk patients to be managed medically. Assigning volunteers to the treatment group and those who do not volunteer to the control group is also likely to result in a biased comparison—volunteers may be different in many respects from patients who do not volunteer.[17] The criticism has also been advanced against allocation to treatment or control groups on an alternate-day basis, through alternating numbers, or with another assigned "preformed" methodology. Even though randomization is believed to ensure that the two groups will differ only by chance, this result is not guaranteed in practice.

Systematic reviews and meta-analyses represent a rigorous method of compiling scientific evidence to answer questions about clinical issues of diagnosis and treatment. In both types of analyses, methodological criteria and controls are crucial. Apart from these two, consensus is also utilized as evidence. However, published studies alone may not provide all the necessary information or complete information regarding details of clinical practice. Consequently, additional sources of information and evidence, as well as consensus, are sought. The consensus is generally obtained from expert committees, but it may also be extended to other experts in the field or obtained through open-forum presentations. Similar to meta-analysis and systematic reviews, health technology assessment (HTA) is another commonly used technique in the evaluation of evidence. HTAs are systematically developed recommendations that assist the practitioner and the patient in making decisions about health care. They may be adapted, modified, or rejected according to healthcare needs or constraints.

Grading the Strength of a Body of Evidence

Systems for grading the strength of a body of evidence are multiple; they are less uniform and less consistent than those for rating study quality.[18] As with the quality rating systems, selecting among the evidence grading systems depends on the reason for measuring evidence strength, the type of studies that are being summarized, and the structure of the review panel. Domains for rating the overall strength of a body of evidence are listed in Table 1–1. The National Health and Medical Research Council (NHMRC)[19] described five key points for considering levels of evidence, which are listed in Table 1–2. Some systems are extremely cumbersome to use, requiring substantial resources, whereas others are incomplete and not comprehensive. Table 1–3 shows the designation of

levels of evidence from level I through level V.[20,21] A further discussion of the value or worth of an individual report or a body of evidence can be found in Chapter 2.

TABLE 1–2	Key Points in Consideration of the Level of Evidence

- Resolution of differences in the conclusions reached about effectiveness from studies at differing levels of evidence or within a given level of evidence.
- Resolution of the discrepancies is an important task in the compilation of an evidence summary.
- Inclusion of biostatistical and epidemiological advice on how to search for possible explanations for the disagreements before data are rejected as being an unsuitable basis on which to make recommendations.
- Recognition of the fact that it may not be feasible to undertake randomized controlled trials in all situations. Guidelines should be used on the best available evidence.
- Recognition of the fact that it may be necessary to use evidence from different study designs for different aspects of the treatment effect.

Adapted from How to Use the Evidence: Assessment and Application of Scientific Evidence. Canberra, Commonwealth of Australia, National Health and Medical Research Council, 2000, pp 1–84.

TABLE 1–1	Domains for Rating the Overall Strength of a Body of Evidence	
Domain	**Definition**	
Quality	The quality of all relevant studies for a given topic, where "quality" is defined as the extent to which a study's design, conduct, and analysis have minimized selection, measurement, and confounding biases	
Quantity	The magnitude of treatment effect The number of studies that have evaluated the given topic The overall sample size across all included studies	
Consistency	For any given topic, the extent to which similar findings are reported from work using similar and different study designs	

Adapted from West S, King V, Carey TS, et al: Systems to Rate the Strength of Scientific Evidence. Evidence Report/Technology Assessment No. 47; AHRQ Publication No. 02-E016. Rockville, Md, University of North Carolina and Agency for Healthcare Research and Quality, 2002.

TABLE 1–3	Designation of Levels of Evidence
Level I	*Conclusive:* Research-based evidence with multiple relevant and high-quality scientific studies or consistent reviews of meta-analyses.
Level II	*Strong:* Research-based evidence from at least one properly designed randomized controlled trial; or research-based evidence from multiple properly designed studies of smaller size or from multiple low-quality trials.
Level III	*Moderate:* (a) Evidence obtained from well-designed pseudo-randomized controlled trials (alternate allocation or some other method); (b) evidence obtained from comparative studies with concurrent controls and allocation not randomized (cohort studies, case-controlled studies, or interrupted time series with a control group); (c) evidence obtained from comparative studies with historical control, two or more single-arm studies, or interrupted time series without a parallel control group.
Level IV	*Limited:* Evidence from well-designed non-experimental studies from more than one center or research group; or conficting evidence with inconsistent findings in multiple trials.
Level V	*Indeterminate:* Opinions of respected authorities, based on clinical evidence, descriptive studies, or reports of expert committees.

Adapted and modified from Australian and New Zealand College of Anaesthetists and Faculty of Pain Medicine: Acute Pain Management: Scientific Evidence, 2nd ed. Canberra, Australia, National Health and Medical Research Council, 2005, pp v–vii.

Conclusion

The practice of evidence-based medicine is performed by evaluating and synthesizing the best available evidence. Subsequently, practice guidelines, parameters, or clinical pathways are systematically developed, on the basis of an unbiased literature synthesis, to help the practitioner and the patient make decisions about healthcare. Practice recommendations may be adapted, modified, or rejected according to clinical needs and constraints. Consequently, the practice of evidence-based medicine offers the possibility of transcending individual limitations, such as narrow clinical experience, distorted memory that assigns greater weight to remarkable if anecdotal responses to certain interventions, and building on a myriad of clinical observations that may discern a "signal" between treatment groups only after thousands of patients are studied. Publication of the first explicitly evidence-based clinical practice guideline on postoperative acute pain management[22] was a sentinel event marking the application of such techniques to this field. Just as courts of law debate whether evidence is admissible and how best to weigh it, but will never revert to reaching verdicts in the absence of evidence, clinicians have acknowledged the importance of relying on unbiased clinical evidence in their daily practice. Improved means of accessing repositories of evidence on the Internet will only accelerate this already robust trend.

REFERENCES

1. McQuay H, Moore A (eds): An Evidence Based Resource for Pain Relief. New York, Oxford University Press, 1998.
2. Tunis SR, Stryer DB, Clancy CM: Practical clinical trials: Increasing the value of clinical research for decision making in clinical and health policy. JAMA 2003;290:1624–1632.
3. Wennberg J, Gittelsohn A: Small area variation in health care delivery. Sci Am 1973;182:1102–1108.
4. Schuster MA, McGlynn EA, Brook RH: How good is the quality of health care in the United States? Milbank Q 1998;76:517–563.
5. Eddy DM, Billings J: The quality of medical evidence: Implications for quality of care. Health Aff (Milwood) 1988;7:19–32.
6. McNeil BJ. Shattuck lecture—Hidden barriers to improvement in the quality of care. N Engl J Med 2001;345:1612–1620.
7. Hatala R, Guyatt G: Evaluating the teaching of evidence-based medicine. JAMA 2002;288:1110–1112.
8. Medical Research Council: Streptomycin treatment of pulmonary tuberculosis. BMJ 1948;2:769–782.
9. Byar DP, Simon RM, Friedewald WT, et al: Randomized clinical trials: Perspectives on some recent ideas. N Engl J Med 1976;295:74–80.
10. Feinstein AR: Current problems and future challenges in randomized clinical trials. Circulation 1984;70:767–774.
11. Abel U, Koch A: The role of randomization in clinical studies: Myths and beliefs. J Clin Epidemiol 1999;52:487–497.
12. Sacks H, Chalmers TC, Smith H Jr: Randomized versus historical controls for clinical trials. Am J Med 1982;72:233–240.
13. Kjaergard LK, Als-Nielsen B: Association between competing interests and authors' conclusions: Epidemiological study of randomized clinical trials published in the BMJ. BMJ 2002;325:1–4.
14. Djulbegovic B, Lacevic M, Cantor A, et al: The uncertainty principle and industry sponsored research. Lancet 2000; 356:635–638.
15. Kane RL: Approaching the outcome question. In Kane RL (ed): Understanding Health Care Outcomes Research. Gaithersburg, Md, Aspen Publishers, 1997, pp 1–15.
16. Concato J, Shah N, Horwitz RI: Randomized, controlled trials, observational studies, and the hierarchy of research designs [see comment]. N Engl J Med 2000;342:1887–1892.
17. Daly LE, Bourke GJ: Epidemiological and clinical research methods. In Daly LE, Bourke GJ (eds): Interpretation and Uses of Medical Statistics. Oxford, Blackwell Science, 2000, pp 143–201.
18. West S, King V, Carey TS, et al: Systems to Rate the Strength of Scientific Evidence. Evidence Report/Technology Assessment No. 47; AHRQ Publication No. 02-E016. Rockville, Md, University of North Carolina and Agency for Healthcare Research and Quality, 2002.
19. How to Use the Evidence: Assessment and Application of Scientific Evidence. Canberra, Australia, National Health and Medical Research Council, 2000, pp 1–84.
20. Australian and New Zealand College of Anaesthetists and Faculty of Pain Medicine: Acute Pain Management: Scientific Evidence, 2nd ed. Canberra, Australia, National Health and Medical Research Council, 2005, pp v–vii.
21. Manchikanti L, Heavner JE, Racz GB, et al; Methods for evidence synthesis in interventional pain management. Pain Physician 2003;6: 89–111.
22. Carr DB, Jacox AK, Chapman CR, et al: Acute Pain Management: Operative or Medical Procedures and Trauma. Clinical Practice Guidline No. 1; AHCPR Publication No. 92-0023. Rockville, Md, AHCPR, 1992.

2 Accessing and Assessing Medical Evidence

MARCUS MÜLLNER • DANIEL B. CARR

When caring for our patients, each of us makes countless decisions every day: Shall I use this diagnostic procedure? How do I interpret these results? What is the best treatment for this particular patient? The bedside decision-making process involves focusing on specific knowledge about a particular situation and an individual patient. Such working knowledge applied to individual patients on a daily basis is often amalgamated with general conclusions drawn from large populations or, at least, from groups of patients who were studied in one or more clinical trials.[1] Thus, in practice, qualitative knowledge is integrated with quantitative knowledge in a fashion that is subject to clinician bias.[2] This chapter focuses on the quantitative knowledge that, increasingly, directs clinical decision-making. In the present era of evidence-based practice as well as in other clinically linked dimensions, such as persuading insurers to pay for the treatments we provide and juries to conclude that we practiced appropriately, we are expected to inform our decisions with measurable quantities. To make individualized and patient-tailored decisions, we first need to know some general facts. Here are some typical examples: What effect can I expect on average from a particular treatment? What are the risks of a particular treatment? Will I detect a condition with this diagnostic procedure? Does a negative test result really mean that a patient does not have the condition?

This chapter addresses how to access and assess the scientific literature, particularly that relevant to acute pain, but for conciseness we focus only on therapeutic interventions. Other issues, such as those related to prognosis, the value of diagnostic tests, and economic analyses, are very well discussed on the website of the National Health Services Centre for Evidence Based Medicine in Oxford.[1] We use the term "therapeutic intervention" in the broadest sense, ranging from drug treatment to surgical interventions to behavioral interventions—indeed, to mean any intervention that aims to influence the course of a disease beneficially.

We first describe how to assess the literature before we discuss how to access it, because certain types of research are not suitable for evidence-based practice and there is no need for a busy practicing physician to access such studies.

How Much Can We Learn from Research?

Before delving into methodological details we must first raise a philosophical point. Where one of the authors (MM) studied medicine, in Vienna, students are not exposed to the philosophy of science during medical school; perhaps this is true in many medical schools worldwide. This fact is most unfortunate, because the discipline forces us to appreciate how little we know and understand in reality, and how much uncertainty necessarily surrounds what we call "knowledge."[2] In fact, we must acknowledge that the full depth of clinical truth will always remain unknown. The truth is so vast that nobody can know it, not even the most famous specialist practicing solely within his or her specialty. We must accept that we will never know whether, say, diclofenac (and many other nonsteroidal analgesics) really reduces pain in osteoarthritis. The available evidence, however, is so convincing that we—and society at large—do not doubt its efficacy. The next problem arises when we ask ourselves, "How large is the average effect of diclofenac in patients with osteoarthritis?" And the final problem arises with the question, "What adverse effects may occur in patients taking diclofenac for arthritis pain over months to years?" Research can answer none of these questions with perfect precision, but if we have enough evidence (in terms of quality and quantity), we may conclude that our results must be reasonably close to the true state of nature, the clinical truth.

Unfortunately, much of the medical research is of poor quality or flawed.[3] Poor-quality research not only wastes resources but also leads us away from the truth. More often than not, flawed trials exaggerate the effectiveness of an intervention,[4] and occasionally, harmful effects may be masked.[5–7] When one applies quality tools, which are discussed later, it becomes obvious that only a small proportion—far less than 10%—of published studies are suitable for medical decision-making.[8] This disappointing state of affairs is particularly true of pain management, although within this broad area the literature on acute pain treatment contains a larger proportion of high-quality clinical evidence than that on the control of cancer pain or chronic noncancer pain.[9]

Considering the delicate and elusive nature of "knowledge" and the high chances that any given article is flawed, the reader may appreciate that thorough critical assessment of research is compulsory before he or she allows such reports to influence clinical practice.

Assessing the Medical Literature

THE HIERARCHY OF EVIDENCE

Before going into details, we introduce the famous hierarchy of levels of evidence. Various forms of this hierarchy have been proposed, some with slightly differing numbers of strata. There are various stages of sophistication to these levels,[1] but a brief and simple outline is more helpful at this stage (Fig. 2–1).

When one is interested to know whether an intervention is effective, the lowest level of evidence is *expert opinion*. Knowledge that is based on opinion and individual experience is very often flawed. Most of the incremental benefits of new medical treatments are now so small that a single individual or even a group (e.g., one department) cannot perceive them. For example, thousands of patients need to be studied for one to discern the life-saving effect of thrombolytic treatment for acute myocardial infarction. Expert opinion is followed by *case reports and case series*. These are often biased in terms of selecting patients and thus are not representative; further, there is no comparison group. *Observational studies with control groups*, such as case-controlled studies and cohort studies, are clearly better than opinion alone or case series but still rank low. There are various possible problems with these designs, but the main problem is that there usually is a reason (often not apparent) for one patient to receive an intervention and another not to. A comparison between treated and untreated patients is fair if, and only if, allocation of every patient to treatment or no treatment is a random event. Random allocation alone ensures that there are no hidden features that may explain the "effect" of the intervention. In fact, we know that nonrandomized studies often greatly exaggerate the effect of an intervention.[10] Accordingly, a *randomized controlled trial* (RCT) ranks fairly high on

this hierarchy. We need to be aware, however, that a single trial is only a snapshot of the situation. Could one man figure out what the city of London looks like if shown only a picture of the relatively famous Swiss Re Building (Fig. 2–2)?

Would the man know London better if shown a series of pictures a friend took during her last visit to the city? Imagine what the pictures would reveal. Most likely they would be a selection of places she considers attractive, memorable, or both. These would certainly persuade the man that London is an interesting city, but he clearly would not get a representative overall picture. Here a more objective and systematic approach would be required—a comprehensive street map, supplemented by economic and sociological data as to how the city's dwellers earn their living, mingle with one another, and organize a multicultural society. This approach leads us to the highest level of the hierarchy: the *systematic review* of RCTs. Sometimes it is possible to combine the results of several systematically identified trials mathematically; this process is called a *meta-analysis*. The way we informally collect evidence is actually very close to how we take pictures on a holiday trip. We gather evidence that best suits us, either because of ease of access or because we simply like what we see (usually we have preferences that are reinforced when we see them confirmed).

CRITICAL APPRAISAL OF RANDOMIZED CONTROLLED TRIALS

To determine whether an intervention is effective, the study to test it should meet the following two criteria: (1) there should be an intervention group and a control group, and (2) allocation of patients to the various groups should be random. A person with great experience, sophistication, and lots of time could also assess nonrandomized controlled studies as additional evidence. Unfortunately, clinicians are usually very busy and their expertise lies in the practice of medicine, not detailed methodological knowledge. Absent the time to scrutinize such studies, one should ignore any study that is not randomized.

Though crucial, random allocation is just a prerequisite, and further quality criteria should also influence assessment of the results of a trial. The following discussion contains

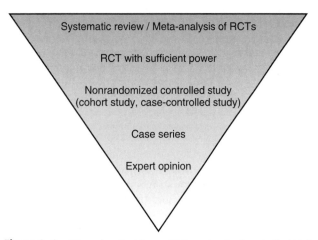

Figure 2–1   Hierarchy of evidence. RCT, randomized controlled trial.

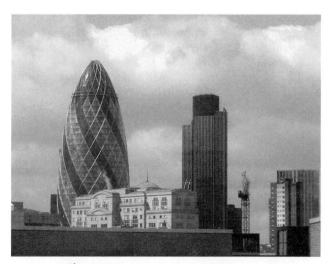

Figure 2–2   Swiss Re Building in London.

a list of questions the reader should pose when assessing an RCT of the efficacy of a treatment.

Does the Intervention Resemble the Intervention I Am Interested In?

The question appears to be self-evident, but there are many situations in which one may evaluate interventions that are similar to the intervention one is interested in but still are not the same. This may happen if there is no evidence on the particular intervention. For example, a surgeon must decide whether to offer epidural infusions of a mixture of hydromorphone and bupivacaine postoperatively after thoracic or upper abdominal surgery, with the goal of improving respiratory outcomes for her patients.[11] She is thinking of implementing this technique in her operating theater and postsurgical ward, but her initial literature search found only RCTs that employed bupivacaine with other morphine-like opioids.[12,13] Still, it seems plausible to draw some inferences from such studies to predict the likely effects of administering an essentially similar epidural solution.

Is There a Control Group?

This crucial point was already discussed.

Was Treatment Allocated Randomly?

This crucial point was already discussed.

Was the Method of Randomization Such that Group Allocation Could Not Be Foreseen?

This question addresses what is also called "allocation concealment." It is a tricky concept. As mentioned previously, people always have preferences. Use of allocation methods such as alternating days, even versus odd birthday dates, and randomization lists posted on the departmental refrigerator allows anticipation of group assignment. This may still lead to an allocation sequence that is as good as random; the problem is that the recruiting physicians might selectively steer patients to one group or another. There is strong evidence that a lack of allocation concealment is associated with an exaggerated estimate for treatment effect.[14] We will never know for any given individual trial whether inflation of the apparent therapeutic effect occurs and how large it is, but such inflation can increase the effect size by 30% to 40% on average.[14] Unfortunately, many studies do not make clear to the reader whether allocation was concealed. If this information is lacking, the reader should assume the worst—that allocation was not concealed—until proven otherwise. A default posture of pessimism is also appropriate for most of the remaining points discussed here.

Was the Person Who Assessed the Outcome Blinded as to Whether Each Patient Was in the Intervention or Control Group?

This point is closely related to those that precede and follow it. Imagine a situation in which the patient is recording pain on a visual analogue scale and the study is not placebo controlled.

Clearly, the outcome assessor (i.e., the patient) is not blind to the intervention. This might influence the effect size, generally to increase it. Blinding is a tricky issue when it comes to reporting. Ideally, every party involved (the patient, the treating physician, the outcome assessor, and the statistician) should not be aware of the allocation. If a study is reported to be "double-blind" but with no specifics as to how this was accomplished, the reader might find entertainment in guessing who did and who did not know. For a more in-depth discussion, see Schultz and Grimes.[15]

Was the Endpoint "Soft" or "Hard"?

In the field of pain treatment, most endpoints are subjective and so may be considered to be "soft." A soft endpoint is acceptable when blinding is assured but becomes very problematic in open-label studies. If, for example, a pharmaceutical company wants to achieve marketing authorization for a drug in Europe or the United States, an open-label study would usually not be acceptable.

Hard endpoints are endpoints for which unblinding cannot lead to a misinterpretation of an effect. The hardest endpoint available is overall mortality. Many technical measurements, such as laboratory parameters, also qualify as hard, but all subjective endpoints are equally soft. The rating of pain intensity on a scale of 0 to 100, either verbally or by means of a line placed by the patient on a 100-mm horizontal scale, is the best-studied and best-validated measure, at least for conscious adults with otherwise normal mental status.[16] Patient global satisfaction with pain treatment received in the hospital, however, may be influenced by many interpersonal factors in addition to effective pain relief per se and is notoriously forgiving of clearly suboptimal acute pain management.[17]

What Did the Control Group Receive?

Ideally, the control group receives a placebo, a pseudo-drug without any effects. Such a placebo should resemble the active drug in appearance, texture, and taste, to ensure that some effects are not caused by wishful thinking on the part of both the patient and the outcome assessor. Certain pain trials have even employed a paradoxically termed "active placebo," meaning an analgesically inactive drug selected as a placebo because it has a known side effect, such as dry mouth or drowsiness, that is expected to occur with the active study drug. The care with which analgesic trials are constructed so as to include a placebo arm (whenever ethically and practically possible) reflects the profound importance and quantitative importance of placebo effects in pain trials. Some pain control interventions clearly cannot be placebo controlled, such as the morphine in a patient-controlled analgesia device that patients in a trial of some other perioperative medication may use for "rescue" medication. Even though placebo acupuncture needles[18] and sham operations,[19] for example, have been used, there are situations in which a study must be open label (i.e., with no placebo control). For example, a continuation study that patients may enter if they have shown a positive response to an active drug during a prior blinded study phase may usefully continue on an open-label basis to gather necessary data on the adverse effects associated with prolonged use of the same agent.

Is the Study Population Sufficiently Similar to My Patients?

This is also an obvious point. Nevertheless it is sometimes quite tricky to compare a study population with one's own patients. Age, gender, ethnicity, comorbidity, and other important baseline features should match. This concept is also known as *external validity*. If a study was conducted in a university hospital but the clinician is working in a nonteaching or nonresearch unit, he or she must be aware that the study patients may be very different from his or her own patients. We know that patients recruited for clinical trials conducted in teaching hospitals are younger and have fewer comorbidities and a much higher adherence to treatment regimens. We also know that the treatment of hypertension is more effective in teaching hospital studies than in primary care studies. In the field of pain treatment, clinical trials customarily exclude patients who have an important comorbidity, are very elderly, or receive potentially confounding multidrug regimens. However, such patients constitute a growing proportion of those treated for acute postoperative pain in the hospital and home settings.

Were Patients Finally Analyzed as Randomized?

This issue is the "intention-to-treat" principle. The intention-to-treat analysis is also a difficult concept. It means that all patients are analyzed according to the group they were originally allocated to, no matter what they really received.

To illustrate this issue, let us use the previous example of epidural opioids to improve postoperative pulmonary function.[20,21] Often, patients who have excellent postsurgical pain control using epidural opioids experience side effects sufficiently severe that they might require an intervention (e.g., low-dose naloxone infusion to reverse hypoventilation or treat refractory pruritus, or insertion of a urinary catheter to treat urinary retention). Such interventions may exclude them from further participation in a trial. Commonly, pain intensity scores from patients who drop out of a trial and scores that were not recorded for some other reason are scored as the last-recorded value carried forward. In theory, carrying the last observation forward at a time when pain is well controlled but at the expense of unsatisfactory side effects may create a distorted picture of the benefits of an intervention, without sufficient weight being given to its risks. Maintaining such patients in a postoperative analgesic trial might augment the aggregate scores for pain intensity if the patients required naloxone to treat side effects, or reduce patient satisfaction if other interventions, such as insertion of a urinary catheter, were necessary. Even though keeping such patients in a trial may decrease the apparent analgesic effect of the intervention, such an approach allows assessment of the effectiveness in real-world circumstances. In daily clinical practice, our devices—in this case, the epidural catheter—also fail sometimes, and a device that is theoretically effective but practically ineffective because it fails too often should simply not be used. If one analyzes data from only those patients who followed the protocol—called the *per protocol analysis*—the effect is much larger. The per protocol analysis mirrors the biological effect, whereas the intention-to-treat analysis mirrors the clinical effect.

Appraisal of the Study

An experienced assessor needs about 1 hour to assess all of the preceding types of information from a study report. The reader is probably now thinking that he or she will not be able to apply these criteria because of lack of time and possibly lack of experience. Fortunately, there is an acceptable shortcut. There are three major quality determinants of RCTs: (1) allocation concealment, (2) intention-to-treat analysis, and (3) blinded outcome assessment. If time is scarce, one should ask these three questions only.

CRITICAL APPRAISAL OF SYSTEMATIC REVIEWS

The authors of a good systematic review will have done all of the previously mentioned quality assessments for the reader, who then must "simply" have to assess whether they did a good job. This means that the appraisal of a systematic review may even be trickier, and the discussion focuses only on key issues. The reader's job should rather be to sort out whether a particular systematic review is really useful. Following are the questions to ask when appraising a systematic review and meta-analysis.

Does the Review Have an Explicit Hypothesis or Aim?

This is one of the key issues that distinguish a conventional review from a systematic review.

Does the Review Include Studies that Were Not Randomized?

A systematic review of the effectiveness of a medical intervention ideally should include only RCTs; if nonrandomized studies are included, they should be analyzed and presented separately because they offer only supportive evidence. I recommend that the clinician who is able to make only a quick appraisal should not consider systematic reviews further if they included nonrandomized studies, even though at times it may make sense to include so-called quasi-randomized trials (e.g., allocation according to alternating days).

Is the Intervention Explicitly Described?

The purpose of this question is obvious.

Are the Endpoints Explicitly Described?

The purpose of this question is obvious.

Is the Target Population Explicitly Defined?

The purpose of this question is obvious.

Is the Search Strategy Explicitly Described?

Ideally, the search is described in such detail that anyone should be able to repeat it and achieve the same results. This means that both the search terms and the databases to which they were applied should be detailed.

How Are the Data Extracted?

All of our actions are riddled with errors (both qualitative and quantitative), and one can anticipate that up to 5% of all data entries are incorrect. This imprecision worsens when judgments are involved.[2] A great deal of judgment may be required in conducting a systematic review, particularly when it comes to trial quality (see next question). Therefore, data should always be extracted by two people independently and then compared. Disagreement should be resolved by discussion and, perhaps, by involving a more experienced methodologist.

Do the Investigators Look at Trial Quality?

As mentioned, a systematic review should specify at least three key issues of trial quality: allocation concealment, intention-to-treat analysis, and blinded outcome assessment. There are several ways for conductors of a systematic review to deal with trial quality by methods collectively termed "sensitivity analysis." A common method is to repeat the analysis after excluding trials with low reporting quality. Ideally, the results should remain unchanged, which means they are robust to this quality bias. Unfortunately, most of the currently available trials fail in one or more of these points, and once they are eliminated, there are hardly any trials left to evaluate.

The Assessment

Many more issues are involved in the assessment of systematic reviews and meta-analysis, but for a quick assessment, the previously mentioned issues are sufficient. Further, these additional issues require more methodological detail that is outside the scope of this brief review. In fact, methods to rate the quality of systematic reviews now number in the dozens.[22]

For the reader interested in learning more, we recommend the excellent self-teaching materials provided by the Cochrane Collaboration.[23] A key issue to be aware of is that not every RCT is of higher quality, and more valuable for clinical decision making, than all nonrandomized trials.[24] An RCT that enrolled a dozen patients in each of two arms and measured pain intensity after a single dose of a drug that might be used clinically for weeks or months, with results for not only pain intensity but also quality of life and functionality, may be less informative than a careful case-controlled study that assesses pain intensity and function during 3 months of therapy in thousands of patients per arm. Unfortunately, the former study in this example is not atypical for clinical trials of acute, cancer-related, or chronic pain. Further, in addition to the nature or type of evidence about a specific clinical question, one must bear in mind the strength and consistency of the available evidence.[25]

An experienced assessor needs a half to 1 hour to extract information about these further issues from a study report. As with analysis of RCTs, the reader is probably now thinking that he or she will not be able to apply these criteria because of lack of time and maybe also lack of experience. So the reader may decide to use sources in which the assessment has already been done by others, which is the next topic.

Accessing Medical Evidence

Ideally, clinicians do not perform literature searches on their own unless they want to do a proper systematic review. Anyone who does perform literature searches for purposes of a systematic review needs much more background information, and this chapter is not sufficient. In many instances it is a waste of resources for a practicing clinician to retrieve primary clinical trials bearing on a clinical question, and the worst-case scenario is the misguided application of a specific trial to a clinical situation where it does not quite fit. It is important to use sources in which a critical appraisal has already been performed by others. There is a large and growing number of evidence-based products—resources in which a critical appraisal has been performed according to a predefined quality procedure. Table 2–1 lists a few general sources that operate with high standards detailed on their respective websites.

Consider the following scenario from a practicing emergency physician describing a search for evidence:

A young man comes to the emergency department after a bicycling accident. He has a humerus fracture that was reduced but has residual pain of moderate to severe intensity. The patient had been given a short-acting intravenous anesthetic (propofol) during closed reduction of the fracture and had vomited "because of the pain" shortly afterwards. He described having vomited previously when given several types of oral opioids after dental extractions.

How should he be treated now? Shall he be given (1) an oral nonsteroidal anti-inflammatory drug (NSAID), (2) an oral opioid, (3) a parenteral NSAID, (4) a parenteral opioid, (5) anti-emetic therapy, or (5) nondrug therapy involving behavioral and physical measures (e.g., ice)? His recent episodes of vomiting prompt avoidance of the oral route until he has shown his ability to take at least clear liquids by mouth, and his history of nausea with opioids prompts the physician to rely on NSAIDs to control his pain. Because of the physician's concern that the patient's pain be well controlled before he leaves the emergency department, the physician decides to check whether published evidence favors keeping him in the emergency department for ongoing parenteral NSAID administration, or whether oral treatment after an anti-emetic would suffice.

TABLE 2–1	General-Purpose Sources for Evidence-Based Medicine	
Database	**Web Address**
Cochrane Library	http://www.cochrane.org
ACP Journal Club	http://www.acpjc.org
Evidence Based Medicine	http://ebm.bmjjournals.com
Evidence Based Nursing	http://ebn.bmjjournals.com
Clinical Evidence	http://www.clinicalevidence.com
Trip Database	http://www.tripdatabase.com
Agency for Healthcare Research and Quality (previously, Agency for Health Care Quality and Research)	http://www.ahrq.gov

The physician finds a systematic review that addresses this question by using Google Scholar Search.[26] After entering the words "NSAID," "efficacy," and "route" into the search field, the physician finds a systematic review at the Oxford Bandolier website[27] that indicates an absence of evidence that NSAIDs given parenterally are superior to those given orally for any condition except renal colic.[5] On the other hand, the authors of that review caution that the absence of evidence does not equal evidence for no effect—that is, they cannot conclusively state that no route-dependent difference in efficacy exists for conditions besides renal colic.

The physician decides that at the moment, given the patient's recent nausea and vomiting, he might best be treated with an injection of an NSAID; the physician then wants to know which one is most efficacious. By going again to the Oxford Bandolier website,[27] and clicking on the "Acute Pain" tab, the physician finds a "league table" of efficacy of NSAIDs in acute pain that arrays nonselective NSAIDs and cyclooxygenase-2 (Cox-2) inhibitors according to their efficacy. That table indicates that in a single-dose study in acute postoperative pain, valdecoxib, 40 mg, is the most efficacious parenteral agent (including comparison with parenteral opioids). One of the physician's colleagues asks whether it is safe to give this "coxib" in view of adverse cardiac events, surgical site bleeding, and other side effects, such as poor bone healing, that she has heard about recently. The physician queries the Oxford Bandolier website and discovers that there is little evidence for impairment of bone healing with NSAID or coxib use, certainly if used for a short time. The same review mentions that smoking is a well-proven risk factor for poor bone healing; the physician finds that the patient is a smoker and conveys the risk to him. The physician recalls a recent controversy surrounding the safety of coxibs and that there was a public hearing of an advisory panel to the U.S. Food and Drug Administration (FDA) to weigh the evidence for and against the safety of coxib use. The physician goes to PubMed[28] and types in "coxib cardiovascular safety." This second search result describes an FDA hearing on this topic in 2005. Five minutes have elapsed so far during the scan of the Internet. The physician clicks on that article but finds that because he is not a subscriber to the journal in which it appeared, and there is no abstract, he is given only the first 100 words. Those words suggest that there is increased risk of cardiovascular complications from coxibs but do not say over what period of administration the risk becomes evident or in what specific setting. The physician then returns to Google Scholar Search and types in "NSAID safety surgery." The first listing obtained is a literature synthesis on the safety of coxibs conducted in 2005 by physicians at a major orthopedic surgery center.[29] To the physician's surprise, he learns that clinical and animal studies, although limited, suggest that the use of both traditional NSAIDs and coxibs may impede fracture healing.

The physician orders ice bags to be applied to the fracture site and notes that as the patient's pain improves, his nausea does, too. He now is sipping clear liquids without nausea. The physician returns to Google Scholar Search and types in "pain cause nausea." The first two listings—one an article by McQuay[30] of the Oxford group—support such a connection. The physician advises the patient to continue applying ice packs, and he writes a prescription for 48 hours'

worth of tramadol, a weak opioid that also has nonopioid actions. The total search time for this information, taken intermittently, is 15 minutes.

Conclusion

Accessing and assessing medical evidence is no mean feat. Ideally, one should use resources providing only articles that have already passed critical appraisal. Presciently, in his 1906 play *The Doctor's Dilemma*, George Bernard Shaw addressed the ethical issues raised by the need to allocate a scarce yet potentially curative medical treatment. Shaw, who had undergone numerous operations for chronic tibial osteomyelitis, wrote that even after the introduction of general anesthesia had rendered operations painless, "the patient pays for anesthesia with hours of wretched sickness; and when that is over there is the pain of the wound made by the surgeon, which has to heal like any other wound." He further observed, "Doctors are not trained in the use of evidence, nor biometrics, nor in the psychology of human credulity, nor in the incidence of economic pressure. They must believe, on the whole, what their patients believe…. That is why all changes come from the laity."

Over 2000 years ago, the earliest recorded clinical trial was described in the Old Testament of the Bible in the Book of Daniel. (The biblical trial was a nonrandomized parallel cohort trial without a placebo group that found a simple vegetarian diet superior to one rich in fancier foods.) Today, the clinical trial is universally recognized as a powerful tool that is accepted in clinical practice and by society at large. Although controversies about many specific questions in evidence-based practice will no doubt continue, the fact that regulators, policymakers, insurers, and patients can now quickly conduct extensive searches of the medical evidence has irreversibly changed clinical practice. To practice high-quality pain medicine in the 21st century, practitioners must now access and assess the evidence on a daily basis, if only to meet the expectations of patients and their families.

REFERENCES

1. National Health Service (NHS) Center for Evidence-Based Medicine. Available at www.cebm.net/
2. Carr DB: On the silent "l" in "qualntitative." In Carr DB, Loeser J, Morris D (eds). Narrative, Pain and Suffering. Seattle, IASP Press, 2005, pp 325–354.
3. Altman DG: The scandal of poor medical research. BMJ 1994;308:283–284.
4. Kjaergard LL, Villumsen J, Gluud CL: Reported methodologic quality and discrepancies between large and small randomized trials in meta-analyses. Ann Intern Med 2001;135:982–989.
5. Tramer MR, Moore RA, Reynolds DJM, McQuay HJ: Quantitative estimation of rare adverse events which follow a biological progression: A new model applied to chronic NSAID use. Pain 2000;85:169–182.
6. Koreny M, Riedmuller E, Nikfardjam M, et al: Arterial puncture closing devices compared with standard manual compression after cardiac catheterization: Systematic review and meta–analysis. JAMA 2004;291:350–357.
7. Edwards JE, McQuay HJ, Moore RA, Collins SL: Reporting of adverse effects in clinical trials should be improved: Lessons from acute postoperative pain. J Pain Symptom Manage 1999;18:427–437.
8. Haynes B: Bridging the Gaps between The Cochrane Collaboration and Clinical Practice. Plenary session presentation at Cochrane Colloquium, Oct. 2–6, 2004, Ottawa, Canada. Available at www.cochrane.mcmaster.ca/Colloquium/PPTs/Oct3/Plenary1_CCConHallABEF_1100_Haynes.ppt#1 (accessed November 22, 2004).

9. Carr DB, Goudas LC, Balk EM, et al: Evidence report on the treatment of pain in cancer patients. J Natl Cancer Inst Monogr 2004;32:23–31.

10. Ioannidis JP, Haidich AB, Pappa M, et al: Comparison of evidence of treatment effects in randomized and nonrandomized studies. JAMA 2001;286:821–830.

11. Ballantyne JC, Carr DB, deFerranti S, et al: The comparative effects of postoperative analgesic therapies on pulmonary outcome: Cumulative meta-analyses of randomized, controlled trials. Anesth Analg 1998; 86:598–612.

12. Block BM, Liu SS, Rowlingson AJ, et al: Efficacy of postoperative epidural analgesia: A meta-analysis. JAMA 2004;291:1197–1198.

13. Choi PT, Bhandari M, Scott J, Douketis J: Epidural analgesia for pain relief following hip or knee replacement (Cochrane Review). In The Cochrane Library, issue 2. Chichester, UK, John Wiley & Sons, 2005.

14. Schulz KF, Chalmers I, Hayes RJ, Altman DG: Empirical evidence of bias: Dimensions of methodological quality associated with estimates of treatment effects in controlled trials. JAMA 1995;273:408–412.

15. Schulz KF, Grimes DA: Blinding in randomised trials: Hiding who got what. Lancet 2002;359:696–700.

16. Carr DB, Goudas LC, Lawrence D, et al: Management of Cancer Symptoms: Pain, Depression, and Fatigue. Evidence Report/Technology Assessment No. 61. AHRQ Publication No. 02-E032. Rockville, Md, Agency for Healthcare Research and Quality, 2002.

17. Miaskowski, C, Nichols R, Brody R, Synold T: Assessment of patient satisfaction utilizing the American Pain Society's Quality Assurance Standard on acute and cancer-related pain. J Pain Symptom Manage 1994;9:5–11.

18. Streitberger K, Kleinhenz J: Introducing a placebo needle into acupuncture research. Lancet 1998;352:364–365.

19. Moseley JB, O'Malley K, Petersen NJ, et al: A controlled trial of arthroscopic surgery for osteoarthritis of the knee. N Engl J Med 2002;347:81–88.

20. Dolin, SJ, Cashman JN, Bland JM: Effectiveness of acute postoperative pain management: I. Evidence from published data. Br J Anaesth 2002;89:409–423.

21. Viscusi ER, Gavia M, Hartrick CT, et al: Forty-eight hours of postoperative pain relief after total hip arthroplasty with a novel, extended-release epidural morphine formulation. Anesthesiology 2005;102:1014–1022.

22. West S, King V, Carey TS, et al: Systems to date the strength of scientific evidence. Evidence Report/Technology Assessment No. 47. AHRQ Publication No. 02-E016. Rockville, Md, Agency for Healthcare Research and Quality, 2002.

23. Cochrane Collaboration Open Learning Material. Available at www.cochranenet.org/openlearning/HTML/mod0.htm/

24. Jadad AR, Cepeda MS: Clinical trials in pain relief: 10 challenges. Pain Clinical Updates 1999;7:1–4.

25. Jacox AK, Carr DB, Payne R, et al: Management of Cancer Pain. Clinical Practice Guideline No. 9; AHCPR Pub. No. 94-0592. Rockville, Md, Agency for Health Care Policy and Research, 1994.

26. Google Scholar Search. Available at http://scholar.google.com/

27. Oxford Pain Internet Site. Available at http://www.jr2.ox.ac.uk/bandolier/booth/painpag/

28. PubMed. Available at http://www.ncbi.nlm.nih.gov/entrez/query.fcgi?CMD=Limits&DB=pubmed/

29. Urban MK, Markenson JA, Lane JM: HSS physicians review literature on the safety of COX-2 inhibitors. Available at http://www.hss.edu/Professionals/Conditions/Arthritis/Safety-of-Cox-2-Inhibitors.

30. McQuay H: Opioids in pain management. Lancet 1999;353:2229–2232.

3 Guidelines, Recommendations, Protocols, and Practice

JEFFREY UPPINGTON

A number of terms fit into the general vocabulary of guidelines. In addition to *recommendations* and *protocols,* one can use *policies, standards, parameters, advisories, alerts, algorithms, options,* and *bulletins.* The definitions and usage overlap, and many terms are used interchangeably.

Eddy[1] uses the overarching term *practice policy* and defines three types on the basis of their flexibility (Box 3–1). The American Society of Anesthesiologists (ASA) has defined certain terms they use in a Policy Statement on Practice Parameters (Box 3–2).[2] There is an implied obligation to follow the "rules" or "requirements" of practice standards. The Institute of Medicine defines guidelines as "systematically developed statements to assist practitioner and patient decisions about appropriate healthcare for specific clinical circumstances,"[3] and this definition has been accepted and used by a number of authorities.[4–6] Because this definition has guidelines "assisting" decisions rather than making them, the guidelines do not have the mandatory quality attached to standards and protocols. This chapter confines itself to discussing protocols (standards) and guidelines as defined by Eddy[1] and the Institute of Medicine.[3] Other terms are considered interchangeable with these terms.

History of Guideline Development and Use

A brief review of the history of guideline development will assist an understanding of the current position of guidelines in practice today. Plato (4th century BC) discussed the difference between doctors practicing with skills grounded in practical expertise and those practicing by following rigid rules.[7] In Plato's view, important hallmarks of expertise include responsiveness and improvisatory ability, an approach to practice endangered by the use of guidelines.[7] Although Plato was prepared to concede the potential of guidelines, he considered their use a debased practice because it did not take into consideration an individual patient but rather presupposed an average one.[8] This criticism of guidelines remains to this day (see later). In more modern times the armed forces have used clinical algorithms to provide corpsmen with guidance to diagnose and stabilize injured soldiers on the front line before transfer to more complete facilities.[9] Guidelines later became viewed as offering advice to doctors in training and to physician extenders.[10]

In the United States in the 1980s, however, the following three major factors played a role in a rapid change of events[11]:
1. Rising healthcare costs, including physician payments.[12–14]
2. Practice variations. There are well-documented instances of variation in clinical practice.[15–20] Although it was not certain that some of these could be explained by difference in patient populations, local resources, and patient preference,[21–23] the issue of practice variations has continued,[24–26] remains to this day,[27] and is still at the forefront of Medicare expense reduction efforts.[28,29]
3. Reports of inappropriate care and of unnecessary medical procedures. The RAND Corporation studies were most commonly cited,[30] but extrapolations claimed a very large incidence.[31,32]

The U.S. Department of Health and Human Services (DHHS) launched an effectiveness initiative,[33] and other federal health departments developed assessment teams that worked with academic researchers to study the appropriateness and effectiveness of procedures with significant variation.[11] By 1988, practice guidelines were specifically suggested as a means of reducing practice variations.

A number of Public Health services began issuing guidelines,[34–36] as have nonfederal panels convened by the government.[37,38] Reports of the Physician Payment Review Commission often include practice guidelines as a focus for implementation,[39] and physician organizations have worked on guideline development.[40] Many specialty societies offer practice guidelines (Box 3–3).[11,41] State and local governments also issue guidelines,[42] as have health maintenance organizations.[43]

BOX 3–1	PRACTICE POLICIES

Standards: Applied rigidly. They must be followed in virtually all cases.
Guidelines: More flexible. They should be followed in most cases.
Options: Neutral with respect to recommendation. They merely note that different options are available.

Adapted from Eddy DM: Designing a practice policy: Standards, guidelines and options. JAMA 1990;263:3077–3084.

BOX 3–2	POLICY STATEMENT ON PRACTICE PARAMETERS*

Practice Parameters: Developed to provide guidance or direction for the diagnosis and management and treatment of specific problems. May refer to Standards, Guidelines, or Alerts.

Practice Standards: Rules or minimum requirements for clinical practice, representing generally accepted principles for sound patient management. May include statements of practice policy or protocol or specific recommendations for patient management.

Practice Guidelines: Systematically developed recommendations for patient care that describe a basic management strategy or a range of basic management strategies.

Practice Advisories: Systematically developed reports intended to assist in decision-making in areas of patient care in which scientific evidence is insufficient.

Practice Alerts: Reports intended to assist decision-making in areas of patient care, facilitating awareness of a specific problem.

Statements, Positions, Protocols: Representing opinions of the House on a variety of subjects, not being subjected to the same level of scientific review as Standards, Guidelines, Advisories, and Alerts.

*Approved by House of Delegates October 13, 1993, and last amended October 27, 2004.
Adapted from American Society of Anesthesiologists: Policy Statement on Practice Parameters. Available at http://www.asahq.org/publicationsAndServices/sgstoc.htm (accessed March 2, 2005).

BOX 3–3	EXAMPLES OF SPECIALTY SOCIETIES WITH EXPERIENCE IN DEVELOPING PRACTICE GUIDELINES

American Academy of Allergy and Immunology
American Academy of Child and Adolescent Psychiatry
American Academy of Ophthalmology
American Academy of Orthopedic Surgeons
American Academy of Otolaryngology–Head and Neck Surgery
American Academy of Pediatrics
American Association of Electromyography and Electrodiagnosis
American College of Cardiology
American College of Emergency Physicians
American College of Obstetricians and Gynecologists
American College of Occupational Medicine
American College of Physicians
American College of Preventive Medicine
American College of Radiology
American College of Rheumatology
American College of Surgeons
American Geriatrics Society
American Medical Association
American Psychiatric Association
American Society for Gastrointestinal Endoscopy
American Society of Anesthesiologists
American Urological Society
College of American Pathologists

Adapted from the Office of Quality Assurance, American Medical Association: Listings of Practice Parameters, Guidelines, and Technology Assessments. Chicago, American Medical Association, 1989; and Woolf SH: Practice guidelines: A new reality in medicine. 1: Recent developments. Arch Intern Med 1990;150:1811–1818.

International Guidelines

There is now an internationally based interest in guidelines and their development (Box 3–4).[44] In Britain, interest in guideline development using evidence assessment,[45] including nursing practice,[46] is growing, and the Scottish Intercollegiate Guideline Network uses a systematic multidiscipline approach to produce and disseminate evidence-based guidelines.[47] Their website contains links to other international Internet sites. The Australasian IMPACT (Interdisciplinary Maternal Perinatal Australasian Clinical Trials) Network is a source of many guideline development efforts.[48] Journals around the world are now dedicated to evidence-based healthcare.[49–51]

Benefits of Guidelines

The main benefit touted for the use of guidelines is better quality of patient care. However, different groups (doctors, payers, and managers) define quality differently,[44] as discussed later. There is general agreement, at least among their proponents, that guidelines have several potential benefits.

BENEFITS TO PATIENTS

Proven guidelines have the potential, by encouraging effective practice, to reduce morbidity and mortality and improve the quality of life in some conditions.[44] They have the potential to reduce the variation in care. This will have benefit if

Archie Cochrane's observation that "if practice varies so widely, you cannot all be right"[52] is correct. Without good experimental evidence that variation promotes good care, the assumption of many people and government agencies is that his observation is correct. Guidelines also have the potential to improve outcomes.[53–56] They help patients if accompanied by leaflets, audiotapes, or other educational materials, especially those with estimates of various outcome probabilities.[57] These items help physicians and patients reach informed healthcare choices. Patients can also be helped when guidelines influence public policy by calling attention to unrecognized or underfunded health problems.

BENEFITS TO HEALTHCARE PROVIDERS

The quality of clinical decisions can be improved with good guidelines. They can be of benefit when there is uncertainty about proper care, can help overturn outmoded practices, can provide reassurance of the appropriateness of clinical actions, and can improve the consistency of care.[44] If supported by evidence-based practice, guidelines alert clinicians to interventions supported by good scientific evidence. Guidelines also can support quality improvement activities. Medical researchers are aided by guidelines that show gaps in the medical literature. Clinicians and payers can use guidelines

BOX 3–4	OVERVIEW OF INTERNATIONAL ACTIVITIES ON GUIDELINES

EUROPE

United Kingdom—Guidelines have existed for decades, encouraged by the National Health Service, professional bodies, and researchers. Mostly consensus conferences; there is an increasing interest in developing explicit methods.

The Netherlands—The Dutch College of General Practitioners has produced guidelines since 1987, at a rate of 8–10 a year. Guidelines figure prominently in Dutch health policy.

Finland and Sweden—Finland has produced more than 700 guidelines since 1989. Development of evidence-based guidelines has started. Swedish guidelines appear in reports by the Swedish Council on Technology Assessment in Health Care and in recommendations from other government bodies.

France—The Agence Nationale de l'Accréditation et d'Évaluation en Santé has published more than 100 guidelines based on consensus conferences or modifications of guidelines from other countries. The guidelines are disseminated through networks of general practitioners and evaluated by audits.

Germany, Italy, and Spain—Guidelines are on the rise in these countries. In Spain, the Catalan Agency for Health Technology is preparing guidelines and teaches methods of guideline development.

NORTH AMERICA

United States—Guidelines, protocols, and care pathways are common in American hospitals and health plans, in which they are used for quality improvement and cost containment. Although some evidence-based guidelines have received prominent attention, many healthcare organizations purchase commercially produced guidelines that emphasize shortened hospital stay and other resource savings.

Canada—Canadian healthcare is largely state funded, but the proportion of organizations using guidelines is similar to that in the United States.

AUSTRALIA AND NEW ZEALAND

Australia—Guidelines in Australia date to the late 1970s, when the state health authority began endorsing guideline booklets. There is a greater emphasis on the need for evidence-based guidelines.

New Zealand—Guidelines emanate directly from national health policy. New Zealand's choosing to restrict services at the point of service through guidelines received international attention in debates on rationing. One guideline on hypertension and subsequent cholesterol control from New Zealand Heart Foundation broke new ground methodologically by linking recommendations to patients' absolute risk probabilities rather than to generic treatment criteria.

Adapted from Woolf SH, Grol R, Hutchinson A, et al: Potential benefits, limitations, and harms of clinical guidelines. BMJ 1999;318:527–530.

for their own benefits, such as medicolegal protection and leverage in "turf wars."[44] Of course, these last benefits verge into undesirable qualities.

BENEFITS FOR HEALTHCARE SYSTEMS

By standardizing care, clinical guidelines may be effective in improving efficiency and value for money.[44,58,59] Guidelines play a major role in the development of critical pathways, management plans that consist of patient goals and the sequence and timing necessary to achieve them.[60] They have been used as yet another tool to improve efficiency and improve quality.[61] Guidelines and critical pathways may reduce costs and have the added advantage of improving the public image of those using them by sending messages about quality of care and commitment to excellence.[44]

Downsides of Guidelines

A number of criticisms have been raised about the use of guidelines. Guidelines can be flawed in the following ways:

- Scientific evidence about what to recommend may be lacking, misleading, or misinterpreted.[44]
- Recommendations are influenced by opinions of the guideline development team, which may be based on misconceptions.[62]
- Patients may not be the only priority of guidelines; recommendations may instead concentrate on controlling

costs or protecting special interests (those of doctors, managers, or politicians, for example) to the detriment of patient needs.[44]

The potential of flawed guidelines to do harm is discussed in the following sections.

HARM TO PATIENTS

The greatest danger of flawed guidelines is harm to patients. There is a risk of reducing individualized care for patients by ignoring their preferences or special circumstances.[63] There are uncertainties in applying disease-specific guidelines to patients with multiple conditions, for which more than one guideline may apply.[64] There is also the risk that guidelines may be ineffective.[65–67] Evidence that guidelines can alter practice has been reported,[68,69] although the effects may be small and short-lasting.[70]

HARM TO HEALTHCARE PROVIDERS

Flawed guidelines can compromise the quality of care delivered by providers. The quality of clinical guidelines development may not be as rigorous as it should be,[71,72] leading to calls for improvement.[73] Guidelines may conflict,[74,75] a situation that can confuse and hamper proper care. A plethora of guidelines is now available, creating difficulties in information dissemination and clarity of intention.[76,77] Clinicians may be adversely affected as professionals. The practice of perceived "cookbook medicine"[78] is not appealing, although guidelines are not cookbook medicine.[5] Many physicians distrust guidelines and believe they can increase costs, can be used to discipline physicians, and can create less satisfaction in practicing medicine.[79]

HARM TO HEALTHCARE SYSTEMS

Harm may result if guidelines lead to higher costs, reduced efficiency, or waste of limited resources.[44]

Legal Considerations of Guidelines

The definition of *medical negligence* involves a number of essential elements (Box 3–5),[80] and clinical guidelines could influence the definition of standard of care. Clinicians fear that guideline proliferation will increase their medicolegal exposure.[81] However, at least in 1995, only in a minority of malpractice actions in the United States did guidelines play a pivotal role.[82] Nevertheless, the picture is not a simple one. France has produced many mandatory practice guidelines under a 1993 statute. Once published, the guidelines are an enforceable agreement between physicians and the country's social security administration.[83,84] Formal complaints have been sent to the French fraud investigation group, alleging improper conduct by participants in the guidelines program.[83]

The legal standard of care in the United Kingdom was defined by the Bolam doctrine as follows: "the test is the standard of the ordinary skilled man exercising and professing to have that special skill."[85] The standard in the United States is similar, in that it involves the concept of the "reasonable and prudent" physician.[86] Although guidelines can be introduced into the courts by expert witnesses as evidence of "accepted and customary standards of care," they cannot yet be introduced as a substitute for expert witnesses.[79] Guidelines that do not meet quality standards[87] should not become legal standards, but because the courts do not generally call experts to assess the robustness of guidelines, this possibility could eventually materialize.[88]

For the moment, however, guidelines do not play a major role in court cases in the United States.[81] In one well-publicized U.S. case, a clinic was held responsible for a physician's not ordering a prostate-specific antigen (PSA)

BOX 3–5	MEDICAL NEGLIGENCE

Medical negligence is a composite legal finding comprising three essential elements. The person bringing the action, the complainant (plaintiff), must show that
1. The defendant doctor owed the complainant a duty of care.
2. The doctor breached this duty of care by failing to provide the required standard of medical care.
3. This failure actually caused the plaintiff harm, a harm that was both foreseeable and reasonably avoided.
   Evidence-based guidelines could influence the manner in which the courts establish the second element.

Adapted from Hurwitz B: How does evidence-based guidance influence determinations of medical negligence? BMJ 2004;328:1024–1028.

test even though he followed national clinical guidelines, and the physician himself was held not liable.[89] This ruling has generated further comments among physicians,[90,91] but a reasonable approach is that following guidelines may not always ensure good clinical care and that diverging from them may not constitute poor care.[92] Hurwitz[80] sums up the present legal position as follows: "Guidelines do not set legal standards for clinical care but they do provide the courts with a benchmark by which to judge clinical conduct."[80]

Evidence-Based Medicine

The definition of evidence-based medicine has been explored in Chapter 2, but a brief review as it pertains to guidelines is appropriate here. *Evidence-based medicine* (EBM) is the "conscientious, explicit, and judicious use of current best evidence in making decisions about the care of individual patients."[93] The term first appeared in the literature in the early 1990s[94,95] and was originally designed for the teaching of medical residents.[96] Such authorities as Archie Cochrane, Alvan Feinstein, and David Sackett[97] laid the foundations for EBM, however, and David Eddy had been writing about similar issues the previous decade. There are many proponents of EBM[97–100] as well as many detractors[101–103] and some doubters.[104] Some writers have expressed their opposition in satire and humor,[105,106] and others have offered humorous alternatives.[107] Still others have expressed caution about applying EBM to health policy[108] and how it can apply to hospital management and ethical decision-making.[109] EBM can be applied to individual patients,[110] but the application of EBM in guideline development concerns this chapter.[111] Although there are proponents of EBM in anesthesia,[111] others have emphasized the difficulties of applying it to anesthesia practice.[112–114] The use of EBM in pain management is becoming established,[115–117] although it may not be used often enough. Merrill[118] has attempted to assess the literature on interventional procedures for pain relief as a source of evidence-based guidelines for the management of chronic noncancer pain.

Development of Guidelines

Evidence-based guidelines are the natural progression of EBM, in that they seek to apply the lessons learned. However, guidelines predated EBM, and many of the guidelines promulgated today are a mixture of the old style of guideline development with the new. Eddy[119] has described the traditional and new approaches to practice policies and has compared them in regard to the specific tasks he identifies that guidelines should cover (Box 3–6). It thus naturally follows that there are a number of key components, one suggestion for which is shown in Box 3–7.[120] It has been suggested that guidelines should include a specific balance sheet, comparing the benefits and harms, which physicians can then use to tailor the information in the balance sheet to individual patients.[121] Woolf[122] has suggested a number of types of guidelines that are similar to Eddy's (Box 3–8). Those practitioners reading a guideline should be able to understand how the guideline was developed. They can then have a

BOX 3–6	GUIDELINE TASKS AND APPROACHES

TASKS FOR GUIDELINES

Identify important health outcomes.

Analyze evidence for the effects of the practice on those outcomes.

Estimate the magnitude of those outcomes (benefits and harms).

Compare the benefits and harms.

Estimate the costs.

Compare the health outcomes with the costs.

Compare alternative practices to determine which deserve priority.

TRADITIONAL APPROACH

Identify practices that are standard and accepted.

Practices are necessarily in common use.

Policies are not designed, but evolve through textbooks, speeches, letters, chairpersons, and conversations.

The seven tasks are not explicitly addressed but occur implicitly.

There is no formal analysis of outcomes.

NEW APPROACHES

Global Subjective Judgment

Opinions (judgments) of policy-makers attempting to consider all factors (global) in their heads (subjective).

No attempt to do any of the guideline tasks.

Very close to the traditional approach.

Simplest, fastest, cheapest.

Used by Diagnostic & Therapeutic Technology Assessment project of the American Medical Association.

Evidence-Based

Describes the available evidence.

Ties the policy to evidence.

Does not explicitly estimate magnitude.

Does not explicitly compare benefits and harms.

Used by Technology Coverage program of Blue Cross Blue Shield Association and U.S. Preventative Services Taskforce.

Outcomes-Based

Anchors the policy to available evidence.

Explicitly estimates the outcomes of alternative procedures.

Focuses on the *quantification* of whether evidence of effectiveness exists.

Used in some policies of the Congressional Office of Technology Assessment.

Preference-Based

Performs all of the tasks explicitly.

Includes assessment of patient preferences.

Adapted from Eddy DM: Practice policies: Where do they come from? JAMA 1990;263:1265, 1269, 1272, 1275.

BOX 3–7	KEY COMPONENTS OF A USEFUL CLINICAL GUIDELINE

IDENTIFICATION OF THE KEY DECISIONS AND THEIR CONSEQUENCES

Making a diagnosis

Estimating prognosis

Assessing relevant outcomes:
- Benefits
- Costs
- Risks of alternative treatment options

REVIEW OF THE RELEVANT, VALID EVIDENCE NECESSARY TO MAKE INFORMED DECISIONS AT EACH OF THE KEY DECISION POINTS

Evidence is relevant to individual patients.

The guideline developer should be guided when possible by absolute risks and benefits.

Measured in events per 100 patients treated (or untreated) per year.

Incorporate cost-effectiveness where data available.

Explicit statements can be weighed by patient preference and available resources.

PRESENTATION: EVIDENCE AND RECOMMENDATIONS ARE PRESENTED IN A CONCISE AND ACCESSIBLE FORM

Form should be flexible and format applicable to specific patients or circumstances.

Information must be retrievable and assimilated quickly.

Adapted from Jackson R, Feder G: Guidelines for clinical guidelines. BMJ 1998;317:427–428.

BOX 3–8	METHODS FOR DEVELOPING PRACTICE GUIDELINES

INFORMAL CONSENSUS DEVELOPMENT

Same as global subjective development (see Box 3–6).[119]

FORMAL CONSENSUS DEVELOPMENT

Expert panel in closed session over a few days' conference.

Used by National Institutes of Health Consensus Development Program.

Used by RAND Corporation.

EVIDENCE-BASED GUIDELINE DEVELOPMENT

Same as evidence-based approach (see Box 3–6).[119]

EXPLICIT GUIDELINE DEVELOPMENT

Harms and benefits specified.

Costs of intervention estimated.

Explicit estimates of probability of outcomes.

Estimates also generated by expert opinion, but source of the estimate is documented.

Assumptions tabulated on a balance sheet.

Making judgments, involving patient preference—same as preference-based guidelines (see Box 3–6).[119]

Adapted from Woolf SH: Practice guidelines, a new reality in medicine. II: Methods of developing guidelines. Arch Intern Med 1992;152:946–952.

| BOX 3–9 | POLICY STATEMENTS: THE EXPLICIT APPROACH |

1. Summary of the policy:
   • Short concise statement, sufficiently accurate so it can be understood alone.
2. Background:
   • Any information needed to understand the policy.
   • Answer the question "Why is this policy being written?"
3. Health question:
   • Define the clinical question and the health problem being addressed.
   • The intervention that is the object of the policy and alternative intervention(s) with which it was compared.
   • Any restrictions on the type of practitioner (e.g., training) or settings for application (e.g., facilities).
4. Health and economic outcomes:
   • List the health outcomes.
   • List the economic costs considered.
5. Evidence:
   • Description of the evidence on which policy is based.
   • How it was interpreted.
   • What subjective judgments were used?
6. Effect on health and economic outcomes:
   • Quantitative estimates of health and economic outcomes.
   • Range of uncertainties if applicable.
7. Methods used to derive the estimates of outcomes:
   • How were the above estimates made?
   • Include statistic methods and models if applicable.
8. Preference judgments:
   • Judgments made about desirability of outcomes.
   • Compare benefits and harms.
   • Describe degree of unanimity.
   • Describe sources of preference judgments (e.g., patient surveys).
9. Instructions for tailoring guidelines—those policies that can be flexible:
   • Describe factors to consider when applying guideline.
   • Instructions for applying to different patients and settings.
10. Conflicts with other policies:
   • Explain and resolve conflict with any other policies on same health problems.
11. Comparisons with other interventions:
   • Policy set in context with other interventions.
12. Caveats:
   • No policy is final; describe expected developments that might alter it.
   • Suggest a date for review and renewing.
13. Authors of the policy:
   • Names and any conflicts of interest.

Adapted from Eddy DM: Guidelines for policy statement: The explicit approach. JAMA 1990;263:2239–2240, 2243.

basis for accepting it as valid and applying it correctly.[123] Thus, the guideline or policy statement should allow for this process and ideally should contain the information listed in Box 3–9.

One method for guideline development is summarized in Box 3–10.[122] Other methods are essentially similar[45,124] and contain the same steps.[125–129] Some differences have developed, however, in how the evidence that guidelines are based on should be evaluated and how the recommendations derived from such evidence should be categorized on the basis of strength and validity. The U.S. Agency for Health Care Policy and Research (now the U.S. Agency for Healthcare Research and Quality [AHRQ]) has developed a hierarchy of study types that is widely accepted (Box 3–11).[130]

| BOX 3–10 | METHODOLOGICAL ISSUES IN GUIDELINE DEVELOPMENT |

1. INTRODUCTORY DECISIONS

Selection of topic:
• May be conditions, complaints (e.g., pain) or procedures (e.g., epidurals).
• Formal methods have been developed to set priorities.[124]
Selection of panel members:
• Various specialty physicians.
• Others, including methodologists, health economists, patients, consumer representatives.
Clarification of purpose:
• Define topic, settings, types of providers.

2. ASSESSMENT OF CLINICAL APPROPRIATENESS

Assessment of clinical benefits and harms
Assessment of clinical evidence:
• Retrieval of evidence from articles, books,[125,126] or electronic sources.[126]
• Evaluation of individual studies.
• Synthesis of evidence.

3. ASSESSMENT OF EXPERT OPINION

Informal methods, discussion, voting
Formal methods, such as Nominal Group Technique and Delphi method[127]
Summary of benefits and harm[121]
Determinations of appropriateness; many policies are in the "gray zone"

4. ASSESSMENT OF PUBLIC POLICY ISSUES

Resource limitation
Feasibility issues

5. GUIDELINE DOCUMENT DEVELOPMENT AND EVALUATION

Peer review and pretesting
Recommendations for dissemination, evaluation and updating
Recommendations for research

Adapted from Woolf SH: Practice guidelines, a new reality in medicine. II: Methods of developing guidelines. Arch Intern Med 1992;152:946–952.

BOX 3–11	HIERARCHY OF STUDY TYPES

1. Systematic reviews and meta-analyses of randomized controlled trials
2. Randomized controlled trials
3. Nonrandomized interventional studies
4. Observational studies
5. Nonexperimental studies
6. Expert opinion

Adapted from Carr DB, Jacox AK, Chapman CR, et al: Acute Pain Management: Operative or Medical Procedures and Trauma. (Clinical Practice Guideline No 1; AHCPR Publication No 92-0023.) Rockville, MD, Agency for Health Care Policy Research, 1993, p 107.

The Canadian Task Force on the Periodic Health Examination has developed a classification of recommendations and study designs[131] that many authorities accept (Table 3–1). These approaches have been adapted and modified by other authorities, as shown in Tables 3–2 through 3–4.[45,129,132]

Numerous sources of information on evidence, EBM, reviews, meta-analyses, and guidelines are available through the Internet.[99,127,133] Sources for evidence-based guidelines are listed in Table 3–5, and those for EBM in Table 3–6.

Any data source and the data generated from that source should be looked at critically and thoroughly. It is important to distinguish a *systematic review*—a concise summary of the best available evidence from primary studies using explicit, reproducible methods to synthesize the evidence[134–136]— from a *meta-analysis*, which uses statistical methods to combine the results of many studies of similar design.[137]

Each randomized controlled trial must be assessed for rigor and accuracy. Similarly, each meta-analysis must be scrutinized thoroughly because common problems have been reported,[138] including bias.[139] Another common problem is that two or more meta-analyses on the same subject have arrived at different conclusions.[140–143] Also, Lelorier et al[144] have reported finding that the outcomes of large randomized controlled trials were not predicted accurately 35% of the time by meta-analyses.

Evaluation of Guidelines

When one is assessing a guideline for implementation, it is important to evaluate it rigorously. The methods used to assess a guideline can be the same as those used to assess the evidence on which it is based.[132,145,146] Older established guidelines have been shown to be less rigorous and thorough than modern guidelines should be,[147,148] as discussed by other writers.[149]

Implementation of Guidelines

There are two stages in putting a guideline to use, dissemination and implementation.[46] Strategies for dissemination include professional journals; educational efforts such as meetings, bulletins, and advisories; and sending guidelines to targeted individuals. These strategies can be used at both the local and national levels. Dissemination by publications or direct mailing alone is not very successful,[150–152] but including specifically directed education has more positive benefits.[153]

TABLE 3–1	Canadian Task Force Classification of Recommendations and Study Designs	
Category	**Descriptions**	
Recommendations		
A	There is good evidence to support the recommendation that the condition be specifically considered in the periodic health examination.	
B	There is fair evidence to support the recommendation that the condition be specifically considered in the periodic health examination.	
C	There is poor evidence regarding the inclusion of the condition in the periodic health examination, but recommendations may be made on other grounds.	
D	There is fair evidence to support the recommendation that the condition be excluded from consideration in the periodic health examination.	
E	There is good evidence to support the recommendation be excluded from consideration in the periodic health examination.	
Study Designs		
I	Evidence obtained from at least 1 properly designed randomized controlled trial.	
II-1	Evidence obtained from well-designed controlled trials without randomization.	
II-2	Evidence obtained from well-designed cohort or case-controlled analytic studies, preferably from more than 1 center or research group.	
II-3	Evidence obtained from comparisons between times or places with or without intervention; dramatic results in uncontrolled experiments.	
III	Opinion of respected authorities, based on clinical experience, descriptive studies, or reports of expert committees.	

Adapted from The periodic health examination. Canadian Task Force on the Periodic Health Examination. Can Med Assoc J 1979;121:1193–1254; and Woolf SH: Practice guidelines, a new reality in medicine. II: Methods of developing guidelines. Arch Intern Med 1992;152:946–952.

TABLE 3–2	Classification Schemes

Categories of Evidence

Ia	Evidence for meta-analysis of randomized controlled trials
Ib	Evidence from at least one randomized controlled trial
IIa	Evidence from at least one controlled study without randomization
IIb	Evidence from at least one other type of quasi-experimental study
III	Evidence from nonexperimental descriptive studies, such as comparative studies, correlation studies, and case-controlled studies
IV	Evidence from expert committee reports or opinions, clinical experience of respected authorities, or both

Strength of Recommendation

A	Directly based on category I evidence
B	Directly based on category II evidence or extrapolated recommendation from category I evidence
C	Directly based on category III evidence or extrapolated recommendation from category I or II evidence
D	Directly based on category IV evidence or extrapolated recommendation from category I, II, or III evidence

Adapted from Shekelle PG, Woolf SH, Eccles M, Grimshaw J: Clinical guidelines: Developing guidelines. BMJ 1999;318:593–596.

TABLE 3–3	Other Classification Schemes for Evidence and Recommendations

Categories of Evidence

I	Based on well-designed randomized controlled trials, meta-analyses, or systematic reviews
II	Based on well-designed cohort or case-controlled studies
III	Based on uncontrolled studies or consensus

Strength of Recommendation

A	Directly based on category I evidence
B	Directly based on category II evidence or extrapolated recommendation from category I evidence
C	Directly based on category III evidence or extrapolated recommendation from category I or II evidence

Adapted from Eccles M, Clapp Z, Grimshaw J, et al: North of England evidence based guidelines development project: Methods of guideline development. BMJ 1996;312:760–762.

TABLE 3–4	Revised* Grading System for Recommendations in Evidence Based Guidelines

Levels of Evidence		Grades of Recommendations	
1++	High quality meta-analyses, systematic reviews of RCTs, or RCTs with a very low risk of bias	A	At least one meta-analysis, systematic review, or RCT rated as 1++ and directly applicable to the target population _or_ A systematic review of RCTs or a body of evidence consisting principally of studies rated as 1+ directly applicable to the target population and demonstrating overall consistency of results
1+	Well-conducted meta-analyses, systematic reviews of RCTs, or RCTs with a very low risk of bias		
1–	Meta-analyses, systematic reviews of RCTs, or RCTs with a high risk of bias		
2++	High-quality systematic reviews of case-control or cohort studies _or_ High-quality case-controlled or cohort studies with a very low risk of confounding bias or chance, and a high probability that the relationship is causal	B	A body of evidence consisting principally of studies rated as 2++ directly applicable to the target population and demonstrating overall consistency of results _or_ Extrapolated evidence from studies rated as 1++ or 1+
2+	Well-conducted case-controlled or cohort studies with a low risk of confounding bias or chance, and a moderate probability that the relationship is causal	C	A body of evidence consisting principally of studies rated as 2+ directly applicable to the target population and demonstrating overall consistency of results _or_ Extrapolated evidence from studies rated as 2++
2–	Case-controlled or cohort studies with a high risk of confounding bias or chance, and a significant risk that the relationship is not causal		
3	Nonanalytic studies, e.g., case reports, case series	D	Evidence level 3 or 4 _or_ Extrapolated evidence from studies rated as 2+
4	Expert opinion		

RCT, randomized controlled trial.
*Revised from Agency for Health Care Policy and Research System.
Adapted from Harbour R, Miller J: A new system for grading recommendations in evidence based guidelines. BMJ 2001;323:334–336.

TABLE 3–5	Data Sources for Evidence-Based Guidelines: Guideline Database

Database	Web Address
AGREE (Appraisal of Guidelines, Research and Evaluation for Europe)	http://www.agreecollaboration.org
American Association of Clinical Endocrinologists	http://www.aace.com/clin/
American College of Chest Physicians	http://www.chestnet.org
American College of Physicians	http://www.acponline.org
Australian National Health and Medical Research Council (NHMRC)	http://www.health.gov.au/nhmrc/publications
Center for Health Services Research (CHSR)	http://www.ncl.ac.uk.pahs/research/services
Clinical Efficacy Assessment Project (CEAP)	http://www.acponline.org/sci-policy/guidelines/ceap.htm
CDC Task Force on Community Preventative Services	thecommunityguide.org
Clinical Practice Guidelines	http://www.kurucz.ca/sue/clinicalpracticeguidleines.com/
Clinical Practice Guidelines	http://www.cam.ca/cpgs
European Society of Cardiology	http://www.escardio.org
Finnish Guidelines (in English)	http://www.ebm-guidelines.com
German Agency for Quality in Medicine	www.aezq.de
Guideline Information Service	www.leitlinien.de
Guidelines-International-Network	http://www.g-i-n.net
Health Services Technology Assessment	http://hstat.nlm.nih.gov/hq/Hquest
Health Technology Assessment databases	http://www.hta.nhsweb.nhs/htapubs.htm
	http://www.inahta.org
	http://www.shef.ac.uk/~scharr/ir/htaorg.html
New Zealand Guidelines Group	http://www.nzgg.org.nz
NHS National Institute for Clinical Excellence	http://www.nice.org.uk
SCHARR database	http://www.shef.ac.uk/~scharr/ir/guidelin/html
Scottish Intercollegiate Guidelines Network (SIGN)	http://www.sign.ac.uk
U.S. Agency for Healthcare Research and Quality	http://www.ahrq.com
U.S. National Guideline Clearing House	http://www.guideline.gov
U.S. Preventative Services Task Force	http://www.ahspr.gov/clinic/cps3dix.htm#Background

Adapted from Oosterhuis WP, Bruns DE, Watine J, et al: Evidence-based guidelines in laboratory medicines: Principles and methods. Clin Chem 2004;50:806–818; and Hunt DL, Jaeschke R, McKibbon KA: User's guides to the medical literature. XXI: Using electronic health information resources in evidence-based practice. Evidence-Based Medicine Group. JAMA 2000;283:1875–1879.

Specific feedback on patient outcomes can improve compliance with guidelines.[154] Where guidelines are to be implemented in hospitals, substantial administrative support, strong persistent leadership, shared goals for improvement, and credible data feedback can improve the rate of compliance.[155] Also in the hospital setting, the use of a nurse facilitator has been a successful approach.[156]

There are many impediments to guideline adherence and practice change.[151,157] They include lack of awareness of or familiarity with the guidelines, lack of agreement on their effectiveness, a lack of self-efficacy, the inertia of previous practice, and various external barriers, such as patient and environmental factors.[158] Patient choices, which may not conform to a rigid guideline, can also reduce compliance.[159] In general practice or primary care, decisions are made using "mindlines"—collectively reinforced, internalized, tacit guidelines[160]—that are well entrenched.

Implementation strategies must take these factors into account by exploiting them,[160,161] focusing on barriers as a means of removing them,[158] including the institution in the implementation plan,[155] and concentrating on their implementation at the local level.[151] One implementation plan consists of developing a concrete proposal for change, analyzing the target setting and group to identify obstacles, linking interventions to needs, and using facilitators to develop a plan and monitor progress.[162]

Enforcement is an implementation strategy that has been advocated for some guidelines. For example, some state legislatures have required adherence to anesthesia-monitoring policies.[163,164] Some malpractice insurers have mandated compliance with guidlines.[165] Practice guidelines have been introduced as quality indicators,[166,167] and Centers for Medicare and Medicaid Services (CMS) and other payers have developed methods of differential payments to hospitals and physicians based partly on adherence to clinical guidelines.[168]

Maintenance of Guidelines

Guideline development processes are now well established and have been described above. When guidelines should be reviewed and updated and what process should be used to accomplish that task are less clear. Box 3–12 lists some situations that might require updating of a guideline.[169] In a 2001 report, Shekelle et al[170] reviewed 17 guidelines of the AHRQ using a focused literature review; they found that 7 needed a major update and 6 a minor one, that 3 were still valid, and that the validity of 1 was uncertain. They recommended that guidelines should be assessed every 3 years. Others have wondered whether a more pragmatic approach should be considered, whereby guidelines based on more

TABLE 3–6	Data Resources for Evidence-Based Medicine: Systematic Review and Evidence-Based Resources
Database	**Web Address**
ACP Journal Club	http://www.hiru.mcmaster.ca/acpjc/default.htm
Australasian Cochrane's Center	http://som.Flinders.edu.au/FUSA/COCHRANE
Bandolier: Evidence-Based Healthcare	http://www.ebandolier.com
Best Evidence	http://www.acponline.org/catalog/electronic/best_evidence.htm
Clinical Evidence	http://www.evidence.org/index-welcome.htm
Cochrane Library	http://www.cochrane.org
Cochrane Methods Working Group on Systematic Review of Screening and Diagnostic Tests	http://www.cochrane.org/cochrane/sadtdoc1.htm
Database of Abstracts of Reviews of Effectiveness (DARE)	http://www.agatha.york.ac.uk
EBMR Reviews (OVID)	http://www.ovid.com/products/cip/ebmr.cfm
EMedicine	http://www.emedicine.com
Evidence-Based Medicine	http://www.bmjpg.com/template.cfm?name=specjou_be
Harrison's Online: Best Evidence	http://www.harrisonsonline.com
IFCC Committee on Evidence-Based Laboratory Medicine (C-EBLM) database	http://www.ckchlmb.nl/ifcc
Internet Grateful Med	http://www.igm.nlm.nih.gov
MD Consult	http://www.mdconsult.com
Medical Matrix	http://www.medmatrix.org/info/medlinetable.asp
Medical World Search	http://www.mwsearch.com
MEDION database	http://www.mediondatabase.nl
National Health Service (NHS) Center for Evidence-Based Medicine	http://www.cebm.net
Levels of evidence and grades of recommendations	http://www.cebm.net/levels_of_evidence.asp
National Library for Health	http://www.nelh.nhs.uk/guidelinesdb/html/glframes.htm
National Library of Medicine	http://text.nlm.nih.gov
NHS Center for Reviews and Dissemination	http://www.york.ac.uk/inst/crd
NHS Research and Development Center for Evidence-Based Medicine	http://www.cebm.jr2.ox.ac.uk
PubMed	http://www.ncbi.nlm.nih.gov/PubMed
SCHARR database	http://www.shef.ac.uk/~scharr/ir/netting
University of Alberta EBM Toolkit	http://www.med.ualberta.ca/ebm
UpToDate	http://www.uptodate.com

Adapted from Oosterhuis WP, Bruns DE, Watine J, et al: Evidence-based guidelines in laboratory medicines: Principles and methods. Clin Chem 2004;50:806–818; Hunt DL, Jaeschke R, McKibbon KA: User's guides to the medical literature. XXI: Using electronic health information resources in evidence-based practice. Evidence-Based Medicine Group. JAMA 2000;283:1875–1879; and McQueen MJ: Overview of evidence-based medicine: Challenge for evidence-based laboratory medicine. Clin Chem 2001;47:1536–1546.

robust (level I) evidence might need less frequent updates.[171]

Gartlehner et al[172] have compared methods of guideline review. The traditional approach, developed by the RTI International–University of North Carolina Evidence-Based Practice Center, consists of searching for studies that answer critical questions, meet eligibility criteria, and are methodologically sound.[172] The investigators compared this approach with the revised approach already described.[170] The revised approach, which provided a more time-efficient model, is shown in Box 3–13.

Effectiveness of Clinical Guidelines

Whether guidelines are effective or not depends on who is judging success and how he or she defines it.[173] Guidelines offer different benefits for physicians, patients, payers, politicians, administrators, and lawyers. Table 3–7 listed four related categories of potential benefits of guidelines—knowledge, attitudes, behavior, and outcomes.

Some surveys have shown that a majority of physicians are aware of national guidelines,[174,175] but in other surveys only a small minority were able to name even one of the recommended practices.[176] There is little evidence that clinicians' attitudes to guidelines can be changed by mere distribution of the guidelines.[151,175] The previous section on guideline implementation has already discussed how physicians often fail to follow guidelines. There have been doubts that guidelines can improve clinical outcomes,[177] but outcome researchers have demonstrated improvement in some studies.[178–180] In general, the hope that guidelines will improve clinical outcome remains.[181]

PRACTICE GUIDELINES ON ACUTE PAIN

One of the early guidelines developed by the AHCPR (now AHRQ) was on acute pain management.[130] Its aims were to improve the treatment of acute pain after surgical and medical procedures and to reduce variation in management. The agency used the existing knowledge base, evaluated papers, and used the expert opinion of the panel members even

BOX 3–12	SITUATIONS THAT MIGHT REQUIRE CLINICAL GUIDELINES TO BE UPDATED

CHANGES IN EVIDENCE ON THE EXISTING BENEFITS AND HARMS OF INTERVENTIONS

New information about the magnitude of benefits and harms. Information about new benefits or harms.

CHANGES IN OUTCOMES CONSIDERED IMPORTANT

New evidence may identify outcomes previously under-appreciated or unexpected.
New evidence on patient preferences (e.g., end-of-life care).

CHANGES IN THE AVAILABLE INTERVENTIONS

New preventative, diagnostic, or treatment interventions.

CHANGES IN EVIDENCE THAT CURRENT PRACTICE IS OPTIMAL

Guidelines are developed to help narrow the gap between ideal and current practice. This gap could shrink until a guideline is no longer needed.

CHANGES IN VALUES PLACED ON OUTCOMES

Economic issues may change.
Ethics issues may be redefined.

CHANGES IN RESOURCES AVAILABLE FOR HEALTHCARE

There may be an increase in available resources.
There may be a decrease in available resources.

Adapted from Shekelle P, Eccles MP, Grimshaw JM, Woolf SH: When should clinical guidelines be updated? BMJ 2001;323:155–157.

BOX 3–13	REFINED REVIEW APPROACH FOR GUIDELINE UPDATE

1. Conduct literature search:
   - Search MEDLINE for Abridged Index Medicus (AIM).
   - Limit to review articles, editorials, guidelines, and commentaries.
   - Search PreMEDLINE, Health Services Technology Assessment Text (HSTAT), the Cochrane Library, and selected National Institutes of Health (NIH) websites.
2. Create database of all found citations.
3. Reviewer 1 reads all abstracts, accepts relevant ones.
4. Reviewer 2 reads all abstracts rejected by reviewer 1.
5. If rejected by both reviewers, mark rejected abstracts in database.
6. Accept all others.
7. Reviewer 1 skims all full-text articles, identifies relevant ones.
8. Reviewer 2 reads full-text articles rejected by reviewer 1, identifies relevant ones.
9. If both reviewers reject articles, mark articles as rejected in database.
10. Accept all others.
11. Compile accepted full-text articles and studies identified from bibliography.
12. Reviewer 1 reads and accepts relevant studies using the eligibility criteria.
13. Reviewer 2 reads and accepts relevant studies using the eligibility criteria.
14. Consensus meeting between reviewers. Accept studies if two reviewers agree.
15. Refine guideline as necessary using agreed studies.

Adapted from Gartlehner G, West SL, Lohr KN, et al: Assessing the need to update prevention guidelines: A comparison of two methods. Int J Qual Health Care 2004;16:399–406.

when there was no unanimity of opinion. Panel members came from a wide variety of backgrounds. This guideline was one of the guidelines reviewed by Shekelle et al,[170] discussed earlier, and found to need a minor update in 2001. However, in 2005 it is "no longer viewed as guidance for current medical practice."[182] The principles guiding development of this guideline, as well as a number of others worldwide that addressed pain treatment, have been summarized elsewhere.[183]

The American Society of Anesthesiologists (ASA) has developed a practice guideline for acute pain management in the perioperative setting.[184] It was first published in 1995 and last amended in 2003. The panel consisted essentially of anesthesiologists and pain physicians, and input was asked from ASA members. Evidence was evaluated and assigned to supportive, suggestive, equivocal, and silent categories. The guidelines are published on the ASA website.[184]

Of the growing number of evidence reviews that have appeared on the topic of acute pain, that prepared by the Australian National Health and Medical Research Council in 1998 and updated in 2005 stands out by virtue of its comprehensiveness and integration with preclinical knowledge.[185] It, too, is available on the Council's website.

TABLE 3–7	Potential Benefits of Practice Guidelines

Category	Benefits
Knowledge	Enhanced medical education (medical school, residency, continuing medical education); illustration of how to perform critical appraisal of evidence; definition of research agenda for future effectiveness studies
Attitudes	Acceptance of new "standard of care"; enforced credibility of technologies, specialty, health condition*
Behavior	Increased compliance with recommended practices; decreased practice variation*
Outcomes	Improved clinical outcomes (e.g., mortality, morbidity); decreased costs,* enhanced value of health care; increased reimbursement for services*; decreased medicolegal liability*

*Benefits sought predominantly by specific parties, such as clinicians (increased reimbursement, decreased medicolegal liability), specialist societies (increased recognition of the field), payers (decreased costs), and policy-makers (decreased practice variations).

Adapted from Woolf SH: Practice guidelines: A new reality in medicine. III: Impact on patient care. Arch Intern Med 1993;153:2646–2655.

Summary

Evidence-based guidelines are here to stay and will proliferate despite the controversies. It is important for practicing physicians and pain specialists to understand where the guidelines come from, how to assess and develop them, and how to use and implement them. This chapter has attempted to help readers do that.

REFERENCES

1. Eddy DM: Designing a practice policy: Standards, guidelines and options. JAMA 1990;263:3077–3084.
2. Policy Statement on Practice Parameters. Available at www.asahq.org/publicationsAndServices/sgstoc.htm (accessed March 2, 2005).
3. Field MJ, Lohr KN (eds): Guidelines for Clinical Practice: From Development to Use. Washington, DC, National Academy Press, 1992.
4. Woolf SH, Grol R, Hutchinson A, et al: Potential benefits, limitations, and harms of clinical guidelines. BMJ 1999;318:527–530.
5. Heffner JE: The overarching challenge. Chest 2000;118:1S–3S.
6. Cluzeau FA, Littlejohns P: Appraising clinical practice guidelines in England and Wales: The development of a methodologic framework and its application to policy. Jt Comm J Qual Improv 1999;25:514–521.
7. Annas J, Waterfield R (eds): Plato: Statesman. Cambridge, Cambridge University Press, 1995.
8. Hurwitz B: Legal and political considerations of clinical practice guidelines. BMJ 1999;318:661–664.
9. Bargar RJ: Introduction. In Casanova JE (ed): Tools for the Task: The Role of Clinical Guidelines. Tampa, Fla, American College of Physician Executives, 1997, pp 1–2.
10. Farmer A: Medical practice guidelines: Lessons from the United States. BMJ 1993;307:313–317.
11. Woolf SH: Practice guidelines: A new reality in medicine. 1: Recent developments. Arch Intern Med 1990;150:1811–1818.
12. Vicenzio JV: Trends in medical care costs: A look at the 1990s. Stat Bull Metrop Insur Co. 1990;January–March:28–35.
13. Iglehart JK: Payment of physicians under Medicare. N Engl J Med. 1988;318:863–868.
14. Iglehart JK: The recommendation of the Physician Payment Review Commission. N Engl J Med 1989;320:1156–1160.
15. Wennberg JE, Gittelsohn A: Small-area variation in health care delivery. Science 1973;182:1102–1108.
16. Wennberg JE, Freeman JL, Culp WJ: Are hospital services rationed in New Haven or over-utilized in Boston? Lancet 1987;1(8543):1185–1189.
17. Perrin JM, Homer CJ, Berwick DM, et al: Variation in rates of hospitalization of children in three urban communities. N Engl J Med 1989;320:1183–1187.
18. Lewis CE: Variations in the incidence of surgery. N Engl J Med 1969; 281:880–885.
19. Chassin M, Brook R, Park R, et al: Variations in the use of medical and surgical services by the Medicare population. N Engl J Med 1968; 314:285–290.
20. McLaughlin LF, Wolfe RA, Tedeschi PJ: Variation in hospital admissions among small area: A comparison of Maine and Michigan. Med Care 1989;27:623–631.
21. Eddy DM: The challenge. JAMA 1990;263:287–290.
22. Smits HL: Medical practice variations revisited. Health Aff (Millwood) 1986;5:91–96.
23. Leape LL, Park RE, Solomon DH, et al: Does inappropriate use explain small-area variations in the use of health care services? JAMA 1990; 263:669–672.
24. Blumenthal D: The variation phenomenon in 1994. N Engl J Med 1994;331:1017–1018.
25. Fisher ES, Wennberg JE, Stukel TA, Sharp SM: Hospital readmission rates for cohorts of Medicare beneficiaries in Boston and New Haven. N Engl J Med 1994;331:989–995.
26. Chassin MR: Explaining geographic variations: The enthusiasm hypothesis. Med Care 1993;31(Suppl 5):YS37–YS44.
27. Wennberg DE, Wennberg JE: Addressing variations: Is there hope for the future? Health Aff (Millwood) 2003;Jul–Dec;Suppl Web Exclusives:W3–614–7.December 10, 2003.
28. Berenson RA: Getting serious about excessive Medicare spending: A purchasing model. Health Aff (Millwood). 2003 Jul–Dec;Suppl Web Exclusives:W3–586–602. December 10, 2003.
29. Lieberman SM, Lee J, Anderson T, Crippen DL: Reducing the growth of Medicare spending: Geographic versus patient-based strategies. Health Aff (Millwood). 2003;Jul–Dec;Suppl Web Exclusives:W3-603-613. December 10, 2003.
30. Chassin MR, Kosecoff J, Park RE, et al: Does inappropriate use explain geographic variations in the use of health care services? A study of three procedures JAMA 1987;258:2533–2537.
31. Holoweiko M: What cookbook medicine will mean for you. Med Econ 1989;66:118–133.
32. National Center for Health Services Research and Health Care Technology Assessment. Research Activities: DHHS Secretary Sullivan Announces NCHRS Grants Totaling $4 Million for Patient Outcomes Research Assessment Teams. Special Release. Publication 241–274–00054. Rockville, Md, National Center for Health Services Research and Health Care Technology Assessment, September 11, 1989.
33. Roper WL, Winkenwerder W, Hackbarth GM, Krakauer H: Effectiveness in health care: An initiative to evaluate and improve medical practice. N Engl J Med 1988;319:1197–1202.
34. Report of the National Cholesterol Education Program Expert Panel on Detection, Evaluation and Treatment of High Blood Cholesterol in Adults. Arch Intern Med 1988;148:36–39.
35. Immunization Practices Advisory Committee: General recommendations on immunization. MMWR Morbid Mortal Wkly Rep 1989;38: 205–214, 219–227.
36. Jacoby I: The consensus development program of the National Institutes of Health: Current practices and historical perspectives. Int J Technol Assess Health Care 1985;1:420–432.
37. US Preventive Services Task Force: Guide to Clinical Preventive Services: An Assessment of the Effectiveness of 169 Interventions. Baltimore, Md, Williams & Wilkins, 1989.
38. Woolf SH, Battista RN, Anderson GM, et al: Assessing the clinical effectiveness of preventive maneuvers: Analytic principles and systematic methods in reviewing evidence and developing clinical practice recommendations. A report by the Canadian Task Force on the Periodic Health Examination. J Clin Epidemiol 1990;43:891–905.
39. Physician Payment Review Commission: Annual Report to Congress. Washington, DC, Physician Payment Review Commission, 1990.
40. Kelly JT, Swartwout JE: Development of practice parameters by physician organizations. QRB Qual Rev Bull 1990;February:54–57.
41. Office of Quality Assurance, American Medical Association: Listings of Practice Parameters: Guidelines, and Technology Assessments. Chicago, American Medical Association, 1989.
42. Pierce EC Jr: The development of anesthesia guidelines and standards. QRB Qual Rev Bull 1990;February:61–64.
43. Schoenbaum SC, Gottlieb LK: Algorithm based improvement of clinical quality. BMJ 1990;301:1374–1376.
44. Woolf SH, Grol R, Hutchinson A, et al: Potential benefits, limitations, and harms of clinical guidelines. BMJ 1999;318:527–530.
45. Eccles M, Clapp Z, Grimshaw J, et al: North of England evidence based guideline development project: Methods of guideline development. BMJ 1996;312:760–762.
46. Thomas L: Clinical practice guidelines. Evidence Based Nursing 1999;2:38–39.
47. Scottish Intercollegiate Guideline Network. Available at www.sign.ac.uk/index.html (accessed March 4, 2005).
48. Bandolier. Available at www.jr2.ox.ac.uk/bandolier/index.html (accessed March 4, 2005).
49. Interdisciplinary Maternal Perinatal Australasian Clinical trials. Available at http://128.250.188.72/psanz/IMPACT/impact_links.htm (accessed March 7, 2005).
50. ACP Journal Club. Available at www.acpjc.org/ (accessed March 4, 2005).
51. EBM on Line. Available at http://ebm.bmjjournals.com/ (accessed March 4, 2005).
52. Cochrane AL: quoted in West RR: Evidence based medicine overviews, bulletins, guidelines and the new consensus. Postgrad Med J 2000; 76:383–389.
53. Grimshaw JM, Russel IT: Effect of clinical guidelines on medical practice: Systematic review of rigorous evaluations. Lancet 1993;342:1317–1322.
54. Grimshaw JM, Russel IT: Achieving health care gains through clinical guidelines. I: Developing scientifically valid guidelines. Qual Health Care 1993;2:243–248.

55. Grimshaw JM, Russell IT: Achieving health care gains through clinical guidelines. II: Ensuring guidelines change medical practice. Qual Health Care 1994;3:45–52.
56. Effective health care. In Implementing Clinical Guidelines. Bulletin No 8. Leeds, UK, University of Leeds, 1994.
57. Entwistle VA, Watt IS, Davis H, et al: Developing information materials to present the findings of technology assessments to consumers: The experience of the NHS Center for Reviews and Dissemination. Int J Tech Assess Health Care 1998;14:47–70.
58. Shapiro DW, Lasker RD, Bindman AB, Lee PR: Containing costs while improving the quality of care: The role of profiling and practice guidelines. Annu Rev Public Health 1993;14:219–241.
59. Eisenberg JM, Williams SV: Cost containment and changing physicians' practice behavior: Can the fox learn to guard the chicken coop? JAMA 1981;246:2195–2201.
60. Pearson SD, Goulart-Fisher D, Lee TH: Critical pathways as a strategy for improving health care: Problems and potential. Ann Intern Med 1995;123:941–948.
61. Nathan RE, Hochman J, Becker R, et al: Critical pathways: A review. Circulation 2000;101:461–467.
62. Kane RL: Creating practice guidelines: The dangers of over-reliance on expert judgment. J Law Med Ethics 1995;23:62–64.
63. Woolf SH: Shared decision-making: The case for letting patients decide which choice is best. J Fam Pract 1997;45:205–208.
64. Tinetti ME, Bogardus ST, Agostini JV: Potential pitfalls of disease specific guidelines for patients with multiple conditions. N Engl J Med 2004;351:2870–2874.
65. Lomas J, Anderson GM, Domnick-Pierre K, et al: Do practice guidelines guide practice? The effect of a consensus statement on the practice of physicians. N Engl J Med 1989;321:1306–1311.
66. Kosecoff J, Kanouse DE, Rogers WH, et al: Effects of the National Institutes of Health Consensus Development Program on physician practice. JAMA 1987;258:2708–2713.
67. Hirani NA, Macfarlance JT: Impact of management guidelines on the outcome of severe community acquired pneumonia. Thorax 1997;52:17–21.
68. Sarasin FP, Maschiangelo M-L, Schaller M-D, et al: Successful implementation of guidelines for encouraging the use of beta blockers in patients after acute myocardial infarction. Am J Med 1999;106:499–505.
69. Weingarten S, Riedinger MAS, Sandhu M, et al: Can practice guidelines safely reduce hospital length of stay? Results from a multicenter interventional study. Am J Med 1998;105:33–40.
70. Grimshaw JM, Russell IT: Effect of clinical guidelines on medical practice: A systematic review of rigorous evaluations. Lancet 1993;342:1317–1322.
71. Graham ID, Beardall S, Carter AO, et al: What is the quality of drug therapy clinical practice guidelines in Canada? CMAJ 2001;165:157–163.
72. Shaneyfelt TM, Mayo-Smith MF, Rothwangl J: Are guidelines following guidelines? The methodological quality of clinical practice guidelines in the peer reviewed medical literature. JAMA 1999;281:1900–1905.
73. Lewis SJ: Further disquiet on the guidelines front. CMAJ 2001;165:180–181.
74. Feder G: Management of mild hypertension: Which guideline to follow? BMJ 1994;308:470–471.
75. Robinson L: Guidelines for the treatment of hypertension: A critical review. Cardiovasc Drugs Ther 1994;8:665–672.
76. Hibble A, Kanka D, Pencheon D, Pooles F: Guidelines in general practice: The new tower of Babel? BMJ 1998;317:862–863.
77. Gray JAM: Data, data, data: Give me peace and knowledge. BMJ 1998;317:832–834.
78. Ellwood PM: Outcomes management, a technology of patient experience. N Engl J Med 1988;318:1549–1556.
79. Tunis SR, Hayward RSA, Wilson MC, et al: Internist's attitudes about clinical practice guidelines. Ann Intern Med 1994;120:956–963.
80. Hurwitz B: How does evidence based guidance influence determinations of medical negligence? BMJ 2004;328:1024–1028.
81. Newton J, Knight D, Woolhead G: General practitioners and clinical guidelines: A survey of knowledge, use and beliefs. Br J Gen Pract 1996;46:513–517.
82. Hyams AL, Brandenberg JA, Lipsitz SR, et al: Practice guidelines and malpractice litigation: A two way street. Ann Intern Med 1995;122:450–455.
83. Maisonneuve H, Codier H, Durocher A, Matillon Y: The French clinical guideline and medical references program: Development of

84. Durand-Zaleski I, Colin C, Blum-Boisgard C: An attempt to save money using mandatory practice guidelines in France. BMJ 1997;315:943–946.
85. Bolam v Friern Hospital Management Committee. 2 All ER 118–28 (1957).
86. Posner KL, Cheney FW, Kroll DA: Professional Liability, Risk Management, and Quality Improvement. In Barash PG, Cullen BF, Stoelting RK (eds): Clinical Anesthesia, 3rd ed. Philadelphia, Lippincott-Raven, 1997, p 93.
87. Grilli R, Magrini N, Penna A, et al: Practice guidelines developed by specialist societies: The need for critical appraisal. Lancet 2000;355:103–106.
88. McDonagh RJ, Hurwitz B: Lying in the bed we've made: Reflections on some unintended consequences of clinical practice guidelines in the courts. J Obstet Gynaecol Can 2003;25:139–143.
89. Merenstein D: Winners and losers. JAMA 2004;291:15–16.
90. Hall MA, Green MD, Hartz A: Evidence-based medicine on trial. Letter. JAMA 2004;291:1697.
91. Fleming M: Evidence-based medicine on trial. Letter. JAMA 2004;291:1697–1698.
92. Mulrow CD, Lohr K: Proof and policy from medical research evidence. J Health Polit Policy Law 2001;26:249–266.
93. Sackett DL, Rosenberg WMC, Muir Gray JA, et al: Evidence based medicine: What it is and what it isn't. BMJ 1996;312;71–72.
94. Guyatt GH: Evidence based medicine. ACP J Club 1991;114:A-16.
95. Evidence-Based Medicine Working Group: Evidence-based medicine: A new approach to teaching the practice of medicine. JAMA 1992:268;2420–2425.
96. Druss B: Evidence based medicine: Does it make a difference? BMJ 2005;330:92.
97. Guyatt G, Cook D, Haynes B: Evidence based medicine has come a long way. BMJ 2004;329:990–991.
98. Straus SE, Jones G: What has evidence based medicine done for us? BMJ 2004;329:987–988.
99. McQueen MJ: Overview of evidence-based medicine: Challenge for evidence-based laboratory medicine. Clin Chem 2001;47:1536–1546.
100. Sackett DL, Haynes RB: Evidence base of clinical diagnosis: The architecture of diagnostic research. BMJ 2002;324:539–541.
101. Saani SI, Gylling HA: Evidence based medicine guidelines: A solution to rationing or politics disguised as science? J Med Ethics 2004;30:171–175.
102. Feinstein AR, Horwitz RI: Problems in the "evidence" of "evidence-based medicine. Am J Med 1997;103:529–535.
103. Grahame-Smith D: Evidence based medicine: Socratic dissent. BMJ 1995;310:1126–1127.
104. Adams CE, Gilbody S: "Nobody ever expects the Spanish Inquisition." Psych Bull 2001;25:291–292.
105. Molesworth N: Down with EBM! BMJ 1998;317:1720–1721.
106. Clinicians for the Restoration of Autonomous Practice (CRAP) Writing Group: EMB: Unmasking the ugly truth. BMJ 2002;325:1496–1498.
107. Isaacs D, Fitzgerald D: Seven alternatives to evidence based medicine. BMJ 1999;319:1618.
108. Black N: Evidence based policy: Proceed with care. BMJ 2001;323:275–279.
109. Biller-Andorno N, Lenk C, Leititis J: Ethics, EBM, and hospital management. J Med Ethics 2004;30:136–140.
110. Pronovost PJ, Berenholtz SM, Dorman T, et al: Evidence-based medicine in anesthesiology. Anesth Analg 2001;92:787–794.
111. Steinberg EP, Luce BR: Evidence based? Caveat emptor! Health Aff 2005;24:80–92.
112. Horan BF: Evidence-based medicine and anaesthesia: Uneasy bedfellows? Anaesth Intensive Care 1997;25:679–685.
113. Goodman NW: Anesthesia and evidence-based medicine. Anaesthesia 1998;53:353–368.
114. Goodman NW: Evidence-based medicine needs proper critical review. Anesth Analg 2002;95:1817–1818.
115. Rathmell JP, Carr DB: The scientific method, evidence-based medicine, and the rational use of interventional pain treatments. Reg Anesth Pain Med 2003;28:498–501.
116. McQuay HJ, Moore A: An Evidence-Based Resource for Pain Relief. Oxford, Oxford University Press, 2002.
117. Tramer MR (ed): Evidence Based Resource in Anaesthesia and Analgesia. London, BMJ Books, 2000.

118. Merrill DG: Hoffman's glasses: Evidence-based medicine and the search for quality in the literature of interventional pain medicine. Reg Anesth Pain Med 2003;28:547–560.

119. Eddy DM: Practice policies: Where do they come from? JAMA 1990;263:1265, 1269, 1272, 1275.

120. Jackson R, Feder G: Guidelines for clinical guidelines. BMJ 1998;317:427–428.

121. Eddy DM: Comparing benefits and harms: The balance sheet. JAMA 1990;263:2493, 2498, 2501, 2505.

122. Woolf SH: Practice guidelines, a new reality in medicine. II: Methods of developing guidelines. Arch Intern Med 1992;152:946–952.

123. Eddy DM: Guidelines for policy statement: The explicit approach. JAMA 1990;263:2239–2240, 2243.

124. Shekelle PG, Woolf SH, Eccles M, Grimshaw J: Clinical guidelines: Developing guidelines. BMJ 1999;318:593–596.

125. Institute of Medicine, Committee on Health and Technology, Priority-Setting Group: National Priorities for the Assessment of Clinical Conditions and Medical Technologies: Report of a Pilot Study. Washington, DC, National Academy Press, 1990.

126. Jaeschke R, Sackett DL: Research methods for obtaining primary evidence. Int J Technol Assess Health Care 1989;5:503–519.

127. Chalmers TC, Hewett P, Reitman D, Sacks HS: Selection and evaluation of empirical research in technology assessment. Int J Technol Assess Health Care 1989;5:521–536.

128. Hunt DL, Jaeschke R, McKibbon KA: Users' guides to the medical literature. XXI: Using electronic health information resources in evidence-based practice. Evidence-Based Medicine Group. JAMA 2000;283:1875–1879.

129. Fink A, Kosecoff J, Chassin M, Brook RH: Consensus methods: Characteristics and guidelines for use. Am J Public Health I 1984; 74:979–983.

130. Carr DB, Jacox AK, Chapman CR, et al: Acute pain management: Operative or medical procedures and trauma. Clinical practice guideline No 1; AHCPR Publication No 92-0023. Rockville, Md, AHCPR, 1993, p 107.

131. The periodic health examination. Canadian Task Force on the Periodic Health Examination. Can Med Assoc J 1979;121:1193–1254.

132. Harbour R, Miller J: A new system for grading recommendations in evidence based guidelines. BMJ 2001;323:334–336.

133. Oosterhuis WP, Bruns DE, Watine J, et al: Evidence-based guidelines in laboratory medicines: Principles and methods. Clin Chem 2004;50:806–818.

134. Chambers I, Altman DG (eds): Systematic Reviews. London, BMJ, 1995.

135. Cook DJ, Mulrow CD, Haynes RB: Systematic reviews: Synthesis of best evidence for clinical decisions. Ann Intern Med 1997;126:376–380.

136. Grennhalgh T: How to read a paper: Papers that summarize other papers (systematic reviews and meta-analysis). BMJ 1997;315:672–675.

137. Glass G: Primary, secondary and meta-analysis of research. Educ Res 1976;5:3–8.

138. Bailar JC III: The practice of meta-analysis. J Clin Epidemiol 1995; 48:149–157.

139. Bailar JC III: The promise and problems of meta-analysis. N Engl J Med 1997;337:559–561.

140. Kerikowske K, Grady D, Rubin SM, et al: Efficacy of screening mammography: A meta-analysis. JAMA 1995;273:149–154.

141. Smart CR, Hendrick RE, Rutledge JH III, Smith RA: Benefit of mammography screening in women ages 40 to 49 years: Current evidence from randomized controlled trials. Cancer 1995;75:1619–1626.

142. Rosenfeld RM, Post JC: Meta-analysis of antibiotics for the treatment of otitis media with effusion. Otolaryngol Head Neck Surg 1992; 106:378–386.

143. Williams RL, Chalmers TC, Strange KC, et al: Use of antibiotics in preventing recurrent acute otitis media and treating otitis media with effusion: A meta-analytic attempt to resolve the brouhaha [erratum in JAMA 1994;271:430]. JAMA 1993;270:1344–1351.

144. Lelorier J, Grégoire G, Benhaddad A, et al: Discrepancies between meta-analysis and subsequent large, randomized, controlled trials. N Engl J Med 1997;337:536–542.

145. Hayward RSA, Wilson MC, Tunis SR, et al: Users' guides to the medical literature. VIII: How to use clinical practice guidelines. A: Are the recommendations valid? The Evidence-Based Medicine Working Group. JAMA 1995;274:570–574.

146. Hayward RSA, Wilson MC, Tunis SR, et al: Users' guides to the medical literature. VIII. How to use clinical practice guidelines. B: What are the recommendations and will they help you in caring for your patients? The Evidence-Based Medicine Working Group. JAMA 1995; 274:1630–1632.

147. Graham ID, Beardall S, Carter AO, et al: What is the quality of drug therapy clinical practice guidelines in Canada? CMAJ 2001;165: 157–163.

148. Grilli R, Magrini N, Penna A, et al: Practice guidelines developed by specialist societies: The need for a critical appraisal. Lancet 2000;355:103–106.

149. Lewis SJ: Further disquiet on the guideline front. CMAJ 2001;165: 180–181.

150. Grol R: Implementing guidelines in general practice care. Quality in Health Care 1992;1:184–191.

151. Lomas J, Anderson GM, Domnick-Pierre K, et al: Do practice guidelines guide practice? The effect of a consensus statement on the practice of physicians. N Engl J Med 1989;321:1306–1311.

152. Freemantle N, Harvey EL, Wolf F, et al: Printed educational materials: Effects on professional practice and health care outcomes (Cochrane Review 2000). In The Cochrane Library, issue 3. Chichester, UK: John Wiley & Sons, 2003.

153. Lomas, J Enkin M, Anderson GM, et al: Opinion leaders vs audit and feedback to implement practice guidelines: Delivery after previous Cesarean section. JAMA 1991;265:2202–2207.

154. Martens WC, Higby DJ, Brown D, et al: Improving the care of patients with regard to chemotherapy-induced nausea and emesis: The effect of feedback to clinicians on adherence to antiemetic prescription guidelines. J Clin Oncol 2003;21:1373–1378.

155. Bradley EH, Holmboe ES, Mattera JA, et al: A qualitative study on increasing β-blocker use after myocardial infarction: Why do some hospitals succeed? JAMA 2001;285:2604–2611.

156. Ansari M, Shlipak MG, Heidenreich PA, et al: Improving guideline adherence: A randomizes trial evaluating strategies to increase β-blocker use in heart failure. Circulation 2003;107:2799–2807.

157. Phillips LS, Branch WT Jr, Cook CB, et al: Clinical inertia. Ann Intern Med 2001;135:825–834.

158. Cabana MD, Rand CS, Powe NR, et al: Why don't physicians follow clinical practice guidelines? A framework for improvement. JAMA 1999;282:1458–1465.

159. Haynes RB, Devereaux PJ, Guyatt GH: Physicians' and patients' choices in evidence based practice: Evidence does not make decisions, people do. BMJ 2002;324:1350.

160. Gabbay J, le May A: Evidence based guidelines or collectively constructed "mindlines"? Ethnographic study of knowledge management in primary care. BMJ 2004;329:1013–1018.

161. Grol R, Dalhuijsen J, Thomas S, et al: Attributes of clinical guidelines that influence use of guidelines on general practice: Observational study. BMJ 1998;317:858–861.

162. Grol R, Grimshaw J: Evidence-based implementation of evidence-based medicine. Jt Comm J Qual Improv 1999;25:503–513.

163. Pierce EC Jr: The development of anesthesia guidelines and standards. QRB Qual Rev Bull 1990;16:61–64.

164. Pomeranz D: Practice parameters: Massachusetts Medical Society studies potential. Penn Med 1991;94:16,18.

165. Holzer JF: The advent of clinical standards for professional liability. QRB Qual Rev Bull 1990;16:71–79.

166. Kelly JT, Kellie SE: Medicare peer review organization preprocedure review criteria. JAMA 1991;265:1265–1270.

167. Larson EB: Evidence-based medicine: Is translating evidence into practice a solution to the cost-quality challenges facing medicine? Jt Comm J Qual Improv 1999;25:480–485.

168. Strunk BC, Hurley RE: Paying for quality: Health plans try carrots instead of sticks. Issue Brief Cent Stud Health Syst Change 2004 May; (82):1–4.

169. Shekelle P, Eccles MP, Grimshaw JM, Woolf SH: When should clinical guidelines be updated? BMJ 2001;323:155–157.

170. Shekelle PG, Ortiz E, Rhodes S, et al: Validity of the Agency for Healthcare Research and Quality clinical guidelines: How quickly do guidelines become outdated? JAMA 2001;286:1461–1467.

171. Bowman GP: Development and aftercare of clinical guidelines: The balance between rigor and pragmatism. JAMA 2001;286:1509–1511.

172. Gartlehner G, West SL, Lohr KN, et al: Assessing the need to update prevention guidelines: A comparison of two methods. Int J Quality Health Care 2004;16:399–406.

173. Woolf SH: Practice guidelines: A new reality in medicine. III: Impact on patient care. Arch Intern Med 1993;153:2646–2655.

174. Hill MN, Levine DM, Whelton PK: Awareness, use and impact of the 1984 Joint National Committee Report on High Blood Pressure. Am J Public Health 1988;78:1190–1194.

175. Stange KC, Kelly R, Chao J, et al: Physician agreement with the US Preventive Task Services Force recommendations. J Fam Pract 1992;34:409–416.

176. Fowler G, Mant D, Fuller A, Jones L: The "Help Your Patient Stop" initiative: Evaluation of smoking prevalence and dissemination of WHO/UICC guidelines in general practice. Lancet 1989;1(8649):1253–1255.

177. Miles A, Bentley P, Polychronis A, Grey J: Evidence-based medicine: Why all the fuss? This is why. J Eval Clin Pract 1997;3:83–85.

178. Krumholz HM, Radford MJ, Ellerbeck EF, et al: Aspirin for secondary prevention after acute myocardial infarction in the elderly: Prescribed use and outcomes. Ann Intern Med 1996;124:292–298.

179. Krumholz HM, Radford MJ, Wang Y, et al: National use and effectiveness of beta-blockers for the treatment of elderly patients after acute myocardial infarction. National Cooperative Cardiovascular Project. JAMA 1998;280:623–629.

180. Wong JH, Findlay JM, Suarez-Almazor ME: Regional performance of carotid endarterectomy: Appropriateness, outcomes and risk factors for complications. Stroke 1997;28:891–898.

181. Straus SE, McAlister FA: Evidence-based medicine: A commentary on common criticisms. CMAJ 2000;163:837–841.

182. Health Services/Technology Assessment Text: Acute pain management: operative or medical procedures and trauma. Available at www.ncbi.nlm.nih.gov/books/bv.fcgi?rid=hstat6.chapter.8991 (accessed November 1, 2005)

183. Carr DB: The development of national guidelines for pain control: Synopsis and commentary. Eur J Pain 2001;5(Suppl A):91–98.

184. Practice guidelines for acute pain management in the perioperative setting. Available at www.asahq.org/publicationsAndServices/pain.pdf (accessed March 14, 2005).

185. National Health and Medical Research Council (Australia): Acute pain management: Scientific evidence. Available at www.nhmrc.gov.au/publications/_files/cp104.pdf (accessed June 20, 2005).

4

The Neurohumoral, Inflammatory, and Coagulation Responses to Surgery

CONOR J. SHIELDS • H. PAUL REDMOND

Surgeons and anesthetists are frequently called on to manage not only the sequelae of patients' illnesses but also the physiological cost of the host metabolic response. This stress response has metabolic, hormonal, immunological, and hematological components. These equip the patient to survive under adverse circumstances and are integral to successful recovery from surgery. Alterations in protein and energy homeostasis are accompanied by fundamental changes in anabolic and catabolic profiles of distant organs. Although these complex and integrated responses are indispensable, an overexuberant response may result in dishomeostasis, predisposing the patient to multiple organ failure syndrome (MOFS) and, ultimately, death.[1]

The response to surgery may be subdivided into a number of distinct phases—either the classic "ebb" and "flow" phases of Cuthbertson[1-3] or Moore's four-phase characterization (injury phase, turning point, anabolic phase, and late anabolism).[4] The longevity of the response is determined in part by the magnitude of the initiating insult.

A number of stimuli provoke the physiological response to injury (Fig. 4–1). Surgery is classically accompanied by anxiety, fasting, anesthetic agents, pain, and immobilization, each of which exerts minor incremental effects on the host stress response. Disruption of tissue, invasion of body cavities, and extracellular fluid loss result in exaggeration of this response, occasionally to a maladaptive extent—hence the utility of minimally invasive and laparoscopic approaches in abrogating a potentially inappropriate response (Table 4–1).[5,6]

The Neurohumoral Response

Neuroafferent signals (such as pain) and the central nervous system (CNS) participate in a neurohumoral reflex arc, in which signaling to the CNS is both neural and endocrinological. Nociceptors, baroreceptors, and chemoreceptors initiate the sympathetic stress response while also attempting to limit injury by provoking avoidance mechanisms.

Activation of the stress system leads to a focused global response, heightening arousal and cognitive function and increasing tolerance of pain.[7,8] Many local inflammatory mediators activate the dual limbs of the stress system, the hypothalamic-pituitary-adrenal axis and the adrenomedullary sympathetic system (Fig. 4–2). These axes respond to a range of diverse signals, including limbic stimuli, circadian stimuli, and blood-borne stimuli, such as tumor necrosis factor-α (TNF-α) and interleukin-1 (IL-1) and IL-6 issuing from the wound.[9]

HYPOTHALAMIC CONTROL

The response to pain is integrated in the cortex via the spinothalamic tracts and the thalamus, coupled with transmission to the hypothalamic and medullary sympathetic centers, resulting in central and regional neuroendocrine activation. Although pain is experienced objectively in the higher centers, the hypothalamus represents the uppermost level of coordination of the autonomic sequelae of surgery. During general anesthesia, pain fibers are activated, generating afferent signals. This activation is attenuated during epidural and spinal anesthesia, but the acute-phase protein response is unimpeded because it is derived from locally secreted inflammatory mediators.[10]

Hypothalamic stimulation results in activation of the autonomic nervous system and influences release of pituitary hormones (Table 4–2). Cumulatively, these agents occasion the downstream liberation of a number of potent effector compounds, including antidiuretic hormone (ADH) from the neurohypophysis, epinephrine from the adrenal medulla, and norepinephrine from sympathetic nerve endings. Release of corticotrophin-releasing hormone (CRH) and ADH is stimulated by firing of the cholinergic and serotonergic systems and is inhibited by benzodiazepines and the opioid systems of the CNS.[11] Activation of the stress system results in increased CRH-mediated secretion of opioid and pro-opiomelanocortin (POMC)–derived peptides, such as β-endorphins and

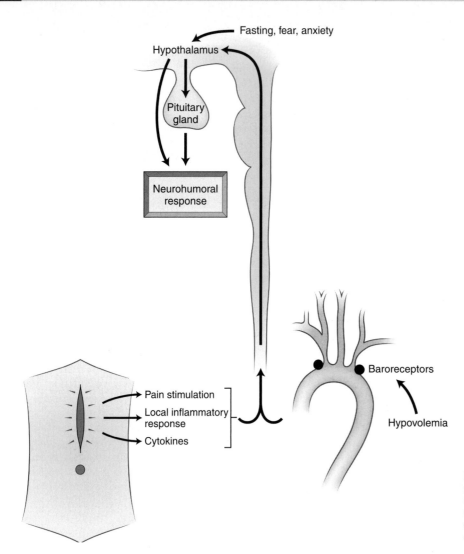

Figure 4–1 The stimuli provoking the host metabolic response to injury and surgery. Baroreceptors, chemoreceptors, and nociceptors initiate the response, which may be exaggerated by immunoregulatory peptides and cytokines issuing from the wound.

TABLE 4–1	Extent of Neurohumoral Response to Surgery	
Procedure	**Stimuli**	**Neurohumoral Response**
Inguinal hernia repair	Anxiety	Response persists for 2–5 days
Laparoscopy	Fear	Focused local inflammatory response, with blunted
Laparoscopic colorectal surgery	Pain	systemic inflammation
	Anesthetic agents	
	Immobilization	
Laparotomy	Fasting	Stress response persists for at least 1 week
Open colorectal surgery	Extracellular fluid loss	Potent, effective, and precise inflammatory response
Elective abdominal aortic aneurysm repair	Invasion of body cavity	Increased circulating carbohydrates, lipids, and proteins
	Blood transfusion	
	Infection	
Laparotomy for visceral perforation	Overwhelming sepsis	Prolonged stress response
Emergency abdominal aortic aneurysm repair	Tissue necrosis	Feed-forward inflammatory response, with continued
	Shock	activation
		Overwhelming protein catabolism
Emergency laparotomy for fulminant colitis	Starvation	May result in multiple organ failure

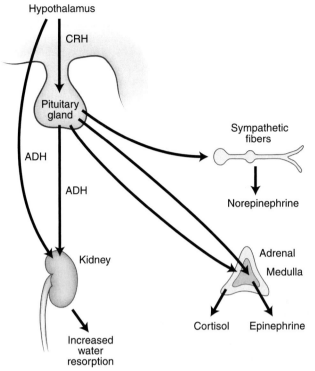

Figure 4–2   The efferent stimuli of the stress system. The hypothalamic-pituitary-adrenal axis *(left)* and the adrenomedullary sympathetic system *(right)*. Hypothalamic activation results in activation of the autonomic nervous system, via release of corticotropin-releasing hormone (CRH) and antidiuretic hormone (ADH), leading to increased water resorption and release of cortisol, epinephrine, and norepinephrine.

enkephalins, in both the arcuate nucleus of the hypothalamus and areas of the hindbrain and spinal cord concerned with pain control, thereby augmenting the analgesic response and attenuating the sympathetic response to noxious stimuli.[12]

PITUITARY HORMONES

Growth hormone (GH) plays an important role in homeostasis, being released in a pulsatile fashion at night; however, its role in the response to injury is less clearly defined. GH stimulates protein synthesis and antagonizes insulin under normal conditions but does not act in this manner in protracted illness, despite elevated concentrations.[13] Although administration of exogenous GH has enjoyed a certain cachet, its efficacy is now disputed, with some reports of increased mortality with its use.[14] Other pituitary hormones appear to have little role in the response to surgery. Secretion of sex hormones, despite their immunomodulatory potential, is moderated in response to elevated CRH, resulting in decreased libido and suppression of menses. Levels of thyroid-stimulating hormone appear unaffected by stress, although inactive thyroxine (reverse tri-iodothyronine) levels rise, causing euthyroid sick syndrome.

GLUCOCORTICOIDS

Glucocorticoid hormone release from the adrenal cortex follows CRH-induced production of adrenocorticotropic hormone (ACTH) by the adenohypophysis. ACTH liberation usually exhibits a circadian variability, which is lost after surgery, when ADH, various catecholamines, aldosterone, and angiotensin II act synergistically to ensure a sustained elevation.[15]

Cortisol plays an important role in generating a nutritive milieu for the wound by increasing circulating carbohydrates, free fatty acids, triglycerides, and protein derived from muscle breakdown, resulting in net nitrogen loss. Glucose tolerance is substantially reduced, an occurrence attributed to greater hepatic gluconeogenesis, insulin resistance, and augmented lipolysis.

The immunomodulatory effects of glucocorticoids, which are well described, make them an important tool in the management of diseases characterized by hyperinflammation,

TABLE 4–2	Hormonal Changes	
Origin	**Hormone**	**Effect(s)**
Hypothalamus	Corticotropin-releasing hormone (CRH)	Stimulates release of adrenocorticotropin hormone (ACTH)
	Growth hormone	No recognized role
	Antidiuretic hormone (ADH)	Preservation of extracellular volume
		Peripheral and splanchnic vasoconstriction
	Substance P	Inhibits CRH secretion
	β-endorphins	Enhance analgesia
Pituitary	Corticotropin	Increased ACTH release
	Follicle-stimulating hormone—luteinizing hormone (FSH-LH)	Decreased secretion; diminished libido, interrupted menses
	Antidiuretic hormone (ADH)	Increased secretion
		Preservation of extracellular volume
		Peripheral and splanchnic vasoconstriction
Adrenal cortex	Cortisol	Immunomodulation
	Aldosterone	Increases extracellular volume
Adrenal medulla	Catecholamines	Increased liberation; hypermetabolism
Pancreas	Insulin	Augments anabolism in presence of insulin resistance
	Glucagon	Increased; results in glucose production for wound

in which their effects provide potential strategies for attenuating inappropriate neutrophil activation. The glucocorticoids exert their effects partly by suppressing gene transcription rates of proinflammatory cytokines such as IL-1β and IL-6 and by compromising the stability of their messenger RNA.[16,17] The benefits extend to the attenuation of receptor-mediated polymorphonuclear cell (PMN) functions, including the downregulation of neutrophil oxidative burst activity and adhesion molecule expression, and the suppression of PMN activation. The inhibition of neutrophil–endothelial cell interactions appears to confer protection against organ injury in inappropriate inflammatory states.

VOLUME REGULATION

Preservation of extracellular volume and osmolarity is a fundamental component of the stress response to surgery and injury. It is served by a number of discrete hormones working in concert. Increased serum osmolarity is the traditional stimulus for ADH secretion, but anxiety, pain, and reduced blood volume act to augment water resorption in the distal renal tubule through hypothalamic stimulation. Maintenance of adequate perfusion is further ensured by ADH-mediated peripheral and splanchnic vasoconstriction. ADH elevations may persist for more than a week. Release of aldosterone from the adrenal cortex is stimulated by ACTH, although angiotensin II has an important adjuvant role in liberation of this mineralocorticoid. Aldosterone acts on the distal tubule to enhance exchange of hydrogen and potassium for sodium and, consequently, acts synergistically with ADH to increase extracellular volume, at the expense of potential metabolic acidosis.

Renin secretion from the juxtaglomerular apparatus is similarly prompted by adverse alterations in the osmolarity of the extracellular milieu. It is promoted by sympathetic system stimulation of the local myoepithelial cells and augmented by ACTH, ADH, and glucagon. Renin activity yields angiotensin I, which is converted by angiotensin-converting enzyme in the pulmonary vasculature to the active angiotensin II. In addition to provoking further release of CRH, ADH, and aldosterone, angiotensin II is a potent vasoconstrictor.

INSULIN

Given the relatively hyperglycemic and insulin-resistant state that occurs after significant injury, one may be inclined to discount the contribution of the pancreatic hormone insulin to modulation of the inflammatory state. However, compelling evidence is emerging that insulin contributes to the generation of a more benign immunological profile by augmenting anabolism, mitigating the effect of TNF-α, and decreasing the production of reactive oxygen species (ROS) by antagonizing nuclear factor κB (NFκB).[18–20] The apotheosis of insulin has been furthered by reports of significantly improved outcome with tight control of plasma glucose through the use of exogenous insulin in critically ill patients.[21]

PSYCHONEUROIMMUNOLOGY

The notion that emotional state and aspects of personality may influence immune responses has now been accepted by many authorities.[22] Signaling to the target glands of the neurohumoral reflex arc is subject to hypothalamic control, which in turn may be influenced by suprahypothalamic stimuli. Pavlovian conditioning has been shown to suppress immune response in animals,[23] whereas medical students have been shown to have diminished natural killer cell activity at examination times.[24] There are critics of the view that fundamental physiological responses may be altered by emotional states, but alterations in pain perception may conceivably affect the magnitude of the neuroendocrine response. Indeed, neuroticism, but not depression or anxiety, is a risk factor for persistent pain after cholecystectomy.[25,26]

The Inflammatory Response

Afferent output from the wound attempts to establish biological preeminence, signaling a greater need for increased nutritive substrate, and provides information on the status of the wound and local environment. Induction of healing through the institution of an acute inflammatory reaction may be attributed to the secretion by the wound of bioactive peptides, especially cytokines. The signaling molecule TNF-α, discharged from activated macrophages, exerts a considerable amplifying influence on the local and systemic inflammatory response. These mediators of inflammation also exert remote proinflammatory effects; hence, within the context of an injury, the wound may be regarded as a distinct organ.[27] The propensity of local inflammation to induce an acute response from the systemic stress system via afferent sensory fibers is predicated on the complex interplay of proinflammatory and anti-inflammatory factors. The afferent neurons may also influence this propensity through secretion of proinflammatory or anti-inflammatory peptides, including somatostatin and substance P.[28]

Increased endothelial permeability within the environment of the wound facilitates the migration of leukocytes and other immune-competent cells from the intravascular compartment. The wound engages in a process of recruitment of immune and accessory cells, each cell serving to enhance the proinflammatory signals. Neutrophils and macrophages are among the most eager recruits (Fig. 4–3).

A variety of immunoactive peptides, including histamine, chemokines, and proteases, is liberated by activated mast cells within the wound. Release of intracellular proteins, such as high-motility group box protein 1 (HMGB1), ensues with cell death and triggers the further release of cytokines, ROS, matrix metalloproteinases, and local vasodilators such as nitric oxide (NO). The perception of pain at a site of inflammation appears to be mediated, at least in part, by NO.[29,30] Whereas high doses of NO may enhance the sensitivity of peripheral nociceptors and induce pain, compounds generating a low NO concentration can serve to reduce incisional pain.[29]

Neutrophil-derived elastase, in conjunction with ROS, activates the matrix metalloproteinases, leading to liberation of transforming growth factor-β (TGF-β), which results in profound local chemoattraction, securing the influx of further neutrophils and macrophages. The induction of the local transcription factor NFκB, and the consequent expression of multiple rapid-response inflammatory genes, culminating in the release of IL-6 and IL-8, TNF-α, and

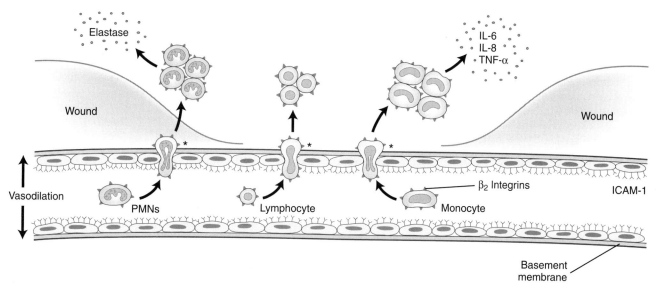

Figure 4–3 The wound with associated inflammatory response. Asterisk (*) indicates increased permeability of endothelium basement membrane. The local inflammatory response results in chemoattraction of a variety of immunocompetent cells with endothelial hyperpermeability. ICAM-1, intercellular adhesion molecule-1; IL, interleukin; PMNs, polymorphonuclear cells; TNF-α, tumor necrosis factor α.

cyclooxygenase-2 (Cox-2), further influences the inflammatory milieu (Table 4–3).[31]

Subsequent neutrophil entrapment within the wound is a consequence of complement activation and cytokine production, culminating in stimulation of adhesion molecule expression.[32] Exposure of neutrophils to these endogenous inflammatory mediators leads to an upregulation of β2 integrin CD11b/CD18 expression and enhanced adhesive potential. The cytokine-driven inflammatory response results in an upregulation of expression of both intercellular adhesion molecule-1 (ICAM-1) on endothelial cells and β2 integrin on leukocytes. This facilitates neutrophil–endothelial cell interaction, in due course provoking endothelial hyperpermeability. The initial step in a process culminating in firm neutrophil–endothelial cell adherence is neutrophil rolling, which involves L-selectin and P-selectin and is mediated by the endothelium (see Fig. 4–3).

Further enhancement of leukocyte accumulation in vascular beds is facilitated by conformational changes in the actin cytoskeleton in conjunction with alterations in the adhesive qualities of neutrophils. Cytoskeletal structures in activated neutrophils are rendered more resolute by polymerization of F-actin filaments and are less inclined to deform,[33] resulting in entrapment of activated leukocytes within capillaries. Phagocytosis of entrapped apoptotic neutrophils at the site of inflammation serves to limit neutrophil-mediated tissue insult.[34] Dysfunction of this regulatory mechanism is a pivotal component in the propagation of the massive inflammatory response evident in systemic inflammatory response syndrome (SIRS).

The initiation of complex intracellular signal transduction pathways leads to increased integrin-binding avidity resulting from tyrosine kinase activation,[35] which is in turn occasioned by redistribution of cytoskeletal proteins.

TABLE 4–3	Wound-Derived Mediators	
Mediator	**Origin(s)**	**Effect(s)**
Tumor necrosis factor-α (TNF-α)	Macrophages	Proinflammatory Proapoptotic Production of interleukin-1β (IL-1β)
Histamine	Mast cells	Vasodilatation
Chemokines	Diverse: macrophages, dendritic cells, T cells	Monocyte and lymphocyte chemoattraction
IL-1β	Macrophages Endothelial cells	Acts synergistically with TNF-α to augment inflammatory response Endogenous pyrogen
IL-6	Macrophages T cells	Mediates hepatic acute phase response Both proinflammatory and anti-inflammatory
IL-8	Macrophages	Leukocyte chemoattraction
IL-10	T cells	Anti-inflammatory; inhibits TNF-α
IL-12	Macrophages Dendritic cells	Proinflammatory Differentiation of type 1 helper T (TH1) cells
Cyclooxygenase-2 (Cox-2)	Membrane phospholipids	Catalyzes conversion of arachidonic acid to prostaglandins

Phosphorylation of various protein tyrosine kinases—including the lipid kinase phosphatidylinositol 3-kinase (PI 3-k),[36] protein kinase C,[37] Src-kinases, and the mitogen-activated protein (MAP) kinases such as p38 MAP kinase, extracellular signal–related kinase (ERK), and Jun N-terminal kinase[38]—is a recurrent theme in signal transduction. The activation of p38 MAP kinase by lipopolysaccharides (LPSs)[39] augments neutrophil immune potential by escalating the liberation of free radicals, enhancing integrin adhesive qualities,[40] and regulating the synthesis of proinflammatory cytokines.[41]

The Coagulation Response

The inflammatory and coagulation systems are highly conserved and tightly integrated defense mechanisms deriving from a common eukaryotic ancestor. They act in tandem to preserve host integrity by preventing loss from the intravascular space and combating microbial entry. Subsequent phagocytosis of any offending microorganism is elicited by the interaction of membrane-bound receptors with particulate ligands on the surface of the pathogen.[42] Concomitant microbial killing results from neutrophil degranulation with release of proteolytic enzymes and generation of ROS.[43] This inflammatory response shifts the balance of coagulation in favor of thrombosis through a number of discrete pathways: upregulation of tissue factors involved in the initiation of clotting and thrombin generation, inhibition of fibrinolysis, and antagonism of anticoagulation through cytokine-mediated downregulation of endothelial cell receptors for protein C within the microvasculature. Thrombin and TNF-α also act synergistically to diminish expression of thrombomodulin, a coactivator of protein C.[44,45] In states of hyperinflammation, the diminished expression of thrombomodulin may lead to manifestations of microvascular dysfunction, such as hypoxia, acidosis, and disseminated intravascular coagulation.

Conclusion

The ability of humans to survive injury and surgery implies that wound healing is a fundamental and teleological biological goal. Afferent signals from pain receptors are among the first intimations of injury, culminating in neuroendocrine activation and the unleashing of a cascade of hypothalamic and pituitary hormones. Peripherally, the immune system is stimulated by antigens, with consequent liberation of immunoregulatory peptides and cytokines such as TNF-α, IL-1, and IL-6, resulting ultimately in diversion of energy from anabolic to catabolic pathways. Peripheral sensory neurons monitor the wound environment and exert an immunomodulatory effect through secretion of substance P and somatostatin.

The intricate and integrated neurohumoral, inflammatory, and coagulation responses to surgery result in an uneasy equilibrium between proinflammatory and anti-inflammatory forces, between procoagulant and anticoagulant tendencies, and between anabolism and catabolism. Various therapeutic endeavors have been proposed to tip the balance from debilitating catabolism, but few exhibit pertinence in the clinical setting.[46] Improved supportive and ventilatory management

of critically ill patients has resulted in a modest decline in overall mortality rate, but the underlying inflammatory processes remain unchecked by medical intervention.[41] Supportive care—specifically, optimizing the extracellular environment, restoring tissue oxygenation, and achieving adequate pain control—remains the principal determinant of outcome.

REFERENCES

1. Boontham P, Chandran P, Rowlands B, Eremin O: Surgical sepsis: Dysregulation of immune function and therapeutic implications. Surgeon 2003;1:187–206.
2. Cuthbertson D: Post-shock metabolic response. Lancet 1942;1:433–437.
3. Sibbald WJ: Shockingly complex: The difficult road to introducing new ideas to critical care. Crit Care 2004;8:419–421.
4. Moore F: Bodily changes in surgical convalescence. 1: The normal sequence-observations and interpretations. Ann Surg 1953;137:289–315.
5. Wu FP, Sietses C, von Blomberg BM, et al: Systemic and peritoneal inflammatory response after laparoscopic or conventional colon resection in cancer patients: A prospective, randomized trial. Dis Colon Rectum 2003;46:147–155.
6. Da Costa ML, Redmond HP, Finnegan N, et al: Laparotomy and laparoscopy differentially accelerate experimental flank tumour growth. Br J Surg 1998;85:1439–1442.
7. Chrousos GP, Gold PW: The concepts of stress and stress system disorders: Overview of physical and behavioral homeostasis. JAMA 1992;267:1244–1252.
8. Chrousos GP: Regulation and dysregulation of the hypothalamic-pituitary-adrenal axis: The corticotropin-releasing hormone perspective. Endocrinol Metab Clin North Am 1992;21:833–858.
9. Johnson JD, O'Connor KA, Watkins LR, Maier SF: The role of IL-1beta in stress-induced sensitization of proinflammatory cytokine and corticosterone responses. Neuroscience 2004;127:569–577.
10. Buyukkocak U, Caglayan O, Oral H, et al: The effects of anesthetic techniques on acute phase response at delivery (anesthesia and acute phase response). Clin Biochem 2003;36:67–70.
11. Grottoli S, Maccagno B, Ramunni J, et al: Alprazolam, a benzodiazepine, does not modify the ACTH and cortisol response to hCRH and AVP, but blunts the cortisol response to ACTH in humans. J Endocrinol Invest 2002;25:420–425.
12. Fukuda Y, Kageyama K, Nigawara T, et al: Effects of corticotropin-releasing hormone (CRH) on the synthesis and secretion of proopio-melanocortin-related peptides in the anterior pituitary: A study using CRH-deficient mice. Neurosci Lett 2004;367:201–204.
13. Shipman J, Guy J, Abumrad NN: Repair of metabolic processes. Crit Care Med 2003;31(Suppl):S512–S517.
14. Takala J, Ruokonen E, Webster NR, et al: Increased mortality associated with growth hormone treatment in critically ill adults. N Engl J Med 1999;341:785–792.
15. Mussi C, Angelini C, Crippa S, et al: Alteration of hypothalamus-pituitary-adrenal glands axis in colorectal cancer patients. Hepatogastroenterology 2003;50(Suppl 2):ccxxviii–ccxxxi.
16. Zitnik RJ, Whiting NL, Elias JA: Glucocorticoid inhibition of interleukin-1-induced interleukin-6 production by human lung fibroblasts: Evidence for transcriptional and post-transcriptional regulatory mechanisms. Am J Respir Cell Mol Biol 1994;10:643–650.
17. Zanker B, Walz G, Wieder KJ, Strom TB: Evidence that glucocorticosteroids block expression of the human interleukin-6 gene by accessory cells. Transplantation 1990;49:183–185.
18. Dandona P, Aljada A, Mohanty P, et al: Insulin inhibits intranuclear nuclear factor kappaB and stimulates IkappaB in mononuclear cells in obese subjects: Evidence for an anti-inflammatory effect? J Clin Endocrinol Metab 2001;86:3257–3265.
19. Satomi N, Sakurai A, Haranaka K: Relationship of hypoglycemia to tumor necrosis factor production and antitumor activity: Role of glucose, insulin, and macrophages. J Natl Cancer Inst 1985;74:1255–1260.
20. Das UN: Is insulin an antiinflammatory molecule? Nutrition 2001;17:409–413.
21. van den Berghe G, Wouters P, Weekers F, et al: Intensive insulin therapy in the critically ill patients. N Engl J Med 2001;345:1359–1367.

22. Carr DJ: Neuroendocrine peptide receptors on cells of the immune system. Chem Immunol 1992;52:84–105.
23. Cohen N, Moynihan JA, Ader R: Pavlovian conditioning of the immune system. Int Arch Allergy Immunol 1994;105:101–106.
24. Malarkey WB, Hall JC, Pearl DK, et al: The influence of academic stress and season on 24-hour concentrations of growth hormone and prolactin. J Clin Endocrinol Metab 1991;73:1089–1092.
25. Borly L, Anderson IB, Bardram L, et al: Preoperative prediction model of outcome after cholecystectomy for symptomatic gallstones. Scand J Gastroenterol 1999;34:1144–1152.
26. Jess P, Jess T, Beck H, Bech P: Neuroticism in relation to recovery and persisting pain after laparoscopic cholecystectomy. Scand J Gastroenterol 1998;33:550–553.
27. Baue AE: Sepsis, systemic inflammatory response syndrome, multiple organ dysfunction syndrome, and multiple organ failure: Are trauma surgeons lumpers or splitters? J Trauma 2003;55:997–998.
28. Coderre TJ, Basbaum AI, Levine JD: Neural control of vascular permeability: Interactions between primary afferents, mast cells, and sympathetic efferents. J Neurophysiol 1989;62:48–58.
29. Prado WA, Schiavon VF, Cunha FQ: Dual effect of local application of nitric oxide donors in a model of incision pain in rats. Eur J Pharmacol 2002;441:57–65.
30. Anbar M, Gratt BM: Role of nitric oxide in the physiopathology of pain. J Pain Symptom Manage 1997;14:225–254.
31. Ardite E, Panes J, Miranda M, et al: Effects of steroid treatment on activation of nuclear factor kappaB in patients with inflammatory bowel disease. Br J Pharmacol 1998;124:431–433.
32. Closa D, Sabater L, Fernandez-Cruz L, et al: Activation of alveolar macrophages in lung injury associated with experimental acute pancreatitis is mediated by the liver. Ann Surg 1999;229:230–236.
33. Skoutelis AT, Kaleridis V, Athanassiou GM, et al: Neutrophil deformability in patients with sepsis, septic shock, and adult respiratory distress syndrome. Crit Care Med 2000;28:2355–2359.
34. Sookhai S, Wang JH, McCourt M, et al: Dopamine induces neutrophil apoptosis through a dopamine D-1 receptor-independent mechanism. Surgery 1999;126:314–322.
35. Yan SR, Berton G: Antibody-induced engagement of beta2 integrins in human neutrophils causes a rapid redistribution of cytoskeletal proteins, Src-family tyrosine kinases, and p72syk that precedes de novo actin polymerization. J Leukoc Biol 1998;64:401–408.
36. Capodici C, Hanft S, Feoktistov M, Pillinger MH: Phosphatidylinositol 3-kinase mediates chemoattractant-stimulated, CD11b/CD18-dependent cell-cell adhesion of human neutrophils: Evidence for an ERK-independent pathway. J Immunol 1998;160:1901–1909.
37. Toker A, Cantley LC: Signalling through the lipid products of phosphoinositide-3-OH kinase. Nature 1997;387(6634):673–676.
38. Scherle PA, Jones EA, Favata MF, et al: Inhibition of MAP kinase kinase prevents cytokine and prostaglandin E2 production in lipopolysaccharide-stimulated monocytes. J Immunol 1998;161:5681–5686.
39. St-Denis A, Chano F, Tremblay P, et al: Protein kinase C-alpha modulates lipopolysaccharide-induced functions in a murine macrophage cell line. J Biol Chem 1998;273:32787–32792.
40. Nick JA, Avdi NJ, Young SK, et al: Common and distinct intracellular signaling pathways in human neutrophils utilized by platelet activating factor and FMLP. J Clin Invest 1997;99:975–986.
41. Denham W, Yang J, Wang H, et al: Inhibition of p38 mitogen activate kinase attenuates the severity of pancreatitis-induced adult respiratory distress syndrome. Crit Care Med 2000;28:2567–2572.
42. Horwitz AH, Williams RE, Liu PS, Nadell R: Bactericidal/permeability-increasing protein inhibits growth of a strain of Acholeplasma laidlawii and L forms of the gram-positive bacteria Staphylococcus aureus and Streptococcus pyogenes. Antimicrob Agents Chemother 1999;43:2314–2316.
43. Krump E, Sanghera JS, Pelech SL, et al: Chemotactic peptide N-formyl-met-leu-phe activation of p38 mitogen-activated protein kinase (MAPK) and MAPK-activated protein kinase-2 in human neutrophils. J Biol Chem 1997;272:937–944.
44. Conway G, Wooley J, Bibring T, LeStourgeon WM: Ribonucleoproteins package 700 nucleotides of pre-mRNA into a repeating array of regular particles. Mol Cell Biol 1988;8:2884–2895.
45. Moore KL, Esmon CT, Esmon NL: Tumor necrosis factor leads to the internalization and degradation of thrombomodulin from the surface of bovine aortic endothelial cells in culture. Blood 1989;73:159–165.
46. Fulkerson WJ, MacIntyre N, Stamler J, Crapo JD: Pathogenesis and treatment of the adult respiratory distress syndrome. Arch Intern Med 1996;156:29–38.

5 Mechanisms of Postoperative Pain—Nociceptive

HENRY FRIZELLE

Pain is defined by the International Association for the Study of Pain as "an unpleasant sensory and emotional experience associated with actual or potential tissue damage, or described in terms of such damage"[1] (Table 5–1). *Nociception* describes the mechanisms by which pain information is passed to the central nervous system. How this information is finally perceived as pain remains unclear. Classically, the following four processes are described:

Transduction: The conversion of the noxious thermal, mechanical, or chemical stimulus into nerve impulses by sensory receptors called nociceptors.

Transmission: Sending of these signals from the peripheral site of transduction to the brain and spinal cord.

Perception: Appreciation of these signals as pain.

Modulation: The process by which descending signals from the brain change nociceptive transmission at the spinal cord.[2,3]

Transduction

Nociceptors are sensory receptors with a high threshold for activation and are primarily sensitive to tissue trauma or to non-noxious stimuli that would damage tissue if exposure were prolonged.[4] These receptors are the free endings of primary afferent nerve fibers that are distributed throughout the body's periphery. A *noxious stimulus* (one that when prolonged produces damage resulting in the humoral and cellular responses to inflammation) activates myelinated A-δ and unmyelinated C nociceptors. A-δ nociceptors are mechanically sensitive and transduce pricking sensations at 5 to 25 m/sec. C nociceptors are polymodal, conduct at less than 2 m/sec, and convey impulses generated by tissue damage; being polymodal, they respond to thermal, chemical, and mechanical insults (Fig. 5–1).

In addition to direct nociception, surgical trauma produces a neurohumoral inflammatory response resulting in the release of intracellular contents (potassium, bradykinin, prostaglandins) from both damaged and inflammatory cells. This heightens the sensitivity of nociceptors at the site of injury. Consequently, there is a greater response to painful stimulus at the site of trauma (*primary hyperalgesia*). An axon reflex sends impulses toward the spinal cord but also toward other peripheral branches of the nociceptors. This causes release of neuropeptide (substance P, calcitonin gene–related peptide), inducing vasodilatation and mast cell degranulation. Both histamine and serotonin are released after mast cell degranulation.[5] These proinflammatory agents sensitize adjacent A-δ and C nociceptors (*secondary hyperalgesia*). Many nociceptors ("sleeping nociceptors") cannot normally be activated and become excitable only under pathological conditions,[6] such as inflammation.

Transmission

The nerve impulses generated in the periphery are transmitted to the brain and spinal cord in several phases.[7] Sensory nerve impulses travel via the axons of the primary afferent neurons of the dorsal horn of the spinal cord. The dorsal root ganglia (DRG) contain the cell bodies of the A-δ and C nociceptors. After entering the spinal cord, the nociceptors ascend or descend several segments in Lissauer's tract prior to synapsing with second-order neurons in laminae I, II (substantia gelatinosa), and V of the dorsal horn. The main transmitter used by nociceptors synapsing in the dorsal horn is glutamate, and the receptors mostly involved in the sensation of acute pain are AMPA (alpha-amino-3-hydroxy-5-methyl-isoxazole-4-propionic acid) receptors.

The two main classes of second-order neurons are nociceptive-specific (NS) and "wide dynamic range" (WDR) neurons. NS neurons respond only to a specific type of noxious stimulus. Their receptive fields are small, and they are found mostly in lamina I. WDR neurons are nociceptive nonspecific. They respond to a wide range of stimuli, from light touch to noxious stimuli. They have larger receptive fields and are found in all laminae but particularly in lamina V. The second-order neurons can synapse with deep interneurons, facilitating or inhibiting further transmission (Fig. 5–2).

ASCENDING CENTRAL PAIN PATHWAY

There are two major ascending systems, the neospinothalamic pathway and the paleospinoreticulodiencephalic pathway. Pinprick sensation (A-δ afferents) passes via the neospinothalamic pathway to the postcentral gyrus, whereas pain from tissue damage (C afferents) is carried by the paleospinoreticulodiencephalic pathway through the reticular formation to the cortex. En route, the signals pass through the intralaminar nuclei of the thalamus. The neospinothalamic tract, the

TABLE 5–1	Characteristics of Nociceptive Pain		
	Visceral Pain	**Superficial Somatic Pain**	**Deep Somatic Pain**
Location of Nociceptor	Visceral organs	Skin, subcutaneous tissue	Bone, muscle, tendon, and joint
Stimuli	Organ stretching, inflammation, ischemia	Mechanical, thermal, chemical	Mechanical injury, ischemia, inflammation
Localization	Poorly localized	Well localized	Diffuse or radiating
Quality	Aching deep pain, or sharp pain referred cutaneously	Sharp, burning, pricking	Dull, aching, cramping
Symptoms and Signs	Nausea, vomiting, sweating, tenderness, muscle spasm	Skin tenderness, hyperalgesia, hyperesthesia	Tenderness, deep muscle spasm
Examples	Appendicitis, pancreatitis, peptic ulcer disease	Cuts, bruising, burns	Arthritis, tendonitis

most important for the transmission of nociceptive stimuli, is located in the anterolateral quadrant of the spinal cord. Most of the axons cross in the ventral white commissure of the spinal cord to ascend in the opposite anterolateral quadrant, but some remain ipsilateral. Neurons from distal regions are found more laterally, and those from proximal regions tend to be more medial. Spinothalamic tract neurons divide into medial and lateral projections to the thalamus. Those that project to the lateral thalamus from laminae I, II, and V synapse with fibers that project to the somatosensory cortex. These fibers are therefore involved in the sensory and discriminative aspects of pain. Neurons that project to the medial thalamus originate from deeper laminae (VI and X). Projections are sent to the reticular formation, the periaqueductal gray matter (PAG), and the hypothalamus (Fig. 5–3).

The reticular formation contains many nuclei associated with the sensation of pain. The nucleus reticularis giganticocellularis, the nucleus raphe magnus (NRM), and neurons in the PAG form part of the opioid-mediated descending inhibitory system. The limbic system consists of the hypothalamus, hippocampus, amygdala, and cingulum. It is involved in the control of behavioral responses to pain. The frontal cortex has a controlling influence on the nature of pain and memory.

Perception

Negative emotion (threat) and a typically unpleasant sensation produce awareness of the injured part of the body, which is appreciated as pain. Cortical and limbic system structures are involved. Information from some dorsal horn projection neurons travels via the thalamus to the contralateral somatosensory cortex. This input is mapped, preserving information about the location, intensity, and quality of the pain. Other nociceptive input is relayed to the limbic system via the thalamus. This joins input from spinoreticular and spinomesencephalic tracts to mediate affective aspects of pain.[7]

Integration of pain at higher centers is complex. The discriminative component is somatotopically specific and involves the primary and secondary sensory cortices. Integration of somatic pain takes place at this level and allows the brain to locate the site of pain. Integration of the affective component involves various limbic structures, in particular the cingulate cortex.

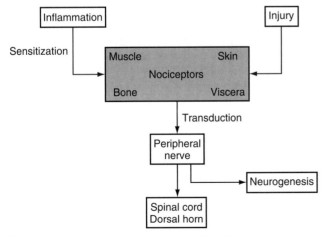

Figure 5–1 Peripheral sources of pain. Stimulation of nociceptors can result from tissue trauma or from prolonged exposure to non-noxious stimuli. Inflammation can sensitize nociceptors, lowering their firing thresholds.

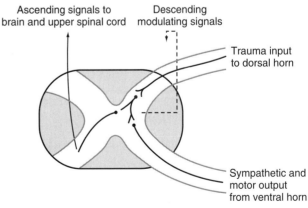

Figure 5–2 Simplified schematic of spinal cord mechanisms. This diagram outlines the basic afferent input to the dorsal horn, with the majority of impulses crossing to the contralateral side, prior to ascending in the anterior spinothalamic tracts. Ipsilateral reflex activity and descending inhibitory influences are also illustrated.

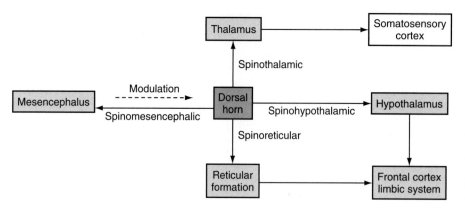

Figure 5–3 Schematic representation of the multiple pathways of transmission of nociceptive impulses from the spinal cord to more central structures. The four main projections (spinothalamic, spinohypothalamic, spinoreticular, and spinomesencephalic) are represented.

Modulation

DESCENDING INHIBITORY PATHWAYS

A number of regions in the brain are involved in the modulation of noxious stimuli—the somatosensory cortex, the hypothalamus, the PAG, and the raphe magnus. Fibers from these structures descend directly or indirectly via the dorsolateral funiculus to the spinal cord and send projections to laminae I and V. There are three major components to the descending system—the opioid system, noradrenergic neurons, and serotonergic neurons. The opioid system is involved in descending analgesia. Opioid precursors and their respective peptides are present in the hypothalamus, amygdala, raphe magnus, and dorsal horn. Noradrenergic neurons project from the locus ceruleus to the dorsolateral funiculus. Serotonergic neurons from the raphe magnus project via the dorsolateral funiculus to the spinal cord.

These pathways appear to have an effect on the spinal gating system. Although the PAG forms part of the opioid-mediated descending inhibitory system, there is a direct connection between the nucleus raphe magnus and the spinal cord—the dorsolateral funiculus, whose inhibitory neuromodulation is mediated by serotonin. Norepinephrine and GABA (gamma-aminobutyric acid) are other inhibitory neurotransmitters involved in these descending pathways. Inhibitory amino acids (e.g., GABA) and neuropeptides (e.g., endogenous opioids) can bind to receptors on primary afferent and dorsal horn neurons and inhibit nociceptive transmission by both presynaptic and postsynaptic mechanisms.[8] Descending inhibitory input from the brain also modulates dorsal horn nociceptive transmission. The inhibitory processes are part of a nociceptive modulating system that counterbalances the nociceptive signaling system.

PERIPHERAL SENSITIZATION

Repeated or prolonged noxious stimuli, exposure to certain inflammatory mediators, or both can sensitize nociceptors. A sensitized nociceptor demonstrates a lowered activation threshold and a higher rate of firing.[9] The typical increase in nociceptor sensitivity following tissue damage is due to one of two mechanisms: Bradykinin may increase the current activated by heat via a mechanism involving protein kinase C, or prostaglandin E_2 alters the voltage threshold of ion channels.[10] There is strong evidence for post-translational modification of ion channels involved in transduction and transmission of nociceptive impulses coincident with biophysical sensitization.[11] The tetrodotoxin-resistant sodium channel Na(v)1.8, present in gut nociceptive primary afferents, is considered the principal cause of the enhanced activity seen with nociceptor sensitization.[12] Peripheral sensitization is important in the development of hyperalgesia, allodynia, and central sensitization (Fig. 5–4).

The phenomenon of *central sensitization* is a state of spinal neuron hyperexcitability. There is increased responsiveness to innocuous stimuli in a zone of secondary hyperalgesia in the uninjured tissue surrounding the injured area. Repeated stimulation of C nociceptors causes a gradual rise in the frequency of dorsal horn neuron firing, known as "wind-up" (Fig. 5–5).[13] Greater amounts of glutamate and substance P are released, stimulating AMPA and neurokinin 1 receptors. This leads to activation of the normally nonfunctional NMDA (*N*-methyl-D-aspartate) receptors, which now also react to glutamate, resulting in an enhanced response.[14] Activation of NMDA receptors causes an inrush of calcium through ion channels (ligand- and voltage-gated), resulting in activation of second messengers (guanosine triphosphate [GTP]–binding

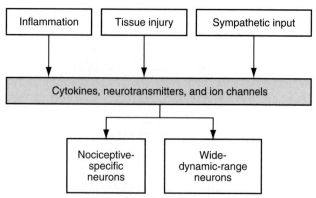

Figure 5–4 Simple outline of the phenomenon of peripheral sensitization. The roles played by cytokines, neurotransmitters, and ion channels are detailed in the text.

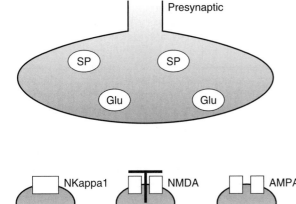

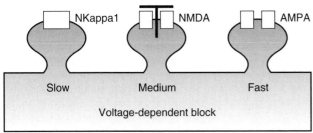

Figure 5–5 Diagram of the increased frequency of dorsal horn neuron firing known as "wind-up." Neurotransmitter release from the afferent terminal activates the slow NK-1 and fast AMPA receptors, ultimately activating second messengers and priming the NMDA receptor. AMPA, alpha-amino-3-hydroxy-5-methyl-isoxazole-4-propionic acid; Glu, glutamate; NMDA, N-methyl-D-aspartate; SP, substance P.

proteins), production of nitric oxide (NO), and induction of oncogenes (*c-fos*) (Figs. 5–6 and 5–7). The second messengers change the excitability of the cell, leading to long-term potentiation (LTP). This is an example of a use-dependent change in synaptic strength. This type of modulation can also happen farther up the nociceptive pathways.

Other changes occurring in the dorsal horn with central sensitization are a reduction in threshold response, an increase in the magnitude and duration of response to stimuli above threshold, and expansion of the dorsal horn

neuron receptive fields.[15] Clinically, these changes manifest in a number of ways: The response to a noxious stimulus is increased (hyperalgesia), a normally innocuous stimulus produces a painful response (*allodynia*), a transient stimulus produces prolonged pain (*persistent pain*), or pain may spread to uninjured tissue (*referred pain*). The phenomenon of sensitization is the most likely cause for continuing pain and hyperalgesia after surgical injury. It can occur after "normal" noxious input from injured inflamed tissue and also because of "abnormal" input from injured nerves or ganglia. In the "normal" situation, sensitization plays an adaptive role, encouraging protection of the injury during healing. Persistence of the processes after healing may give rise to chronic pain. Central sensitization also explains the clinical observation that well-established pain is more difficult to treat than acute pain.

Agonists and Antagonists of Nociception

As discussed, many substances produced by tissue damage, inflammation, or nerve injury may alter the quality of pain experienced, resulting in hyperalgesia and allodynia. These chemical factors can act directly on peripheral fibers to produce pain or may increase the fibers' sensitivity and responsiveness to a variety of exogenous stimuli.

Kinins are of major importance in affecting the excitability of peripheral fibers, because they are produced rapidly after tissue injury and initiate a cascade of chemical interactions affecting peripheral and central neurons. Bradykinin and kallidin (lysyl-bradykinin) are the products of high- and low-molecular-weight kininogens, respectively. They activate the major kinin receptors B1 and B2. The majority of pharmacological effects are due to B2 receptor activation. B2 receptors occur on nociceptors (A-δ and C fibers) in most tissues,[16] and bradykinin-induced pain is produced by direct activation of these receptors. Bradykinin also sensitizes these fibers to physical and chemical stimuli. This sensitization occurs through synergistic interactions with other

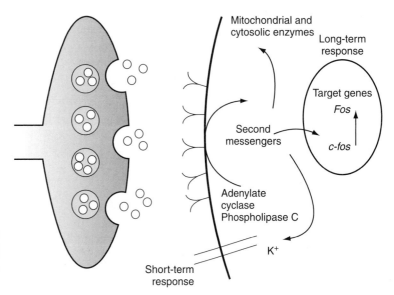

Figure 5–6 Second messenger release and gene activation. Peripheral neurotransmitter release activates postsynaptic receptors. Second messengers such as cAMP and calcium can decrease excitability by reducing K efflux and inducing proto-oncogenes (*c-fos*).

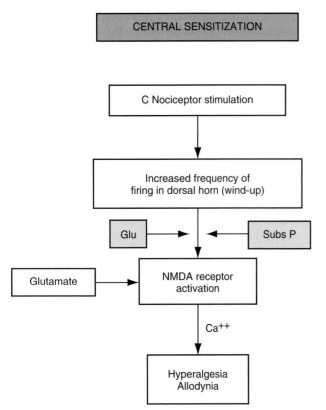

Figure 5–7 Simplified schematic of the processes involved in central sensitization. The importance of the NMDA receptor, the neurotransmitter glutamate, and calcium as a second messenger are illustrated. Glu, glucose; NMDA, N-methyl-D-aspartate; Subs P, substance P.

inflammatory mediators, such as serotonin and cytokines, or by release of histamine from mast cells.

Signal transduction by the B2 receptor occurs through the activation of several second-messenger systems, including receptor-coupled activation of membrane phospholipase C and cleavage of membrane phospholipids. The resultant rise in sodium ion permeability leads to membrane depolarization. This depolarization also causes increased calcium ion permeability, with consequent sensory neuropeptide release, activation of nitric oxide synthetase (NOS), and production of cyclic guanosine monophosphate (cGMP). Bradykinin also excites postganglionic sympathetic nerve fibers, causing release of prostanoids and other inflammatory mediators. B1 receptors are less abundant than B2 receptors, but their expression is increased by inflammatory mediators (interleukins) and growth promoters. B1 receptors appear to have a significant role in the generation of hyperalgesia, but how this action occurs remains unclear.

Nerve growth factor (NGF) is a neurotrophic product of inflammation that changes the excitability of sympathetic and sensory nerves. Its production is stimulated by interleukin-1β and tumor necrosis factor-α (TNF-α) during inflammation. NGF induces a rapid indirect sensitization of nociceptors via mediator release, mast cell degranulation, and increased B1 receptors. Longer-lasting changes are due to the alteration in gene regulation.

ION CHANNEL ACTIVITY

Overexpression of membrane ion channels can account for the increases in membrane excitability seen in sensory neurons during inflammation. These changes can account for hyperesthesia and the spontaneous pain of inflammation. The numbers and roles of the varying ion channels involved in nociception continue to increase as our knowledge evolves. Acid-sensing ion channels (ASICs) are ubiquitous in mammalian nervous systems. Recent strong evidence for their involvement in peripheral nociception has come from experiments involving knockout models. Although the actual mechanisms remain unclear, the role of fluctuations in tissue pH is under scrutiny.[17]

G protein–signaling systems may be a common link between many neurotransmitter systems. G protein–coupled, inwardly rectifying potassium channels (GIRKs) may prove to be a common link between a variety of neurotransmitter receptors and the regulation of synaptic transmission. These receptors include opioid, α-adrenergic, muscarinic cholinergic, GABA B, and cannabinoid receptors; coupled with postsynaptic GIRK2 channels, they account for most antinociceptive effects in males.[18] G protein–signaling systems are common to other ion channels mediating nociception. Modulation of ion channels by proinflammatory mediators occurs largely through G protein–dependent and cGMP–dependent pathways.[19] The nonopioid peptide nociception inhibits voltage-dependent calcium currents (ICa) largely by binding to its own receptor, ORL-1.[20] This receptor is structurally and functionally similar to the opioid receptors and is similarly G protein–coupled.[21]

The opioid receptor system interacts with the NMDA receptor system in modulating nociception. As already discussed, activation of NMDA receptors contributes to the phenomenon of hyperexcitability through second-messenger systems. Among the opioid receptor subtypes, mu and delta receptors may inhibit or potentiate NMDA receptor–mediated events, whereas kappa receptors have an inhibitory effect.[22] Activation of NMDA receptors in some brain areas (thalamus, trigeminal nucleus) is pronociceptive, but activation in other areas (PAG, ventrolateral medulla) is antinociceptive.[23]

Injury to axons in the DRG changes sodium channel expression in these neurons. The SNS/PN3 and NaN sodium channel genes are downregulated, and the previously silent type III sodium channel gene is upregulated. This process changes the electrophysiological characteristics of the DRG neurons, allowing spontaneous firing or firing at inappropriately high frequencies. The relevance of this altered gene expression to the development of analgesic agents remains to be seen.[24]

Conclusion

The level of knowledge about postoperative nociceptive pain mechanisms has risen considerably in recent years. The large number of neurotransmitters and receptors involved suggests many therapeutic possibilities for analgesic agents. However, the presence of large numbers of potential targets, coupled with the capacity of the nervous system to change, means that a single analgesic agent would probably be ineffective.

REFERENCES

1. Merskey H, Bogduk N (eds): Classification of Chronic Pain: Descriptions of Chronic Pain Syndromes and Definitions of Pain Terms, 2nd ed. Seattle, IASP Press, 1994.
2. Besson JM, Chaouch A: Peripheral and spinal mechanisms of nociception. Physiol Rev 1987;67:67–186.
3. Pasero C, Paice JA, McCaffery M: Basic mechanisms underlying the causes and effects of pain. In McCaffery M, Pasero C (eds): Pain Clinic Manual, 2nd ed. St Louis, Mosby Inc, 1999, pp 15–34.
4. Merskey H, Bogduk N: Classification of Chronic Pain: Descriptions of Chronic Pain Syndromes and Definitions of Pain Terms, 2nd ed. Seattle, IASP Press, 1994.
5. Song SO, Carr DB: Pain and Memory. Pain: Clinical Updates 1999;VII:1.
6. Siddal PJ, Cousins MJ: Spinal pain mechanisms. Spine 1997;22:98–104.
7. Willis WD, Westlund KN: Neuroanatomy of the pain system and of the pathways that modulate pain. J Clin Neurophysiol 1997;14:2–31.
8. Terman GW, Bonica JJ: Spinal mechanisms and their modulation. In Loeser JD, Butler SH, Chapman CR, Turk DC (eds): Bonica's Management of Pain, 3rd ed. Baltimore, Lippincott Williams & Wilkins, 2001, pp 73–152.
9. Woolf CJ: Recent advances in the pathophysiology of acute pain. Br J Anaesth 1989;63:139–146.
10. Cesare P, McNaughton P: Peripheral pain mechanisms. Curr Opin Neurobiol 1997;7:493–499.
11. Bhave G, Gereau RW 4th: Posttranslational mechanisms of peripheral sensitization. J Neurobiol 2004;61:88–106.
12. Cervero F, Laird JM: Role of ion channels in mechanisms controlling gastrointestinal pain pathways. Curr Opin Pharmacol 2003;3:608–612.
13. Woolf CJ: Evidence for a central component of post-injury pain hypersensitivity. Nature 1983;306:686–688.
14. Eide PK: Wind up and the NMDA receptor complex from a clinical perspective. Eur J Pain 2000;4:5–17.
15. Dickenson AH: Central acute pain mechanisms. Ann Med 1995;27:223–227.
16. Steranka LR, Manning D, DeHaas CJ, et al: Bradykinin as a pain mediator: Receptors are localized to sensory neurons and antagonists have analgesic actions. Proc Natl Acad Sci U S A 1988;85:3245–3249.
17. Krishtal O: The ASICs: Signalling molecules? Modulators? Trends Neurosci 2003;26:477–483.
18. Blednov YA, Stoffel M, Alva H, Harris RA: A pervasive mechanism for analgesia: Activation of GIRK2 channels. Proc Natl Acad Sci U S A 2003;100:277–282.
19. Liu L, Yang T, Bruno MJ, et al: Voltage-gated ion channels in nociceptors: Modulation by cGMP. J Neurophysiol 2004;92:2323–2332.
20. Yeon KY, Sim MY, Choi SY, et al: Molecular mechanisms underlying calcium current modulation by nociceptin. Neuroreport 2004;15:2205–2209.
21. New DC, Wong YH: The ORL1 receptor: Molecular pharmacology and signalling systems. Neurosignals 2002;11:197–212.
22. Riedel W, Neeck G: Nociception, pain and antinociception: Current concepts. Z Rheumatol 2001;60:404–415.
23. Fundytus ME: Glutamate receptors and nociception: Implications for the drug treatment of pain. CNS Drugs 2001;15:29–58.
24. Waxman SG: The molecular pathophysiology of pain: Abnormal expression of sodium channel genes and its contributions to hyperexcitability of primary sensory neurons. Pain 1999;(Suppl 6):S133–S140.

6 Mechanisms of Postoperative Pain—Neuropathic

RICHARD M. TALBOT • CONNAIL R. McCRORY

Neuropathic pain is typically due to an injury to any part of the nervous system—peripheral nerve, dorsal root ganglion (DRG), dorsal root, or the central nervous system (CNS) (Figs. 6–1 and 6–2). Whereas nociceptive pain is experienced by all postoperative patients, even after minor surgery, the presence of a neuropathic component to the pain complex may be more difficult to diagnose and thus to treat. This difficulty is particularly important because of the potential for neuropathic pain to become chronic. Research has now highlighted the prevalence of chronic pain after surgery. It is estimated that approximately 20% of patients experience chronic postoperative pain.[1] Poorly controlled acute postoperative pain is a major predictor of chronic postoperative pain.[2,3] However, the prevalence and optimal therapy for the management of neuropathic postoperative pain are not well delineated. Compounding factors include difficulty in taking a detailed history from a patient who is already receiving opioid therapy and a paucity of research demonstrating that surgery, as an inflammatory process, induces neuropathic pain or enhances the degree of pain experienced by a patient with preoperative neuropathic pain.

This chapter explores the interaction of the inflammatory surgical response and neuropathic pain, discusses the effect of surgery on preexisting neuropathic pain, and draws evidence-based conclusions about the diagnosis and management of postoperative neuropathic pain.

Definition

Neuropathic pain has been defined by the International Association for the Study of Pain (ISAP)[4] as "pain initiated or caused by a primary lesion or dysfunction in the nervous system." It is produced by an alteration of neurologic structure and/or function and involves central or peripheral neurologic damage.

Prevalence

It is estimated that 8 million people in the United States and 0.5 million in the United Kingdom suffer from neuropathic pain.[5] There are currently no prospective data defining the prevalence of pure neuropathic pain after surgery. There are data, however, regarding the commonly recognized postoperative neuropathic pain states such as post-thoracotomy pain and postmastectomy pain.

Etiology

The traumatic event leading to the patient's presence in the operating room may be the principal cause of the nerve injury and, hence, neuropathic pain. Box 6–1 lists the etiologies of neuropathic pain syndromes. Postoperative neuropathic pain may occur from surgical, anesthetic, or nonsurgical trauma. Included in this box are conditions associated with the development of neuropathic pain syndromes, which may contribute to the development of postoperative neuropathic pain or previously existing (preoperative) neuropathic pain.

Mechanisms

Neuropathic pain is caused by trauma or a lesion to the peripheral or central nervous system.

Mechanisms of pain are as follows[6-11] (Figs. 6–3 through 6–6):
- Nociception
- Peripheral sensitization
- Phenotypic switches and ectopic excitability
- Central sensitization
- Neuroimmune system modulation
- Augmented facilitation
- Structural reorganization
- Decreased inhibition (disinhibition)
- Other proteins expressed in nerve injury

No one mechanism is specific to a given pain state. All postoperative pain, including postoperative neuropathic pain, originates from contributions of each mechanism (Table 6–1).

The relationship among etiology, mechanisms, and clinical features of neuropathic pain is complex (see Fig. 6–3).

Peripheral neuropathic pain after nerve injury manifests as either spontaneous pain (stimulus-independent pain) or pain hypersensitivity in response to a stimulus (stimulus-evoked pain) (see Fig. 6–4).[11]

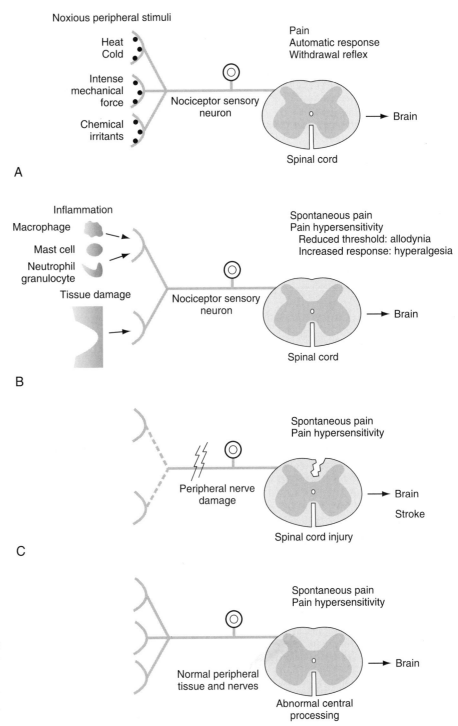

Figure 6–1 The four principal types of pain. **A,** Nociceptive pain. **B,** Inflammatory pain. **C,** Neuropathic pain. **D,** Functional pain. (Modified from Woolf CJ: Pain: Moving from symptom control toward mechanism-specific pharmacologic management. Ann Intern Med 2004;140: 441–451.)

NOCICEPTION

Nociception is the perception of noxious stimuli; it is initiated by stimuli that activate the peripheral terminals of nociceptors. A *nociceptor* is "a receptor preferentially sensitive to a noxious stimulus or to a stimulus that would become noxious if prolonged."[4] Nociception consists of transduction, transmission, and perception.

Transducer ion channels are generally sodium or nonselective cation channels that are gated not by voltage but by temperature, chemical ligands, and mechanical forces. Several voltage-gated sodium channels expressed on sensory neurons mediate conduction of action potentials, two of which are unique to nociceptors—$Na_v1.8$ and $Na_v1.9$.[12,13]

PERIPHERAL SENSITIZATION

Pain hypersensitivity, both after injury and postoperatively, is primarily the effect of central and peripheral sensitization.

Distribution of lesions

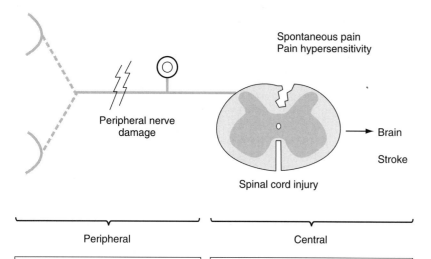

Figure 6–2 Distribution of lesions in neuropathic pain. (Modified from Woolf CJ: Pain: Moving from symptom control toward mechanism-specific pharmacologic management. Ann Intern Med 2004;140:441–451.)

Tissue injury and resultant inflammation leads to the release of intracellular contents such as K^+ ions and adenosine triphosphatase (ATPase) to the extracellular space and leads to the biosynthesis of cytokines, chemokines, and growth factors by recruited inflammatory cells.[14] These factors may cause either activation or sensitization of nociceptors. *Peripheral sensitization* refers to the increased sensitivity and excitability of the nociceptor terminal. Peripheral sensitization produces increases in pain sensitivities that are restricted to the site of inflammation.

An example of an activation factor would be ATPase and its activation of the ligand-gated $P2X_3$ purine nociceptor, which allows immediate nociceptor detection of tissue damage.[15]

Sensitizing factors, such as prostaglandin E_2, bind to specific receptors expressed on the membrane of nociceptor terminals, which are coupled to intracellular kinases.

BOX 6–1   ETIOLOGIES OF NEUROPATHIC PAIN SYNDROMES

Peripheral nerve injury
Surgical trauma:
- Post amputation
- Retractor injury
- Nerve ligation
- Compression or traction injuries

Anesthetic trauma:
- Complications of regional anesthesia/analgesia techniques causing direct and indirect nerve injury

Nonsurgical trauma:
- Nerve entrapment
- Carpal tunnel syndrome
- Tarsal tunnel syndrome
- Cubital tunnel syndrome
- Radial tunnel syndrome
- Meralgia paresthetica (lateral femoral cutaneous nerve)
- Thoracic outlet syndrome

Metabolic diseases:
- Diabetes mellitus
- Hypothyroidism
- Uremic neuropathy
- Amyloidosis
- Multiple myeloma
- Porphyria (hereditary and acquired)
- Wilson's disease
- Hemochromatosis

Ischemic insults:
- Peripheral vascular disease
- Central nervous system infarct

Nutritional:
- Beriberi (thiamine deficiency)
- Alcoholism (multiple vitamin deficiencies)
- Pellagra (niacin deficiency)

Vascular compression:
- Aberrant arterial loop—chronically injured nerve in some cases of trigeminal neuralgia

Malignancy:
- Direct tumor compression
- Toxic effects of chemotherapeutic agents—cisplatin, vincristine, paclitaxel
- Postradiation fibrosis—chronic nerve compression and ischemia
- Associated metabolic disturbances
- Paraneoplastic effects—sensorimotor neuropathy:
  —Associated with carcinoma (nonspecific)
  —Associated with dysproteinemia (e.g., multiple myeloma)
  —Subacute sensory neuronopathy (small cell carcinoma most commonly)

Toxic:
- Isoniazid (pyridoxine vitamin B_6 antagonist)
- Gold
- Thallium
- Arsenic
- Cyanide
- Lead

Infectious:
- Acquired immunodeficiency syndrome
- Post-herpetic neuralgia
- Acute inflammatory polyneuropathy (Guillain-Barré syndrome)
- Lyme disease

Autoimmune diseases:
- Polyarteritis
- Systemic lupus erythematosus

Genetic (rare):
- Fabry's disease
- Hereditary sensory neuropathy

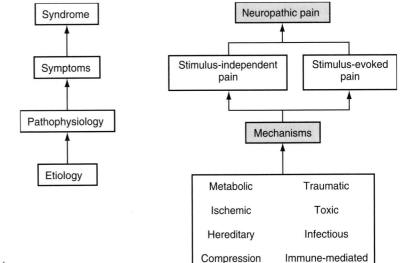

Figure 6–3   Etiologies, mechanisms, and symptoms of neuropathic pain. (Modified from Woolf CJ, Mannion RJ: Neuropathic pain: Aetiology, symptoms, mechanisms and management. Lancet 1999;353:1959–1964.)

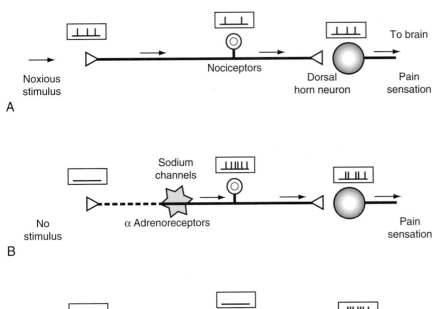

Figure 6–4 Spontaneous pain mechanism after nerve injury. **A,** Normal sensory function. **B,** Sensory function after nerve injury with spontaneous firing along axon. **C,** Sensory function after nerve injury with spontaneous firing of dorsal horn neurons in spinal cord. (Modified from Woolf CJ, Mannion RJ: Neuropathic pain: Aetiology, symptoms, mechanisms and management. Lancet 1999; 353:1959–1964.)

Activation of adenylyl cyclase by prostaglandin E_2 raises levels of cyclic adenosine monophosphate (cAMP), which activates cAMP-dependent protein kinase A. Calcium either is released from microsomes in the terminal or enters through membrane channels and activates the calcium-activated protein kinase C.[15] Intracellular kinases such as protein kinase A and protein kinase C phosphorylate the amino acids serine and threonine in many proteins. Phosphorylation alters the protein structure (post-translation change) and hence the activity of receptors and ion channels and their activation thresholds. For example, after phosphorylation, the heat-sensitive transducer transient receptor potential V1 channel, TRPV1, has a lower threshold of activation, from 42° C to close to normal body temperature,[16] as typified by the burning pain experienced by a sunburn victim in response to a warm shower. Some receptors are constitutive, for example, bradykinin B_2 receptor, which is activated and sensitized by bradykinin[17]; others are induced after inflammation or injury, such as bradykinin B_1 receptor.

Tumor necrosis factor-α (TNF-α) and interleukin-1β (IL-1β) induce cyclooxygenase-2 (Cox-2) enzyme a number of hours after the inflammatory insult.[18] Accordingly, nonsteroidal anti-inflammatory drugs (NSAIDs) or Cox-2–selective agents have an immediate analgesic action in conditions in which there is chronic Cox-2 enzyme expression, such as rheumatoid arthritis, but not in acute situations, such as nociceptive pain and immediate inflammatory pain. Several sensitizing factors may be present (prostaglandin E_2, nerve growth factor [NGF], and bradykinin); therefore, impeding the production of one factor does not eradicate peripheral sensitization. This redundancy of sensitizing factors leads to the limited effects of analgesic agents such as Cox-2 inhibitors.

PHENOTYPIC SWITCHES AND ECTOPIC EXCITABILITY

After peripheral nerve injury, hundreds of genes are upregulated or downregulated.[19,20] Initially, activation of the sensory neuron intracellular transduction cascade occurs in response to inflammatory mediators, NGF, and other factors and ligands binding to receptors and ion channels. Transcription factors that modulate gene expression are controlled by these transduction cascades. Alteration in gene expression leads to changes in levels of receptors, ion channels, and other functional proteins, thus leading to alterations in excitability of neurons, transduction, and transmitter properties which may summate to switching the phenotype of the neuron.

For example, C fibers normally express the neuromodulators brain-derived neurotrophic factor and substance P; however, A fibers also begin to express the same neuromodulators after peripheral nerve injury.[21,22] The implication is that A fibers may be able to induce central sensitization, which is normally produced only by C fibers.[23]

As another example, after peripheral inflammation, the level of heat-sensitive TRPV1 channels rises in the peripheral terminals of nociceptors, increasing heat sensitivity peripherally[24] and altering levels of synaptic modulators, substance P, and brain-derived neurotrophic factor,[25] amplifying central input to the spinal cord. Such modifications are the consequence of increased production of NGF in inflamed tissue. This peripheral NGF is transported to the cell body of the sensory neuron in the dorsal root ganglion. Here, it activates intracellular signaling pathways. These pathways include NGF–induced activation of p38 mitogen–activated protein kinase, which increases the expression and peripheral

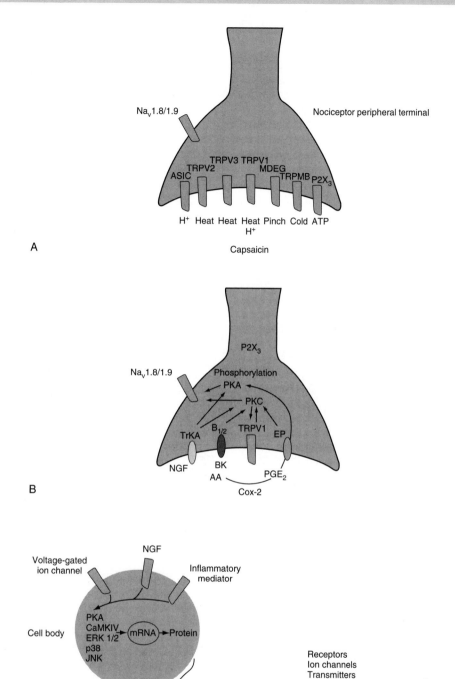

Figure 6–5   Contributions of primary sensory neurons to pain. **A,** A nociceptor neuron peripheral terminal. Ion channels that respond to thermal, mechanical, and chemical stimuli are shown. The receptive abilities of the sensory neuron are dictated by which transducing ion channels are expressed. **B,** Inflammatory mediators prostaglandin E₂ (PGE₂), bradykinin (BK), and nerve growth factor (NGF) are released during tissue injury and inflammation. Intracellular kinases are activated by these mediators, which phosphorylate transducer channels, reducing their threshold or increasing the excitability of sodium channels. **C,** Activation of sensory neuron intracellular transduction cascades occurs in response to inflammatory mediators, activity, and growth factors. Transcription factors that modulate gene expression are under the control of these cascades. This causes changes in levels of gene expression, leading to changes in the levels of receptors, ion channels, and other functional proteins. The change in gene expression leads to changes in proteins, which may lead to a phenotypic switch in the neuron. AA, arachidonic acid; ASIC, acid-sensing ion channel; ATP, adenosine triphosphate; B$_{1/2}$, bradykinin B₁ and B₂ receptors; BK, bradykinin; CaMKIV, camkinase IV; Cox-2, cyclooxygenase-2; DRG, dorsal root ganglion; EP, prostaglandin E receptor; ERK, extracellular signal-regulated kinase; JNK, jun kinase; MDEG, mammalian degenerin; mRNA, messenger RNA; Na$_v$1.8/1.9, voltage-gated sodium channels 1.8/1.9; NGF, nerve growth factor; PKA, protein kinase A; P2X₃, ligand-gated purine nociceptor for ATP; PKC, protein kinase C; TRP, transient receptor potential receptor. (From Woolf CH: Pain: Moving from symptom control toward mechanism-specific pharmacologic management. Ann Intern Med 2004;140;441–451.)

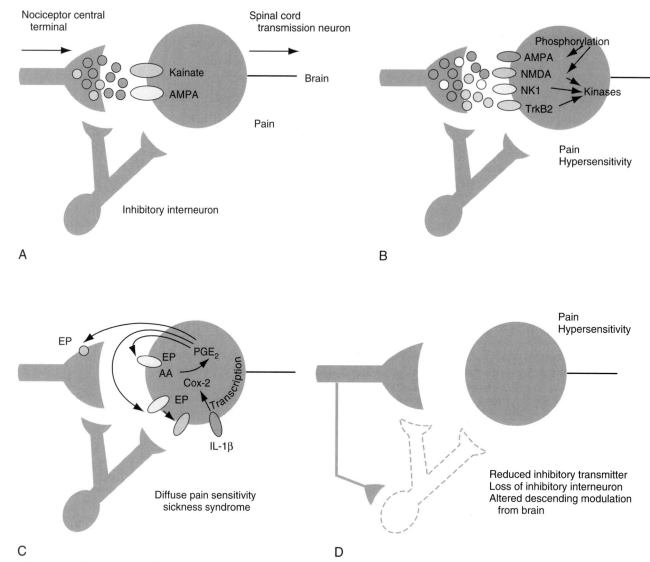

Figure 6–6   Contribution of spinal cord dorsal horn neurons to pain. **A,** Nociceptive transmission. **B,** The acute phase of central sensitization. **C,** The late phase of central sensitization. Changes in the expression of some genes are activity driven and have restricted regional effects, e.g., dynorphin, whereas changes in the expression of others are widespread and result in global changes in function, e.g., induction of cyclo-oxygenase-2 (Cox-2) in central neurons after peripheral inflammation. **D,** Disinhibition. AA, arachidonic acid; AMPA, alpha-amino-3-hydroxy-5-methyl-4-isoxazole propionate; EP, prostaglandin E receptor; IL-1β, interleukin-1β; NK1, neurokinin-1; NMDA, N-methyl-D-aspartic acid; PGE$_2$, prostaglandin E$_2$; TrkB2, tyrosine kinase B2. (From Woolf CH: Pain: Moving from symptom control toward mechanism-specific pharmacologic management. Ann Intern Med 2004;140;441–451.)

TABLE 6–1	Pain Mechanisms as Associated with Pain States						
	Nociception	Peripheral Sensitization	Phenotypic Switches	Central Sensitization	Ectopic Excitability	Structural Reorganization	Decreased Inhibition
Nociceptive pain	•	•		•			
Inflammatory pain		•		•			
Neuropathic pain		•	•	•	•	•	•
Functional pain				•		•	

Adapted from text in Woolf CJ: Pain: Moving from symptom control toward mechanism-specific pharmacologic management. Ann Intern Med 2004;140:441–451.

transport of TRPV1 in primary sensory neurons after peripheral inflammation, thus exacerbating heat hyperalgesia.[24]

After peripheral axonal injury, μ opiate receptors decrease in number as DRG $\alpha_2\delta$ calcium channel subunits increase, underlying the respective reduction in sensitivity to morphine and increase in sensitivity to gabapentin.[26] After nerve injury, altered expression and dissemination of potassium and sodium ion channels increase membrane excitability, leading to spontaneous ectopic excitability, a prime contributing factor to spontaneous neuropathic pain.[27]

CENTRAL SENSITIZATION

Central sensitization is a term used to describe the greater synaptic efficacy established in somatosensory neurons in the dorsal horn of the spinal cord. It occurs after intense peripheral noxious stimuli such as a surgical incision, but it may also be induced by sensitized nociceptors during inflammation or by spontaneous ectopic activity generated in sensory neurons after nerve injury. Central sensitization was originally described 20 years ago.[28,29] It performs a primary function in the development of acute postoperative, posttraumatic, and neuropathic pain.[11,30–34]

There are two forms of central sensitization.[34] The first (acute phase), an activity-dependent form, occurs in response to afferent nociceptor activity, which modifies synaptic transfer via phosphorylation and alteration of voltage, and to ligand-gated ion channel receptors; it is induced in seconds and lasts minutes. The second (late phase), a transcription-dependent form, is induced over some hours and outlives the initiating stimulus.[9,35] The mechanisms of central sensitization—activation of intracellular kinases, phosphorylation of proteins, and induction of genes—are similar to those of peripheral sensitization.

The release of transmitters from nociceptor central terminals initiates an increase in activity in the dorsal horn of the spinal cord, leading to changes in receptor properties (density, threshold, kinetics, distribution, and activation), which is the early, activity-dependent form of central sensitization. A major role in activity-dependent central sensitization is attributed to the glutamate-activated NMDA (N-methyl-D-aspartate) receptor.[36] The phosphorylation of the NMDA receptor during central sensitization increases its synaptic membrane distribution from intracellular stores. Removal of the Mg^+ NMDA channel blockade and longer channel opening time lead to greater responsiveness to glutamate and increased excitability.[9,37] The implications of such increased excitability include activation at previously subthreshold levels (*allodynia*), exaggerated responses at normal stimulation levels (*hyperalgesia*), and possible spread to noninjured areas (*secondary hyperalgesia*).

Ketamine, a competitive NMDA receptor antagonist, has been demonstrated to reduce the early phase of central sensitization and resultant pain hypersensitivity[31,36] and to have a role in the treatment of chronic neuropathic pain.[38] Efforts to find other NMDA receptor antagonists have had some success; for example, amantadine, an antiviral and anti-parkinsonian agent, was shown to act as a noncompetitive NMDA receptor antagonist and to reduce surgical neuropathic pain in patients with cancer.[39] The extensive distribution of NMDA receptors throughout the nervous system and a poor therapeutic index have limited the clinical use of such agents.

The later, transcription-dependent form of central sensitization involves activation of transcription factors and alterations in transcription and gene expression. It may be initiated by synaptically mediated activation of intracellular transduction pathways or by humoral signals. The former changes in gene expression are restricted to parts of the nervous system that receive inputs from injured tissue. For example, the endogenous opioid peptide dynorphin is regulated by mitogen-activated protein kinases.[40] The latter, humoral-type activation of genes has effects that are more widespread.

The principal example of the later form is the expression of cyclooxygenase-2 (Cox-2) in many areas of the central nervous system several hours after a localized peripheral tissue injury. This occurs in response to a circulating humoral cytokine released by inflammatory cells that stimulates endothelial cells of the cerebral vasculature to produce IL-1β, which enters cerebrospinal fluid and binds to neuronally expressed IL-1β receptors, which then produce Cox-2.[41] The ensuing prostaglandin E_2 has presynaptic and postsynaptic effects, yielding multiple extensive actions.

The clinical implications of this finding are that both peripherally and centrally induced Cox-2 must be targeted to treat pain. In addition to reducing sensory traffic in to the central nervous system with regional anesthesia/analgesia techniques, one must also target the centrally induced, humorally mediated Cox-2 induction with selective Cox-2 inhibitors.[6]

NEUROIMMUNE SYSTEM MODULATION

There is growing evidence for a role of the immune system in neuropathy and neuropathic pain.[42] It has been estimated that half of all clinical cases of neuropathic pain are associated with infection or inflammation of peripheral nerves rather than with nerve trauma.[43] The roles of the immune system in pain have been reviewed[44]; they can be summarized as follows:

- Painful neuropathy involving nerve trauma and inflammation
- Painful neuropathy from antibody attack on peripheral nerves
- Painful neuropathy from immune attack on peripheral blood vessels
- Pain from immune effects on DRGs and dorsal roots

Animal models of both traumatic and inflammatory neuropathies have shown that the key immune cells involved at the level of the peripheral nerve are neutrophils and macrophages recruited into the affected area from the general circulation, together with a host of local cells. Cells normally found within peripheral nerves are fibroblasts, endothelial cells, Schwann cells, mast cells, macrophages, and dendritic cells.[45] The released proinflammatory cytokines nitric oxide and reactive oxygen species kill invading pathogens but can also directly increase nerve excitability, damage myelin, and alter the blood-nerve barrier.[46] Immune activation is not restricted to the periphery; spinal cord immune involvement also occurs, in the form of glial activation.[47]

Two distinctive antibody-mediated attacks on nerves exist. First, antibodies attach to nerve cell membranes and alter ion channel function; Second, immunoglobulin (Ig) M, IgG1, and IgG3 antibodies activate the complement cascade. Activation of the complement cascade leads to disruptions of the blood-nerve barrier, recruitment of macrophages and neutrophils into the nerve, Schwann cell function disruption, the creation of membrane attack complexes that create lesions in nerves, and facilitation of macrophage destruction of antibody-bound sites.[48] Such antibodies are believed to arise by "molecular mimicry," because antibodies are generated to recognize segments ("epitopes") of the external surface of viruses, bacteria, and cancer cells but may also attack similarly shaped regions on the surface of normal nerves.[49] These antibodies may also arise after nerve trauma exposes peripheral nerve protein[50] because of either the initial trauma or iatrogenic trauma. Finally, antibodies may also be directed against pathogens that have invaded the nerve. At least 70% of patients with Guillain-Barré syndrome experience neuropathic pain.[51,52]

Immune attack on peripheral blood vessels leading to painful neuropathy is called *vasculitic neuropathy*.[53] Commonly, it is a diffuse attack on vessels throughout the body. It is believed to occur because of ischemia resulting from blood vessel injury, intravascular clotting, and necrosis.[54]

DRGs contain many immune cells near the cell bodies of sensory neurons that can release excitatory amino acids and L-arginine, the substrate for neuronal nitric oxide production. Additionally, peripheral nerve injury stimulates activated satellite cells to release proinflammatory cytokines and a variety of growth factors near DRG neurons.[42] Immune-derived substances such as proinflammatory cytokines may contribute to pain through activation of receptors or may excite sensory nerve fibers and spinal roots through a direct effect.[55]

There is a speculative relationship between the postoperative stress response and neuroimmune modulation.

AUGMENTED FACILITATION

The descending inhibitory and facilitatory influences of the brain on sensory processing in the spinal cord are poorly understood. It has been theorized that facilitatory controls are triggered or augmented after both inflammatory and peripheral nerve injuries.[56] Animal experiments have indicated the presence of descending serotonergic bulbospinal facilitatory pathways that are susceptible to blockade by 5-hydroxytryptamine-3 (5-HT$_3$) antagonists such as ondansetron, and 5-HT$_3$ receptor antagonism has been demonstrated to yield a reduction in behavioral and electrical indications of nociception.[57,58] An analgesic effect has been reported with administration of 5-HT$_3$ antagonists in patients with neuropathic pain and in patients with fibromyalgia.[59–62]

STRUCTURAL REORGANIZATION

Nociceptive afferent fibers from the periphery terminate in a highly organized fashion in the dorsal horn. Animal experiments examining the dorsal horn of the spinal cord after peripheral injury have shown sprouting of central terminals of the low-threshold afferents into the zones normally occupied by the nociceptor terminals.[63] Confirmation of such structural reorganization in humans would help explain some of the nonresponsive neuropathic pain conditions.

DECREASED INHIBITION (DISINHIBITION)

Both presynaptic and postsynaptic inhibition fine-tunes incoming sensory input to a limited transitory appropriate response. Inhibitory neurons in the spinal cord release the inhibitory neurotransmitters glycine and gamma-aminobutyric acid (GABA). Peripheral nerve injury has been shown to result in selective loss of GABAergic inhibition,[64] and administration of GABA receptor agonists reduces neuropathic pain.[65] It has been postulated that loss of inhibition (*disinhibition*) contributes to the pain hypersensitivity seen in neuropathic pain sufferers.

OTHER PROTEINS EXPRESSED IN NERVE INJURY

Glypican-1 is a protein widely expressed in developing and adult nervous systems as well as in cultured Schwann cells. Glypican-1 acts as a co-receptor for numerous ligands, including slit axonal guidance proteins. A study reported by Bloechlinger et al[66] provides evidence that the expression of the proteoglycan glypican-1 is regulated in DRG neurons in a growth-dependent and injury-induced manner, with reported changes lasting for more than 1 month in the case of peripheral injury but for a shorter duration after central axotomy. The presence of slit 1, robo 2, and glypican-1 in adult DRGs indicates that these molecules could form a functional complex that may regulate axonal growth in the adult nervous system when glypican-1 is presented at the cell surface.[66] It is believed that robos may form a receptor complex that renders neurons responsive to the actions of slits, guiding axonal growth and direction.

SUMMARY

The understanding of pain mechanisms is evolving steadily with the discovery of more proteins and the complex interactions among varying inflammatory cascades, immune processes, and gene expression. Expression, distribution, and modification of proteins occur both in parallel and in series, underscoring the difficulties in understanding and successfully treating the various clinical pain entities.

Anesthetist's Role

The role of the anesthetist in treatment of neuropathic pain consists of the following steps:
- Identify patients at possible risk
- Assess patients for preoperative pain
- Develop a preemptive strategy
- Make a diagnosis

DIAGNOSIS

Diagnosis of neuropathic pain is achieved through the following maneuvers:
- History and physical examination
- Clinical diagnosis

There are no test results pathognomonic for neuropathic pain, although some ancillary tests may be useful.

History

The history should elicit information about spontaneous pain and lancinating or burning pain as well as about evoked pain (see Fig. 6–3).

The following are symptoms of neuropathic pain[4]:

- Dysesthesia—an unpleasant abnormal sensation, whether spontaneous or evoked.
- Allodynia—pain due to a stimulus that does not normally provoke pain.
- Hypoalgesia—diminished sensitivity to noxious stimulation.
- Hyperalgesia—an increased response to a stimulus that is normally painful.
- Hypoesthesia—diminished sensitivity to stimulation, excluding special senses.
- Hyperesthesia—increased sensitivity to stimulation, excluding special senses.
- Hyperpathia—a painful syndrome, characterized by increased reaction to a stimulus, especially a repetitive stimulus, as well as an increased threshold.

Physical Examination

There may also be focal neurologic deficits—weakness or focal autonomic changes (swelling, vasomotor instability) and trophic changes (skin, subcutaneous tissues or hair and nails).

Ancillary tests that are sometimes used include electrodiagnostic studies (electromyogram and nerve conduction velocities can be helpful in confirming existence of neurologic lesion) and thermography (occasionally useful to confirm autonomic dysregulation). In the assessment of a potential case of complex regional pain syndrome (CRPS) or sympathetically mediated pain, observations of resting or evoked sudomotor asymmetry (quantitative sudomotor axon reflex [QSART]), response to systemic α-adrenergic antagonist infusion, tourniquet ischemia testing, laser Doppler cutaneous blood flow measurement, and measurements of percutaneous oxygen partial-pressure differences have been advocated.

However useful these tests may be, this is a clinical diagnosis, and careful interpretation of any test result is paramount to prevent overzealous interpretation and misdiagnosis. Magnetic resonance imaging coupled with nerve conduction studies can identify specific sites of a lesion, which may indicate cause in cases of intraoperative nerve injury.

PREVENTIVE MEASURES

The anesthetist's role in prevention of neuropathic pain includes the following:

1. Risk assessment (Box 6–2 and Table 6–2).
2. Medical optimization of diabetes mellitus,[67] thyroid disease, vitamin deficiencies, and other medical conditions that may predispose to nerve dysfunction and neuropathy.
3. Prevention of iatrogenic nerve injury.

The following mechanisms of perioperative nerve injury may occur alone or in combination[68,69]:

- Direct trauma by needles, sutures, instruments, and intraneural injection
- Injection of neurotoxic material or direct neurotoxic effects of local anesthetic, which is concentration and dose dependent
- Mechanical stretch and compression, due to surgical access and perioperative positioning or compression from hematoma, secondary to congenital and, more specifically, acquired coagulation abnormalities (i.e., administration of anticoagulants and deep venous thrombosis prophylaxis agents)
- Ischemia, secondary to compression or prolonged and severe hypotension compromising the blood supply

Nerves that traverse a long distance are susceptible to stretch injury, and nerves that pass over or adjacent to bony processes are vulnerable to compression injury. The American

BOX 6–2	SPECIFIC CONSIDERATIONS FOR DEVELOPMENT OF POSTOPERATIVE NEUROPATHIC PAIN

Preoperative neuropathic pain
Elderly
Female
Working status (employed versus unemployed)
Diabetes
Alcohol abuse
Uremia
Acquired immunodeficiency syndrome or other immunocompromise
Malignancy, e.g., osteosarcoma
Neoadjuvant chemo/radiotherapy
Fibromyalgia
Trauma
Drugs or toxins—painful polyneuropathies (isoniazid, gold, misonidazole, nitrofurantoin, vincristine, cis-platinum, paclitaxel, arsenic, cyanide, thallium)
Nutritional, specific vitamin deficiency (e.g., niacin, B_{12}, pyridoxine)
Depression

TABLE 6–2	Predictive Factors for Chronic Pain	
Preoperative factors	Pain, moderate to severe, lasting more than 1 month	
	Repeat surgery	
	Psychological vulnerability	
	Workers' compensation	
Intraoperative factors	Surgical approach with risk of nerve damage	
Postoperative factors	Pain (acute, moderate to severe)	
	Radiation therapy to area	
	Neurotoxic chemotherapy	
	Depression	
	Psychologic vulnerability	
	Neuroticism	
	Anxiety	

Adapted from Perkins FM, Kehlet H: Chronic pain as an outcome of surgery: A review of predictive factors. Anesthesiology 2000;93: 1123–1133.

Society of Anesthesiologists (ASA) Closed Claims Project (www.asaclosedclaims.org) is an in-depth investigation of closed malpractice claims designed to identify major areas of loss in anesthesia, patterns of injury, and strategies for prevention."Loss" implies all incidences leading to malpractice claims, not just sensory loss. Sixteen percent of the 4183 claims the Project studied were for anesthesia-related nerve injury. These claims, in order of decreasing frequency, were for the ulnar nerve (28%), brachial plexus (20%), lumbosacral nerve root (16%), and spinal cord (13%).[70] Neural damage is a possible consequence of general anesthesia, central nervous system blockade, and regional anesthesia/analgesia techniques.[71,72]

The three types of nerve injury are as follows[68,69]:

- Neurapraxic injury occurs where myelin is damaged and the axon is intact, leading to a loss of nerve function. This is the type most commonly seen with anesthesia. Prognosis is good, although recovery may take weeks to months.
- Axonotmesis occurs from disruption of the axon with preservation of the nerve sheath. Function may gradually return as the axon regenerates, at a rate of 1 mm per day.
- Neurotmesis occurs when the nerve is completely severed, thus disrupting axon, sheath, and connective tissue. A nerve so injured does not usually recover, and the patient may experience chronic neuropathic pain.

Symptoms can occur within a day but may not be present for 2 to 3 weeks. The severity of injury varies the intensity and duration of symptoms.[69]

Preventive measures include performing regional anesthesia/analgesia techniques with the patient awake whenever possible, using a nerve stimulator and not eliciting paresthesia, and understanding anatomy. The most important preventive measure is to ensure proper patient positioning with respect to avoiding nerve and nerve plexus stretch and compression.

Recognized Postoperative Neuropathic Pain States

POST-THORACOTOMY PAIN

Post-thoracotomy pain syndrome may have an incidence of approximately 50%.[73] A review of six studies totaling 878 patients reported that 47% had post-thoracotomy pain syndrome.[3] The etiology may depend on nerve damage as reflected by the increased severity after chest wall resection[74] and the noted higher probability of post-thoracotomy pain syndrome associated with the loss of superficial abdominal reflexes.[75,76] Tumor recurrence must form part of the possible contributing differential.[74] Two studies reported that patients undergoing thoracotomy via the anterior approach have a lower incidence of intercostal nerve dysfunction and post-thoracotomy pain syndrome than those having the posterolateral approach; however, both studies were small and did not include chronic postoperative pain as a primary outcome parameter.[76,77] Other studies have noted the presence of preoperative pain but have not qualified it as an independent risk factor, although intensity of postoperative pain has been identified as a predictor of post-thoracotomy pain syndrome.[78]

A 2004 review reported that video-assisted thoracic surgery (VATS) is associated with better outcomes and seems to have a complication profile comparable to that of thoracotomy for the treatment of pneumothorax and minor resections.[79] Shortened hospital stay and lower analgesic medication consumption were also noted advantages.

Combining intraoperative and postoperative epidural analgesia, as opposed to using postoperative epidural analgesia alone, has been found to reduce the incidence of pain at 6 months from 67% to 33%.[80]

POSTMASTECTOMY PAIN

Postmastectomy pain is described as a chronic neuropathic pain syndrome that can affect women who have undergone lumpectomy or mastectomy. The incidence of pain 1 year after breast surgery for cancer is approximately 50%. Chronic postoperative breast pain is found in 27% of breast cancer survivors.[81] Women who have undergone breast surgery may suffer chest wall, breast, or scar pain (11% to 57%), phantom breast pain (13% to 24%), and arm or shoulder pain (12% to 51%).[3] Postoperative neuropathic pain may be experienced around the scar and may radiate to the axilla.

A prospective study did not find preoperative breast pain to be a predictive factor as previously indicated,[82–84] and preoperative depression and anxiety were reported as being more common, although statistical significance was not obtained.[83] The type and extent of surgery may affect the incidence of pain. For example, the extent of axillary dissection correlated with the incidence of arm pain and symptoms,[85,86] and mastectomy combined with implantation of prosthesis resulted in a higher incidence of pain (53%) than mastectomy alone (31%).[87]

The extent of acute postoperative pain and analgesic dosages needed has been demonstrated to be the best predictor of persistent breast and ipsilateral arm pain. In addition, postoperative adjuvant radiotherapy and chemotherapy were risk factors for chronic neuropathic pain in the breast and arm.[88,89]

Nerve damage has been credited with most of pain after breast surgery.[89–92] Altered sensation in the distribution of the intercostobrachial nerve has been reported in 48% to 84% of women undergoing axillary dissection; 25% to 50% of women with altered sensation experienced intercostobrachial neuralgia.[93,94]

POST–INGUINAL HERNIA REPAIR PAIN

The incidence of chronic pain after inguinal hernia repair surgery ranges between 0% and 37% with an overall incidence of 11.5%.[3] One investigator demonstrated that chronic pain occurred in 30% of patients after open inguinal hernia repair (pain persisting beyond 3 months).[95] A description of neuropathic pain was reported by 46% of this study group. Risk factors identified as being associated with chronic pain included younger age, outpatient surgery, presence of preoperative pain, and operation for recurrent hernia.

Postoperative pain intensity at 1 week and 4 weeks is predictive of pain at 1 year after inguinal hernia repair.[96] Nerve injury is proposed as a principal factor in this postoperative neuropathic pain syndrome.[97–99]

There is no convincing evidence to date demonstrating that either anesthesia or surgical hernia repair techniques make any significant difference in postoperative neuropathic pain after inguinal hernia repair.[100]

PHANTOM PAIN AND STUMP PAIN

The classic description of phantom pain is that following limb amputation, but the term *phantom pain* is applied to pain that occurs after amputation of any body part; it has been described after both mastectomy and dental extraction. Phantom pain is commonly considered a type of deafferentation pain. *Deafferentation pain* is defined as "pain due to loss of sensory input into the central nervous system, as occurs with avulsion of the brachial plexus or other types of lesions of peripheral nerves or due to pathology of the central nervous system."[4] Central sensitization has been postulated as the sustaining pathophysiology for deafferentation pain. The reported incidence of phantom limb pain varies from 30% to 81%; stump pain was noted in 66% of patients with phantom pain and in half of those without phantom pain, implying that the incidence of stump pain can exceed 60%.[3]

Not all epidemiological surveys distinguish phantom pain from nonpainful phantom sensations and stump pain. Phantom sensations include exteroceptive sensations (perception of touch, temperature, pressure, itch, and pain), kinesthetic sensations (perception of posture, length, and volume), and kinetic sensation (perception of intended and spontaneous movement). The onset of phantom pain and sensations typically occurs soon after nerve injury, although symptoms may develop at any time after denervation. The incidence and frequency of painful episodes of phantom limb pain decline during the first year after amputation,[101,102] but approximately half of the individuals with long-term phantom pain do not report a decrease in intensity.[103]

Documented predictors of phantom pain are preamputation pain and persistent stump pain (acute and chronic),[103–105] and there is an association between nonpainful phantom sensation and phantom pain. Chemotherapy is associated with a higher incidence of phantom pain.[105] Traditional predictors were older age, proximal amputations, upper limb lesions, sudden amputations, and preexisting psychological disturbances; however, later studies have not confirmed these factors as predictors.[106] A review of phantom limb pain has listed other internal and external factors that may have a role in the modulation of phantom limb pain (Table 6–3).[107]

Stump pain is most probably related to the development of a neuroma at the end of the severed nerve and is therefore considered peripheral neuropathic pain. The onset is typically delayed for months, and stump pain has a lower incidence than phantom pain. Of note, many patients have both stump and phantom pain after limb amputation.

A small number of studies have looked at perioperative epidural infusion and incidence of stump and phantom pain. Preoperative commencement of epidural analgesia (combination of bupivacaine, clonidine, and diamorphine) has been demonstrated as effective in reducing phantom pain after amputation[108]; however, a subsequent study did not confirm this finding.[109] Both of these studies had small sample sizes.

TABLE 6–3	Factors That May Modulate the Experience of Phantom Pain
Internal factors	Genetic predisposition
	Anxiety/emotional distress
	Attention/distraction
	Urination/defecation
	Other diseases (cerebral hemorrhage, prolapsed intervertebral disc)
External factors	Weather change
	Touching the stump
	Use of prosthesis
	Spinal anesthesia
	Rehabilitation
	Treatment

Adapted from Nikolajsen L, Jensen TS: Phantom limb pain. Br J Anaesth 2001;87:107–116.

The use of nerve sheath infusions of local anesthetic solutions was also studied to determine whether continuous infusion of bupivacaine hydrochloride reduced the use of narcotics for the relief of pain after an amputation and affected the incidence of phantom pain. One study demonstrated efficacy,[110] whereas the other did not demonstrate prevention of residual or phantom limb pain in patients undergoing amputation of the lower extremity.[111] A study comparing perioperative epidural block (started 24 hours before the amputation) with infusion of local anesthetic via a perineural catheter did not demonstrate the epidural technique as superior in preventing phantom pain but did show better relief of stump pain in the immediate postoperative period in the group receiving epidural anesthesia.[112] These studies also had small sample sizes.

POSTCHOLECYSTECTOMY PAIN

Chronic abdominal pain after cholecystectomy, also known as the postcholecystectomy syndrome, is common (3% to 56%).[3] There are many components in addition to abdominal pain, and there may be multiple causes. The causes include postoperative somatic incisional pain, pain secondary to sphincter of Oddi dysfunction, pain due to bile duct stone, pain due to a preoperatively undiagnosed disease other than gallstones, and other preoperative factors—psychological vulnerability, female sex, and preoperative long-standing symptoms.[113–118] It is worth noting that a history yielding classic symptoms of cholelithiasis is associated with reduced risk of chronic pain.[119–121] There appears to be no difference between laparoscopic and open cholecystectomy in long-term outcome for abdominal pain.[122,123]

It is recognized that port site pain after laparoscopic cholecystectomy may be severe. A prospective randomized study comparing two-port versus four-port laparoscopic cholecystectomy reported that overall pain score, analgesia requirements, hospital stay, and patient satisfaction score on surgery and scars were similar in the two patient groups, even though two-port laparoscopic cholecystectomy resulted in less individual port site pain.[124]

Prospective studies of postcholecystectomy syndrome have not separated neuropathic pain and scar pain from other causes of chronic visceral pain and symptoms.

POSTOPERATIVE COMPLEX REGIONAL PAIN SYNDROME

Complex regional pain syndrome is a term used for the description of a syndrome of pain and vasomotor instability after injury, typically preceded by an initial noxious event in the periphery, that is not limited to distribution of a single nerve and that is disproportionate to the inciting event.[125,126] Two types have been recognized (Box 6–3 and Table 6–4).

Patients with CRPS I or CRPS II may have sympathetically maintained pain[127] or sympathetically independent pain, as determined by response to sympathetic blockade or interventions. Patients may present with components of either or, commonly, both types.[128]

CRPS is not an uncommon postsurgical complication. The incidence varies according to type and site of surgery, setting, and period of patient assessment. Postoperatively, the incidence of CRPS has been noted to diminish in the first 3 months and to stabilize at 6 months.[129] A review of 140 cases of CRPS reported that 16.4% were the result of surgery.[130] Most of CRPS cases occur after orthopedic surgery, implicating both cause and effect, because it has been previously stated that the development of CRPS can be expected in 5% of all trauma cases.[131]

According to a review of the prevention of development of CRPS, the areas of intervention are timing of surgery, regional anesthetic techniques, preemptive multimodal analgesia, and pharmacological therapies.[132]

Timing of Surgery

The optimal time to perform surgery in patients with a history of CRPS remains unknown owing to a lack of evidence-based medical research. One view is that surgery in the presence of active CRPS may cause deterioration in a patient's preoperative CRPS.[133,134] Thus, if possible, surgery should be delayed until symptoms of CRPS are well controlled.[135]

Preoperative pain has been shown to be a predictor of chronic pain after a variety of surgical procedures.[3] Therefore,

TABLE 6–4	Complex Regional Pain Syndrome (CRPS) and Orthopedic Surgery Procedures

Orthopedic Surgical Procedure	Estimated Incidence of CRPS (%)
Arthroscopic knee surgery	2.3–4
Carpal tunnel surgery	2.1–5
Ankle surgery	13.6
Total knee arthroplasty	0.8–13
Wrist fractures	7–37
Fasciectomy for Dupuytren's contracture	4.5–40

Data from Reuben SS: Preventing the development of complex regional pain syndrome after surgery. Anesthesiology. 2004;101:1215–1224.

it may be valuable to assess pain intensity preoperatively as a marker of potentially severe postoperative pain.[129]

Regional Anesthetic Techniques

There have been case reports of patients with previous CRPS undergoing surgical procedures, in whom CRPS was reactivated when a general anesthetic technique was used but was not reactivated when a regional anesthetic was used.[136,137] A study prospectively examined the effects of 23 inductions of spinal anesthesia in 17 patients with previous lower limb amputations; only one patient had clinically significant phantom limb pain, which lasted only minutes.[138] Techniques reported as having potential in decreasing the incidence of postoperative CRPS include stellate ganglion blockade, intravenous regional anesthesia, and epidural anesthesia.

Stellate Ganglion Blockade. Not all upper limb regional anesthetic techniques result in sympathectomy. A retrospective study demonstrated that a perioperative stellate ganglion blockade reduced the occurrence of CRPS.[139] To date, however, no published study has demonstrated this reduction in patients without a history of CRPS.

Intravenous Regional Anesthesia. Technically less demanding than stellate ganglion blockade, intravenous regional anesthesia techniques have a lower complication rate. Drugs examined for efficacy of pain relief in reflex sympathetic dystrophy in prospective randomized controlled clinical trials include guanethidine,[140–144] reserpine,[141,142] droperidol,[145] atropine,[146] bretylium,[147] and ketanserin.[148] The suggestions of critical reviews of these trials[143,149,150] have been summarized as follows: (1) confirmation of the effective analgesia of intravenous regional blockade with bretylium and ketanserin is limited, (2) consistent data indicate the ineffectiveness of intravenous regional techniques using guanethidine and reserpine, and (3) data indicating the ineffectiveness of intravenous regional droperidol and atropine are limited.[132] Both a study and a review have advocated the use of intravenous lignocaine and the α_2-adrenergic agonist clonidine (1 µg/kg) as an effective technique for managing acute postoperative pain and symptoms of upper limb CRPS.[151–153]

BOX 6–3	COMPLEX REGIONAL PAIN SYNDROMES (CRPSs) I AND II

Type I CRPS (formerly known as reflex sympathetic dystrophy) develops after an initiating noxious event.
Type II CRPS (formerly known as causalgia) develops after a nerve injury.
Both type I and type II have the following characteristics:
- Spontaneous pain or allodynia/hyperalgesia occurs and is not limited to the territory of a single peripheral nerve (and, in CRPS type I, is disproportionate to the inciting event).
- There is or has been evidence of edema, skin blood flow abnormality, or abnormal sudomotor activity in the region of the pain since the inciting event.
- This diagnosis is excluded by the existence of conditions that would otherwise account for the degree of pain or dysfunction.

Epidural Anesthesia. Case reports have recommended epidural anesthesia as the anesthetic technique of choice for patients with lower extremity CRPS who are undergoing surgery.[136,137,154] The lack of prospective studies means that optimal timing, treatment duration, safety, efficacy, and appropriate analgesic combinations (if any) are all unknown. Clonidine may have a leading role in such drug infusion regimens.[155]

Preemptive Multimodal Analgesia

Inferred pathophysiology of CRPS suggests that peripheral nociception leads to central sensitization. Analgesic techniques are aimed at reducing central sensitization, which occurs

TABLE 6–5	Treatment Options for Neuropathic Pain
Treatment Modality	**Examples**
Surgical interventions directed at etiology	Peripheral nerve decompression (e.g., carpal tunnel release)
	Nerve root decompression (e.g., intervertebral discectomy)
Systemic pharmacotherapy	Tricyclic antidepressants (e.g., amitriptyline)
	Antiepileptic drugs (e.g., gabapentin, pregabalin)
	Sympatholytic drugs (e.g., guanethidine, phentolamine)
	Opiates (e.g., oxycodone, morphine)
	Sodium channel–blocking drugs (e.g., lidocaine, mexiletine)
	N-Methyl-D-aspartate antagonists (e.g., ketamine)
Regional pharmacotherapy	Topical medications (e.g., capsaicin, lidocaine)
	Peripheral:
	Conduction blockade
	Steroid injection
	Sympathectomy
	Neuraxial:
	Conduction blockade
	Steroid injection
	Sympatholytics
	Opiates
Electrical stimulation	Transcutaneous nerve stimulation
	Direct peripheral nerve stimulation
	Spinal cord stimulation
	Deep brain stimulation
Functional therapies	Physical therapy
	Occupational therapy
Behavioral modifications/ psychotherapies	Biofeedback
	Relaxation techniques
Destructive nervous system techniques	Peripheral neurolysis
	Peripheral neurectomy
	Chemical and surgical rhizotomy
	Cordotomy
	Stereotactic brain lesions

Adapted from Panlilio LM, Tella P, Raja SN: Neuropathic pain: Outcome studies on the role of nerve blocks. In Prithvi RJ (ed): Textbook of Regional Anesthesia. Philadelphia, Churchill Livingstone 2002, p 972.

from noxious input not only from the incision (preemptive analgesia) but also during the entire postoperative period (preventative analgesia).[156,157] It is recommended that multimodal analgesia using combined analgesics with differing mechanisms of action be used.[158] Studies have shown this technique to be efficacious.[159–161]

Pharmacological Therapies

Varieties of drugs have been administered perioperatively to reduce incidence of CRPS postoperatively. Free radical scavengers have been studied, on the assumption that CRPS is induced by an exaggerated inflammatory response to tissue injury, mediated by an excessive production of toxic oxygen radicals. Dimethylsulfoxide,[162,163] mannitol,[164] N-acetylcysteine,[163] carnitine,[165] and vitamin C[166,167] have been investigated in the treatment of CRPS. To date, only vitamin C has been the subject of a prospective, randomized, placebo-controlled, double-blind trial to assess the efficacy of administration of a free radical scavenger in reducing CRPS.[166] Of note, this trial involved the conservative nonsurgical treatment of wrist fractures and showed a significant reduction in the incidence of CRPS at 1 year. A later prospective nonrandomized study of surgical treatment (intrafocal pinning) of wrist fractures confirmed the benefits of vitamin C.[167]

Other pharmacological therapies studied are calcitonin and ketanserin therapy. Calcitonin is a polypeptide hormone produced by the thyroid gland that regulates blood concentrations of calcium and bone calcium metabolism. With the discovery of calcitonin-binding sites in the central nervous system, questions about its antinociceptive actions were raised.[168] The proposed mechanisms of action include Ca^{2+} fluxes, catecholaminergic and serotoninergic mechanisms, protein phosphorylation, β-endorphin production, cyclooxygenase inhibition, and histamine interference.[168,169] A later study quantified and confirmed the important role of calcitonin gene–related peptide in patients with CRPS.[170] Large-scale randomized prospective studies are required to establish the efficacy of calcitonin administration in the perioperative period in reducing both the incidence and the recurrence of CRPS after high-risk orthopedic surgical procedures.[132]

Ketanserin is a serotonin type-2 receptor antagonist that may possess analgesic properties that can be of benefit to patients with CRPS.[143,148]

Management of Postoperative Neuropathic Pain

Once postoperative neuropathic pain is diagnosed, the same management principles apply as for chronic neuropathic pain. Table 6–5 lists the various treatments used, although the optimal treatment for neuropathic pain remains to be defined. Antiepileptic drugs, tricyclic antidepressants, and opioid analgesics form the pharmacological basis of treatment. Neuropathic pain is difficult to treat and sometimes does not respond to treatment or intervention. The lists and dosing regimens of pharmacologic agents that appear in this chapter (Tables 6–6 through 6–8; Box 6–4) are only guides,

TABLE 6-6 Antiepileptic Drugs Used in the Treatment of Neuropathic Pain

Drug	Intravenous Dose	Oral Dose	Systemic Side Effects	Neurotoxic Side Effects	Rare Side Effects
Carbamazepine (Tegretol; Tegretol-XR; Carbatrol)	Not applicable	Start at 2 to 3 mg/kg/day; increase dose every 5 days to 10 mg/kg/day; dose may need to be further increased to 15–20 mg/kg/day after 2 to 3 months because of hepatic autoinduction; maximum 1.6 g/day	Nausea, vomiting, diarrhea, hyponatremia, rash, pruritus	Drowsiness, dizziness, blurred or double vision, lethargy, headache	Agranulocytosis, Stevens-Johnson syndrome, aplastic anemia, hepatic failure, dermatitis/rash, serum sickness, pancreatitis
Gabapentin (Neurontin)	Not applicable	300 mg on the first day, 300 mg twice daily on the second day, 300 mg three times daily on the third day; increase as needed to 1800 mg/day in 3 divided doses; lower doses recommended in patients with renal insufficiency	None known	Sommolence, dizziness, ataxia	Unknown
Lamotrigine (Lamictal)	Not applicable	For patients taking an enzyme-inducing antiepileptic drug: 25 mg twice a day, titrated upward by 5-mg increments every 1–2 weeks as needed. For patients taking valproate: 25 mg every other day, with increases of 25–50 mg every 2 weeks as needed to a maximum of 300–500 mg/day	Rash, nausea	Dizziness, sommolence	Stevens-Johnson syndrome, hypersensitivity
Oxcarbazepine (Trileptal)	Not applicable	Start at 300 to 600 mg/day in two or three divided doses; increase by 600 mg/day weekly to a total dose of 900–3000 mg per day in two or three divided doses	Nausea, rash, hyponatremia	Sedation, headache, dizziness, vertigo, ataxia, diplopia	Unknown

Drug	Dose	Dose			
Phenytoin (Dilantin), fosphenytoin (Cerebyx)	15 mg/kg (not > 50 mg/min): dose expressed as phenytoin equivalents Status epilepticus: 15–20 mg/kg at 100–150 mg/min Nonemergency loading: intravenous or intramuscular 10–20 mg/kg Maintenance dose: 4–6 mg/kg per day	15 mg/kg in 3 divided doses over 9–12 hours; 5 mg/kg/day maintenance	Gingival hypertrophy, body hair increase, rash, lymphadenopathy	Confusion, slurred speech, double vision, ataxia, neuropathy (with long-term use)	Agranulocytosis, aplastic anemia, Stevens-Johnson syndrome, hepatic failure, dermatitis/rash, serum sickness
Tiagabine (Gabitril)	Not applicable	4 mg once daily; in adults, titrate at weekly increments of 4–8 mg/day until clinical response, or up to 56 mg/day in divided doses	None known	Dizziness, lack of energy, somnolence, nausea, nervousness, tremor, difficulty concentrating, abdominal pain	Unknown
Topiramate (Topamax)	Not applicable	50 mg/day for 1 week; titrate at weekly increments of 50 mg to an effective dose Recommended total daily dose as adjunctive therapy is 200 mg twice daily	Weight loss, renal stones, paresthesias	Fatigue, nervousness, difficulty concentrating, confusion, depression, anorexia, language problems, anxiety, mood problems, tremor	Acute myopia and glaucoma; oligohidrosis and hyperthermia, which occur primarily in children
Valproate (Depakote [oral]; Depacon [IV])	Infuse over 60 minutes at 20 mg/min as needed to a maximum dose of 2500 mg/day in 2–4 divided doses Rapid infusion: up to 15 mg/kg over 5–10 minutes (1.5–3 mg/kg per minute)	15 mg/kg/day in 2–4 divided doses; increase by 5–10 mg/kg/day every week as needed	Weight gain, nausea, vomiting, hair loss, easy bruising	Tremor	Agranulocytosis, Stevens-Johnson syndrome, aplastic anemia, hepatic failure, dermatitis/rash, serum sickness, pancreatitis

Modified from Bajwa ZH, Sami N, Ho CC: Antiepileptic drugs in the treatment of neuropathic pain. In UpToDate February 17, 2004. Available at www.uptodate.com/

TABLE 6–7	Tricyclic Antidepressant Drugs Used in the Treatment of Neuropathic Pain			
Drug	Dose	Mechanism of Action	Side Effects	Further Comments
Amitriptyline	10–150 mg/day	Norepinephrine and serotonin reuptake inhibitor	Anticholinergic effects, sedation, orthostatic hypotension	Caution in patients with glaucoma, those taking monoamine oxidase inhibitors (MAOIs; serotonin syndrome), and those unable to tolerate anticholinergic or sedative side effects
Nortriptyline (active metabolite of amitriptyline)	25 mg three or four times a day Maximum: 150 mg/day	Norepinephrine and serotonin reuptake inhibitor	Anticholinergic effects, sedation, orthostatic hypotension	Fewer side effects than amitriptyline; use with caution in patients with cardiovascular disease
Imipramine	25 mg three times a day: increase up to 150 mg/day	Norepinephrine and serotonin reuptake inhibitor	Anticholinergic effects, sedation, orthostatic hypotension, tremor	Caution in patients with glaucoma, those taking MAOIs (serotonin syndrome), or those unable to tolerate anticholinergic or sedative side effects
Desipramine (active metabolite of imipramine)	100–200 mg/day	Norepinephrine and serotonin reuptake inhibitor	Anticholinergic effects, sedation, tremor	Has one of the lowest rates of anticholinergic side effects

From Namaka M, Gramlich CR, Ruhlen D, et al: A treatment algorithm for neuropathic pain. Clin Ther 2004;26:951–979.

TABLE 6–8   Opioid Analgesics Used in the Treatment of Neuropathic Pain

Drug Name	Dose	Mechanism of Action	Side Effects	Further Comments
Morphine	Variable	μ Opioid receptor agonist	Physical dependence, respiratory depression, nausea, vomiting, sedation	Gold standard
Methadone	5–10 mg every 4–8 hours In prolonged use, not to be given more frequently than every 12 hours	μ Opioid receptor agonist in descending pathway	Side effects same as those of morphine	Can be used in patients who experience exacerbation of pain or excitation with morphine
Tramadol	50–100 mg every 4 to 6 hours as required, orally or intramuscularly May be given by slow infusion (over 2–3 minutes)	Weak opioid receptor agonist, norepinephrine reuptake inhibitor, and enhances serotonin release	Physical dependence, stomach pain, dizziness, drowsiness, rash, nausea	Convulsions reported (usually after rapid intravenous administration)
Fentanyl	Topical patch: 25 μg to 300 μg per hour for 72 hours Lozenge: initially 200 μg over 15 mins; repeat if necessary 15 minutes after first dose; no more than 2 dose units per pain episode Maximum: 4 dose units per day	μ Opioid receptor agonist	Side effects same as those of morphine With patches, local reactions such as rash, erythema, pruritus	Monitor patients for increased side effects if febrile as increased absorption possible External heat exposure to application site may also increase absorption Long duration of action
Buprenorphine	Topical patch: 35 μg to 70 μg per hour for 72 hours Sublingual: 200 to 400 μg 6-8 hourly	Partial agonist which dissociates slowly from μ opioid receptor leading to prolonged analgesia	Side effects same as those of morphine With patches, local reactions such as rash, erythema, pruritus, delayed local allergic reactions with severe inflammation Buprenorphine has opioid agonist and antagonist properties, may precipitate withdrawal symptoms in patients dependent on other opioids; its effects are only partially reversed by naloxone	Monitor patients for increased side effects if febrile as increased absorption possible External heat exposure to application site may also increase absorption Long duration of action Severe respiratory depression has occurred when benzodiazepines have been co-administered
Oxycodone hydrochloride	Orally: 5 mg every 4–6 hours as required; maximum usually 400 mg daily Intravenously: 1–10 mg every 4 hours as required Subcutaneously: 5 mg every 4 hours as required	Opioid receptor agonist	Side effects same as those of morphine	Avoid in porphyria

Adapted from Namaka M, Gramlich CR, Ruhlen D, et al: A treatment algorithm for neuropathic pain. Clin Ther 2004;26:951–979; further data from British National Formulary 48, September 2004. London, British National Association and Pharmaceutical Society of Great Britain. www.bnf.org.

<table>
<tr><td>

BOX 6–4

</td><td>

TOPICAL DRUGS USED IN THE TREATMENT OF NEUROPATHIC PAIN

</td></tr>
</table>

Lidocaine gel and lidocaine 5% patch
Capsaicin cream 0.025% and 0.075%
Ether/aspirin

---

as the dosages and side effects will differ because of the variability of patient responses. Treatment of neuropathic pain was not the primary role of several drugs commonly used in the management of neuropathic pain. Drugs developed for the treatment of neuropathic pain include pregabalin, gabapentin, and capsaicin.

ANTIEPILEPTIC DRUGS

Antiepileptic drugs have analgesic effects in patients with neuropathic pain (see Table 6–6). Owing to the differing mechanisms of action of these drugs, failure with one agent does not eliminate the potential effectiveness of another antiepileptic drug.

Pregabalin is structurally related to gabapentin but has a much greater binding affinity for the $\alpha_2\delta$ subunit protein associated with voltage-gated calcium channels, which have a role in neuropathic pain.[171,172] Pregabalin modulates these Ca^{2+} channels, reduces neurotransmitter release, and has been shown to have analgesic effects in neuropathic pain.[173,174]

TRICYCLIC ANTIDEPRESSANT DRUGS

In patients with neuropathic pain, tricyclic antidepressants (TCAs) have analgesic effects[175-180] that may not be directly related to their antidepressant properties, and a dose-response relationship may exist.[181,182] TCAs affect norepinephrine and serotonin release and reuptake, potentiating the inhibitory and antinociceptive effects of the descending serotonergic and noradrenergic systems (see Table 6–7).[183-185]

OPIOID ANALGESICS

Opioid analgesics (morphine, methadone, tramadol, fentanyl, buprenorphine, and oxycodone) have been shown to have an analgesic effect in neuropathic pain (see Table 6–8).[186-195] Opioids bind to opioid receptors and have a noncompetitive antagonistic effect at the NMDA receptor, including an action on calcium channels on nociception neurons.[196,197]

TOPICAL AGENTS

Lidocaine (lignocaine) patches have been shown to be effective in the treatment of postherpetic neuralgia,[198,199] and further evidence suggests a role in the treatment of other neuropathic pain conditions.[200,201] A review of topical capsaicin concluded that this agent may be useful as an adjunctive or sole treatment for patients who show no response to other treatments.[202] Topical aspirin/diethyl ether mixture has been shown to have analgesic benefits in the treatment of acute herpetic and postherpetic neuralgia (see Box 6–4).[203-205]

POSSIBLE TREATMENT STRATEGY FOR POSTOPERATIVE NEUROPATHIC PAIN

The following are agents or combinations that may be used to treat postoperative neuropathic pain:

- TCA—Amitriptyline
- Pregabalin
- Oxycodone and TCA
- Ketamine during general anesthesia
- Tramadol
- Local anesthesia
- Preemptive—no data to support this approach, although the concept is attractive

---

Conclusion

Postoperative neuropathic pain is probably underdiagnosed. One in four patients with cancer has neuropathic pain, and a significant number of such cases may be due to iatrogenic nerve injury.[206] Until the pathophysiology is more clearly understood, an optimal therapeutic strategy remains to be defined. Optimization of preoperative neuropathic pain therapy and early intervention in newly diagnosed cases of postoperative neuropathic pain are recommended.

REFERENCES

1. Davies HT, Crombie IK, Macrae WA, Rogers KM: Pain clinic patients in northern Britain. Pain Clin 1992;5:129–135.
2. Carr DB, Goudas LC: Acute pain. Lancet 1999;353:2051–2058.
3. Perkins FM, Kehlet H: Chronic pain as an outcome of surgery: A review of predictive factors. Anesthesiology 2000;93:1123–1133.
4. Merskey H, Bogduk N (eds): Classification of Chronic Pain, 2nd ed. IASP Task Force on Taxonomy. Seattle, IASP Press, 1994. See also IASP website: www.iasp-pain.org/terms-p.html/
5. Melton L: Taking a shot at neuropathic pain. Lancet Neurol 2003; 2:719.
6. Woolf CJ. Pain: Moving from symptom control toward mechanism-specific pharmacologic management. Ann Intern Med 2004;140: 441–451.
7. Scholz J, Woolf CJ: Can we conquer pain? Nat Neurosci 2002; 5(Suppl):1062–1067.
8. Julius D, Basbaum AI: Molecular mechanisms of nociception. Nature 2001;413: 203–210.
9. Woolf CJ, Salter MW: Neuronal plasticity: Increasing the gain in pain. Science 2000;288:1765–1769.
10. Mogil JS, Yu L, Basbaum AI: Pain genes? Natural variation and transgenic mutants. Ann Rev Neurosci 2000;23:777–811.
11. Woolf CJ, Mannion RJ: Neuropathic pain: Aetiology, symptoms, mechanisms and management. Lancet 1999;353:1959–1964.
12. Waxman SG, Wood JN: Sodium channels from mechanisms to medicines? Brain Res Bull 1999;50:309–310.
13. Amaya F, Decosterd I, Samad TA, et al: Diversity of expression of the sensory neuron-specific TTX-resistant voltage-gated sodium ion channels SNS and SNS2. Mol Cell Neurosci 2000;15:331–342.
14. Levine JD, Reichling DB: Peripheral mechanisms of inflammatory pain. In Wall PD, Melzack R (eds): Textbook of Pain, 4th ed. Edinburgh, Churchill Livingstone, 1999, pp 59–84.
15. McCleskey EW, Gold MS: Ion channels of nociception. Annu Rev Physiol 1999;61:835–856.
16. Numazaki M, Tominaga T, Toyooka H, Tominaga M: Direct phosphorylation of capsaicin receptor VR1 by protein kinase Cepsilon and identification of two target serine residues. J Biol Chem 2002;277:13375–13378.
17. Walker K, Perkins M, Dray A: Kinins and kinin receptors in the nervous system. Neurochem Int 1995;26:1–16.
18. Vane JR, Bakhle YS, Botting RM: Cyclooxygenases 1 and 2. Annu Rev Pharmacol Toxicol 1998;38:97–120.

19. Costigan M, Befort K, Karchewski L, et al: Replicate high-density rat genome oligonucleotide microarrays reveal hundreds of regulated genes in the dorsal root ganglion after peripheral nerve injury. BMC Neurosci 2002;3:16.

20. Xiao HS, Huang QH, Zhang FX, et al: Identification of gene expression profile of dorsal root ganglion in the rat peripheral axotomy model of neuropathic pain. Proc Natl Acad Sci U S A 2002;99:8360–8365.

21. Noguchi K, Kawai Y, Fukuoka T, et al: Substance P induced by peripheral nerve injury in primary afferent sensory neurons and its effect on dorsal column nucleus neurons. J Neurosci 1995;15:7633–7643.

22. Fukuoka T, Kondo E, Dai Y, et al: Brain-derived neurotrophic factor increases in the uninjured dorsal root ganglion neurons in selective spinal nerve ligation model. J Neurosci 2001;21:4891–4900.

23. Decosterd I, Allchorne A, Woolf CJ: Progressive tactile hypersensitivity after a peripheral nerve crush: Non-noxious mechanical stimulus-induced neuropathic pain. Pain 2002;100:155–162.

24. Ji RR, Samad TA, Jin SX, et al: p38 MAPK activation by NGF in primary sensory neurons after inflammation increases TRPV1 levels and maintains heat hyperalgesia. Neuron 2002;36:57–68.

25. Mannion RJ, Costigan M, Decosterd I, et al: Neurotrophins: Peripherally and centrally acting modulators of tactile stimulus-induced inflammatory pain hypersensitivity. Proc Natl Acad Sci U S A 1999;96:9385–9390.

26. Luo ZD, Chaplan SR, Higuera ES, et al: Upregulation of dorsal root ganglion (alpha)2(delta) calcium channel subunit and its correlation with allodynia in spinal nerve-injured rats. J Neurosci 2001;21:1868–1875.

27. Liu CN, Devor M, Waxman SG, Kocsis JD: Subthreshold oscillations induced by spinal nerve injury in dissociated muscle and cutaneous afferents of mouse DRG. J Neurophysiol 2002;87:2009–2017.

28. Woolf CJ: Evidence for a central component of post-injury pain hypersensitivity. Nature 1983;306:686–688.

29. Woolf CJ, Wall PD: Relative effectiveness of C primary afferent fibers of different origins in evoking a prolonged facilitation of the flexor reflex in the rat. J Neurosci 1986;6:1433–1442.

30. Eliav E, Teich S, Benoliel R, et al: Large myelinated nerve fiber hypersensitivity in oral malignancy. Oral Surg Oral Med Oral Pathol Oral Radiol Endod 2002;94:45–50.

31. Stubhaug A, Breivik H, Eide PK, et al: Mapping of punctuate hyperalgesia around a surgical incision demonstrates that ketamine is a powerful suppressor of central sensitization to pain following surgery. Acta Anaesthesiol Scand 1997;41:1124–1132.

32. Campbell JN, Raja SN, Meyer RA, Mackinnon SE: Myelinated afferents signal the hyperalgesia associated with nerve injury. Pain 1988;32:89–94.

33. Koltzenburg M, Scadding J: Neuropathic pain. Curr Opin Neurol 2001;14:641–647.

34. Woolf CJ: Dissecting out mechanisms responsible for peripheral neuropathic pain: Implications for diagnosis and therapy. Life Sci 2004;74:2605–2610.

35. Ji RR, Kohno T, Moore KA, Woolf CJ: Central sensitization and LTP: Do pain and memory share similar mechanisms? Trends Neurosci 2003;26:696–705.

36. South SM, Kohno T, Kaspar BK, et al: A conditional deletion of the NR1 subunit of the NMDA receptor in adult spinal cord dorsal horn reduces NMDA currents and injury-induced pain. J Neurosci 2003;23:5031–5040.

37. Ji RR, Woolf CJ: Neuronal plasticity and signal transduction in nociceptive neurons: Implications for the initiation and maintenance of pathological pain. Neurobiol Dis 2001;8:1–10.

38. Felsby S, Nielsen J, Arendt-Nielsen L, Jensen TS: NMDA receptor blockade in chronic neuropathic pain: A comparison of ketamine and magnesium chloride. Pain 1996;64:283–291.

39. Pud D, Eisenberg E, Spitzer A, et al: The NMDA receptor antagonist amantadine reduces surgical neuropathic pain in cancer patients: A double blind, randomized, placebo controlled trial. Pain 1998;75:349–354.

40. Ji RR, Befort K, Brenner GJ, Woolf CJ: ERK MAP kinase activation in superficial spinal cord neurons induces prodynorphin and NK-1 upregulation and contributes to persistent inflammatory pain hypersensitivity. J Neurosci 2002;22:478–485.

41. Samad TA, Moore KA, Sapirstein A, et al: Interleukin-1beta-mediated induction of Cox-2 in the CNS contributes to inflammatory pain hypersensitivity. Nature 2001;410:471–475.

42. Watkins LR, Maier SF: Beyond neurons: Evidence that immune cells and glial cells contribute to pathological pain states. Physiol Rev 2002;82:981–1011.

43. Said G, Hontebeyrie-Joskowicz M: Nerve lesions induced by macrophage activation. Res Immunol 1992;143:589–599.

44. Watkins LR, Maier SF: Neuropathic pain: The immune connection. Pain: Clin Updates 2004;12:1.

45. Olsson Y: Microenvironment of the peripheral nervous system under normal and pathological conditions. Crit Rev Neurobiol 1990;5:265–311.

46. Stoll G, Jander S, Myers RR: Degeneration and regeneration of the peripheral nervous system: From Augustus Waller's observations to neuroinflammation. J Peripher Nerv Syst 2002;7:13–27.

47. Watkins LR, Milligan ED, Maier SF: Glial activation: A driving force for pathological pain. Trends Neurosci 2001;24:450–455.

48. Koski CL: Mechanisms of Schwann cell damage in inflammatory neuropathy. J Infect Dis 1997;176:S169–S172.

49. Quarles RH, Weiss MD: Autoantibodies associated with peripheral neuropathy. Muscle Nerve 1999;22:800–822.

50. Koski CL: Humoral mechanisms in immune neuropathies. Neurol Clin 1992;10:629–649.

51. Moulin DE, Hagen N, Feasby TE, et al: Pain in Guillain-Barré syndrome. Neurology 1997;48:328–331.

52. Nguyen DK, Agenarioti-Belanger S, Vanasse M: Pain and the Guillain-Barré syndrome in children under 6 years old. J Paediatr 1999;134:773–776.

53. Hawke SH, Davies L, Pamphlett R, et al: Vasculitic neuropathy: A clinical and pathological study. Brain 1991;114:2175–2190.

54. Heuss D, Probst-Cousin S, Kayser C, Neundorfer B: Cell death in vasculitic neuropathy. Muscle Nerve 2000;23:999–1004.

55. Sorkin LS, Xiao WH, Wagner R, Myers RR: Tumour necrosis factor-alpha induces ectopic activity in nociceptive primary afferent fibres. Neuroscience 1997;81:255–262.

56. Porreca F, Ossipov MH, Gebhart GF: Chronic pain and medullary descending facilitation. Trends Neurosci 2002;25:319–325.

57. Suzuki R, Morcuende S, Webber M, et al: Superficial NK1-expressing neurons control spinal excitability through activation of descending pathways. Nat Neurosci 2002;5:1319–1326.

58. Zeitz KP, Guy N, Malmberg AB, et al: The 5-HT3 subtype of serotonin receptor contributes to nociceptive processing via a novel subset of myelinated and unmyelinated nociceptors. J Neurosci 2002;22:1010–1019.

59. McCleane GJ, Suzuki R, Dickenson AH: Does a single intravenous injection of the 5HT3 receptor antagonist ondansetron have an analgesic effect in neuropathic pain? A double-blinded, placebo-controlled cross-over study. Anesth Analg 2003;97:1474–1478.

60. Farber L, Stratz TH, Bruckle W, et al; German Fibromyalgia Study Group: Short-term treatment of primary fibromyalgia with the 5-HT3-receptor antagonist tropisetron: Results of a randomized, double-blind, placebo-controlled multicenter trial in 418 patients. Int J Clin Pharmacol Res 2001;21:1–13.

61. Haus U, Varga B, Stratz T, et al: Oral treatment of fibromyalgia with tropisetron given over 28 days: Influence on functional and vegetative symptoms, psychometric parameters and pain. Scand J Rheumatol Suppl 2000;113:55–58.

62. Stratz T, Farber L, Varga B, et al: Fibromyalgia treatment with intravenous tropisetron administration. Drugs Exp Clin Res 2001;27:113–118.

63. Woolf CJ, Shortland P, Coggeshall RE: Peripheral nerve injury triggers central sprouting of myelinated afferents. Nature 1992;355:75–78.

64. Moore KA, Kohno T, Karchewski LA, et al: Partial peripheral nerve injury promotes a selective loss of GABAergic inhibition in the superficial dorsal horn of the spinal cord. J Neurosci 2002;22:6724–6731.

65. Hwang JH, Yaksh TL: The effect of spinal GABA receptor agonists on tactile allodynia in a surgically-induced neuropathic pain model in the rat. Pain 1997;70:15–22.

66. Bloechlinger S, Karchewski LA, Woolf CJ: Dynamic changes in glypican-1 expression in dorsal root ganglion neurons after peripheral and central axonal injury. Eur J Neurosci 2004;19:1119–1132.

67. The effect of intensive diabetes therapy on the development and progression of neuropathy. The Diabetes Control and Complications Trial Research Group. Ann Intern Med 1995;122:561–568.

68. Werrett G: Nerve injuries. In Allman KG, Wilson IH (eds): Oxford Handbook of Clinical Anaesthesia. Oxford, Oxford University Press, 2001, pp 947–953.

69. Sawyer RJ, Richmond MN, Hickey JD, Jarrratt JA: Peripheral nerve injuries associated with anaesthesia. Anaesthesia 2000;55:980–991.

70. Cheney FW, Domino KB, Caplan RA, Posner KL: Nerve injury associated with anesthesia: A closed claims analysis. Anesthesiology 1999; 90:1062–1069.

71. Ben-David B: Complications of regional anesthesia: An overview. Anesthesiol Clin North Am 2002;20:665–667.

72. Borgeat A, Ekatodramis G: Nerve injury associated with regional anesthesia. Curr Top Med Chem 2001;1:199–203.

73. Katz J, Jackson M, Kavanagh BP, Sandler AN: Acute pain after thoracic surgery predicts long-term post-thoracotomy pain. Clin J Pain 1996; 12:50–55.

74. Keller SM, Carp NZ, Levy MN, Rosen SM: Chronic post thoracotomy pain. J Cardiovasc Surg 1994;35(Suppl 1):161–164.

75. Benedetti F, Vighetti S, Ricco C, et al: Neurophysiologic assessment of nerve impairment in posterolateral and muscle-sparing thoracotomy. J Thorac Cardiovasc Surg 1998;115:841–847.

76. Benedetti F, Amanzio M, Casadio C, et al: Postoperative pain and superficial abdominal reflexes after posterolateral thoracotomy. Ann Thorac Surg 1997;64:207–210.

77. Nomori H, Horio H, Fuyuno G, Kobayashi R: Non-serratus-sparing antero-axillary thoracotomy with disconnection of anterior rib cartilage: Improvement in postoperative pulmonary function and pain in comparison to posterolateral thoracotomy. Chest 1997;111: 572–576.

78. Perttunen K, Tasmuth T, Kalso E: Chronic pain after thoracic surgery: A follow-up study. Acta Anaesthesiol Scand 1999;43:563–567.

79. Sedrakyan A, van der Meulen J, Lewsey J, Treasure T: Video assisted thoracic surgery for treatment of pneumothorax and lung resections: Systematic review of randomised clinical trials. BMJ 2004;329(7473): 1008.

80. Obata H, Saito S, Fujita N, et al: Epidural block with mepivacaine before surgery reduces long-term post-thoracotomy pain. Can J Anaesth 1999;46:1127–1132.

81. Carpenter JS, Andrykowki MA, Sloan P, et al: Postmastectomy/postlumpectomy pain in breast cancer survivors. J Clin Epidemiol 1998;51:1285–1292.

82. Kroner K, Krebs B, Skov J, Jorgensen HS: Immediate and long-term phantom breast syndrome after mastectomy: Incidence, clinical characteristics and relationship to pre-mastectomy breast pain. Pain 1989; 36:327–334.

83. Tasmuth T, Estlanderb AM, Kalso E: Effect of present pain and mood on the memory of past postoperative pain in women treated surgically for breast cancer. Pain 1996;68:343–347.

84. Tasmuth T, von Smitten K, Kalso E: Pain and other symptoms during the first year after radical and conservative surgery for breast cancer. Br J Cancer 1996;74:2024–2031.

85. Maunsell E, Brisson J, Deschenes L: Arm problems and psychological distress after surgery for breast cancer. Can J Surg 1993;36:315–320.

86. Keramopoulos A, Tsionou C, Minaretzis D, et al: Arm morbidity following treatment of breast cancer with total axillary dissection: A multivariate approach. Oncology 1993;50:445–449.

87. Wallace MS, Wallace AM, Lee J, Dobke MK: Pain after breast surgery: A survey of 282 women. Pain 1996;66:195–205.

88. Tasmuth T, Kataja M, Blomqvist C, et al: Treatment-related factors predisposing to chronic pain in patients with breast cancer—a multivariate approach. Acta Oncol 1997;36:625–630.

89. Tasmuth T, von Smitten K, Hietanen P, et al: Pain and other symptoms after different treatment modalities of breast cancer. Ann Oncol 1995; 6:453–459.

90. Watson CP, Evans RJ, Watt VR: The post-mastectomy pain syndrome and the effect of topical capsaicin. Pain 1989;38:177–186.

91. Killer HE, Hess K: Natural history of radiation-induced brachial plexopathy compared with surgically treated patients. J Neurol. 1990;237:247–250.

92. Vecht CJ, Van de Brand HJ, Wajer OJ: Post-axillary dissection pain in breast cancer due to a lesion of the intercostobrachial nerve. Pain 1989; 38:171–176.

93. Abdullah TI, Iddon J, Barr L, et al: Prospective randomized controlled trial of preservation of the intercostobrachial nerve during axillary node clearance for breast cancer. Br J Surg 1998;85:1443–1445.

94. Bratschi HU, Haller U: [Significance of the intercostobrachial nerve in axillary lymph node excision] Geburtshilfe Frauenheilkd 1990;50: 689–693.

95. Poobalan AS, Bruce J, King PM, et al: Chronic pain and quality of life following open inguinal hernia repair. Br J Surg 2001;88:1122–1126.

96. Callesen T, Bech K, Kehlet H: Prospective study of chronic pain after groin hernia repair. Br J Surg 1999;86:1528–1531.

97. Seid AS, Amos E: Entrapment neuropathy in laparoscopic herniorrhaphy. Surg Endosc 1994;8:1050–1053.

98. Starling JR, Harms BA: Diagnosis and treatment of genitofemoral and ilioinguinal neuralgia. World J Surg 1989;13:586–591.

99. Heise CP, Starling JR: Mesh inguinodynia: A new clinical syndrome after inguinal herniorrhaphy? J Am Coll Surg 1998;187:514–518.

100. Callesen T: Inguinal hernia repair: Anaesthesia, pain and convalescence. Dan Med Bull 2003;50:203–218.

101. Krane EJ, Heller LB: The prevalence of phantom sensation and pain in pediatric amputees. J Pain Symptom Manage 1995;10:21–29.

102. Jensen TS, Krebs B, Nielsen J, Rasmussen P: Immediate and long-term phantom limb pain in amputees: Incidence, clinical characteristics and relationship to pre-amputation limb pain. Pain 1985;21: 267–278.

103. Sherman RA, Sherman CJ, Parker L: Chronic phantom and stump pain among American veterans: Results of a survey. Pain 1984;18: 83–95.

104. Nikolajsen L, Ilkjaer S, Kroner K, et al: The influence of preamputation pain on postamputation stump and phantom pain. Pain 1997;72: 393–405.

105. Smith J, Thompson JM: Phantom limb pain and chemotherapy in pediatric amputees. Mayo Clin Proc 1995;70:357–364.

106. Portenoy RK: Neuropathic pain. In Kanner R (ed): Pain Management Secrets, 2nd ed. Philadelphia, Hanley & Belfus, 2003, pp 147–170.

107. Nikolajsen L, Jensen TS: Phantom limb pain. Br J Anaesth 2001; 87:107–116.

108. Jahangiri M, Jayatunga AP, Bradley JW, Dark CH: Prevention of phantom pain after major lower limb amputation by epidural infusion of diamorphine, clonidine and bupivacaine. Ann R Coll Surg Engl 1994; 76:324–326.

109. Nikolajsen L, Ilkjaer S, Christensen JH, et al: Randomised trial of epidural bupivacaine and morphine in prevention of stump and phantom pain in lower-limb amputation. Lancet 1997;350: 1353–1357.

110. Fisher A, Meller Y: Continuous postoperative regional analgesia by nerve sheath block for amputation surgery—a pilot study. Anesth Analg 1991;72:300–303.

111. Pinzur MS, Garla PG, Pluth T, Vrbos L: Continuous postoperative infusion of a regional anesthetic after an amputation of the lower extremity: A randomized clinical trial. J Bone Joint Surg Am 1996; 78:1501–1505.

112. Lambert AW, Dashfield AK, Cosgrove C, et al: Randomized prospective study comparing preoperative epidural and intraoperative perineural analgesia for the prevention of postoperative stump and phantom limb pain following major amputation. Reg Anesth Pain Med 2001; 26:316–321.

113. Jorgensen T, Teglbjerg JS, Wille-Jorgensen P, et al: Persisting pain after cholecystectomy. A prospective investigation. Scand J Gastroenterol 1991;26:124–128.

114. Jess P, Jess T, Beck H, Bech P: Neuroticism in relation to recovery and persisting pain after laparoscopic cholecystectomy. Scand J Gastroenterol 1998;33:550–553.

115. Borly L, Anderson IB, Bardram L, et al: Preoperative prediction model of outcome after cholecystectomy for symptomatic gallstones. Scand J Gastroenterol 1999;34:1144–1152.

116. Middelfart HV, Kristensen JU, Laursen CN, et al: Pain and dyspepsia after elective and acute cholecystectomy. Scand J Gastroenterol 1998; 33:10–14.

117. Bates T, Ebbs SR, Harrison M, A'Hern RP: Influence of cholecystectomy on symptoms. Br J Surg 1991;78:964–967.

118. Stefaniak T, Vingerhoets A, Babinska D, et al: Psychological factors influencing results of cholecystectomy. Scand J Gastroenterol 2004; 39:127–132.

119. Fenster LF, Lonborg R, Thirlby RC, Traverso LW: What symptoms does cholecystectomy cure? Insights from an outcomes measurement project and review of the literature. Am J Surg 1995;169:533–538.

120. Gilliland TM, Traverso LW: Modern standards for comparison of cholecystectomy with alternative treatments for symptomatic cholelithiasis with emphasis on long-term relief of symptoms. Surg Gynecol Obstet 1990;170:39–44.

121. Gui GP, Cheruvu CV, West N, et al: Is cholecystectomy effective treatment for symptomatic gallstones? Clinical outcome after long-term follow-up. Ann R Coll Surg Engl 1998;80:25–32.

122. Vander Velpen GC, Shimi SM, Cuschieri A: Outcome after cholecystectomy for symptomatic gall stone disease and effect of surgical access: Laparoscopic v open approach. Gut 1993;34:1448–1451.

123. Ros A, Nilsson E: Abdominal pain and patient overall and cosmetic satisfaction one year after cholecystectomy: Outcome of a randomized trial comparing laparoscopic and minilaparotomy cholecystectomy. Scand J Gastroenterol 2004;39:773–777.

124. Poon CM, Chan KW, Lee DW, et al: Two-port versus four-port laparoscopic cholecystectomy. Surg Endosc 2003;17:1624–1627.

125. Stanton-Hicks M, Janig W, Hassenbusch S, et al: Reflex sympathetic dystrophy: Changing concepts and taxonomy. Pain 1995;63:127–133.

126. Benzon HT: Taxonomy: Definitions of pain terms and chronic pain syndromes. In Eds; Benzon HT, Raja SN, Borsook D, et al (eds): Essentials of Pain Medicine and Regional Anesthesia. Philadelphia, Churchill Livingstone, 1999, pp 10–11.

127. Roberts WJ: A hypothesis on the physiological basis for causalgia and related pains. Pain 1986;24:297–311.

128. Boas RA: Sympathetic nerve blocks: In search of a role. Reg Anesth Pain Med 1998;23:292–305.

129. Harden RN, Bruehl S, Stanos S, et al: Prospective examination of pain-related and psychological predictors of CRPS-like phenomena following total knee arthroplasty: A preliminary study. Pain 2003;106:393–400.

130. Pak TJ, Martin GM, Magness JL, Kavanaugh GJ: Reflex sympathetic dystrophy: Review of 140 cases. Minn Med 1970;53:507–512.

131. Bonica JJ: Causalgia and other reflex sympathetic dystrophies. In Bonica JJ, Liebeskind JC, Albe-Fressard D, et al (eds): Advances in Pain Research and Therapy, vol 3. New York, Raven Press, 1979, pp 141–166.

132. Reuben SS: Preventing the development of complex regional pain syndrome after surgery. Anesthesiology 2004;101:1215–1224.

133. Katz MM, Hungerford DS: Reflex sympathetic dystrophy affecting the knee. J Bone Joint Surg Br 1987;69:797–803.

134. Veldman PH, Goris RJ: Surgery on extremities with reflex sympathetic dystrophy. Unfallchirurg 1995;98:45–48.

135. Katz MM, Hungerford DS, Krackow KA, Lennox DW: Reflex sympathetic dystrophy as a cause of poor results after total knee arthroplasty. J Arthroplasty 1986;1:117–124.

136. Rocco AG: Sympathetically maintained pain may be rekindled by surgery under general anesthesia. Anesthesiology 1993;79:865.

137. Viel EJ, Pelissier J, Eledjam JJ: Sympathetically maintained pain after surgery may be prevented by regional anesthesia. Anesthesiology 1994;81:265–266.

138. Tessler MJ, Kleiman SJ: Spinal anaesthesia for patients with previous lower limb amputations. Anaesthesia 1994;49:439–441.

139. Reuben SS, Rosenthal EA, Steinberg RB: Surgery on the affected upper extremity of patients with a history of complex regional pain syndrome: A retrospective study of 100 patients. J Hand Surg [Am] 2000;25:1147–1151.

140. Glynn CJ, Basedow RW, Walsh JA: Pain relief following post-ganglionic sympathetic blockade with I.V. guanethidine. Br J Anaesth 1981;53:1297–1302.

141. Rocco AG, Kaul AF, Reisman RM, et al: A comparison of regional intravenous guanethidine and reserpine in reflex sympathetic dystrophy: A controlled, randomized, double-blind crossover study. Clin J Pain 1989;5:205–209.

142. Blanchard J, Ramamurthy S, Walsh N, et al: Intravenous regional sympatholysis: A double-blind comparison of guanethidine, reserpine, and normal saline. J Pain Symptom Manage 1990;5:357–361.

143. Jadad AR, Carroll D, Glynn CJ, McQuay HJ: Intravenous regional sympathetic blockade for pain relief in reflex sympathetic dystrophy: A systematic review and a randomized, double-blind crossover study. J Pain Symptom Manage 1995;10:13–20.

144. Ramamurthy S, Hoffman J: Intravenous regional guanethidine in the treatment of reflex sympathetic dystrophy/causalgia: A randomized, double-blind study. Guanethidine Study Group. Anesth Analg 1995;81:718–723.

145. Kettler RE, Abram SE: Intravenous regional droperidol in the management of reflex sympathetic dystrophy: A double-blind, placebo-controlled, crossover study. Anesthesiology 1988;69:933–936.

146. Glynn CJ, Stannard C, Collins PA, Casale R: The role of peripheral sudomotor blockade in the treatment of patients with sympathetically maintained pain. Pain 1993;53:39–42.

147. Hord AH, Rooks MD, Stephens BO, et al: Intravenous regional bretylium and lidocaine for treatment of reflex sympathetic dystrophy: A randomized, double-blind study. Anesth Analg 1992;74:818–821.

148. Hanna MH, Peat SJ: Ketanserin in reflex sympathetic dystrophy: A double-blind placebo controlled cross-over trial. Pain 1989;38:145–150.

149. Kingery WS: A critical review of controlled clinical trials for peripheral neuropathic pain and complex regional pain syndromes. Pain 1997;73:123–139.

150. Perez RS, Kwakkel G, Zuurmond WW, de Lange JJ: Treatment of reflex sympathetic dystrophy (CRPS type 1): A research synthesis of 21 randomized clinical trials. J Pain Symptom Manage 2001;21:511–526.

151. Reuben SS, Steinberg RB, Klatt JL, Klatt ML: Intravenous regional anesthesia using lidocaine and clonidine. Anesthesiology 1999;91:654–658.

152. Reuben SS, Steinberg RB, Madabhushi L, Rosenthal E: Intravenous regional clonidine in the management of sympathetically maintained pain. Anesthesiology 1998;89:527–530.

153. Reuben SS, Rosenthal EA, Steinberg RB, et al: Surgery on the affected upper extremity of patients with a history of complex regional pain syndrome: The use of intravenous regional anesthesia with clonidine. J Clin Anesth 2004;16:517–522.

154. Cramer G, Young BM, Schwarzentraub P, et al: Preemptive analgesia in elective surgery in patients with complex regional pain syndrome: A case report. J Foot Ankle Surg 2000;39:387–391.

155. Rauck RL, Eisenach JC, Jackson K, et al: Epidural clonidine treatment for refractory reflex sympathetic dystrophy. Anesthesiology 1993;79:1163–1169.

156. Kissin I: Preemptive analgesia: Terminology and clinical relevance. Anesth Analg 1994;79:809–810.

157. Katz J: Pre-emptive analgesia: evidence, current status and future directions. Eur J Anaesthesiol Suppl 1995;10:8–13.

158. Kehlet H, Dahl JB: The value of "multimodal" or "balanced analgesia" in postoperative pain treatment. Anesth Analg 1993;77:1048–1056.

159. Gatt CJ Jr, Parker RD, Tetzlaff JE, et al: Preemptive analgesia: Its role and efficacy in anterior cruciate ligament reconstruction. Am J Sports Med 1998;26:524–529.

160. Reuben SS, Sklar J: Pain management in patients who undergo outpatient arthroscopic surgery of the knee. J Bone Joint Surg Am 2000;82:1754–1766.

161. Reuben SS, Makari-Judson G, Lurie SD: Evaluation of efficacy of the perioperative administration of venlafaxine XR in the prevention of postmastectomy pain syndrome. J Pain Symptom Manage 2004;27:133–139.

162. Zuurmond WW, Langendijk PN, Bezemer PD, et al: Treatment of acute reflex sympathetic dystrophy with DMSO 50% in a fatty cream. Acta Anaesthesiol Scand 1996;40:364–367.

163. Perez RS, Zuurmond WW, Bezemer PD, et al: The treatment of complex regional pain syndrome type I with free radical scavengers: A randomized controlled study. Pain 2003;102:297–307.

164. Zyluk A: The reasons for poor response to treatment of posttraumatic reflex sympathetic dystrophy. Acta Orthop Belg 1998;64:309–313.

165. De Grandis D, Minardi C: Acetyl-L-carnitine (levacecarnine) in the treatment of diabetic neuropathy: A long-term, randomised, double-blind, placebo-controlled study. Drugs R D 2002;3:223–231.

166. Zollinger PE, Tuinebreijer WE, Kreis RW, Breederveld RS: Effect of vitamin C on frequency of reflex sympathetic dystrophy in wrist fractures: A randomised trial. Lancet 1999;354:2025–2028.

167. Cazeneuve JF, Leborgne JM, Kermad K, Hassan Y: [Vitamin C and prevention of reflex sympathetic dystrophy following surgical management of distal radius fractures.] Acta Orthop Belg 2002;68:481–484.

168. Braga PC: Calcitonin and its antinociceptive activity: Animal and human investigations 1975-1992. Agents Actions 1994;41:121–131.

169. Yoshimura M: Analgesic mechanism of calcitonin. J Bone Miner Metab 2000;18:230–233.

170. Birklein F, Schmelz M, Schifter S, Weber M: The important role of neuropeptides in complex regional pain syndrome. Neurology 2001;57:2179–2184.

171. Jones DL, Sorkin LS: Systemic gabapentin and S(+)-3-isobutyl-gamma-aminobutyric acid block secondary hyperalgesia. Brain Res 1998;810:93–99.

172. Field MJ, Hughes J, Singh L: Further evidence for the role of the alpha(2)delta subunit of voltage dependent calcium channels in models of neuropathic pain. Br J Pharmacol 2000;131:282–286.

173. Fink K, Dooley DJ, Meder WP, et al: Inhibition of neuronal Ca(2+) influx by gabapentin and pregabalin in the human neocortex. Neuropharmacology 2002;42:229–236.

174. Lesser H, Sharma U, LaMoreaux L, Poole RM: Pregabalin relieves symptoms of painful diabetic neuropathy: A randomized controlled trial. Neurology 2004;63:2104–2110.

175. Watson CP, Evans RJ, Reed K, et al: Amitriptyline versus placebo in postherpetic neuralgia. Neurology 1982;32:671–673.

176. Bowsher D: Acute herpes zoster and postherpetic neuralgia: Effects of acyclovir and outcome of treatment with amitriptyline. Br J Gen Pract 1992;42:244–246.

177. Kvinesdal B, Molin J, Froland A, Gram LF: Imipramine treatment of painful diabetic neuropathy. JAMA 1984;251:1727–1730.

178. Max MB, Lynch SA, Muir J, et al: Effects of desipramine, amitriptyline, and fluoxetine on pain in diabetic neuropathy. N Engl J Med 1992; 326:1250–1256.

179. Watson CP, Vernich L, Chipman M, Reed K: Nortriptyline versus amitriptyline in postherpetic neuralgia: A randomized trial. Neurology 1998;51:1166–1171.

180. Sawynok J, Esser MJ, Reid AR: Antidepressants as analgesics: An overview of central and peripheral mechanisms of action. J Psychiatry Neurosci 2001;26:21–29.

181. Max MB, Culnane M, Schafer SC, et al: Amitriptyline relieves diabetic neuropathy pain in patients with normal or depressed mood. Neurology 1987;37:589–596.

182. Sindrup SH, Gram LF, Skjold T, et al: Concentration-response relationship in imipramine treatment of diabetic neuropathy symptoms. Clin Pharmacol Ther 1990;47:509–515.

183. Botney M, Fields HL: Amitriptyline potentiates morphine analgesia by a direct action on the central nervous system. Ann Neurol 1983;13: 160–164.

184. Ansuategui M, Naharro L, Feria M: Noradrenergic and opioidergic influences on the antinociceptive effect of clomipramine in the formalin test in rats. Psychopharmacology 1989;98:93–96.

185. McCleane G: Pharmacological strategies in relieving neuropathic pain. Expert Opin Pharmacother 2004;5:1299–1312.

186. Rowbotham MC, Twilling L, Davies PS, et al: Oral opioid therapy for chronic peripheral and central neuropathic pain. N Engl J Med 2003; 348:1223–1232.

187. Kalman S, Osterberg A, Sorensen J, et al: Morphine responsiveness in a group of well-defined multiple sclerosis patients: A study with i.v. morphine. Eur J Pain 2002;6:69–80.

188. Raja SN, Haythornthwaite JA, Pappagallo M, et al: Opioids versus antidepressants in postherpetic neuralgia: A randomized, placebo-controlled trial. Neurology 2002;59:1015–1021.

189. Gimbel JS, Richards P, Portenoy RK: Controlled-release oxycodone for pain in diabetic neuropathy: A randomized controlled trial. Neurology 2003;60:927–934.

190. Duhmke RM, Cornblath DD, Hollingshead JR: Tramadol for neuropathic pain. Cochrane Database Syst Rev 2004;(2):CD003726.

191. Kouya PF, Hao JX, Xu XJ: Buprenorphine alleviates neuropathic pain-like behaviors in rats after spinal cord and peripheral nerve injury. Eur J Pharmacol 2002;450:49–53.

192. Watson CP, Moulin D, Watt-Watson J, et al: Controlled-release oxycodone relieves neuropathic pain: A randomized controlled trial in painful diabetic neuropathy. Pain 2003;105:71–78.

193. Zhao C, Tall JM, Meyer RA, Raja SN: Antiallodynic effects of systemic and intrathecal morphine in the spared nerve injury model of neuropathic pain in rats. Anesthesiology 2004;100:905–911.

194. Sartain JB, Mitchell SJ: Successful use of oral methadone after failure of intravenous morphine and ketamine. Anaesth Intensive Care 2002; 30:487–489.

195. Mancini I, Lossignol DA, Body JJ: Opioid switch to oral methadone in cancer pain. Curr Opin Oncol 2000;12:308–313.

196. Yamakura T, Sakimura K, Shimoji K: Direct inhibition of the N-methyl-D-aspartate receptor channel by high concentrations of opioids. Anesthesiology 1999;91:1053–1063.

197. McDowell TS: Fentanyl decreases Ca^{2+} currents in a population of capsaicin-responsive sensory neurons. Anesthesiology 2003;98:223–231.

198. Galer BS, Rowbotham MC, Perander J, Friedman E: Topical lidocaine patch relieves postherpetic neuralgia more effectively than a vehicle topical patch: Results of an enriched enrollment study. Pain 1999;80: 533–538.

199. Davies PS, Galer BS: Review of lidocaine patch 5% studies in the treatment of postherpetic neuralgia. Drugs 2004;64:937–947.

200. Galer BS, Jensen MP, Ma T, et al: The lidocaine patch 5% effectively treats all neuropathic pain qualities: Results of a randomized, double-blind, vehicle-controlled, 3-week efficacy study with use of the neuropathic pain scale. Clin J Pain 2002;18:297–301.

201. Argoff CE, Galer BS, Jensen MP, et al: Effectiveness of the lidocaine patch 5% on pain qualities in three chronic pain states: Assessment with the Neuropathic Pain Scale. Curr Med Res Opin. 2004; 20(Suppl 2):21–28.

202. Mason L, Moore RA, Derry S, et al: Systematic review of topical capsaicin for the treatment of chronic pain. BMJ 2004;328(7446):991.

203. Bareggi SR, Pirola R, De Benedittis G: Skin and plasma levels of acetylsalicylic acid: A comparison between topical aspirin/diethyl ether mixture and oral aspirin in acute herpes zoster and postherpetic neuralgia. Eur J Clin Pharmacol 1998;54:231–235.

204. De Benedittis G, Lorenzetti A: Topical aspirin/diethyl ether mixture versus indomethacin and diclofenac/diethyl ether mixtures for acute herpetic neuralgia and postherpetic neuralgia: A double-blind crossover placebo-controlled study. Pain 1996;65:45–51.

205. De Benedittis G, Besana F, Lorenzetti A: A new topical treatment for acute herpetic neuralgia and post-herpetic neuralgia: The aspirin/diethyl ether mixture. An open-label study plus a double-blind controlled clinical trial. Pain 1992;48:383–390.

206. Marchettini P, Formaglio F, Lacerenza M: Iatrogenic painful neuropathic complications of surgery in cancer. Acta Anaesthesiol Scand 2001;45:1090–1094.

7 Postoperative Pain—Genetics and Genomics

ULRIKE M. STAMER • FRANK STÜBER

The Human Genome Project has revealed nearly complete genomic sequence data, which provide the basis for further research on genomic variations influencing nociceptive sensitivity and susceptibility to pain conditions as well as the response to the pharmacotherapy of pain. Candidate genes involved in pain perception, pain processing, and pain management, such as opioid receptors, transporters, and other targets of pharmacotherapy, are currently under investigation. Furthermore, screening for variations in expression of drug-metabolizing enzymes has been suggested as a potential diagnostic tool for improving patient therapy. Genetic polymorphisms altering expression of metabolizing enzymes are supposed to be a major factor in adverse drug reactions, possibly influencing duration of hospital stay and total costs of care.

The Basics of Genetics

Mendel published his "laws of heredity" in 1866 and demonstrated with pea plant experiments that parents pass discrete elements of heredity to their offspring. Specific characteristics, visible as the so-called phenotype, such as color of flowers and color of mammalian skin, are determined by genes that exist in a variety of forms, or *alleles*. Black and white mice have different alleles of the same gene, depending on the dominance relationship of the inherited parent alleles.

Not all characteristics are inherited according to mendelian traits, however. A variety of genetic factors might modulate complex diseases such as diabetes, hypertension, coronary artery disease, schizophrenia, and migraine. Distinct genetic characteristics such as individual variations in the base sequence of genes most often occur as low informative markers. A few are highly informative markers, which are major causes for inherited diseases (i.e., Huntington's chorea, cystic fibrosis). Genomic variations occur as single-base variations or SNPs (single-nucleotide polymorphisms), as insertion/deletion variants, or as more complex variants involving longer stretches of DNA and larger allele numbers. These complex variants comprise microsatellites, minisatellites, and variable numbers of tandem repeats (Fig. 7–1). Even alleles defined by different copy numbers of a whole functioning gene are targets for genotyping, because the number of gene copies may closely relate to protein expression levels.

These genetic variations, whereby individuals differ in their DNA sequence at a certain point of the genome, are called polymorphisms or mutations. The term *polymorphism* refers to variations with allele frequencies higher than 1% in a population, whereas the term *mutation* refers to variations with allele frequencies less than 1%.

Much work has been performed in experimental pain settings, investigating, for example, inbred mouse strains or knockout or transgenic mice in their behavioral response to acute and chronic pain.[1,2] In contrast, mechanistic studies in humans are difficult to perform, and results from animal experiments are not always transferable to humans.

Genetics and Genomics

The genomic era offers a new kind of medicine focusing on predictive rather than preventive or curative medicine.[3] Searching for genetic variations that predispose an individual to development of an illness or that protect an individual from disorders such as chronic pain has become a major concern and will individualize and personalize medical treatment in the future. Which patient is at risk for development of a chronic pain syndrome after a surgical procedure such as thoracotomy, mastectomy, or limb amputation? Which patient needs very large doses of opioids and will not comply with a standard regimen of postoperative pain management? A 2004 epidemiologic study set out to examine potential associations between candidate gene variants and neuropathic pain.[4] The literature was screened for 200 genes that are assumed to be involved. On the basis of previously published studies, 20 genes are likely to influence neuropathic pain. The scientific community is looking forward to the results of this first large-scale genetic epidemiologic trial.

The interindividual variability in the severity and persistence of pain has been attributed to the severity of the injury, to the patient's age, personality traits, social background, emotional and psychological factors, and economic status, and to other environmental influences. Molecular mediators of pain processing, such as inflammatory mediators (serotonin, histamine, bradykinin, cytokines), second messengers, receptors, and endogenous neurotransmitters, are under investigation, which, it is hoped, will reveal new strategies for individualized pain management in the future.

Pharmacotherapy occasionally confronts the clinician with drugs that unexpectedly have no effect or have serious adverse effects. This situation can be life-threatening for some patients. A meta-analysis of 39 prospective studies estimated

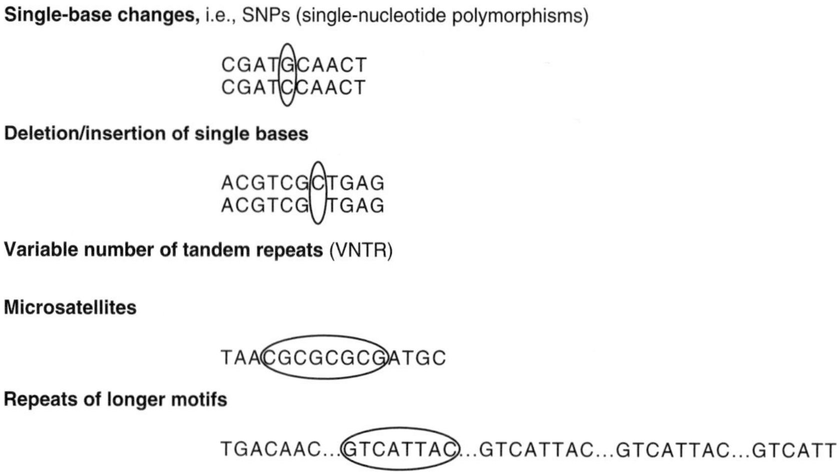

Single-base changes, i.e., SNPs (single-nucleotide polymorphisms)

CGAT**G**CAACT
CGAT**C**CAACT

Deletion/insertion of single bases

ACGTCG**C**TGAG
ACGTCG TGAG

Variable number of tandem repeats (VNTR)

Microsatellites

TAA**CGCGCGCG**ATGC

Repeats of longer motifs

TGACAAC...**GTCATTAC**...GTCATTAC...GTCATTAC...GTCATT

Figure 7–1   Genomic variations.

an overall incidence for serious adverse drug reactions (ADRs) of 6.7%. *Serious events* were defined as those either requiring hospitalization or resulting in permanent disability or death.[5]

The occurrence of ADRs is associated with morbidity, mortality, and substantial medical care costs. Potential risk factors for ADR or therapeutic failure include the patient's age, sex, comorbidities, co-medication, organ function (especially of the liver and kidneys), and diet as well as some lifestyle variables such as smoking habits and alcohol intake (Fig. 7–2). Furthermore, genetic variables can modify pharmacokinetics and pharmacodynamics of drugs and, therefore, can predispose to adverse drug reactions or reduced drug efficacy. Variations in DNA sequences may influence the sensitivity of a subject to a drug and his or her regulation of metabolic pathways. The effector side of analgesics also varies among subjects. Polymorphisms of receptors, ion channels, drug transporters, and other targets of pharmacotherapy are well recognized and explain some of the variation in response to analgesics and coanalgesics. Other confounding variables are the intensity of pain, the kind of pain or pain syndrome (acute postoperative pain after abdominal surgery versus bone surgery, chronic nonmalignant pain versus cancer pain, visceral versus neuropathic pain, etc.), and environmental influences as well as psychological aspects.

Pharmacogenetics describes genetically determined variability in the metabolism of drugs. These genetic variations

can lead to ADRs, toxicity, or therapeutic failure of a drug. The German pediatrician Friedrich Vogel introduced this term in 1958, when he realized that metabolism of drugs is influenced by heredity. The term *pharmacogenomics* is a newer, much broader term referring to the advances achieved by molecular biology and related technologies. Instead of focusing on single-base exchanges only, we now consider the complexity of the genome, encompassing the dynamic structure of the genes, their expression, the transcriptome, the translatome, and the proteome. Pharmacogenomics encompasses all aspects of drug behavior, including drug absorption, distribution, metabolism, excretion, and receptor-target affinity. Furthermore, the term also refers to the development and discovery of new pharmacological agents based on the growing knowledge of the genome. The potential of pharmacogenetics/pharmacogenomics to improve the clinical outcome of multiple-drug therapy is already realized and represents an important biomedical advance in the genomic era.

Genetics of Drug Metabolism

Alterations in drug effects can be caused by polymorphisms. These polymorphisms can occur within the systems of drug uptake, drug transport, the effector molecules (e.g., a receptor or an ion channel), the metabolism, and excretion.

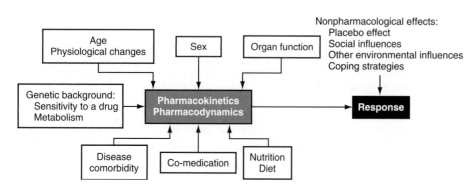

Figure 7–2 Variables determining response to a drug/analgesic. (Modified from Spina E, Scordo MG: Clinically significant drug interactions with antidepressants in the elderly. Drugs Aging 2002; 19:299–320.).

Extended pharmacological effect, ADR, toxicity, absence of prodrug activation, increased or decreased effective dose, and greater drug-drug interaction are potential effects of genetic variability.[6]

Drug metabolism involves two steps. In phase I metabolism, functional groups of the substrate are modified by oxidation, oxygenation, reduction, and hydrolysis to generate specific functional groups in a drug molecule. These may serve as conjugation sites for glucuronic acid, sulfate, or glutathione catalyzed by phase II enzymes (e.g., N-acetyltransferase, UDP-glucuronosyltransferase, glutathione-S-transferase). The cytochrome P450 gene family (CYP), which metabolizes endogenous and exogenous substrates, plays a pivotal role in phase I metabolism. These enzymes are available in all living beings. Numerous subfamilies evolved during phylogenetic development over billions of years. Depending on environmental influences and selection pressure, each species and subpopulation formed new CYP genes as part of an adaptation process.

CYTOCHROME P450 2D6

The polymorphic cytochrome P450 enzymes metabolize numerous drugs (Table 7–1) and exhibit considerable interindividual variability in their catalytic activity. Critical base changes or deletions result in defective messenger RNA (mRNA) and proteins, with consequences for their metabolizing capacity.

CYP2D6 is a highly polymorphic isoenzyme of the cytochrome P450 system. More than 50 different variants for CYP2D6 exist, leading to a wide spectrum of metabolic capacity within populations.[7,8] A detailed list of all known cytochrome alleles is available at the gene nomenclature website.[9]

Individuals displaying normal enzyme activity are known as extensive metabolizers (EMs). In contrast, individuals with a decreased or absent enzyme activity, poor metabolizers (PMs), present single-base exchanges or deletions within the 2D6 gene locus. PMs display two inactive alleles and are characterized by deficient hydroxylation of several classes of commonly used drugs, such as beta-blockers, antiarrhythmics, antidepressants, neuroleptics, and analgesics (see Table 7–1).

The genetic variability of this drug-metabolizing capacity is of clinical importance because about 10% of the white population is affected by this autosomal recessive trait of nonfunctional alleles.[7,10] In contrast, duplication or multiduplication of the CYP2D6 gene is related to an ultrarapid metabolism of certain drugs. "Ultrarapid metabolizers" (UMs) have significantly greater enzyme activity, resulting in subtherapeutic blood levels of their substrates. Up to 4% to 5% of white persons are UMs. However, patients of other ethnic origins display different frequencies. The number of individuals carrying multiple CYP2D6 gene copies is highest in Ethiopia and Saudi Arabia, amounting to 21% and 25%, respectively (Table 7–2).

Diverse frequencies among individuals from various racial and ethnic backgrounds can lead to modification of therapeutic strategies. Whereas the CYP2D6*4 allele is present in high frequency (allele frequency 20%) in white persons, accounting for more than 75% of the mutant CYP2D6 alleles, it is almost absent in the Chinese population (see Table 7–2).

Codeine

Codeine is a prodrug without analgesic properties. It is eliminated primarily by glucuronidation, with O-demethylation to morphine and N-demethylation to norcodeine as minor elimination pathways. The O-demethylation of codeine to

TABLE 7–1 Selected Drugs Metabolized by Specific Cytochrome P450 Isoforms: CYP2C9, CYP2C19, and CYP2D6*

Isoenzymes	Drugs Metabolized	Drugs: Examples	Adverse Effects on Case of Altered Enzyme Activity
CYP2C9	Warfarin		Bleeding
	Phenytoin		Ataxia
	NSAIDs	Ibuprofen, diclofenac, naproxen, meloxicam, celecoxib	Gastrointestinal bleeding
	Oral antidiabetics	Tolbutamide, glipizide	Hypoglycemia
	Angiotensin II blockers	Losartan, irbesartan	No data
CYP2C19	Proton pump inhibitors	Omeprazole, pantoprazole	No data
	Anti-epileptics	Diazepam, phenytoin	Sedation
CYP2D6	Antidepressants	Amitriptyline, clomipramine, desipramine, imipramine, paroxetine	Sedation, cardiotoxicity
	Beta-blockers	Metoprolol, timolol	Overdose
	Antiarrhythmic drugs	Propafenone, mexiletine, flecainide, ajmaline	Arrhythmia
	Antipsychotics	Haloperidol	Parkinsonism
	5HT$_3$-Antagonists	Ondansetron, tropisetron	Nausea, emesis
	Antiemetics	Metoclopramide	No data
	Analgesics	Codeine, tramadol, oxycodone, dextromethorphan	No/reduced analgesia
	Amphetamine	Ecstasy	No data; toxicity?

*For more detailed information, see http://medicine.iupi.edu/flockart

TABLE 7–2	Distribution of Variant *CYP2D6* Alleles by Allele Frequencies (%) in Different Ethnic Populations				
Allele Variants	Enzyme Function	Caucasian	Asian	Black-African	Ethiopian, Saudi-Arabian
*2×N	Gene duplication: Increased enzyme activity	1–5	0–2	2	10–16
*4	Splicing defect: inactive enzyme	12–21	1	2	1–4
*5	Deletion: no enzyme	2–7	6	4	1–3
*10	Unstable enzyme	1–2	51	6	3–9
*17	Reduced affinity to substrate	0	No data	34	3–9

From Ingelman-Sundberg M, Oscarson M, McLellan RA: Polymorphic human cytochrome P450 enzymes: An opportunity for individualized drug treatment. Trends Pharmacol Sci 1999;20:342–349.

the active metabolite morphine depends on CYP2D6 activity,[11] accounting for the relative deficiency in PMs.

Codeine is widely administered for treatment of postoperative pain, especially in pediatric patients. In contrast to practice in the United States and United Kingdom, codeine is not routinely used as a monoanalgesic in Germany. However, codeine is a component of various drug combinations (e.g., paracetamol/acetaminophen plus codeine) and is widely used for acute and chronic pain management. The relative deficiency in analgesic efficacy of codeine in PMs has been demonstrated in several investigations.[10,12] Williams et al[13,14] studied the analgesic efficacy of codeine in children undergoing adenotonsillectomy. Plasma morphine concentrations were very low and were correlated with the metabolizing phenotype, with no morphine or metabolite (morphine-6-glucuronide [M6G] or morphine-3-glucuronide [M3G]) measurable in the two PMs and some heterozygous patients with declining metabolic capacity. In clinical practice, there is a large interindividual variation in efficacy of codeine; about 10% of white patients derive little or no benefit from its use.[13,15]

Tramadol

Tramadol is a synthetic opioid, and studies document its analgesic efficacy with a low potential for depression of respiration and for development of tolerance, dependence, and abuse. This racemic mixture produces analgesia through a synergistic action of its two enantiomers, (+)-tramadol and (−)-tramadol, and their metabolites. Hepatic cytochrome P450 metabolizes tramadol to 11 desmethylated compounds, of which M1 (O-desmethyltramadol) predominates and possesses analgesic properties.(+)-O-Desmethyltramadol has been demonstrated to have an affinity for μ-opioid receptors that is approximately 200 times greater than that of the parent compound. Thus, it is largely responsible for opioid receptor–mediated analgesia, whereas (+)-tramadol and (−)-tramadol inhibit reuptake of the neurotransmitters serotonin and noradrenaline.[16,17] O-Desmethylation to M1 requires *CYP2D6* for its formation.

Pharmacogenetics may explain some of the varying responses to pain medication in postoperative patients.[18] A prospective clinical study in patients recovering from abdominal surgery demonstrated that CYP2D6 genotype influenced tramadol analgesia. In this study, 300 patients were assigned to postoperative pain management by patient-controlled analgesia (PCA). Patients' genotypes were analyzed for the PM-associated *CYP2D6* mutations. Demographic and surgery-related factors were similar in EMs and PMs. Tramadol loading dose, subsequent tramadol consumption, and need for rescue medication were greater in PMs than in patients carrying at least one wild-type allele. The proportion of nonresponders was greater in the PM group than in the EM group. One can conclude that in the postoperative setting, PMs experience less analgesia after tramadol administration than EMs.

Serotonin-3-Receptor Antagonists

Postoperative nausea and vomiting (PONV) occurs in approximately 30% of all surgical patients. Volatile anesthetic agents and opioids (administered as components of the anesthetic technique or for postoperative pain management) are important etiological factors in PONV. Serotonin-3 ($5HT_3$) receptor antagonists, which were originally introduced for prophylaxis of chemotherapy-induced nausea and vomiting, are now also widely used for prophylaxis and therapy of PONV. Kaiser et al[19] demonstrated that the efficacy of tropisetron and ondansetron to prevent nausea and vomiting in patients with cancer depends on a patient's number of active *CYP2D6* genes. In a study of tropisetron pharmacokinetics in healthy Korean subjects, serum levels correlated with selected genotypes; UMs displayed the lowest serum concentrations.[20] Later results from a trial in postoperative patients confirmed that individuals with multiple functional copies of the *CYP2D6* allele and UM status had a higher incidence of ondansetron failure.[21] From these results, it can be concluded that efficacy of antiemetic treatment with the $5HT_3$-antagonists ondansetron and tropisetron depends on the patient's CYP2D6 enzyme activity, with UMs showing a low response.

Drug Interactions

Genetic polymorphisms can also influence drug interactions. Inhibition or induction of enzyme activity is a possible reason for a variable pharmacological effect. Inhibitors of specific enzyme activity produce pharmacologically determined poor

CYP2D6 INHIBITORS*

Amiodarone
Cimetidine, ranitidine
Celecoxib
Clinidine
Cocaine
Paroxetine
Propafenone
Methadone
Histamine h1-receptor antagonists
Fluoxetine
Haloperidol

*A continuously updated version is available online at http://medicine.iupi.edu/flockart/

metabolizers—for example, *CYP2D6* inhibition by amiodarone, metoclopramide, haloperidol, celecoxib, and several other drugs (Box 7–1). *CYP2D6* inhibition by celecoxib, 2×200 mg/day for 7 days, and amiodarone, 1.2 g/day for 6 days, was demonstrated by elevated plasma concentrations of the concurrently administered CYP2D6 substrate metoprolol.[22,23] Owing to reduced metabolism, plasma concentrations of the beta-blocker were doubled on average. In individual patients, the extent of this drug interaction depended on *CYP2D6* genotype.[23]

It can be concluded that postoperative analgesia with codeine and tramadol is not a good choice if patients are concurrently receiving celecoxib, cimetidine, or ranitidine on a long-term basis (see Box 7–1).

Opioid Receptors

Opioids are the mainstay of pharmacological treatment in patients with severe acute and chronic pain. Cloning of the opioid receptor genes has initiated discussion of the genetic determinants that control the expression of the opioid receptors. Transcriptional factors such as cytokines can regulate these genes. Post-transcriptional events involve alternative splicing and variation in mRNA stability and translation efficiency. Furthermore, these receptors show polymorphic regions that might influence expression and function of the binding sites.

Several polymorphisms and mutations of the μ-opioid receptor have been described so far. The allelic variation *T802C* (*S268P*) affects both desensitization and G protein coupling of the μ-opioid receptor.[24] The loss of function of the human μ-opioid receptor may influence opioid-regulated behaviors or drug addiction in vivo.[25]

The *A118G* polymorphism in exon 1 of the μ-opioid receptor causes an exchange of asparagines for aspartate at position 40 and has been shown to decrease the pupil constrictory effects of M6G, a major active metabolite of morphine.[26] Carriers of two *G118* alleles experienced a lower potency of M6G than subjects carrying only one copy and subjects carrying two wild-type alleles.

This finding was confirmed in a case report of two patients receiving morphine for control of cancer pain.[27] M6G is eliminated via the kidneys and accumulates in patients with renal failure. In contrast to the patient with the mutation at position 118, only the patient with the wild-type receptor experienced central nervous system side effects such as sedation, drowsiness, and reduced vigilance. Accumulation of M6G proved to be a risk factor for opioid toxicity, especially of central nervous system side effects during morphine treatment. However, patients with the wild-type receptor seem to be at particular risk for these adverse events. Thus, it is hypothesized that the *118G* genotype is protective against M6G-related opioid toxicity.[27]

Klepstad et al[28] correlated μ-opioid receptor genotype with opioid requirements in patients with pain due to malignant diseases. Patients homozygous for the *118G* allele ($n = 4$) needed larger morphine doses to achieve pain control than those heterozygous for the allele ($n = 17$) or homozygous for the wild-type allele ($n = 78$). To date, however, the sample sizes in the studies performed have been low; larger studies are needed to confirm these results and exclude possible "chance" findings.[4,29]

Potential associations exist between μ-opioid receptor polymorphisms and the development of tolerance, drug abuse, and efficacy of opioids in pain management. To date, results are conflicting, perhaps owing to variations in the populations and number of patients studied. Current research now focuses on analysis of extended haplotypes (a combination of alleles at closely linked loci on a single chromosome) and genotype-phenotype associations.[30]

ALTERNATIVE SPLICING OF THE μ-OPIOID RECEPTOR

The analgesic potencies of opioids such as fentanyl, hydromorphone, oxycodone, and methadone in relation to morphine are well described. However, these standard conversion ratios are average values, and individual subjects might react quite differently and have much lower or higher requirements. A patient who needs escalating doses of morphine, indicating tolerance, or is suffering from morphine-dependent side effects is usually switched to another opioid, such as oxycodone, hydromorphone, or methadone. This opioid rotation often demonstrates that much lower doses are sufficient than those expected from the relative potencies of the drugs. In case of highly tolerant patients, incomplete cross-tolerance can be often observed. There seems to be a differential relative sensitivity to various μ-opioid agonists.

Meanwhile, there is evidence for the existence of multiple μ-opioid receptor subtypes. A number of splice variants of the gene differing at the intracellular carboxy-terminus have been identified.[31] They all contain the same first three exons. However, exon 4, present in μ-opioid receptor-1 (MOR-1), is replaced by a combination of further exons. These splicing changes result in differences in the amino acid sequences in the intracellular 3′ end having influence on efficacy and trafficking of the receptor.[32] The regional distribution of the splice variants is unique, and splicing mechanisms seem to be cell- and region-specific.[33,34] Finally, pharmacological function of opioid receptor subtypes has to be elucidated, and evidence for the link between splicing variables and differential response to opioids among patients and the clinical finding of incomplete cross-tolerance has yet to be elucidated.

Nonopioid Analgesics

Nonopioid analgesics are widely used in the treatment of acute postoperative pain after minor surgery or in combination with opioids after major surgery. They are an essential part of multimodal pain management, because analgesics with different mechanisms of action should be combined to increase efficacy of treatment and reduce adverse effects, such as opioid-dependent nausea and vomiting and respiratory depression.

A number of investigations demonstrated clear-cut genetic influences on the efficacy of nonopioid analgesia. In animal models, specific traits (mice species) seem to be particularly sensitive to nonsteroidal anti-inflammatory drugs (NSAIDs) or acetaminophen, whereas others showed a degree of resistance to these drugs.[1,35] It is supposed that similar differences in efficacy of nonopioids can also be found in humans.

NSAIDs such as diclofenac, ibuprofen, naproxen, and piroxicam are metabolized by CYP2C9. Polymorphisms for this cytochrome that are associated with a deficiency in enzyme activity have been identified. One percent to 3% of white persons are PMs. The CYP2C9 polymorphism might play a significant role in the analgesic efficacy and toxicity of NSAIDs. A more than two-fold reduced clearance after oral intake of celecoxib was observed in homozygous carriers of CYP2C9*3 compared with carriers of the wild-type genotype CYP2C9*1/*1, and the clearance rates in heterozygous carriers of one *3 allele were in between.[36] Tang et al[37] reported celecoxib concentrations in plasma after a single oral dose (calculated as area under the curve [AUC] from 2 to 24 hours) to be increased 2.2-fold in two CYP2C9*1/*3 subjects and one *3/*3 subject. Decreased concentrations of carboxy-celecoxib and hydroxy-celecoxib were detected in heterozygous and homozygous carriers of CYP2C9*3, supporting the proposition that CYP2C9 polymorphisms influence celecoxib pharmacokinetic variability. Homozygous carriers of the CYP2D9*3 allele will have greatly increased internal exposure to celecoxib with extensive accumulation of this cyclooxygenase-2 inhibitor in blood and tissues. It remains to be shown whether this difference is associated with greater efficacy or with a higher incidence and severity of adverse events such as renal impairment and other dose-related adverse outcomes.[36]

Ibuprofen pharmacokinetics and ibuprofen-mediated inhibition of cyclooxygenases 1 and 2 are significantly influenced by CYP2D9 genotype.[38] Clearance of racemic ibuprofen and S-ibuprofen was reduced in carriers of two CYP2C9*3 alleles. The reduced clearance of S-ibuprofen accompanied by greater pharmacodynamic activity may be clinically important in patients receiving this NSAID.

Dextromethorphan, an N-methyl-D-aspartate (NMDA) antagonist, as well as antidepressants that are regularly used in chronic pain management as coanalgesics, are substrates of CYP2D6. For trimipramine, bioavailability and systemic clearance significantly depend on CYP2D6 genotype. High bioavailability with low systemic clearance in CYP2D6 PMs results in high exposure to trimipramine with the risk of adverse drug reactions. On the other hand, carriers of CYP2D6 gene duplications experience ultrarapid metabolization of tricyclic antidepressants, which may result in subtherapeutic drug concentrations with a high risk of poor therapeutic response.[39] Similar findings are reported for other antidepressants and antipsychotics. Genetically caused differences in blood concentrations make dose adjustments advisable.[40]

Gender Differences

Studies on experimental pain and chronic pain in humans indicate a greater prevalence of pain in females than males.[41,42] Few randomized trials have examined the gender specificity of acute postoperative pain. Women were found to experience greater intensity of pain after anterior arthroscopic cruciate ligament reconstruction[43] and in a cohort study involving various surgical procedures.[44] Furthermore, women in the cohort study required 30% more morphine on a per-weight basis to achieve a similar level of analgesia.[44]

Specifically, κ-receptor–mediated analgesia seems to be different in males and females. κ-Agonists like nalbuphine and pentazocine produced pronounced analgesia in women but not in men.[45,46] Mogil et al[47] demonstrated that the melanocortin-1 receptor (MC1R) mediates κ-opioid receptor–induced sensitivity in mice, but only females. In humans, two mutant alleles of the MC1R gene are associated with fair skin and red hair. Women with this genotype displayed robust pentazocine analgesia in contrast to men.[47] Other results indicated that redheads are more sensitive to thermal pain and are resistant to the analgesic effect of subcutaneous lidocaine. In addition, women with red hair required 19% more desflurane to suppress movement response to noxious electrical stimuli.[48,49]

Other Candidate Genes

Numerous other candidate genes that are supposed to be involved in pain perception, modulation, and therapy are under investigation. Catechol-O-methyltransferase (COMT) is one promising candidate, metabolizing catecholamines and thereby acting as a key modulator of dopaminergic and adrenergic/noradrenergic neurotransmission. The val158met polymorphism reduces COMT activity by three- to four-fold. Using a standardized human pain model, Zubieta et al[50] linked this polymorphism to altered pain response. Individuals with a homozygous met158 genotype showed diminished regional μ-opioid system response to pain, signified by decreased radiolabeled carfentanil binding to opioid receptors tracked by positron emission tomography. Additionally, methionine homozygotes reported greater sensory and affective ratings of pain.

Besides metabolizing enzymes, cannabinoid-, NMDA-, dopamine- and serotonin-adrenergic receptors, ion channels, interleukins, endogenous opioids, and other substances are specific targets involved in pain and pain management.[4] Genes coding for transporters may play an important role in determining drug concentrations at specific regions—for example, central nervous system and synaptic cleft. Candidate genes are the P-glycoprotein that is expressed at the blood-brain barrier and the serotonin and dopamine transporters, which regulate reuptake of these neurotransmitters from the synaptic cleft.

Conclusions

Research in the field of pain has been undertaken to elucidate genomic variations influencing pain mechanisms and perception as well as transmission and spinal processing of pain signals. Preclinical animal models are well-established, and therapeutic potential of novel analgesics is under investigation. Owing to the development of faster and better techniques of genotyping, the number of identified polymorphisms in genes encoding drug-metabolizing enzymes, drug transporters, and receptors is rapidly growing. In many cases these genetic factors have a major impact on the pharmacokinetics and pharmacodynamics of a particular drug, especially in the setting of a narrow therapeutic index. Specific dosage recommendations based on genotypes will be a future tool for clinicians.

Because interindividual and interpopulation variation is likely to be high, sophisticated high-throughput techniques for genetic analysis and large patient numbers are needed. Pharmacogenetic DNA chips for use at the bedside or in the clinic or office to determine a patient's drug sensitivity are technologies already under investigation. Such development will lead to a more patient-tailored drug therapy that, one hopes, will result in fewer adverse drug reactions and greater efficacy of analgesic pharmacotherapy.

REFERENCES

1. Mogil JS, Wilson SG, Bon K, et al: Heritability of nociception I: Responses of 11 inbred mouse strains on 12 measures of nociception. Pain 1999;80:67–82.
2. Seitzer Z, Wu T, Max MB, Diehl SR: Mapping a gene for neuropathic pain-related behaviour following peripheral neurectomy in the mouse. Pain 2000;93:101–106.
3. Dausset J: Journal of Biomedicine and Biotechnology [editorial]. J Biomed Biotechnol 2001;1:1-2.
4. Belfer I, Wu T, Kingman A, et al: Candidate gene studies of human pain mechanisms. Anesthesiology 2004;100:1562–1572.
5. Lazarou J, Pomeranz BH, Corey PN: Incidence of adverse drug reactions in hospitalized patients: A meta-analysis of prospective studies. JAMA 1998;279:1200–1205.
6. Tsai YJ, Hoyme HE: Pharmacogenomics: The future of drug therapy. Clin Genet 2002;62:257–264.
7. Daly AK, Brockmoller J, Broly F, et al: Nomenclature for human CYP2D6 alleles. Pharmacogenetics 1996;6:193–201.
8. Marez D, Legrand M, Sabbagh N, et al: Polymorphism of the cytochrome P450 CYP2D6 gene in a European population: Characterization of 48 mutations and 53 alleles, their frequencies and evolution. Pharmacogenetics 1997;7:193–202.
9. Human Cytochrome P450 (CYP) Allele Nomenclature Committee: Home page. Available at http://www.imm.ki.se/CYPalleles/
10. Sachse C, Brockmoller J, Bauer S, Roots I: Cytochrome P450 2D6 variants in a Caucasian population: Allele frequencies and phenotypic consequences. Am J Hum Genet 1997;60:284–295.
11. Poulsen L, Brosen K, Arendt-Nielsen L, et al: Codeine and morphine in extensive and poor metabolizers of sparteine: Pharmacokinetics, analgesic effect and side effects. Eur J Clin Pharmacol 1996;51:289–295.
12. Eckhardt K, Li S, Ammon S, et al: Same incidence of adverse drug events after codeine administration irrespective of the genetically determined differences in morphine formation. Pain 1998;76:27–33.
13. Williams DG, Hatch DJ, Howard RF: Codeine phosphate in paediatric medicine. Br J Anaesth 2001;86:413–421.
14. Williams DG, Patel A, Howard RF: Pharmacogenetics of codeine metabolism in an urban population of children and its implications for analgesic reliability. Br J Anaesth 2002;89:839–845.
15. Fagerlund TH, Braaten Ø: No pain relief from codeine...? An introduction to pharmacogenomics. Acta Anaesthesiol Scand 2001;68:140–149.
16. Raffa RB, Friderichs E, Reimann W, et al: Complementary and synergistic antinociceptive interaction between the enantiomers of tramadol. J Pharmacol Exp Ther 1993;267:331–340.
17. Poulsen L, Arendt-Nielsen L, Brosen K, Sindrup SH: The hypoalgesic effect of tramadol in relation to CYP2D6. Clin Pharmacol Ther 1996;60:636–644.
18. Stamer UM, Lehnen K, Höthker F, et al: Impact of CYP2D6 genotype on postoperative tramadol analgesia. Pain 2003;105:231–238.
19. Kaiser R, Sezer O, Papies A, et al: Patient-tailored antiemetic treatment with 5-hydroxytryptamine type 3 receptor antagonists according to cytochrome P-450 2D6 genotypes. J Clin Oncol 2002;20:2805–2811.
20. Kim M-K, Cho J-Y, Lim H-S, et al: Effect of the CYP2D6 genotype on the pharmacogenetics of tropisetron in healthy Korean subjects. Eur J Clin Pharmacol 2003;9:111–116.
21. Candiotti KA, Birnbach DJ, Lubarsky DA, et al: The impact of pharmacogenomics on postoperative nausea and vomiting: Do CYP2D6 allele copy number and polymorphisms affect the success or failure of ondansetron prophylaxis? Anesthesiology 2005;102:543–549.
22. Werner U, Werner D, Rau T, et al: Celecoxib inhibits metabolism of cytochrome P450 2D6 substrate metoprolol in humans. Clin Pharmacol Ther 2003;74:130–137.
23. Werner D, Wuttke H, Fromm MF, et al: Effect of amiodarone on the plasma levels of metoprolol. Am J Cardiol 2004;94:1319–1321.
24. Koch T, Kroslak T, Averbeck M, et al: Allelic variation S268P of the human mu-opioid receptor affects both desensitization and G protein coupling. Mol Pharmacol 2000;58:328–334.
25. Befort K, Filliol D, Decaillot FM, et al: A single nucleotide polymorphic mutation in the human mu-opioid receptor severely impairs receptor signaling. J Biol Chem 2001;276:3130–3137.
26. Lötsch J, Skarke C, Grosch S, et al: The polymorphism A118G of the human mu-opioid receptor gene decreases the pupil constrictory effect of morphine-6-glucuronide but not that of morphine. Pharmacogenetics 2002;12:3–9.
27. Lötsch J, Zimmermann M, Darimont J, et al: Does the A118G polymorphism at the mu-opioid receptor gene protect against morphine-6-glucuronide toxicity? Anesthesiology 2002;97:814–819.
28. Klepstad P, Rakvag TT, Kaasa S, et al: The 118 A→G polymorphism in the human micro-opioid receptor gene may increase morphine requirements in patients with pain caused by malignant disease. Acta Anaesthesiol Scand 2004;48:1232–1239.
29. Eisenach JC: Fishing for genes: Practical ways to study polymorphisms for pain. Anesthesiology 2004;100:1343–1344.
30. Hoehe MR, Kopke K, Wendel B, et al: Sequence variability and candidate gene analysis in complex disease: Association of mu-opioid receptor gene variation with substance dependence. Hum Mol Genet 2000;9:2895–2908.
31. Pasternak GW, Pan YX: Alternative splicing of mu-opioid receptors. In Mogil JS (ed): The Genetics of Pain. Seattle, IASP Press, 2004, pp 85–103.
32. Koch T, Schulz S, Pfeiffer M, et al: C-terminal splice variants of the mouse mu-opioid receptor differ in morphine-induced internalization and receptor resensitization. J Biol Chem 2001;276:31408–31414.
33. Abbadie C, Pan YX, Pasternak GW: Differential distribution in rat brain of mu opioid receptor carboxy terminal splice variants MOR-1C-like and MOR-1-like immunoreactivity: Evidence for region-specific processing. J Comp Neurol 2000;419:244–256.
34. Abbadie C, Pasternak GW, Aicher SA: Presynaptic localization of the carboxy-terminus epitopes of the mu opioid receptor splice variants MOR-1C and MOR-1D in the superficial laminae of the rat spinal cord. Neuroscience 2001;106:833–842.
35. Pick CG, Cheng J, Paul D, Pasternak G: Genetic influences in opioid analgesic sensitivity in mice. Brain Res 1991;556:295–298.
36. Kirchheiner J, Störmer E, Meisel C, et al: Influence of CYP2C9 genetic polymorphisms on pharmacokinetics of celecoxib and its metabolites. Pharmacogenetics. 2003;13:473–480.
37. Tang C, Shou M, Rushmore TH, et al: In-vitro metabolism of celecoxib, a cyclooxygenase-2 inhibitor, by allelic variant forms of human liver microsomal cytochrome P450 2C9: Correlation with CYP2C9 genotype and in-vivo pharmacokinetics. Pharmacogenetics 2001;11:223–235.
38. Kirchheiner J, Meineke I, Freytag G, et al: Enantiospecific effects of cytochrome P450 2C9 amino acid variants on ibuprofen pharmacokinetics and on the inhibition of cyclooxygenases 1 and 2. Clin Pharmacol Ther 2002;72:62–75.

39. Kirchheiner J, Sasse J, Meineke I, et al: Trimipramine pharmacogenetics after intravenous and oral administration in carriers of CYP2D6 genotypes predicting poor, extensive and ultrahigh activity. Pharmacogenetics 2004;13:721–728.

40. Kirchheiner J, Nickchen K, Bauer M, et al: Pharmacogenetics of antidepressants and antipsychotics: The contribution of allelic variations to the phenotype of drug response. Mol Psychiatry 2004;9:442–473.

41. Unruh AM: Gender variations in clinical pain experience. Pain 1996;65:23–67.

42. Riley J, Robinson MG, Wise EA, et al: Sex differences in the perception of noxious experimental stimuli: A meta-analysis. Pain 1998;74:180–187.

43. Taenzer AH, Clark C, Curry CS: Gender affects report of pain and function after arthroscopic anterior cruciate ligament reconstruction. Anesthesiology 2000;53:670–675.

44. Cepeda MS, Carr DB: Women experience more pain and require more morphine than men to achieve a similar degree of analgesia. Anesth Analg 2003;97:1464–1468.

45. Gear RW, Miaskowski C, Gordon NC, et al: Kappa-opioids produce significantly greater analgesia in women than in men. Nat Med 1996;2:1248–1250.

46. Gear RW, Miaskowski C, Gordon NC, et al: The kappa opioid nalbuphine produces gender- and dose-dependent analgesia and antianalgesia in patients with postoperative pain. Pain 1999;83:339–345.

47. Mogil JS, Wilson SG, Chesler EJ, et al: The melanocortin-1 receptor gene mediates female-specific mechanisms of analgesia in mice and humans. Proc Natl Acad Sci USA 2003;100:4867–4872.

48. Liem EB, Lin CM, Suleman MI, et al: Anesthetic requirement is increased in redheads. Anesthesiology 2004;101:279–283.

49. Liem EB, Joiner TV, Tsueda K, Sessler DI: Increased sensitivity to thermal pain and reduced subcutaneous lidocaine efficacy in redheads. Anesthesiology 2005;102:509–514.

50. Zubieta JK, Heitzeg MM, Smith YR, et al: COMT val158met genotype affects mu-opioid neurotransmitter responses to a pain stressor. Science 2003;299(5610):1240–1243.

8 Postoperative Pain Management and Patient Outcome

CHRISTOPHER L. WU • ROBERT W. HURLEY

Over the past few decades, our knowledge of the neurobiology of nociception, adverse acute and chronic effects of postoperative pain, and various treatment modalities for postoperative pain has grown several-fold. These advances have coincided with increasing recognition of the undertreatment of postoperative pain, as reflected by the development of a national (U.S.) acute pain management practice guideline by the Agency for Healthcare Quality and Research and of clinical practice guidelines for acute pain management by professional societies.[1-3] In addition, the Joint Commission on Accreditation of Healthcare Organizations (JCAHO), which accredits hospitals in the United States, has implemented new pain management standards.[4] Finally, the development of postoperative pain services has optimized delivery of postoperative analgesia.

Although *outcomes* have traditionally been viewed in terms of major morbidity and mortality, the term also incorporates nontraditional endpoints, such as patient satisfaction, quality of life, and quality of recovery. It is unclear, however, whether postoperative pain per se actually affects patient outcomes. Certainly, postoperative pain has a wide range of detrimental physiological and psychological effects that may ultimately lead to a rise in patient morbidity and mortality. Human and animal studies suggest that controlling postoperative pain may attenuate some of these detrimental effects, thus potentially improving postoperative patient outcomes. In addition, different analgesic regimens, which confer different levels of analgesia, may variously influence patient outcomes. Finally, the organization of postoperative pain delivery itself (i.e., "acute pain services") may affect patient outcomes.

Acute and Chronic Consequences of Postoperative Pain

An understanding of the range of acute and chronic effects of postoperative pain, including the neurobiology of nociception, is necessary to a comprehension of how postoperative pain and its treatment may ultimately affect patient outcomes. Postoperative pain has a wide range of detrimental acute and chronic effects on both traditional and nontraditional patient outcomes.

ACUTE EFFECTS

The trauma from surgery is associated with a variety of pathophysiological responses that may be potentiated by nociceptive input and may increase patient morbidity and mortality. The neuroendocrine stress response, mediated by local inflammatory and systemic mediators, results in part from the transmission of nociceptive information to the central nervous system (CNS). The neuroendocrine stress response, in essence, is a hypermetabolic, catabolic state with increased levels of metabolism and oxygen consumption resulting in sodium and water retention and elevations in blood glucose, free fatty acids, ketone bodies, and lactate. Other organ systems and areas of the body may be affected by the neuroendocrine stress response. There may be enhancement of coagulation (including inhibition of fibrinolysis, increased platelet reactivity, and greater plasma viscosity),[5] postoperative immunosuppression,[6] and poor wound healing.[7]

Uncontrolled postoperative pain, primarily via activation of the sympathetic nervous system, may contribute to morbidity or mortality. Sympathetic activation may worsen myocardial ischemia and infarction by raising myocardial oxygen consumption or diminishing myocardial oxygen supply through coronary vasoconstriction.[8] An increase in sympathetic efferent activity from uncontrolled postoperative pain may also further reduce gastrointestinal activity and delay return of gastrointestinal function. In addition, postoperative pain may activate several detrimental spinal reflex arcs that may lead to a decrease in postoperative respiratory function, especially after upper abdominal and thoracic surgery,[9] as well as an inhibition of gastrointestinal function.[10,11]

CHRONIC EFFECTS

The development of chronic pain after surgery may result from poor control of postoperative pain.[12,13] Although the causality of this relationship is unclear, evidence suggests that the change from acute postoperative pain to chronic pain occurs much earlier than previously thought.[14] Chronic pain is relatively common after certain procedures, including limb amputation (up to 83%), thoracotomy (up to 67%), sternotomy (27%), breast surgery (up to 57%), and gallbladder surgery (up to 56%).[12,15] The severity of acute postoperative pain may be an important predictor of the development of chronic pain after thoracic surgery,[16–18] hernia repair,[19] breast surgery,[20] amputation,[21] and gallbladder surgery.[12,22] In addition, controlling the severity of postoperative pain may improve long-term patient-oriented outcomes.[23–25]

Pain Pathways and the Neurobiology of Nociception

Because control of postoperative pain may be important in the development of chronic pain after surgery, understanding the neurobiology of nociception may help us appreciate the importance of various pathways and their roles in the transition from acute to chronic pain. Tissue injury from surgery leads to a release of inflammatory mediators that activate peripheral nociceptors. Small-diameter A-δ and C fibers transmit the nociceptive information to the dorsal horn of the spinal cord, neurotransmission being performed by numerous peptides and amino acids, including substance P, calcitonin gene–related protein, galanin, vasoactive intestinal polypeptide, and somatostatin. These neurotransmitters activate second-order spinal cord projection neurons that possess a wide variety of receptors, a subset of which increase nociceptive pain transmission. These include the excitatory amino acid receptors, N-methyl-D-aspartate (NMDA), alpha-amino-3-hydroxy-5-methyl-isoxazole-4-propionic acid (AMPA)/kainite, mGluR, and the substance P (SP) and neurokinin receptors (NK-1).

The dorsal horn of the spinal cord is one of the more important locations for the integration of nociceptive information, because it receives input from both the peripheral nociceptors and descending modulatory sites. Continuous input of nociceptive stimuli from the periphery results in spinal cord or central sensitization, whereby nociceptors have a reduced threshold for activation, a higher discharge rate with activation, and an increased rate of basal or even spontaneous discharge.[14] Although the precise role of the various neurotransmitters in the process of nociception has not been fully elucidated, it seems that certain receptors (e.g., NMDA) may be especially important for the development of chronic pain after an acute injury.[26] NMDA receptors, which are found both presynaptically and postsynaptically within the superficial and deep dorsal horns, increase nociceptive pain transmission.[27] Thus, on the basis of the current understanding of the neurobiology of nociception, it is clear that continued peripheral nociceptive input from surgical injury could maintain central sensitization and chronic pain, and that attenuation or even prevention of central sensitization and postoperative pain might lower the incidence of chronic pain.[28,29]

Preemptive Analgesia

Using an antinociceptive treatment to prevent or attenuate central sensitization and hyperexcitability after surgery (i.e., preemptive analgesia) may have both short-term (e.g., reduction in postoperative pain) and long-term (e.g., reduction in chronic pain) benefits in patient recovery after surgery (Fig. 8–1). Even though experimental studies indicate that preemptive analgesia would be efficacious in decreasing postsurgical pain, the results of clinical trials are equivocal.[30–33]

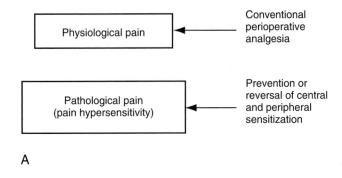

A

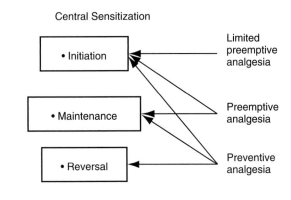

B

Figure 8–1   Central sensitization and postoperative pain. **A,** Treatment of postoperative pain. In contrast to conventional perioperative analgesia, preemptive analgesia is focused only on the prevention of pathological pain. **B,** Different scope of the approaches designed to exclude the contribution of central sensitization to postoperative pain (i.e., prevent pain hypersensitivity). (From Kissin I: Preemptive analgesia. Anesthesiology 2000;93:1138–1143.)

One of the reasons for the controversy about whether preemptive analgesia is clinically relevant relates to the precise definition of *preemptive analgesia*. Several definitions have been offered, and they typically fall into a "narrow" (i.e., intraoperative) category or a "broader" (i.e., perioperative) category.[30] The narrow definition for preemptive analgesia focuses primarily on the timing of the intervention (i.e., before or after incision) and does not account for postoperative pain that may cause central sensitization after the intervention has lost its efficacy. As a result, this narrow definition may contribute to the lack of a detectable effect of preemptive analgesia in available clinical trials.

A much broader definition that accounts for other aspects of preemptive analgesia (e.g., intensity and duration of the intervention) may be more clinically relevant to treat both incisional and inflammatory injuries, which are important in initiating and maintaining central sensitization (Fig. 8–2). Thus, the precise timing of the intervention per se may not be as important as its efficacy in preventing central sensitization. A variety of agents and techniques have been used to study this issue and as a whole provide equivocal results about the clinical relevance of preemptive analgesia.[33] Nevertheless, the results of clinical trials using the broader definition of preemptive analgesia indicate that this modality is a clinically relevant phenomenon and that maximal clinical benefit

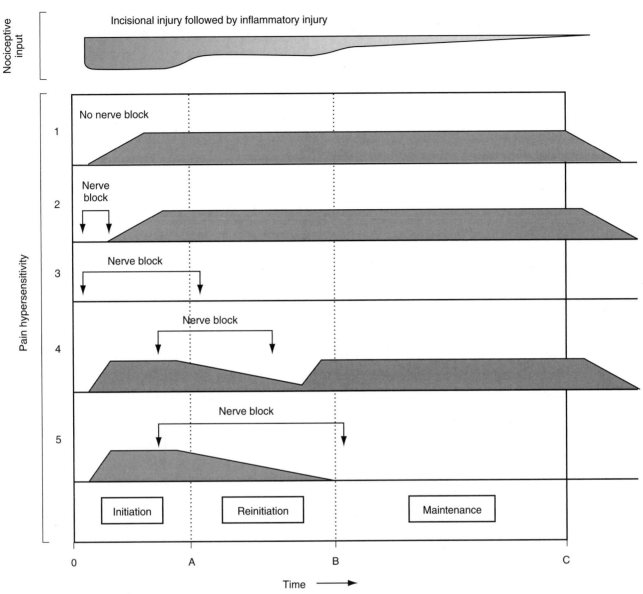

Figure 8–2 A model illustrating hypothetical conditions necessary to preempt or reverse pain hypersensitivity with neural blockade. **Top,** A nociceptive input caused by incisional injury, inflammatory injury, or both, with width of band indicating input intensity. **Bottom,** Five possible variants of pain hypersensitivity generated in response to the afferent input with different nerve block conditions: No block (1), shorter (2) and longer-lasting (3) preinjury blocks, and shorter (4) and longer-lasting (5) blocks administered when pain hypersensitivity is already established. Time A, time after which nociceptive input is unable to initiate pain hypersensitivity yet strong enough to reinitiate it (if it was already established before the block); Time B, time after which the input is unable to reinitiate pain hypersensitivity but can maintain it (until Time C). The effectiveness of a potential preemptive effect is determined by the duration of nociceptive input that can initiate and maintain central hypersensitivity. If the blockade lasts until afferent input subsides to the level at which it cannot trigger central hypersensitivity, the preemptive effect might be clinically meaningful (see variants 2 and 3). The reversal of central hypersensitivity (see variants 4 and 5) is determined by two factors, persistence of central sensitization and continuance of the afferent input that can initiate, reinitiate, and maintain (respectively, in accordance with the declining level of the input intensity) pain hypersensitivity. The blockade should last until central sensitization subsides and the intensity of the afferent input is below the level that could potentially reinitiate central hypersensitivity (variant 5). Because the intensity of afferent input for reinitiation of central hypersensitivity is lower than that for its initiation, blockade for a successful reversal of pain hypersensitivity should be longer (to permit greater input fading) than that for preemptive effect. (From Kissin I: Preemptive analgesia. Anesthesiology 2000;93:1138–1143; modified from Kissin I, Lee SS, Bradley EL Jr: Effect of prolonged nerve block on inflammatory hyperalgesia in rats: Prevention of late hyperalgesia. Anesthesiology 1998;88:224–232.)

accrues when there is complete intraoperative block of noxious stimuli with extension of this block into the postoperative period.[34] Thus, use of preemptive analgesia to prevent central sensitization, especially with intensive multimodal analgesic interventions (see later), may reduce both acute postoperative pain and chronic pain after surgery.[12,28]

The Effect of Different Analgesic Regimens on Outcomes

Although there is a wide range of analgesic options for the treatment of postoperative pain, certain advantages of particular options may improve perioperative patient outcomes. The most common options discussed here are systemic analgesics (opioid and nonsteroidal anti-inflammatory drugs [NSAIDs]) and regional (neuraxial and peripheral) analgesic techniques. The effect of each analgesic technique or agent on patient outcome may be related to many factors, including the level of analgesia provided, whether detrimental perioperative physiological effects are attenuated, and the presence or absence of side effects. In addition, there may be differences in patient outcomes within a specific technique or agent (e.g., epidural analgesia). Despite the apparent benefits of certain analgesic options on patient outcomes, the clinician also must consider possible adverse events, some of which are rare but devastating, in tailoring the analgesic regimen for each patient.

SYSTEMIC ANALGESIA

Several systemic analgesic agents are available for the treatment of postoperative pain; however, the two most commonly used agents are opioids and NSAIDs. Agents in both groups can be administered via the oral or intravenous route, the latter being more frequently used in patients who are unable to tolerate oral intake postoperatively. These agents can provide excellent postoperative analgesia. However, when administered in a systemic fashion alone, these agents may not be able to attenuate perioperative pathophysiology enough to improve traditional patient outcomes.

Systemic Opioids

Although use of opioids for the treatment of postoperative pain may be effective, the analgesic efficacy of opioids is typically limited by the development of tolerance[35] or opioid-related side effects such as nausea, vomiting, sedation, and respiratory depression. Systemic opioids can be administered subcutaneously, intramuscularly, or transdermally, but the most effective route is intravenous, especially via a device that the patient controls (intravenous patient-controlled anesthesia [IV-PCA]). Transdermal fentanyl has been used for acute pain management[36]; however, the traditional steady-release form of transdermal fentanyl cannot be titrated easily for the management of acute pain. Newer, electrically facilitated PCA delivery of transdermal fentanyl has been reported for treatment of acute pain.[37,38]

The optimal route for systemic opioid administration appears to be via a PCA device. This form of administration can be individually tailored to account for the wide interpatient variability in postoperative opioid requirements and minimizes the effects of pharmacokinetic and pharmacodynamic variability among individual patients. Administration of opioids via a PCA device generally provides superior analgesia compared with administration by other routes (intramuscular, subcutaneous) on an "as needed" basis. Transdermal PCA appears to provide levels of analgesia similar to those provided by IV-PCA.[38]

Effect of Systemic Opioids on Patient Outcomes

Compared with other forms of analgesia, systemic opioids do not appear to confer any global advantages in improving patient outcomes postoperatively. There are no significant data suggesting that use of systemic opioids reduces postoperative mortality. However, various patient outcomes are different for different methods of delivery of systemic opioids. Use of a PCA device (whether intravenous or transdermal) is considered the "gold standard" against which delivery of all systemic opioids is evaluated.

Compared with traditional "as needed" analgesic regimens (typically intramuscular or subcutaneous), IV-PCA not only provides superior postoperative analgesia but also improves patient satisfaction and may decrease the risk of pulmonary complications.[39,40] A meta-analysis of 15 randomized trials ("as needed" intramuscular dosing versus IV-PCA) noted significantly greater analgesic efficacy with IV-PCA but no reduction in mortality or major morbidity.[40] A subsequent quantitative systematic review (again comparing IV-PCA with non–IV-PCA for administration of systemic opioids) showed a lower risk for pulmonary complications in patients who received IV-PCA (Fig. 8–3).[39]

Compared with traditional "as needed" analgesic regimens, IV-PCA may also improve patient-oriented outcomes such as patient satisfaction, although the assessment of this outcome is extremely complicated. Patients generally have greater satisfaction with an IV-PCA device and tend to prefer IV-PCA to other modalities such as "as needed" intramuscular or subcutaneous administration of opioids.[39-41] The reasons for the typically higher satisfaction ratings for IV-PCA are not clear but may be related to better analgesia, perceived control over analgesic medication administration, and avoidance of disclosing pain to nurses or having to ask them for analgesic medication.[41-44] Although a difference in the incidence of side effects among techniques may influence patient satisfaction,[45] the incidence of opioid-related side effects from IV-PCA does not appear to differ significantly from those from intramuscular, subcutaneous, or transdermal analgesia.[38]

Nonsteroidal Anti-inflammatory Drugs

NSAIDs, which include aspirin and acetaminophen, exert their analgesic effect through the inhibition of cyclooxygenase and the synthesis of prostaglandins, which are important mediators for peripheral and central sensitization. NSAIDs provide effective analgesia for mild to moderate postoperative pain and are a useful supplement to opioids for treatment of moderate to severe postoperative pain. With the introduction of cyclooxygenase-specific inhibitors (e.g., cyclooxygenase-2 inhibitors), NSAIDs that can be administered either orally or parenterally are considered an integral part of a multimodal analgesic regimen, because they produce analgesia through different mechanisms from those of opioids and local anesthetics.

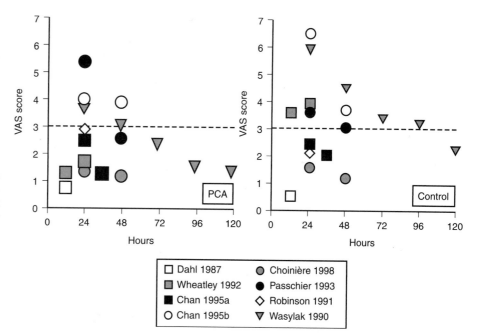

Figure 8–3 Pain intensity scores for patient-controlled analgesia (PCA) **(left)** and controls **(right)**. Data are from eight morphine trials that reported pain intensity on a visual analogue scale (VAS). Symbol sizes are proportional to trial sizes. The *dotted line* represents moderate pain. (From Walder B, Schafer M, Henzi I, Tramer MR: Efficacy and safety of patient-controlled opioid analgesia for acute postoperative pain: A quantitative systematic review. Acta Anaesthesiol Scand 2001;45:795–804.)

Effect on Patient Outcomes

As with opioids, NSAIDs by themselves do not appear to have a significant impact on mortality or major morbidity in comparison with other analgesic agents. However, NSAIDs may improve analgesia and patient-oriented outcomes (e.g., satisfaction), in part by reducing opioid analgesic requirements, decreasing opioid-related side effects, and facilitating patient recovery.[46–48] When given in addition to a systemic opioid, NSAIDs improve postoperative analgesia and reduce opioid requirements by up to 50%—an effect that may diminish opioid-related side effects and nausea, facilitate return of gastrointestinal function, abate respiratory depression, and improve patient satisfaction. However, not all studies report a diminution in opioid-related side effects with concurrent use of an NSAID.[49–51]

REGIONAL AND PERIPHERAL ANALGESIA

A variety of neuraxial (primarily epidural) and peripheral analgesic techniques are effective for the treatment of postoperative pain. Postoperative epidural and peripheral techniques, especially when a local anesthetic–based solution is used, generally provide better analgesia than systemic opioids.[52,53] Unlike systemic opioids, regional analgesic techniques may be associated with physiologic benefits that may attenuate the detrimental perioperative effects of surgery and lead to improvements in patient outcomes, including major morbidity. How the specific regional analgesic technique is used (e.g., catheter location, local versus opioid analgesic regimen, duration of analgesic regimen) influences its level of efficacy in improving patient outcomes.

Neuraxial Opioids

Opioid-based neuraxial analgesia, which may be administered as a single dose or by continuous infusion, effectively controls postoperative pain. Neuraxial opioids can be classified according to their lipophilicity, with lipophilic agents (e.g., fentanyl, sufentanil) having a faster onset but shorter duration of action than lipophobic/hydrophilic agents (e.g., morphine, hydromorphone). In general, in comparison with intravenous infusion, the overall benefit of continuous epidural infusions of lipophilic opioids is minimal[54]; however, epidural infusions of hydrophilic opioids provide better analgesia than traditional "as needed" intravenous administration of opioids.[55,56] Continuous infusion of epidural opioids may provide superior analgesia with fewer side effects compared with intermittent bolus administration.[57,58]

Effect of Neuraxial Opioids on Outcomes

Neuraxial opioids may attenuate perioperative pathophysiology (e.g., neuroendocrine stress response), an effect that typically does not occur with routine clinical doses of systemic opioids and so may influence perioperative outcomes. Even though the analgesia provided by neuraxial opioids (especially morphine) is superior to that from systemic opioids, administration of neuraxial opioids typically achieves only partial attenuation of perioperative pathophysiology. Neuraxial opioids may modify the perioperative stress response, but to a lesser extent than a local anesthetic–based epidural analgesic regimen.[59] This partial, rather than complete, suppression of perioperative pathophysiology may be due to the fact that neuraxial opioids allow transmission of nociceptive information through the central nervous system and so cannot completely suppress the neuroendocrine stress response. Thus, neuraxial opioids may not have as great an effect on patient outcomes as a local anesthetic–based epidural analgesic regimen.

Even though neuraxial opioids only partially attenuate perioperative pathophysiology, some studies indicate that neuraxial opioids, particularly epidural morphine, may achieve better patient outcomes postoperatively than systemic opioids (Table 8–1).[60–67] Randomized studies indicate that perioperative epidural morphine leads to fewer cardiovascular and pulmonary complications than systemic opioids.[61,62,64–67] A meta-analysis of several randomized trials demonstrated

| TABLE 8–1 | Outcomes Studies of Epidural Morphine versus Systemic Opioids for Postoperative Analgesia |

Study	Study Population (n)	Trial Design	Morbidity (EA vs. SYST)	Mortality (EA vs. SYST)
Park et al (2001)[60]	ABD (1021)	RCT	22% vs. 37%*	Combined data
Tsui et al (1997)[61]	ABD-THOR (578)	RCT	EA improved pulmonary (EA: 13% vs. 25%; $P = .002$) and CV (EA: 21% vs. 43%; $P < .001$) outcomes and LOS (EA: 22 ± 20 vs. 30 ± 37; $P = .005$)	EA: 8% vs. 14%; $P = .038$
Major et al (1996)[62]	ABD (65)	OBS	Improvement in EA for CV ($P = .0002$) and pulmonary ($P = .019$) outcomes and LOS ICU ($P = .024$)	None reported
Liu et al (1995)[63]	ABD (54)	RCT	No difference in GI recovery between epidural and systemic opioids	None reported
Beattie et al (1993)[64]	Mixed (55)	RCT	Improvement in EA for CV ischemia (EA: 17.2% vs. 50%; $P = .01$) and tachyarrhythmias (EA: 20.7% vs. 50%; $P < .05$)	None reported
Her et al (1990)[65]	ABD (49)	OBS	Improvement in EA for need for ventilatory support ($P = .0002$), respiratory failure ($P = .018$), and LOS in ICU (EA: 2.7 days vs. 3.8 days; $P = .003$)	None reported
Hasenbos et al (1987)[66]	THOR (129)	RCT	Improvement in EA for pulmonary complications (EA: 12.1% vs. 38%)	None reported
Rawal et al (1984)[67]	ABD	RCT	Improvement in EA for pulmonary complications (EA: 13% vs. 40%), GI function (EA: 56.7 ± 3.1 hours vs. 75.1 ± 3.1 hours; $P < .05$), and LOS (EA: 7 ± 0.5 days vs. 9 ± 0.6 days; $P < .05$)	None reported

*Data represented are from a subgroup (aortic aneurysm repair) of the study that showed no overall difference. Morbidity and mortality data combined.
ABD, undergoing abdominal surgery; CV, cardiovascular; EA, epidural anesthesia; GI, gastrointestinal; ICU, intensive care unit; LOS, length of stay; OBS, observation; RCT, randomized controlled trial; SYST, systemic anesthesia; THOR, undergoing thoracic surgery.
Modified from Casey Z, Wu CL: Epidural opioids for postoperative pain. In Benzon HT, Raja SN, Moloy RE, et al (eds): Essentials of Pain Medicine and Regional Anesthesia, 2nd ed. St. Louis, Churchill Livingstone, 2005.

that compared with systemic opioids, epidural morphine decreased the incidence of postoperative atelectasis.[68] Thus, perioperative neuraxial opioids may be associated with improvement in patient outcome in some cases. Finally, some side effects of neuraxial opioids may affect patient-oriented outcomes.[69] For example, administration of neuraxial opioids results in dose-dependent[70,71] nausea and vomiting for 20% to 50% of patients after a single dose[72] or for 45% to 80% of patients cumulatively.[73] In addition, neuraxial administration of opioids may be associated with pruritus in 60% of patients, compared with 15% to 18% of patients receiving epidural local anesthetics or systemic opioids.[39,74,75]

Local Anesthetic–Based Epidural Analgesia

Local anesthetic–based epidural analgesia (which typically uses a low-dose lipophilic opioid) is an effective method for managing postoperative pain.[76] A local anesthetic–based epidural analgesic regimen provides better analgesia than systemic opioids (Fig. 8–4).[53] Epidural analgesia may be administered either as a continuous infusion or as patient-controlled epidural analgesia (PCEA). Like IV-PCA, PCEA allows for individualization of postoperative analgesic requirements, may have several advantages over a continuous epidural infusion (e.g., lower drug requirement,[77,78] greater patient satisfaction,[79] and superior analgesia[78]), and is a safe and effective technique for postoperative analgesia.[80,81] In general, PCEA provides better analgesia and higher patient satisfaction than IV-PCA.[82,83] The local anesthetic solution in the epidural regimen may have side effects that may influence some patient-oriented outcomes.[69] For example, local anesthetics may cause hypotension (incidence 0.7% to 3%)[54,80,84] or may lead to lower extremity motor block (incidence 2% to 3%).[54,80]

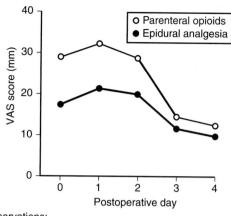

Figure 8–4 Comparison of parenteral opioids versus epidural analgesia for control of postoperative pain. Epidural analgesia provides significantly superior pain control for up to 4 days after surgery. VAS, Visual analogue scale. (From Block BM, Liu SS, Rowlingson AJ, et al: Efficacy of postoperative epidural analgesia: A meta-analysis. JAMA 2003;290:2455–2463.)

No. of patient-observations:					
Parenteral opioids	1104	2635	1496	794	536
Epidural analgesia	1010	2618	1527	822	566

Effect of Epidural Analgesia on Patient Outcomes

A local anesthetic–based epidural analgesic solution can attenuate or even completely suppress perioperative pathophysiology; as a result, it may be associated with lower mortality and morbidity than systemic opioids.[10,11,68,85,86] In addition, the superior analgesia provided by epidural analgesia[53] compared with systemic opioids may contribute to an improvement in patient-oriented outcomes. Use of intraoperative anesthesia with local anesthetic has already been suggested to decrease mortality; a meta-analysis of randomized data (Collaborative Overview of Randomised Trials of Regional Anaesthesia [CORTRA] meta-analysis: 141 trials consisting

of 9559 subjects) demonstrated that neuraxial anesthesia and analgesia reduced 30-day mortality by approximately 30% (Fig. 8–5).[86]

Compared with systemic or even neuraxial opioids in certain instances, use of epidural analgesia with a local anesthetic–based regimen decreases the incidence of postoperative coagulation and gastrointestinal, pulmonary, and cardiac complications (Fig. 8–6).[10,11,86] A local anesthetic–based thoracic epidural analgesic regimen inhibits sympathetic outflow, decreases the total opioid dose, and attenuates a spinal reflex inhibition of the gastrointestinal tract,[10,87] thus facilitating return of gastrointestinal motility. Randomized controlled trials (RCTs) indicate that postoperative thoracic epidural analgesia with a local anesthetic–based analgesic solution allows earlier return of gastrointestinal function and earlier fulfillment of discharge criteria than analgesia with systemic opioids.[63,82,88] In addition, patients who receive local epidural anesthetics have an earlier return of gastrointestinal motility after abdominal surgery than those who receive epidural opioids.[63,89,90] There are no data to indicate whether thoracic epidural analgesia with local anesthetics would contribute to anastomotic bowel dehiscence.[91]

By preserving postoperative pulmonary function, providing superior analgesia, and attenuating a spinal reflex inhibition of diaphragmatic function,[10] a local anesthetic–based epidural regimen may also reduce postoperative pulmonary complications in high-risk patients undergoing abdominal and thoracic surgery.[68,85] Both a meta-analysis of approximately 50 RCTs[68] and a large RCT[85] demonstrate that a local anesthetic–based regimen administered through thoracic epidural analgesia is associated with a lower incidence of pulmonary infections and complications than epidural or systemic opioids (Fig. 8–7).[68] In another meta-analysis examining 15 trials enrolling 1178 patients undergoing coronary artery bypass surgery, thoracic epidural analgesia significantly reduced the risk of dysrhythmias (odds ratio [OR] 0.52) and

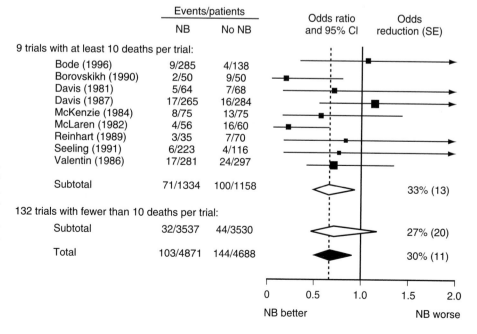

Figure 8–5 Effect of neuraxial blockade (NB) on postoperative mortality within 30 days of randomization. *Diamonds* denote 95% confidence intervals (CI) for odds ratios of combined trial results. The *vertical dashed line* represents the overall pooled result. SE, sampling error. (From Rodgers A, Walker N, Schug S, et al: Reduction of postoperative mortality and morbidity with epidural or spinal anaesthesia: Results from overview of randomised trials. BMJ 2000;321:1493.)

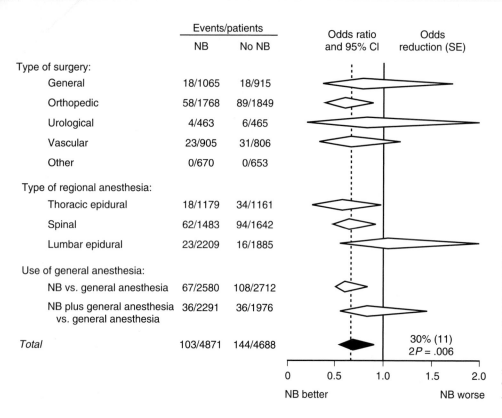

	Events/patients			
	NB	No NB		
Type of surgery:				
General	18/1065	18/915		
Orthopedic	58/1768	89/1849		
Urological	4/463	6/465		
Vascular	23/905	31/806		
Other	0/670	0/653		
Type of regional anesthesia:				
Thoracic epidural	18/1179	34/1161		
Spinal	62/1483	94/1642		
Lumbar epidural	23/2209	16/1885		
Use of general anesthesia:				
NB vs. general anesthesia	67/2580	108/2712		
NB plus general anesthesia vs. general anesthesia	36/2291	36/1976		
Total	103/4871	144/4688	30% (11) 2P = .006	

Figure 8–6 Effects of neuraxial blockade (NB) on postoperative complications. *Diamonds* denote 95% confidence intervals (CI) for odds ratios of combined trial results. The *vertical dashed line* represents the overall pooled result. (From Rodgers A, Walker N, Schug S, et al: Reduction of postoperative mortality and morbidity with epidural or spinal anaesthesia: Results from overview of randomised trials. BMJ 2000;16:321.)

the rate of pulmonary complications (OR 0.41), and shortened the time to tracheal extubation by 4.5 hours (Fig. 8–8).[92]

In addition, intraoperative epidural and spinal anesthesia may result in a decrease in perioperative hypercoagulable events, such as deep venous thrombosis (DVT), pulmonary embolism, and vascular graft failure. The investigators in the CORTRA meta-analysis performed a subgroup analysis on the effect of intraoperative neuraxial anesthesia on perioperative morbidity; they noted that neuraxial anesthesia and analgesia reduced the odds of DVT by 44% and of pulmonary embolism by 55% (see Fig. 8–6).[86] An earlier meta-analysis also showed that intraoperative neuraxial anesthesia lowered the odds of DVT by 31% compared with general anesthesia; the odds ratio for development of DVT was almost four times higher for general anesthesia.[93] In an RCT in patients

undergoing elective vascular reconstruction of the lower extremities, patients who were randomly assigned to receive perioperative epidural anesthesia/analgesia had a lower incidence of regrafting or embolectomy than those assigned to receive general anesthesia.[94] Another RCT in patients undergoing lower extremity revascularization noted a lower incidence of thrombotic events (peripheral arterial graft coronary artery or deep venous thromboses) in patients who were randomly assigned to receive epidural anesthesia–analgesia as part of their anesthetic regimen.[95] Perioperative use of epidural anesthesia may reduce the rate of hypercoagulable events by increasing blood flow and attenuating the perioperative stress response. It should be noted, however, that many of the earlier trials did not use concurrent prophylactic anticoagulants; therefore, it is unclear what additional

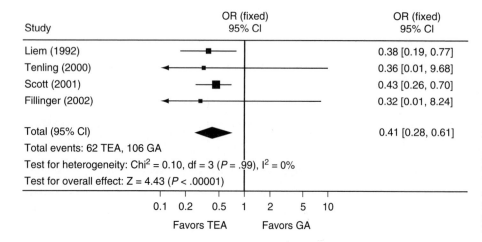

Study	OR (fixed) 95% CI	OR (fixed) 95% CI
Liem (1992)		0.38 [0.19, 0.77]
Tenling (2000)		0.36 [0.01, 9.68]
Scott (2001)		0.43 [0.26, 0.70]
Fillinger (2002)		0.32 [0.01, 8.24]
Total (95% CI)		0.41 [0.28, 0.61]

Total events: 62 TEA, 106 GA
Test for heterogeneity: Chi² = 0.10, df = 3 (P = .99), I² = 0%
Test for overall effect: Z = 4.43 (P < .00001)

Figure 8–7 The effect of perioperative epidural analgesia on the incidence of pulmonary complications in patients undergoing coronary artery bypass. *Diamond* denotes 95% confidence interval (CI) for odds ratios of combined trial results. CI, confidence interval; GA, general anesthesia; OR, odds ratio; TEA, thoracic epidural anesthesia. (Data from Liu SS, Block BM, Wu CL: Effects of perioperative central neuraxial analgesia on outcome after coronary artery bypass surgery: A meta-analysis. Anesthesiology 2004;101:153–161.)

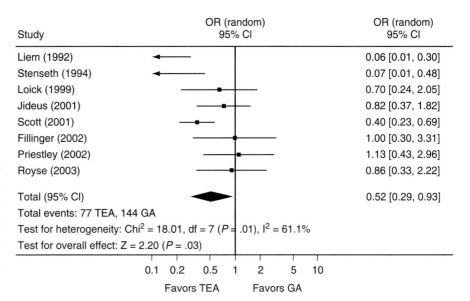

Study	OR (random) 95% CI	OR (random) 95% CI
Liem (1992)		0.06 [0.01, 0.30]
Stenseth (1994)		0.07 [0.01, 0.48]
Loick (1999)		0.70 [0.24, 2.05]
Jideus (2001)		0.82 [0.37, 1.82]
Scott (2001)		0.40 [0.23, 0.69]
Fillinger (2002)		1.00 [0.30, 3.31]
Priestley (2002)		1.13 [0.43, 2.96]
Royse (2003)		0.86 [0.33, 2.22]
Total (95% CI)		0.52 [0.29, 0.93]

Total events: 77 TEA, 144 GA
Test for heterogeneity: Chi^2 = 18.01, df = 7 (P = .01), I^2 = 61.1%
Test for overall effect: Z = 2.20 (P = .03)

Favors TEA   Favors GA

Figure 8–8 The effect of perioperative epidural analgesia on the incidence of dysrhythmias in patients undergoing coronary artery bypass. *Diamond* denotes 95% confidence interval (CI). GA, general anesthesia; OR, odds ratio; TEA, thoracic epidural anesthesia. (Data from Liu SS, Block BM, Wu CL: Effects of perioperative central neuraxial analgesia on outcome after coronary artery bypass surgery: A meta-analysis. Anesthesiology 2004;101:153–161.)

benefit perioperative epidural anesthesia/analgesia might confer beyond that of prophylactic anticoagulation.

Finally, a local anesthetic–based epidural regimen administered via a thoracic, but not a lumbar, epidural catheter may decrease the incidence of postoperative myocardial infarction (Fig. 8–9).[96] The mechanisms of such a benefit are unclear but may involve attenuation of the stress response and hypercoagulability, provision of superior postoperative analgesia, and improvement in coronary blood flow.[5,97] Experimental data also indicate that thoracic epidural analgesia with a local anesthetic–based solution would have physiological benefits, including a reduction in the size of myocardial infarction, attenuation of sympathetically mediated coronary vasoconstriction, and improvement of coronary flow to ischemic areas.[98–100] It is apparent that the benefits of epidural analgesia are maximized with "catheter-incision congruent" analgesia, whereby insertion of the epidural catheter is appropriate to the surgical incision, and may result in delivery of less drug and lower incidence of drug-induced side effects.[80,101–103] Epidural "catheter-incision congruent" analgesia[103] enables an earlier return of gastrointestinal function,[104] a lower incidence of myocardial infarction,[96] and superior analgesia than epidural catheter-incision incongruent" epidural analgesia.[105,106]

Despite the apparent benefits of a local anesthetic–based epidural regimen in decreasing postoperative gastrointestinal, pulmonary, and possibly cardiac morbidity, the effects of epidural analgesia on postoperative coagulation, cognitive dysfunction,[107] and immune function[108] are equivocal. RCTs suggest that intraoperative regional anesthesia reduces the incidence of hypercoagulability-related events such as DVT[86,93–95]; however, the benefits of postoperative epidural analgesia in lowering the incidence of hypercoagulable-related events are not clear.[109] Finally, a local anesthetic–based epidural regimen may be associated with an improvement in patient-oriented outcomes, including patient satisfaction[110] and health-related quality of life,[25] which in part may reflect the fact that a local anesthetic–based epidural regimen consistently provides better analgesia than systemic opioids.[53]

Peripheral Regional Analgesia

Peripheral regional analgesia incorporates a wide variety of techniques (e.g., brachial plexus, lumbar plexus, femoral, sciatic-popliteal) and either may be a one-time injection used primarily for intraoperative anesthesia or as an adjunct to postoperative analgesia or may consist of a continuous infusion of local anesthetics administered through peripheral nerve catheters. The use of peripheral regional analgesic techniques, as either single injections or continuous infusion, can provide better analgesia than systemic opioids[111–113] and may even improve various outcomes.[23,110,114,115] A single-shot peripheral nerve block using a local anesthetic–based regimen provides superior analgesia and is associated with improvements in some outcomes, such as fewer opioid-related side effects—possibly related to decreased opioid use—and better patient satisfaction.[111–115] Compared with systemic opioids, the use of continuous or patient-controlled peripheral infusions for postoperative analgesia also achieves superior analgesia with fewer opioid-related side effects and greater patient satisfaction.[110,116,117] Despite the superior analgesia and possible physiological benefits provided by peripheral nerve blocks, no large-scale randomized trial has been conducted to examine the efficacy of this technique in reducing perioperative mortality or morbidity in surgical patients.

Multimodal Analgesia

Postoperative pain control by itself may not be enough to decrease perioperative morbidity and mortality; however, the effect on patient outcomes of achieving control of postoperative pain is optimized when a multimodal strategy for patient recovery is implemented.[118,119] This type of strategy typically incorporates various aspects of patient care, including control of postoperative pain to allow patient mobilization, early enteral nutrition, patient education, and attenuation of the perioperative stress response, primarily

Comparison: 01 myocardial infarction
Outcome: 01 myocardial infarctions

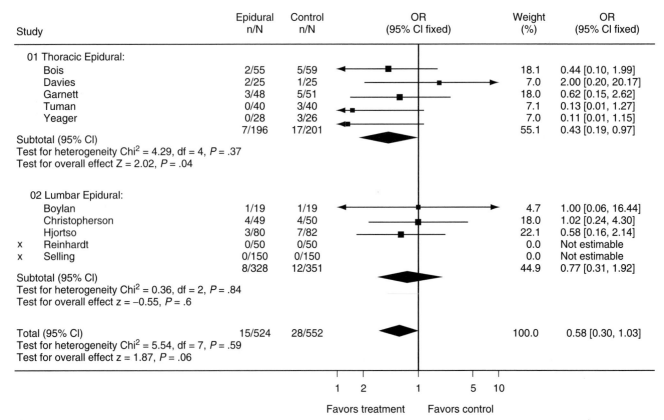

Figure 8–9   The effect of postoperative epidural anesthesia on postoperative myocardial infarction. Note that only thoracic, and not lumbar, epidural analgesia decreases the incidence of postoperative myocardial infarction. *Diamonds* denote 95% confidence interval (CI). OR, odds ratio. (From Beattie WS, Badner NH, Choi P: Epidural analgesia reduces postoperative myocardial infarction: A meta-analysis. Anesth Analg 2001;93:853–858.)

through a combination of local anesthetic–based regional analgesic techniques[120] and other analgesic agents (multimodal analgesia) to facilitate patient recovery.[46] A local anesthetic–based epidural or peripheral analgesic technique is an integral part of the multimodal strategy because of the superior analgesia and physiological benefits it confers.

Some evidence suggests that a multimodal strategy controls postoperative pathophysiology, accelerates patient recovery, and shortens hospitalization.[118] In several studies, patients undergoing abdominal or thoracic surgery who participated in a multimodal strategy had a lower stress response with preservation of total body protein, shorter times to extubation, lower pain scores, earlier return of bowel function, and earlier fulfillment of criteria for discharge from the intensive care unit.[121-124] In one study, the overall complication rate, especially of cardiopulmonary complications, was significantly lower in patients who received multimodal, "fast-track" rehabilitation than in those receiving conventional care, although there was no difference in the rate of readmission.[124] Significant reductions in perioperative morbidity may be possible through the use of a standardized multimodal approach (e.g., fluid restriction and epidural analgesia) in routine clinical practice.[125]

Postoperative Pain Services

Many perioperative pain management programs, commonly called "acute pain services," have been developed since the initial description of an anesthesiology-based acute pain service in 1988.[126] Although there are several models for the development of acute pain services,[127] data suggest that all perioperative pain services positively affect some perioperative patient outcomes, such as pain scores, patient satisfaction, and, possibly, patient morbidity, especially with use of epidural analgesia.[11,128-131] The introduction of an acute pain service may lower postoperative pain scores in many instances, with a reduction of severe pain by more than 50% in some cases.[129,132] These reductions in pain scores occur with the introduction of a nurse-based acute pain service.[133,134] In addition, some studies show that introduction of an acute pain service improves patient satisfaction and may be associated with a decrease in analgesic medication–related side effects such as nausea, sedation, pruritus, and respiratory depression,[128,131] although this finding may not be definitive.[132] One of the potentially most important roles that an acute pain service can play is to establish or coordinate multimodal rehabilitation programs ("fast-track" surgery, clinical pathways), because (1) postoperative mortality and morbidity most likely depend on many factors (e.g., patient education, quality of analgesia, existing programs for postoperative rehabilitation) and (2) pain relief by itself is unlikely to improve postoperative outcome significantly.[132]

Summary

Postoperative pain may have an adverse effect on perioperative patient outcomes. Control of postoperative pain, especially through the use of analgesic options that provide superior analgesia and have physiological benefits in attenuating perioperative pathophysiology—and their use as part of a multimodal regimen for patient recovery—may favorably influence patient outcomes after surgery. Some analgesic techniques, such as epidural analgesia with a local anesthetic–based regimen, appear to attenuate perioperative pathophysiology with a resultant decrease in morbidity and even mortality in some trials. It is important to realize, however, that the techniques themselves may not be as important as how they are used. For example, "epidural analgesia" is not a single generic term; various options within the technique, such as the choice and dose of analgesic agents, the location of catheter placement, and the onset and duration of perioperative analgesia, affect patient outcome differently. Future studies should be directed at comparing the effects of various analgesic regimens and techniques on patient-oriented outcomes (e.g., satisfaction, quality of life, and quality of recovery).

REFERENCES

1. Carr DB, Jacox AK, Chapman RC, et al: Clinical Practice Guideline: Acute Pain Management: Operative or Medical Procedures and Trauma. Rockville, Md, Agency for Health Care Policy and Research, 1992.
2. American Society of Anesthesiologists: Practice guidelines for acute pain management in the perioperative setting: A report by the American Society of Anesthesiologists task force on pain management, acute pain section. Anesthesiology 1995;82:1071–1081.
3. American Pain Society Quality of Care Committee: Quality improvement guidelines for the treatment of acute pain and cancer pain. JAMA 1995;274:1874–1880.
4. Phillips DM: JCAHO pain management standards are unveiled. JAMA 2000;284:428–429.
5. Rosenfeld BA: Benefits of regional anesthesia on thromboembolic complications following surgery. Reg Anesth 1996;21(Suppl):9–12.
6. Desborough JP: The stress response to trauma and surgery. Br J Anaesth 2000;85:109–117.
7. Pomposelli JJ, Baxter JK 3rd, Babineau TJ, et al: Early postoperative glucose control predicts nosocomial infection rate in diabetic patients. JPEN J Parenter Enteral Nutr 1998;22:77–81.
8. Warltier DC, Pagel PS, Kersten JR: Approaches to the prevention of perioperative myocardial ischemia. Anesthesiology 2000;92:253–259.
9. Fratacci MD, Kimball WR, Wain JC, et al: Diaphragmatic shortening after thoracic surgery in humans: Effects of mechanical ventilation and thoracic epidural anesthesia. Anesthesiology 1993;79:654–665.
10. Liu S, Carpenter RL, Neal JM: Epidural anesthesia and analgesia: Their role in postoperative outcome. Anesthesiology 1995;82:1474–1506.
11. Wu CL, Fleisher LA: Outcomes research in regional anesthesia and analgesia. Anesth Analg 2000;91:1232–1242.
12. Perkins FM, Kehlet H: Chronic pain as an outcome of surgery: A review of predictive factors. Anesthesiology 2000;93:1123–1233.
13. Macrae WA: Chronic pain after surgery. Br J Anaesth 2001;87:88–98.
14. Carr DB, Goudas LC: Acute pain. Lancet 1999;353:2051–2058.
15. Kalso E, Mennander S, Tasmuth T, et al: Chronic post-sternotomy pain. Acta Anaesthesiol Scand 2001;45:935–939.
16. Katz J, Jackson M, Kavanagh BP, et al: Acute pain after thoracic surgery predicts long-term post-thoracotomy pain. Clin J Pain 1996;12:50–55.
17. Kalso E, Perttunen K, Kaasinen S: Pain after thoracic surgery. Acta Anaesthesiol Scand 1992;36:96–100.
18. Ochroch EA, Gottschalk A, Augostides J, et al: Long-term pain and activity during recovery from major thoracotomy using thoracic epidural analgesia. Anesthesiology 2002;97:1234–1244.
19. Callesen T, Bech K, Kehlet H: Prospective study of chronic pain after groin hernia repair. Br J Surg 1999;86:1528–1531.
20. Tasmuth T, Kataja M, Blomqvist C, et al: Treatment-related factors predisposing to chronic pain in patients with breast cancer—a multivariate approach. Acta Oncol 1997;36:625–630.
21. Fisher A, Meller Y: Continuous postoperative regional analgesia by nerve sheath block for amputation—a pilot study. Anesth Analg 1991;72:300–303.
22. Borly L, Anderson IB, Bardram L, et al: Preoperative prediction model of outcome after cholecystectomy for symptomatic gallstones. Scand J Gastroenterol 1999;34:1144–1152.
23. Capdevila X, Barthelet Y, Biboulet P, et al: Effects of perioperative analgesic technique on the surgical outcome and duration of rehabilitation after major knee surgery. Anesthesiology 1999;91:8–15.
24. Gottschalk A, Smith DS, Jobes DR, et al: Preemptive epidural analgesia and recovery from radical prostatectomy: A randomized controlled trial. JAMA 1998;279:1076–1082.
25. Carli F, Mayo N, Klubien K, et al: Epidural analgesia enhances functional exercise capacity and health-related quality of life after colonic surgery: Results of a randomized trial. Anesthesiology 2002;97:540–549.
26. Wu CL, Garry MG, Zollo RA, et al: Gene therapy for the management of pain. Part II: Molecular targets. Anesthesiology 2001;95:216–240.
27. Liu H, Wang H, Sheng M, et al: Evidence for presynaptic N-methyl-D-aspartate autoreceptors in the spinal cord dorsal horn. Proc Natl Acad Sci U S A 1994;91:8383–8387.
28. Obata H, Saito S, Fujita N, et al: Epidural block with mepivacaine before surgery reduces long-term post-thoracotomy pain. Can J Anaesth 1999;46:1127–1132.
29. Schug SA, Burrell R, Payne J, et al: Pre-emptive epidural analgesia may prevent phantom limb pain. Reg Anesth 1995;20:256.
30. Kissin I: Preemptive analgesia. Anesthesiology 2000;93:1138–1143.
31. Kissin I: Preemptive analgesia: Why its effect is not always obvious. Anesthesiology 1996;84:1015–1019.
32. Woolf CJ, Chong MS: Preemptive analgesia—treating postoperative pain by preventing the establishment of central sensitization. Anesth Analg 1993;77:362–379.
33. Moiniche S, Kehlet H, Dahl JB: A qualitative and quantitative systematic review of preemptive analgesia for postoperative pain: The role of timing of analgesia. Anesthesiology 2002;96:725–741.
34. Kissin I, Lee SS, Bradley EL Jr: Effect of prolonged nerve block on inflammatory hyperalgesia in rats: Prevention of late hyperalgesia. Anesthesiology 1998;88:224–232.
35. Taylor DA, Fleming WW: Unifying perspectives of the mechanisms underlying the development of tolerance and physical dependence to opioids. J Pharmacol Exp Ther 2001;297:11–18.
36. Lehmann LJ, DeSio JM, Radvany T, et al: Transdermal fentanyl in postoperative pain. Reg Anesth 1997;22:24–28.
37. Chelly JE, Grass J, Houseman TW, et al: The safety and efficacy of a fentanyl patient-controlled transdermal system for acute postoperative analgesia: A multicenter, placebo-controlled trial. Anesth Analg 2004;98:427–433.
38. Viscusi ER, Reynolds L, Chung F, et al: Patient-controlled transdermal fentanyl hydrochloride vs intravenous morphine pump for postoperative pain: A randomized controlled trial. JAMA 2004;291:1333–1341.
39. Walder B, Schafer M, Henzi I, et al: Efficacy and safety of patient-controlled opioid analgesia for acute postoperative pain: A quantitative systematic review. Acta Anaesthesiol Scand 2001;45:795–804.
40. Ballantyne JC, Carr DB, Chalmers TC, et al: Postoperative patient-controlled analgesia: Meta-analyses of initial randomized control trials. J Clin Anesth 1993;5:182–193.
41. Thomas V, Heath M, Rose D, et al: Psychological characteristics and the effectiveness of patient-controlled analgesia. Br J Anaesth 1995;74:271–276.
42. Pellino TA, Ward SE: Perceived control mediates the relationship between pain severity and patient satisfaction. J Pain Symptom Manage 1998;15:110–116.
43. Chumbley GM, Hall GM, Salmon P: Why do patients feel positive about patient-controlled analgesia? Anaesthesia 1999;54:366–369.

44. Jamison RN, Taft K, O'Hara JP, et al: Psychosocial and pharmacologic predictors of satisfaction with intravenous patient-controlled analgesia. Anesth Analg 1993;77:121–125.
45. Morgan PJ, Halpern S, Lam-McCulloch J: Comparison of maternal satisfaction between epidural and spinal anesthesia for elective Cesarean section. Can J Anaesth 2000;47:956–961.
46. Jin F, Chung F: Multimodal analgesia for postoperative pain control. J Clin Anesth 2001;13:524–539.
47. Crews JC: Multimodal pain management strategies for office-based and ambulatory procedures. JAMA 2002;288:629–632.
48. White PF: The role of non-opioid analgesic techniques in the management of pain after ambulatory surgery. Anesth Analg 2002;94:577–585.
49. Ballantyne JC: Use of nonsteroidal antiinflammatory drugs for acute pain management. Problems in Anesthesia 1998;10:23–36.
50. Grass JA, Sakima NT, Valley M, et al: Assessment of ketorolac as an adjuvant to fentanyl patient-controlled epidural analgesia after radical retropubic prostatectomy. Anesthesiology 1993;78:642–648.
51. Schug SA, Sidebotham DA, McGuinnety M, et al: Acetaminophen as an adjunct to morphine by patient-controlled analgesia in the management of acute postoperative pain. Anesth Analg 1998;87:368–372.
52. Dolin SJ, Cashman JN, Bland JM: Effectiveness of acute postoperative pain management. I: Evidence from published data. Br J Anaesth 2002;89:409–423.
53. Block BM, Liu SS, Rowlingson AJ, et al: Efficacy of postoperative epidural analgesia: A meta-analysis. JAMA 2003;290:2455–2463.
54. Wheatley RG, Schug SA, Watson D: Safety and efficacy of postoperative epidural analgesia. Br J Anaesth 2001;87:47–61.
55. Loper KA, Ready LB: Epidural morphine after anterior cruciate ligament repair: A comparison with patient-controlled intravenous morphine. Anesth Analg 1989;68:350–352.
56. Malviya S, Pandit UA, Merkel S, et al: A comparison of continuous epidural infusion and intermittent intravenous bolus doses of morphine in children undergoing selective dorsal rhizotomy. Reg Anesth Pain Med 1999;24:438–443.
57. de Leon-Casasola OA, Lema MJ: Postoperative epidural opioid analgesia: What are the choices? Anesth Analg 1996;83:867–875.
58. Rauck RL, Raj PP, Knarr DC, et al: Comparison of the efficacy of epidural morphine given by intermittent injection or continuous infusion for the management of postoperative pain. Reg Anesth 1994;19:316–324.
59. Gourlay GK, Kowalski SR, Plummer JL, et al: Fentanyl blood concentration-analgesic response relationship in the treatment of postoperative pain. Anesth Analg 1988;67:329–337.
60. Park WY, Thompson JS, Lee KK: Effect of epidural anesthesia and analgesia on perioperative outcome: A randomized, controlled Veterans Affairs cooperative study. Ann Surg 2001;234:560–569.
61. Tsui SL, Law S, Fok M, et al: Postoperative analgesia reduces mortality and morbidity after esophagectomy. Am J Surg 1997;173:472–478.
62. Major CP Jr, Greer MS, Russell WL, Roe SM: Postoperative pulmonary complications and morbidity after abdominal aneurysmectomy: A comparison of postoperative epidural versus parenteral opioid analgesia. Am Surg 1996;62:45–51.
63. Liu SS, Carpenter RL, Mackey DC, et al: Effects of perioperative analgesic technique on rate of recovery after colon surgery. Anesthesiology 1995;83:757–765.
64. Beattie WS, Buckley DN, Forrest JB: Epidural morphine reduces the risk of postoperative myocardial ischaemia in patients with cardiac risk factors. Can J Anaesth 1993;40:532–541.
65. Her C, Kizelshteyn G, Walker V, et al: Combined epidural and general anesthesia for abdominal aortic surgery. J Cardiothorac Anesth 1990;4:552–557.
66. Hasenbos M, van Egmond J, Gielen M, Crul JF: Post-operative analgesia by high thoracic epidural versus intramuscular nicomorphine after thoracotomy. Part III: The effects of peri- and post-operative analgesia on morbidity. Acta Anaesthesiol Scand 1987;31:608–615.
67. Rawal N, Sjostrand U, Christoffersson E, et al: Comparison of intramuscular and epidural morphine for postoperative analgesia in the grossly obese: Influence on postoperative ambulation and pulmonary function. Anesth Analg 1984;63:583–592.
68. Ballantyne JC, Carr DB, deFerranti S, et al: The comparative effects of postoperative analgesic therapies on pulmonary outcome: Cumulative meta-analyses of randomized, controlled trials. Anesth Analg 1998;86:598–612.
69. Wu CL, Richman JM: Postoperative pain and quality of recovery. Curr Opin Anesthesiol 2004;17:455-460.
70. Bailey PL, Rhondeau S, Schafer PG, et al: Dose-response pharmacology of intrathecal morphine in human volunteers. Anesthesiology 1993;79:49–59.
71. Kirson LE, Goldman JM, Slover RB: Low-dose intrathecal morphine for postoperative pain control in patients undergoing transurethral resection of the prostate. Anesthesiology 1989;71:192–195.
72. Chaney MA: Side effects of intrathecal and epidural opioids. Can J Anaesth 1995;42:891–903.
73. Gedney JA, Liu EH: Side-effects of epidural infusions of opioid bupivacaine mixtures. Anaesthesia 1998;53:1148–1155.
74. Kjellberg F, Tramer MR: Pharmacological control of opioid-induced pruritus: A quantitative systematic review of randomized trials. Eur J Anaesthesiol 2001;18:346–357.
75. Bucklin BA, Chestnut DH, Hawkins JL: Intrathecal opioids versus epidural local anesthetics for labor analgesia: A meta-analysis. Reg Anesth Pain Med 2002;27:23–30.
76. Grass JA: Epidural analgesia. Problems in Anesthesia 1998;10:45–67.
77. Ferrante FM, Lu L, Jamison SB, et al: Patient-controlled epidural analgesia: Demand dosing. Anesth Analg 1991;73:547–552.
78. Lubenow TR, Tanck EN, Hopkins EM, et al: Comparison of patient-assisted epidural analgesia with continuous-infusion epidural analgesia for postoperative patients. Reg Anesth 1994;19:206–211.
79. Gambling DR, McMorland GH, Yu P, et al: Comparison of patient-controlled epidural analgesia and conventional intermittent "top-up" injections during labor. Anesth Analg 1990;70:256–261.
80. Liu SS, Allen HW, Olsson GL: Patient-controlled epidural analgesia with bupivacaine and fentanyl on hospital wards: Prospective experience with 1,030 surgical patients. Anesthesiology 1998;88:688–695.
81. Wigfull J, Welchew E: Survey of 1057 patients receiving postoperative patient-controlled epidural analgesia. Anaesthesia 2001;56:70–75.
82. Mann C, Pouzeratte Y, Boccara G, et al: Comparison of intravenous or epidural patient-controlled analgesia in the elderly after major abdominal surgery. Anesthesiology 2000;92:433–441.
83. Blake DW, Stainsby GV, Bjorksten AR, et al: Patient-controlled epidural versus intravenous pethidine to supplement epidural bupivacaine after abdominal aortic surgery. Anaesth Intensive Care 1998;26:630–635.
84. de Leon-Casasola OA, Parker B, Lema MJ, et al: Postoperative epidural bupivacaine-morphine therapy: Experience with 4,227 surgical cancer patients. Anesthesiology 1994;81:368–375.
85. Rigg JR, Jamrozik K, Myles PS, et al: Epidural anaesthesia and analgesia and outcome of major surgery: A randomised trial. Lancet 2002;359:1276–1282.
86. Rodgers A, Walker N, Schug S, et al: Reduction of postoperative mortality and morbidity with epidural or spinal anaesthesia: Results from overview of randomised trials. BMJ 2000;321:1493–1496.
87. Rimback G, Cassuto J, Wallin G, et al: Inhibition of peritonitis by amide local anesthetics. Anesthesiology 1988;69:881–886.
88. Jayr C, Thomas H, Rey A, et al: Postoperative pulmonary complications: Epidural analgesia using bupivacaine and opioids versus parenteral opioids. Anesthesiology 1993;78:666–676.
89. Scheinin B, Asantila R, Orko R: The effect of bupivacaine and morphine on pain and bowel function after colonic surgery. Acta Anaesthesiol Scand 1987;31:161–164.
90. Thoren T, Sundberg A, Wattwil M, et al: Effects of epidural bupivacaine and epidural morphine on bowel function and pain after hysterectomy. Acta Anaesthesiol Scand 1989;33:181–185.
91. Holte K, Kehlet H: Epidural analgesia and risk of anastomotic leakage. Reg Anesth Pain Med 2001;26:111–117.
92. Liu SS, Block BM, Wu CL: Effects of perioperative central neuraxial analgesia on outcome after coronary artery bypass surgery: A meta-analysis. Anesthesiology 2004;101:153–161.
93. Sorenson RM, Pace NL: Anesthetic techniques during surgical repair of femoral neck fractures: A meta-analysis. Anesthesiology 1992;77:1095–1104.
94. Christopherson R, Beattie C, Frank SM, et al: Perioperative morbidity in patients randomized to epidural or general anesthesia for lower extremity vascular surgery. Anesthesiology 1993;79:422–434.
95. Tuman KJ, McCarthy RJ, March RJ, et al: Effects of epidural anesthesia and analgesia on coagulation and outcome after major vascular surgery. Anesth Analg 1991;73:696–704.

96. Beattie WS, Badner NH, Choi P: Epidural analgesia reduces post-operative myocardial infarction: A meta-analysis. Anesth Analg 2001; 93:853–858.

97. Veering BT, Cousins MJ: Cardiovascular and pulmonary effects of epidural anaesthesia. Anaesth Intensive Care 2000;28:620–635.

98. Davis RF, DeBoer LW, Maroko PR: Thoracic epidural anesthesia reduces myocardial infarct size after coronary artery occlusion in dogs. Anesth Analg 1986;65:711–717.

99. Rolf N, Van de Velde M, Wouters PF, et al: Thoracic epidural anesthesia improves functional recovery from myocardial stunning in conscious dogs. Anesth Analg 1996;83:935–940.

100. Kock M, Blomberg S, Emanuelsson H, et al: Thoracic epidural anes-thesia improves global and regional left ventricular function during stress-induced myocardial ischemia in patients with coronary artery disease. Anesth Analg 1990;71:625–630.

101. Magnusdottir H, Kirno K, Rickesten SE, et al: High thoracic epidural analgesia does not inhibit sympathetic nerve activity in the lower extremities. Anesthesiology 1999;91:1299–1304.

102. Chisakuta AM, George KA, Hawthorne CT: Postoperative epidural infusion of a mixture of bupivacaine 0.2% with fentanyl for upper abdominal surgery: A comparison of thoracic and lumbar routes. Anaesthesia 1995;50:72–75.

103. Hodgson PS, Liu SS: Thoracic epidural anaesthesia and analgesia for abdominal surgery: Effects on gastrointestinal function and perfusion. Balliere's Clini Anesthesiol 1999;13:9–22.

104. Scott AM, Starling JR, Ruscher AE, et al: Thoracic versus lumbar epidural anesthesia's effect on pain control and ileus resolution after restorative proctocolectomy. Surgery 1996;120:688–695.

105. Broekema AA, Gielen MJ, Hennis PJ: Postoperative analgesia with continuous epidural sufentanil and bupivacaine: A prospective study in 614 patients. Anesth Analg 1996;82:754–759.

106. Kahn L, Baxter FJ, Dauphin A, et al: A comparison of thoracic and lumbar epidural techniques for post-thoracoabdominal esophagec-tomy analgesia. Can J Anaesth 1999;46:415–422.

107. Wu CL, Hsu W, Richman JM, Raja SN: Postoperative cognitive function as an outcome of regional anesthesia and analgesia. Reg Anesth Pain Med 2004;29:257–268.

108. de Leon-Casasola OA: Immunomodulation and epidural anesthesia and analgesia. Reg Anesth 1996;21(Suppl):24–25.

109. Dalldorf PG, Perkins FM, Totterman S, et al: Deep venous thrombosis following total hip arthroplasty: Effects of prolonged postoperative epidural anesthesia. J Arthroplasty 1994;9:611–616.

110. Wu CL, Naqibuddin M, Fleisher LA: Measurement of patient satisfac-tion as an outcome of regional anesthesia and analgesia. Reg Anesth Pain Med 2001;26:196–208.

111. Allen HW, Liu SS, Ware PD, et al: Peripheral nerve blocks improve analgesia after total knee replacement surgery. Anesth Analg 1998; 87:93–97.

112. Mulroy MF, Larkin KL, Batra MS, et al: Femoral nerve block with 0.25% or 0.5% bupivacaine improves postoperative analgesia following outpatient arthroscopic anterior cruciate ligament repair. Reg Anesth Pain Med 2001;26:24–29.

113. Allen JG, Denny NM, Oakman N: Postoperative analgesia following total knee arthroplasty: A study comparing spinal anesthesia and combined sciatic femoral 3-in-1 block. Reg Anesth Pain Med 1998;23:142–146.

114. Wang H, Boctor B, Verner J: The effect of single-injection femoral nerve block on rehabilitation and length of hospital stay after total knee replacement. Reg Anesth Pain Med 2002;27:139–144.

115. Stevens RD, Van Gessel E, Flory N, et al: Lumbar plexus block reduces pain and blood loss associated with total hip arthroplasty. Anesthesiology 2000;93:115–121.

116. Borgeat A, Schappi B, Biasca N, et al: Patient-controlled analgesia after major shoulder surgery: Patient-controlled interscalene analgesia versus patient-controlled analgesia. Anesthesiology 1997;87:1343–1347.

117. Singelyn FJ, Deyaert M, Joris D, et al: Effects of intravenous patient-controlled analgesia with morphine, continuous epidural analgesia, and continuous three-in-one block on postoperative pain and knee rehabilitation after unilateral total knee arthroplasty. Anesth Analg 1998;87:88–92.

118. Kehlet H, Wilmore DW: Multimodal strategies to improve surgical outcome. Am J Surg 2002;183:630–641.

119. Kehlet H: Multimodal approach to control postoperative pathophysio-logy and rehabilitation. Br J Anaesth 1997;78:606–617.

120. Kehlet H, Holte K: Effect of postoperative analgesia on surgical outcome. Br J Anaesth 2001;87:62–72.

121. Barratt SM, Smith RC, Kee AJ, et al: Multimodal analgesia and intra-venous nutrition preserves total body protein following major upper gastrointestinal surgery. Reg Anesth Pain Med 2002;27:15–22.

122. Brodner G, Pogatzki E, Van Aken H, et al: A multimodal approach to control postoperative pathophysiology and rehabilitation in patients undergoing abdominothoracic esophagectomy. Anesth Analg 1998;86:228–234.

123. Brodner G, Van Aken H, Hertle L, et al: Multimodal perioperative management—combining thoracic epidural analgesia, forced mobi-lization, and oral nutrition—reduces hormonal and metabolic stress and improves convalescence after major urologic surgery. Anesth Analg 2001;92:1594–1600.

124. Basse L, Thorbol JE, Lossl K, Kehlet H: Colonic surgery with acceler-ated rehabilitation or conventional care. Dis Colon Rectum 2004;47: 271–277.

125. Neal JM, Wilcox RT, Allen HW, Low DE: Near-total esophagectomy: The influence of standardized multimodal management and intraop-erative fluid restriction. Reg Anesth Pain Med 2003;28:328–334.

126. Ready LB, Oden R, Chadwick HS, et al: Development of an anesthesiology-based postoperative pain management service. Anesthesiology 1988;68:100–106.

127. Rawal N: 10 years of acute pain services—achievements and challenges. Reg Anesth Pain Med 1999;24:68–73.

128. Brodner G, Mertes N, Buerkle H, et al: Acute pain management: Analysis, implications and consequences after prospective experience with 6349 surgical patients. Eur J Anaesthesiol 2000;17:566–575.

129. Bardiau FM, Braeckman MM, Seidel L, et al: Effectiveness of an acute pain service inception in a general hospital. J Clin Anesth 1999; 11:583–589.

130. Sartain JB, Barry JJ: The impact of an acute pain service on post-operative pain management. Anaesth Intensive Care 1999;27: 375–380.

131. Miaskowski C, Crews J, Ready LB, et al: Anesthesia-based pain services improve the quality of postoperative pain management. Pain 1999; 80:23–29.

132. Werner MU, Soholm L, Rotboll-Nielsen P, Kehlet H: Does an acute pain service improve postoperative outcome? Anesth Analg 2002; 95:1361–1372.

133. Stadler M, Schlander M, Braeckman M, et al: A cost-utility and cost-effectiveness analysis of an acute pain service. J Clin Anesth 2004;16:159–167.

134. Bardiau FM, Taviaux NF, Albert A, et al: An intervention study to enhance postoperative pain management. Anesth Analg 2003;96: 179–185.

9

Opioids: Excitatory Effects— Hyperalgesia, Tolerance, and the Postoperative Period

OLIVER H. G. WILDER-SMITH

It is now well established that the processing of noxious inputs by the nervous system is not hard-wired. A key insight of pain research over the last few decades has been the fact that *nociception* (the processing of noxious inputs) results in alterations of the gain for subsequent sensory processing,[1] a process termed *nociceptive neuroplasticity*. A typical—and undesirable—example is central sensitization due to surgery, which results in hyperalgesia and thus greater pain.[2] Obviously, drugs used for anesthesia and analgesia can be expected to modulate nociceptive inputs and affect subsequent nociceptive processing in their own right. Thus, the infusion of opioids inhibits nociceptive input—manifested by raised pain thresholds[3–5]—and also inhibits central sensitization as a result of surgical noxious inputs.[2]

A later insight is that such drugs can also have undesirable effects on pain processing. The use of opioids can result in excitatory neuroplasticity, particularly expressed as tolerance and hyperalgesia.[6] Other relevant excitatory effects are myoclonus, seizures, and nausea and vomiting. Clearly, such effects are undesirable in the postoperative context. There are two main reasons why hyperalgesia after surgery is unwanted. First, postoperative hyperalgesia results in increased pain, with all of its consequences (more stress, more complications, longer hospitalization, etc.) in the acute postoperative period.[7–9] Second, there is growing evidence that hyperalgesia that is excessive in intensity or duration in the postoperative period may be linked to the subsequent "chronification" of pain. This is because chronic pain after surgery is associated with nerve damage (a cause of hyperalgesia) and signs of persisting and intense postoperative pain (symptoms of hyperalgesia),[10,11] and because abnormal persistence of central sensitization is increasingly accepted to be a significant mechanism for pain "chronification" in general.[1,12]

The aims of this chapter are (1) to supply a brief overview of the mechanisms involved in the production of opioid-induced hyperalgesia (OIH) and tolerance, (2) to summarize evidence from animal research as to the reality of OIH and tolerance, (3) to provide support for the existence of OIH and tolerance in humans from volunteer and clinical research, and (4) to present possible strategies for dealing with OIH and tolerance in the clinical context.

Definitions

In the context of this chapter, *opioid-induced hyperalgesia* is defined as a reduction of pain thresholds below original baseline; it is considered a sign of positive system adaptation, or sensitization. *Tolerance* is defined as the need for more drug to achieve the same analgesic result despite stable levels of pain; it is considered a sign of negative system adaptation, or desensitization. It must be emphasized in this context that the clinical phenomenon of opioid-induced tolerance not only may be the result of a *loss* of drug sensitivity but also may occur because of an *increase* in pain sensitivity—for example, as the result of OIH (discussed later).

Mechanisms of Opioid-Induced Hyperalgesia

The binding of an opioid to the μ-opioid receptor (MOR) has both inhibitory and excitatory effects on pain processing—and this appears to be true even for a single opioid application.[6] Thus, MOR binding initiates both negative (inhibition, tolerance) and positive (excitation, hyperalgesia) feedback loops.

Mechanisms suggested to be implicated in the negative feedback loop are as follows:
- Downregulation of MOR populations; this mechanism has been largely discounted.[6]
- Desensitization of the MOR via uncoupling from inhibitory G-proteins, leading to decreased responsiveness of the associated K^+ channel.[13,14]
- Increased endocytosis of the MOR from the surface of neuronal cells.[15,16] Remifentanil may be particularly effective in this context.[3]
- Spinal cord neurotoxicity due to chronic opioid application. These potentially irreversible changes involve neuronal neuroplasticity and apoptosis mediated by N-methyl-D-aspartate (NMDA) receptor mechanisms, nitric oxide (NO), and poly(adenosine diphosphate–ribose) synthetase (PARS).[17]

Mechanisms proposed to be involved in the positive feedback loop are as follows:

- Phosphorylation and activation of the NMDA receptor via protein kinase Cγ (PKCγ).[6] The fact that NMDA agonism is pronociceptive is well documented.[18] This mechanism provides a positive feedback loop—resulting in an effect similar to that of long-term potentiation—via subsequent increases in intracellular calcium, which further stimulate PKCγ production. The involvement of the NMDA receptor means that there is substantial "cross-talk" between OIH and central sensitization as a result of noxious inputs. A further consequence of activating the NMDA receptor cascade is the calcium-calmodulin–modulated production of NO, which not only has the potential to modulate MOR expression[19] but may also activate glial cells, a process now well linked to the production of central hyperalgesia.[20-23]
- Increase in the excitatory Gs-coupled MOR state, modulated via increases in protein kinase A (PKA).[16] MOR can exist in both inhibitory (Gi/Go-coupled) and excitatory (Gs-coupled) states.[16]
- Release of spinal pronociceptive substances such as dynorphin. Prolonged exposure to opioids has been shown to result in the overproduction of spinal dynorphin, leading to hyperalgesia and loss of efficacy of opioids.[24-26]
- Descending facilitation from the rostral ventromedial medulla (RVM). A network of cells present in the RVM provides both inhibitory and excitatory modulation of spinal nociceptive inputs.[27-30] "On-cells" are considered to facilitate nociceptive input, whereas "off-cells" are believed to be inhibitory. Both of these cell populations are linked to MOR; if the balance of synaptic activity due to MOR activation favors the "on-cell" population, the result is hyperalgesia.
- Other postulated mechanisms for OIH are excitatory metabolites (e.g., morphine-3-glucoronide), possibly acting via antiglycinergic mechanisms.[31,32]

The mechanisms considered to be involved in the production of OIH are summarized in Box 9–1.

Evidence for the Existence of Opioid-Induced Hyperalgesia

ANIMAL DATA

The existence of OIH is now well documented in animal experiments. In 2000, Celerier et al[33] demonstrated dose-dependent hyperalgesia lasting up to 5 days after four injections, 15 minutes apart, of fentanyl in doses from 20 to 100 μg/kg in rats (Fig. 9–1). Other animal studies have shown similar effects.[33-38] Laulin et al[37] reported the important finding that such OIH reduces subsequent morphine analgesia—and that the application of naloxone unmasks this hyperalgesia 10 days later (Fig. 9–2). Other studies from this group using heroin have shown the long-term implications of this phenomenon: Daily application of heroin over 12 days resulted in rising hyperalgesia that took 2 weeks to resolve after cessation of heroin.[35] Application of

---

BOX 9–1

MECHANISMS CONSIDERED TO BE INVOLVED IN THE GENESIS OF OPIOID-INDUCED HYPERALGESIA

Central glutaminergic system: *N*-methyl-D-aspartate receptor
Spinal dynorphin release
Descending/supraspinal facilitation: "on-cells" and "off-cells" in rostral ventromedial medulla
Excitatory Gs-coupled mode μ-opioid-receptor: increased expression/effectiveness
Antiglycinergic effects
Metabolites (morphine-3-glucuronide)

---

a small, single dose of heroin more than a week after resolution of hyperalgesia (and more than a month after the start of the study) again produced marked and long-lasting hyperalgesia (*rekindling*) (Fig. 9–3).[35] Indeed, in a group of rats it proved possible to induce hyperalgesia using naloxone 2 months after cessation of 12 daily doses of heroin.[35] The induction of repeated cycles of heroin-induced hyperalgesia over a month or so demonstrated that the amount of hyperalgesia induced (i.e., area under the curve vs. baseline of each cycle) remained constant. However, in a comparison of the hyperalgesia states produced on day 1 and day 13, it was clear that the baseline from which hyperalgesia had been induced had itself been shifted in the direction of hyperalgesia (Fig. 9–4), thus explaining the phenomenon of (apparent) opioid tolerance.[35] There is now also evidence, based on the use of carrageenan-induced as well as surgery-induced nociception, that OIH and nociception-induced hyperalgesia (NIH) interact positively to produce greater and more extensive hyperalgesia (Fig. 9–5).[39,40]

In summary, studies thus far have shown that OIH in rodents

- Is a real and reliably inducible phenomenon
- Provides at least a partial explanation for opioid tolerance
- May be dose dependent
- Affects subsequent opioid analgesia over long periods
- Can be unmasked or rekindled over long periods
- Appears to produce a long-lasting state change affecting sensory processing
- May interact synergistically with NIH

HUMAN DATA

The evidence on OIH and tolerance in humans is more limited than that in animals. Nevertheless, a number of review articles have been published about OIH, including its possible clinical relevance.[6,41-43] Even before formal studies of this phenomenon were published, occasional case reports appeared in the literature describing its existence.[44-46] In the clinical context, first evidence for human OIH came from studies in opioid addicts, which clearly demonstrated that such persons had lower pain thresholds than unaddicted persons and that addicts showed a smaller analgesic response to opioids (Fig. 9–6).[47] Further (indirect) evidence supporting the reality of altered analgesic responses to opioids comes from a volunteer study involving remifentanil infusion during which pressure pain thresholds

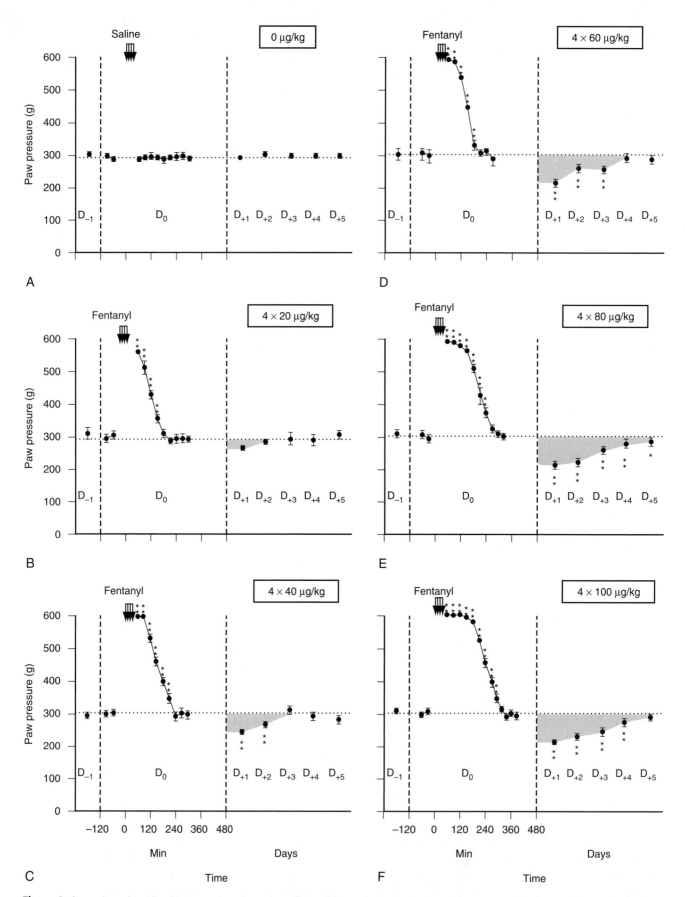

Figure 9–1 **A** through **F,** The short-term dose-dependent effects of fentanyl on pain sensitivity in rats. Pain sensitivity is determined by identifying the paw pressure (grams) at which the animal vocalizes. Values are means and SEM. *Solid circles* are the team time course of the thresholds (± SEM). *Asterisks* signify statistical significance versus baseline values for thresholds. *, $P < .05$; **, $P < .01$. D, day; Min, minutes. (From Celerier E, Rivat C, Jun Y, et al: Long-lasting hyperalgesia induced by fentanyl in rats: Preventive effect of ketamine. Anesthesiology 2000;92:465–472.)

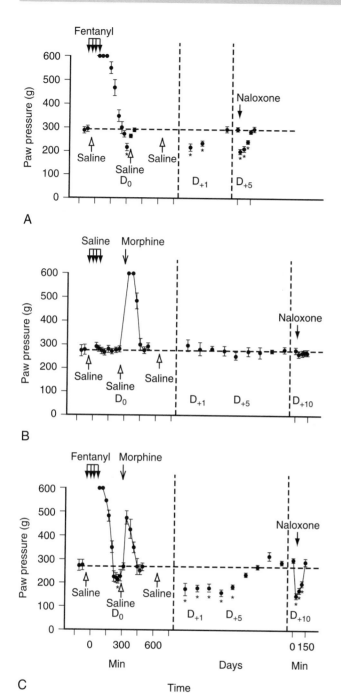

A

B

C

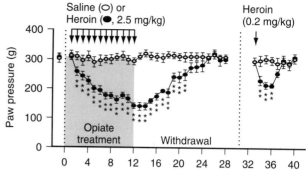

Figure 9–3 The long-term effects of heroin (2.5 mg/kg daily for 12 days) on pain sensitivity in rats. Pain sensitivity is determined by identifying the paw pressure (grams) at which the animal vocalizes. Note the long-lasting and cumulative nature of opioid-induced hyperalgesia and that it can be rekindled long after apparent normalization of pain sensitivity by a single, low-dose heroin injection. Values are means and SEM. *Asterisks* signify statistical significance versus baseline values for thresholds. *, $P < .05$; **, $P < .01$. (From Celerier E, Laulin JP, Corcuff JB, et al: Progressive enhancement of delayed hyperalgesia induced by repeated heroin administration: A sensitization process. J Neurosci 2001;21:4074–4080.)

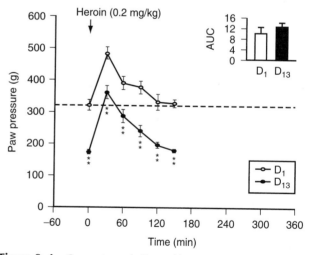

Figure 9–4 Comparison of effects of heroin (0.2 mg/kg given subcutaneously [SC]), given before and after 2.5 mg/kg heroin daily for 12 days, on pain sensitivity in rats, i.e., on day 1 (D_1) and D_{13}. Pain sensitivity is determined by identifying the paw pressure (g) at which the animal vocalizes. Note that the area under the curve (AUC; a measure of analgesic effect) is similar on D_1 and D_{13}. Thus, the reduction in analgesic effect (apparent tolerance) is explained by the reduction in baseline threshold, i.e., by opioid-induced hyperalgesia. Values are means and SEM. *Asterisks* signify statistical significance versus baseline values for thresholds. *, $P < .05$; **, $P < .01$. D, day; min, minutes. (From Celerier E, Laulin JP, Corcuff JB, et al: Progressive enhancement of delayed hyperalgesia induced by repeated heroin administration: A sensitization process. J Neurosci 2001;21:4074–4080.)

Figure 9–2 A through C, The medium-term effects of fentanyl (4 × 60 µg given subcutaneously [SC]) on pain sensitivity and morphine (5 mg/kg SC) analgesia in rats. Pain sensitivity is determined by identifying the paw pressure (g) at which the animal vocalizes. Note the long-lasting nature of opioid-induced hyperalgesia and that opioid hyperalgesia can be (re)produced 10 days later by naloxone injection. Values are means and SEM. *Solid circles* are the team time course of the thresholds (± SEM). *Asterisks* signify statistical significance versus baseline values for thresholds. *, $P < .05$; **, $P < .01$. D, day; Min, minutes. (From Laulin JP, Maurette P, Corcuff JB, et al: The role of ketamine in preventing fentanyl-induced hyperalgesia and subsequent acute morphine tolerance. Anesth Analg 2002;94:1263–1269.)

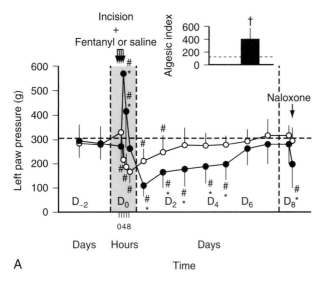

A

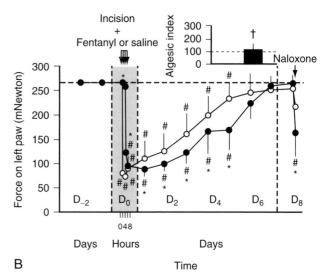

B

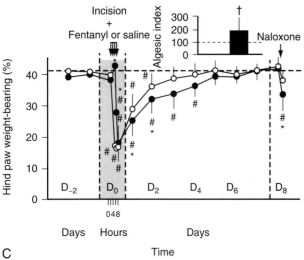

C

Figure 9–5   Synergistic effects of hyperalgesia produced by fentanyl on left rat hind paw plantar incision, in terms of mechanical hyperalgesia (**A**), tactile allodynia (**B**), and weight-bearing changes (**C**). A hind paw plantar incision was made in rats during halothane anesthesia on day 0 (D_0). Four doses of fentanyl (100 µg/kg) or saline injection were given subcutaneously (SC) at 15-minute intervals, resulting in a total dose of 400 µg/kg (n = 12). Surgery was performed just after the second fentanyl injection. The three pain parameters were evaluated before surgery on D_{-2}, D_{-1}, and D_0; at 2, 4, and 6 hours after surgery on D_0; and subsequently once daily for 8 days. At the end of the experiment (D_8), all rats were injected with naloxone (1 mg/kg SC), and the three pain parameters were measured 5 minutes later. *Insets,* Algesic index showing the variations of mechanical hyperalgesia (**A**), tactile allodynia (**B**), and weight-bearing (**C**) on the days after the incision. Pain parameter values and algesic index are expressed as mean ± SD. *Open circles,* saline-treated rats; *filled circles,* fentanyl-treated rats; **#**, Dunnett test, $P < .05$ compared with the D_0 basal value; *, Dunnett test, $P < .05$ for comparison between groups; †, Mann-Whitney test for algesic index comparison, $P < .05$. (From Richebe P, Rivat C, Laulin JP, et al: Ketamine improves the management of exaggerated postoperative pain observed in perioperative fentanyl-treated rats. Anesthesiology 2005;102:421–428.)

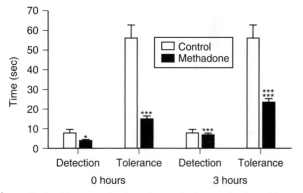

Figure 9–6   Time to pain detection and tolerance in the cold pressor test in patients on a methadone maintenance program compared with matched normal controls. For the patients, the first measurement took place circa 30 minutes before intake of the methadone dose, and the second 3 hours later. Values are means and SEM. *Asterisks* signify statistical significances. *, $P < .05$ for control versus methadone at 0 hr for detection. ***, $P < .001$ for control versus methadone at 0 hr for tolerance; $P < .001$ for control versus methadone at 3 hr for tolerance; $P < .001$ for 0 hr versus 3 hr for methadone for detection and tolerance. (From Doverty M, White JM, Somogyi AA, et al: Hyperalgesic responses in methadone maintenance patients. Pain 2001;90:91–96.)

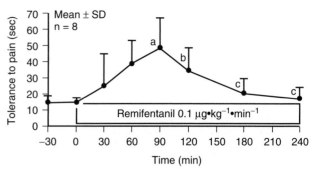

Figure 9–7   Time to pain tolerance in the cold pressor test in volunteers undergoing remifentanil infusion at a constant rate of 0.1 µg/kg/min. a, $P < .0001$ versus time 0; b, $P < .05$ versus 90 min; c, $P < .0001$ versus 90 min. (From Vinik HR, Kissin I: Rapid development of tolerance to analgesia during remifentanil infusion in humans. Anesth Analg 1998;86:1307–1311.)

were regularly measured. This study demonstrated that from 90 minutes of remifentanil infusion at 0.1 µg/kg/min onward, analgesic effect decreased, with no difference of pressure pain thresholds from original baseline values being demonstrable at the end of the study, after 240 minutes of remifentanil infusion (Fig. 9–7).[3]

A small number of placebo-controlled and prospective volunteer studies have formally investigated the presence of OIH in humans.[5,48,49] In all of these studies, some form of formal quantitative sensory testing (pain response to a defined sensory stimulus) was employed to quantify hyperalgesia, and pain report alone was not enough to diagnose hyperalgesia. All three of the cited studies showed evidence of hyperalgesia after the cessation of short-term (up to 30 minutes) remifentanil infusion in clinically typical doses.[5,48,49] One of the studies used pressure pain thresholds as an endpoint for hyperalgesia and demonstrated not only presence of hyperalgesia after the remifentanil infusion was stopped but also reduced analgesic effect (tolerance) during remifentanil infusion (Fig. 9–8).[49]

To date, only one placebo-controlled prospective study demonstrating OIH in the postoperative period has been published.[50] However, the volunteer studies cited can be considered to provide supporting evidence for the existence of this phenomenon in humans, albeit without yet providing any evidence for its significance or relevance in the clinical context.

Evidence for the Modulation of Opioid-Induced Hyperalgesia

ANIMAL DATA

As already mentioned, there is much theoretical evidence linking activation of excitatory amino acid receptor systems

such as the NMDA receptor to OIH and tolerance. Most animal research on the modulation—and hence potential prevention and treatment—of OIH and tolerance has thus focused on the use of NMDA blockers. Opioid tolerance has been shown to be reduced by the use of ketamine to achieve noncompetitive NMDA receptor blockade in rats.[51] Several rat

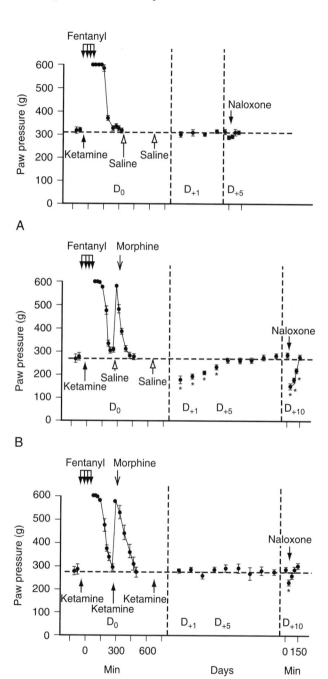

B

C

Time

Figure 9–9 A through C, The effects of single and multiple ketamine doses (10 mg/kg given subcutaneously [SC]) started before fentanyl application (4 × 60 µg/kg SC) on subsequent pain sensitivity and morphine analgesia (5 mg/kg SC) in rats. Pain sensitivity is determined by identifying the paw pressure (grams) at which the animal vocalizes. Values are means and SEM. *Asterisks* signify statistical significances. D, day; Min, minutes. (From Laulin JP, Maurette P, Corcuff JB, et al: The role of ketamine in preventing fentanyl-induced hyperalgesia and subsequent acute morphine tolerance. Anesth Analg 2002;94: 1263–1269.)

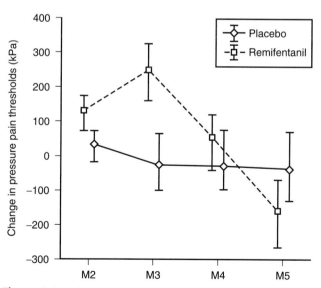

Figure 9–8 Change (compared with baseline) in pressure pain threshold (kPa) during remifentanil or placebo (saline) infusion. At measurement 2 (M2), the target plasma concentration of remifentanil was 1 µg/mL, at M3 it was 2 µg/mL, and at M4 it was 1 µg/kg again. M5 was obtained 10 minutes after the end of the infusion. Values are means and 95% confidence intervals. (Modified from Luginbuhl M, Gerber A, Schnider TW, et al: Modulation of remifentanil-induced analgesia, hyperalgesia, and tolerance by small-dose ketamine in humans. Anesth Analg 2003;96:726–732.)

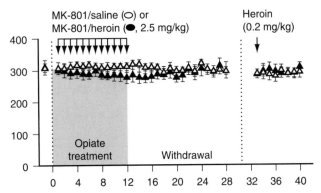

Figure 9–10 How the coapplication of MK-801 (0.15 mg/kg given subcutaneously [SC] 30 minutes before each heroin administration) prevented not only opioid-induced hyperalgesia due to 12 days of heroin (2.5 mg/kg SC) but also rekindling of hyperalgesia by a small dose of heroin given later. Pain sensitivity is determined by identifying the paw pressure (grams) at which the animal vocalizes. Values are means and SEM. Compare with Figure 9–4. (From Celerier E, Laulin JP, Corcuff JB, et al: Progressive enhancement of delayed hyperalgesia induced by repeated heroin administration: A sensitization process. J Neurosci 2001;21:4074–4080.)

studies have demonstrated that NMDA receptor blockade is effective in the prevention of OIH using ketamine[33,37] or MK-801.[34,35] Thus, a single dose of ketamine given before fentanyl dosing reduces subsequent hyperalgesia and improves morphine analgesia, with repeated dosing resulting in better effects (Fig. 9–9).[37] Equally, repeated dosing with MK-801 in the context of long-term heroin application not only prevents production of rising hyperalgesia but also inhibits subsequent late rekindling of hyperalgesia by further opioid or opioid antagonist dosing (Fig. 9–10).[35] Of particular importance is the fact that NMDA antagonism by ketamine also depresses the synergism between OIH and NIH (Fig. 9–11).[39,40]

In summary, we now possess good animal evidence that establishment of NMDA receptor blockade by ketamine before opioid application is able to strongly inhibit subsequent induction of hyperalgesia. These effects are visible in both

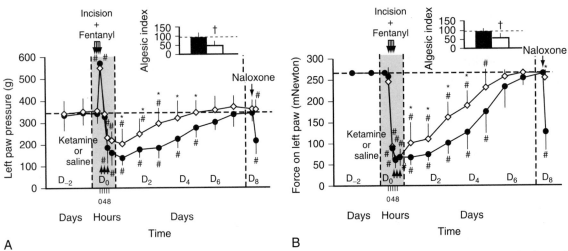

Figure 9–11 Effects of ketamine on the fentanyl enhancement of mechanical hyperalgesia (**A**), tactile allodynia (**B**), and weight-bearing changes (**C**) induced by hind paw plantar incision. A hind paw plantar incision was made in rats during halothane anesthesia on day 0 (D_0). Four doses of fentanyl (100 µg/kg) or saline injection were given subcutaneously (SC) at 15-minute intervals, resulting in a total dose of 400 µg/kg (n = 12). Surgery was performed just after the second fentanyl injection. Three ketamine (3 × 10 mg/kg; n = 12) or saline boluses (n = 12) were subcutaneously administered. The first one was performed 30 minutes before surgery, and the following injections were performed every 5 hours. The three pain parameters were evaluated before surgery on D_{-2}, D_{-1}, and D_0; at 2, 4, 6, and 10 hours after the surgery on D_0; and subsequently once daily for 8 days. At the end of the experiment (D_8), all rats were injected with naloxone (1 mg/kg SC), and the three pain parameters were measured 5 minutes later. *Insets,* Algesic index showing the variations of mechanical hyperalgesia (**A**), tactile allodynia (**B**), and weight-bearing (**C**) on the days after the incision. Pain parameter values and algesic index are expressed as mean ± SD. *Filled circles,* saline-fentanyl-treated rats; *open diamonds,* ketamine-fentanyl-treated rats; #, Dunnett test, $P < .05$ compared with the D_0 basal value; *, Dunnett test, $P < .05$ for comparison between groups; †, Mann-Whitney test for algesic index comparison, $P < .05$. (From Richebe P, Rivat C, Laulin JP, et al: Ketamine improves the management of exaggerated postoperative pain observed in perioperative fentanyl-treated rats. Anesthesiology 2005;102:421–428.)

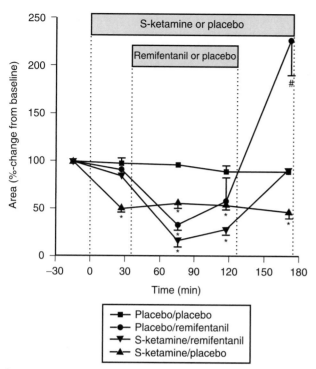

Figure 9–12 The infusion of the *N*-methyl-D-aspartate (NMDA) receptor antagonist *S*-ketamine, the μ-opioid agonist remifentanil (Remi), and the combination of *S*-ketamine and remifentanil significantly decreased the area of mechanical hyperalgesia by 50% to 75%(*). However, once the infusion was stopped (#), the area of mechanical hyperalgesia exceeded the preinfusion value by about 130% for remifentanil administered alone. Coadministration of *S*-ketamine abolished the expansion of mechanical hyperalgesia associated with administration of remifentanil alone. The area of mechanical hyperalgesia remained stable throughout the experiment if saline placebo was infused (two-way repeated measures, analysis of variance, *P* < .01 for all comparisons). Values are means and SD. (From Angst MS, Koppert W, Pahl I, et al: Short-term infusion of the mu-opioid agonist remifentanil in humans causes hyperalgesia during withdrawal. Pain 2003;106:49–57.)

the short and long term, with NMDA receptor blockade preventing the state change responsible for late uncovering and rekindling of OIH. These effects are more marked if NMDA receptor blockade is continued beyond the initial dose. We have no hard evidence at the moment as to the effectiveness of post hoc NMDA blockade, as would be practiced in the therapeutic—as opposed to prophylactic—context. Of great potential consequence in the surgical context is the demonstration that NMDA receptor blockade inhibits the synergism between OIH and NIH.

HUMAN DATA

Quite a bit of evidence from the literature indirectly supports the positive effect of NMDA receptor blockade on OIH and tolerance via its effect on human postoperative pain and opioid consumption.[52–56] The effect of prophylactic NMDA receptor blockade in the prevention of OIH has, to date, been investigated formally in only three prospective placebo-controlled human volunteer studies.[5,48,49] In two studies using a model involving hyperalgesia induced and maintained by transcutaneous stimulation, Koppert et al[5,48] were able to demonstrate that ketamine infusion started before remifentanil infusion prevented the increases in hyperalgesic area seen after remifentanil infusion alone (Fig. 9–12). Interestingly, in one of these studies, the group demonstrated that although ketamine has more effect on objective measures of altered sensory processing (area of hyperalgesia), the α_2-receptor agonist clonidine had a greater effect on subjective pain experience, suggesting differential effects on various aspects of OIH (Fig. 9–13).[5] The third study, using pressure pain thresholds and conducted by Luginbuhl et al,[49] was unable to demonstrate a significant effect of ketamine, probably owing to the short duration of remifentanil infusion in combination with relatively low plasma ketamine concentrations. One recent study has demonstrated positive

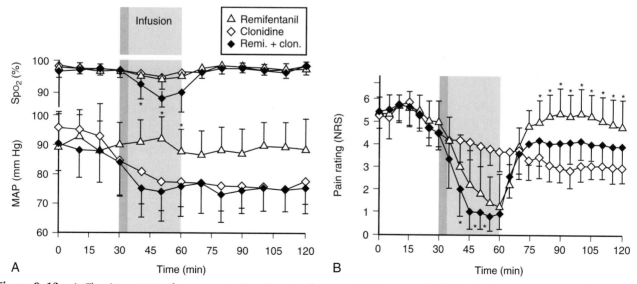

Figure 9–13 **A,** The time course of oxygen saturation (SpO_2) and mean arterial pressure (MAP) during the experiment. Coadministration of clonidine (2 μg/kg over a period of 5 minutes before remifentanil) with remifentanil (0.1 μg/kg/min) shortened the onset of remifentanil-induced analgesia and decreased remifentanil-induced postinfusion antianalgesia (*P* < .001 by analysis of variance [ANOVA]) (**B**) and

Continued

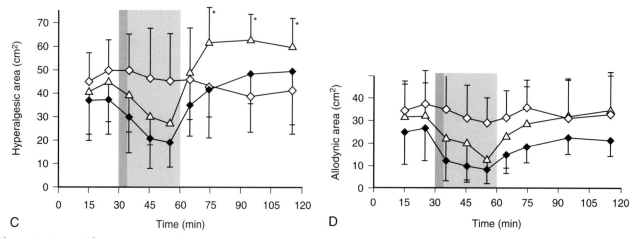

Figure 9–13, cont'd punctate hyperalgesia ($P < .001$ by ANOVA) (**C**). Areas of touch-evoked allodynia were not affected (**D**) (P is not significant by ANOVA for each). Data are expressed as mean ± SD (n = 13). *, $P < .05$, planned comparisons corrected with the Bonferroni procedure. NRS, numerical rating scale. (From Koppert W, Sittl R, Scheuber K, et al: Differential modulation of remifentanil-induced analgesia and postinfusion hyperalgesia by S-ketamine and clonidine in humans. Anesthesiology 2003;99:152–159.)

effects of ketamine supplementation on remifentanil-induced hyperalgesia after major abdominal surgery.[50]

At present, the human evidence for the preventive effects on OIH of NMDA receptor blockade using ketamine must be regarded as limited but promising. Clearly, further studies are needed, in particular with regard to establishing the clinical reality and significance of this effect.

Summary and Conclusions

Convincing animal evidence is now available about the mechanisms of OIH and tolerance. This evidence suggests that the underlying state change can be long lasting, that it affects subsequent opioid analgesia, and that it can be unmasked or rekindled a considerable length of time later by substances interacting with the opioid receptor. Human evidence for the reality and nature of OIH and tolerance— in essence concordant with animal-derived data—is now also available, albeit based on only a few human studies. There is thus a need for further research to establish and define the clinical relevance of this phenomenon in the postoperative context.

As could be expected from the experimental link between opioid and NMDA receptors, animal evidence now also exists as to the effectiveness of NMDA receptor blockade by ketamine or MK-801 in inhibiting the establishment of OIH and tolerance. Although the animal evidence can be regarded as convincing, the human evidence for such therapy is limited to a few (well-designed and well-realized) volunteer and clinical studies. Therefore, much further research is needed to substantiate these first studies in humans to establish the clinical significance and relevance of these findings.

As detailed earlier in the chapter, it is evident that postoperative hyperalgesia is highly undesirable, with both short- and long-term potential to significantly worsen outcomes after surgery. Thus, the available evidence that our current analgesic management may be causing or worsening the very situation we are trying to avoid is troubling and in need of urgent attention. Clearly, there is a need for well-designed and clinically relevant studies on this topic.

How should the evidence presented here affect the daily practice of the clinician? Managing postoperative hyperalgesia may yet prove the key to substantially improving pain management after surgery. Admittedly, specific, definitive, high-level clinical evidence about OIH and its modulation by NMDA receptor blockade is not yet available. However, the strongly suggestive supporting evidence available, in combination with the existing convincing, high-level information about the positive nonspecific effects of low-dose ketamine on postoperative pain outcomes,[51,54–56] should lead every clinician to consider the possibility of adding this concept to his or her repertoire of clinical practice while awaiting the definitive evidence.

REFERENCES

1. Woolf CJ, Salter MW: Neuronal plasticity: Increasing the gain in pain. Science 2000;288:1765–1769.
2. Wilder-Smith OH, Tassonyi E, Crul BJ, Arendt-Nielsen L: Quantitative sensory testing and human surgery: Effects of analgesic management on postoperative neuroplasticity. Anesthesiology 2003;98:1214–1222.
3. Vinik HR, Kissin I: Rapid development of tolerance to analgesia during remifentanil infusion in humans. Anesth Analg 1998;86:1307–1311.
4. Leung A, Wallace MS, Ridgeway B, Yaksh T: Concentration-effect relationship of intravenous alfentanil and ketamine on peripheral neurosensory thresholds, allodynia and hyperalgesia of neuropathic pain. Pain 2001;91:177–187.
5. Koppert W, Sittl R, Scheuber K, et al: Differential modulation of remifentanil-induced analgesia and postinfusion hyperalgesia by S-ketamine and clonidine in humans. Anesthesiology 2003;99:152–159.
6. Simonnet G, Rivat C: Opioid-induced hyperalgesia: Abnormal or normal pain? Neuroreport 2003;14:1–7.
7. Kehlet H: Postoperative pain relief—what is the issue? Br J Anaesth 1994;72:375–378.
8. Carli F, Mayo N, Klubien K, et al: Epidural analgesia enhances functional exercise capacity and health-related quality of life after colonic surgery: Results of a randomized trial. Anesthesiology 2002;97:540–549.
9. Rodgers A, Walker N, Schug S, et al: Reduction of postoperative mortality and morbidity with epidural or spinal anaesthesia: Results from overview of randomised trials. BMJ 2000;321:1493.

10. Macrae WA: Chronic pain after surgery. Br J Anaesth 2001;87:88–98.
11. Perkins FM, Kehlet H: Chronic pain as an outcome of surgery: A review of predictive factors. Anesthesiology 2000;93:1123–1133.
12. Coderre TJ, Katz J, Vaccarino AL, Melzack R: Contribution of central neuroplasticity to pathological pain: Review of clinical and experimental evidence. Pain 1993;52:259–285.
13. Christie MJ, Williams JT, North RA: Mechanisms of tolerance to opiates in locus coeruleus neurons. NIDA Res Monogr 1987;78:158–168.
14. Christie MJ, Williams JT, North RA: Cellular mechanisms of opioid tolerance: Studies in single brain neurons. Mol Pharmacol 1987;32:633–638.
15. Whistler JL, Chuang HH, Chu P, et al: Functional dissociation of mu opioid receptor signaling and endocytosis: Implications for the biology of opiate tolerance and addiction. Neuron 1999;23:737–746.
16. Crain SM, Shen KF: Antagonists of excitatory opioid receptor functions enhance morphine's analgesic potency and attenuate opioid tolerance/dependence liability. Pain 2000;84:121–131.
17. Mao J, Mayer DJ: Spinal cord neuroplasticity following repeated opioid exposure and its relation to pathological pain. Ann N Y Acad Sci 2001;933:175–184.
18. Aanonsen LM, Wilcox GL: Nociceptive action of excitatory amino acids in the mouse: Effects of spinally administered opioids, phencyclidine and sigma agonists. J Pharmacol Exp Ther 1987;243:9–19.
19. Cadet P, Mantione K, Bilfinger TV, Stefano GB: Real-time RT-PCR measurement of the modulation of Mu opiate receptor expression by nitric oxide in human mononuclear cells. Med Sci Monit 2001;7:1123–1128.
20. Watkins LR, Milligan ED, Maier SF: Glial activation: A driving force for pathological pain. Trends Neurosci 2001;24:450–455.
21. Watkins LR, Milligan ED, Maier SF: Glial proinflammatory cytokines mediate exaggerated pain states: Implications for clinical pain. Adv Exp Med Biol 2003;521:1–21.
22. DeLeo JA, Tanga FY, Tawfik VL: Neuroimmune activation and neuroinflammation in chronic pain and opioid tolerance/hyperalgesia. Neuroscientist 2004;10:40–52.
23. Wieseler-Frank J, Maier SF, Watkins LR: Immune-to-brain communication dynamically modulates pain: Physiological and pathological consequences. Brain Behav Immun 2005;19:104–111.
24. Vanderah TW, Ossipov MH, Lai J, et al: Mechanisms of opioid-induced pain and antinociceptive tolerance: Descending facilitation and spinal dynorphin. Pain 2001;92:5–9.
25. Gardell LR, Wang R, Burgess SE, et al: Sustained morphine exposure induces a spinal dynorphin-dependent enhancement of excitatory transmitter release from primary afferent fibers. J Neurosci 2002;22:6747–6755.
26. Ossipov MH, Lai J, Vanderah TW, Porreca F: Induction of pain facilitation by sustained opioid exposure: Relationship to opioid antinociceptive tolerance. Life Sci 2003;73:783–800.
27. Fields HL, Vanegas H, Hentall ID, Zorman G: Evidence that disinhibition of brain stem neurones contributes to morphine analgesia. Nature 1983;306:684–686.
28. Schnell C, Ulucan C, Ellrich J: Atypical on-, off- and neutral cells in the rostral ventromedial medulla oblongata in rat. Exp Brain Res 2002;145:64–75.
29. McGaraughty S, Reinis S, Tsoukatos J: Two distinct unit activity responses to morphine in the rostral ventromedial medulla of awake rats. Brain Res 1993;604:331–333.
30. Heinricher MM, Neubert MJ: Neural basis for the hyperalgesic action of cholecystokinin in the rostral ventromedial medulla. J Neurophysiol 2004;92:1982–1989.
31. Yaksh TL, Harty GJ: Pharmacology of the allodynia in rats evoked by high dose intrathecal morphine. J Pharmacol Exp Ther 1988;244:501–507.
32. Smith MT: Neuroexcitatory effects of morphine and hydromorphone: Evidence implicating the 3-glucuronide metabolites. Clin Exp Pharmacol Physiol 2000;27:524–528.
33. Celerier E, Rivat C, Jun Y, et al: Long-lasting hyperalgesia induced by fentanyl in rats: Preventive effect of ketamine. Anesthesiology 2000;92:465–472.
34. Celerier E, Laulin J, Larcher A, et al: Evidence for opiate-activated NMDA processes masking opiate analgesia in rats. Brain Res 1999;847:18–25.
35. Celerier E, Laulin JP, Corcuff JB, et al: Progressive enhancement of delayed hyperalgesia induced by repeated heroin administration: A sensitization process. J Neurosci 2001;21:4074–4080.
36. Laulin JP, Celerier E, Larcher A, et al: Opiate tolerance to daily heroin administration: An apparent phenomenon associated with enhanced pain sensitivity. Neuroscience 1999;89:631–636.
37. Laulin JP, Maurette P, Corcuff JB, et al: The role of ketamine in preventing fentanyl-induced hyperalgesia and subsequent acute morphine tolerance. Anesth Analg 2002;94:1263–1269.
38. Laulin JP, Larcher A, Celerier E, et al: Long-lasting increased pain sensitivity in rat following exposure to heroin for the first time. Eur J Neurosci 1998;10:782–785.
39. Rivat C, Laulin JP, Corcuff JB, et al: Fentanyl enhancement of carrageenan-induced long-lasting hyperalgesia in rats: Prevention by the N-methyl-D-aspartate receptor antagonist ketamine. Anesthesiology 2002;96:381–391.
40. Richebe P, Rivat C, Laulin JP, et al: Ketamine improves the management of exaggerated postoperative pain observed in perioperative fentanyl-treated rats. Anesthesiology 2005;102:421–428.
41. Koppert W: [Opioid-induced hyperalgesia. Pathophysiology and clinical relevance.] Anaesthesist 2004;53:455–466.
42. Mao J: Opioid-induced abnormal pain sensitivity: Implications in clinical opioid therapy. Pain 2002;100:213–217.
43. Mercadante S, Ferrera P, Villari P, Arcuri E: Hyperalgesia: An emerging iatrogenic syndrome. J Pain Symptom Manage 2003;26:769–775.
44. Twycross R: Paradoxical pain. BMJ 1993;306:793.
45. Hanks GW, O'Neill WM, Fallon MT: Paradoxical pain. BMJ 1993;306:793.
46. Bowsher D: Paradoxical pain. BMJ 1993;306:473–474.
47. Doverty M, White JM, Somogyi AA, et al: Hyperalgesic responses in methadone maintenance patients. Pain 2001;90:91–96.
48. Angst MS, Koppert W, Pahl I, et al: Short-term infusion of the mu-opioid agonist remifentanil in humans causes hyperalgesia during withdrawal. Pain 2003;106:49–57.
49. Luginbuhl M, Gerber A, Schnider TW, et al: Modulation of remifentanil-induced analgesia, hyperalgesia, and tolerance by small-dose ketamine in humans. Anesth Analg 2003;96:726–732.
50. Joly V, Richebe P, Guignard B, et al: Remifentanil-induced postoperative hyperalgesia and its prevention with small-dose ketamine. Anesthesiology 2005;103:147–155.
51. Kissin I, Bright CA, Bradley EL Jr: The effect of ketamine on opioid-induced acute tolerance: Can it explain reduction of opioid consumption with ketamine-opioid analgesic combinations? Anesth Analg 2000;91:1483–1488.
52. Schmid RL, Sandler AN, Katz J: Use and efficacy of low-dose ketamine in the management of acute postoperative pain: A review of current techniques and outcomes. Pain 1999;82:111–125.
53. De Kock M, Lavand'homme P, Waterloos H: 'Balanced analgesia' in the perioperative period: Is there a place for ketamine? Pain 2001;92:373–380.
54. McCartney CJ, Sinha A, Katz J: A qualitative systematic review of the role of N-methyl-D-aspartate receptor antagonists in preventive analgesia. Anesth Analg 2004;98:1385–1400.
55. Raith K, Hochhaus G: Drugs used in the treatment of opioid tolerance and physical dependence: A review. Int J Clin Pharmacol Ther 2004;42:191–203.
56. Subramaniam K, Subramaniam B, Steinbrook RA: Ketamine as adjuvant analgesic to opioids: A quantitative and qualitative systematic review. Anesth Analg 2004;99:482–495.

10 Defining Pain Management Objectives

PETER G. MOORE

Rationale for Compassionate Care

In recent years, widespread concerns about the misdiagnosis and undertreatment of pain have drawn the attention of legislators, state and federal regulatory agencies, and the healthcare industry.[1-5] This attention has led to the establishment of regulations and standards for healthcare providers and healthcare organizations on the recognition and treatment of pain as a primary objective of patient care.[4,6,7]

In setting a national agenda, Dennis S. O'Leary, MD, president of the Joint Commission on Accreditation of Healthcare Organizations (JCAHO), said: "Unrelieved pain has enormous physiological and psychological effects on patients. The Joint Commission believes the effective management of pain is a crucial component of good care." He continued, "Research clearly shows that unrelieved pain can slow recovery, create burdens for patients and their families, and increase costs to the health care system."[8]

Postoperative pain is defined primarily as acute pain caused by tissue injury associated with surgery. Although surgery and the attendant trauma in themselves result in acute pain, they may not be the only causes of postoperative pain; considerable pain may result from patient positioning or pressure effects owing to prolonged immobility. Furthermore, many patients may suffer chronic pain from underlying illness or injury, such as degenerative diseases or malignancy, that may contribute significantly to the intensity of the postoperative pain they experience.

The fundamental principle of postoperative pain management is founded on the notion that pain relief is a basic human right[9] and in itself is an achievable endpoint that promotes healing and recovery. By accepting this principle, we reject the notion that pain is an inevitable consequence of the tissue trauma and surgery. Thus, the goals of postoperative pain management are to alleviate pain and suffering and to promote healing and recovery.

The JCAHO, in setting goals for healthcare organizations, has set out to define the fundamental principles for reform (Table 10–1).[8] Those goals demand that healthcare organizations and all care providers commit to and believe in the fundamental principles of patient care and patient rights.

The JCAHO standard begins with a statement as to the rights of patients to appropriate assessment and management. The basic concept is that pain management, rather than being an adjuvant therapy, is an intrinsic and indivisible component of therapy. The fundamental principles of compassionate care are derived from the following principles that guide all therapies:

- The primacy of patient welfare—an obligation to heal and relieve pain and suffering despite the physical harm of surgery.

TABLE 10–1	Joint Commission on Accreditation of Healthcare Organizations Recommendations for Pain Management
Rights and ethics	Recognize the right of patients to appropriate assessment and management of pain
Assessment of pain	Assess the existence and, if so, the nature and intensity of pain in all patients
	Record the results of the asessment in a way that facilitates regular reassessment and follow-up
Patient care	Establish policies and procedures that support the appropriate prescription or ordering of effective pain medications
Patient education	Educate patients and their families about effective pain management
Continuum of care	Address patient needs for symptom management in the discharge planning process
Quality improvement and organization performance	Determine and assure staff competency in pain assessment and management, and address pain assessment and management in the orientation of all new staff

Adapted from Joint Commission on Accreditation of Healthcare Organizations: Joint Commission focuses on pain management. Aug 3, 1999. Available at www.jcaho.org/news+room/health+care+issues/jcaho+focus+on+pain+management.htm

- Patient autonomy and informed consent—recognition of the right of the patient to make informed decisions as to the care he or she will receive.
- Social justice and equitable care—commitment to a standard of care based on patient need.

By adopting these fundamental tenets, we accept the right of our patients (1) to know about their condition and the various treatment options, including risks, and (2) to be informed about, participate in, and concur with the formation of a perioperative management plan.

Evidence for Preoperative Patient Education

Despite the recent focus on the undertreatment of pain, there is good evidence that pain during postoperative recovery may be inadequately treated in up to half of all surgical procedures; the overall incidence of moderate to severe pain in surgical patients is about 25% to 40% despite the availability of pain treatment.[10–12] Whereas this is a substantial improvement over results of previous studies of hospitalized medical and surgical patients, which reported an 87% incidence of moderate to severe pain and a 41% incidence of delay in drug treatment,[13] pain remains a substantial problem that is often masked by a patient's acceptance of pain as a natural consequence of surgery.[12]

It would seem obvious that an episode of uncontrollable and/or poorly managed pain, regardless of its brevity, would be sufficient to color a patient's whole perspective of the care he or she has received, but this impression may not be borne out through patient surveys.[14–16]

Patient satisfaction alone, however, may be an insufficient measure of the effectiveness of pain treatment.[14–16] That is, the assessment of effectiveness of pain treatment can be determined only when pain assessment measures are used and patients are specifically surveyed as to the severity of pain experienced during hospitalization.[15,17–22]

The beneficial effects of preoperative patient education are realized through the alleviation of anxiety, apprehension, and fear and the understanding therein that pain control is an expected goal of postoperative care.[23–40] Common patient barriers include cultural and language barriers,[17] stoicism and/or opiophobia, and personal experience or the experiences of friends and relatives.[17,25,37,41–45] These barriers may be removed through patient education and counseling as well as by changing attitudes of caregivers.[40,45–47] There is good evidence that an active educational program carried out by informed physicians and nurses directed at preoperative patient preparation results in a better postoperative outcome.[26,34,35,48–63]

Evidence for Preoperative Pain Intervention for Preexisting Pain

It is estimated that most patients presenting for elective surgery have moderate to severe chronic and/or disabling pain from an underlying disease.[24,25,31,49,64,65] The implementation of active preoperative pain management programs is successful in improving postoperative pain and recovery for patients with degenerative joint diseases who undergo joint arthroplasty.[20,24,26,27,34,35,39,49,54,64,66–75] The September 2004 withdrawal of rofecoxib from the market and concerns about the cyclooxygenase-2 (Cox-2) class of drugs as a whole are of particular concern.[76–86] As this is still a rapidly evolving story, the impact of the withdrawal of Cox-2 pain therapies on perioperative pain management is unknown.[87,88]

Evidence for Preemptive Analgesia

The concept of preemptive analgesia is based on laboratory studies showing that preoperative analgesic intervention reduces the intensity of postoperative pain by blocking or attenuating the neurophysiological and neurotransmitter changes evoked by nociceptive stimuli—in other words, preemptive analgesia inhibits the "wind-up" phenomenon.[89–91] The experimental evidence, largely from animal models, is sound, but the implementation of preemptive analgesia in clinical practice has met with mixed results. Although ketamine,[92–94] neuraxial analgesia,[89,92,95–97] local agents,[98–100] nonsteroidal anti-inflammatory drugs (NSAIDs),[101–117] and parenteral opioids, alone or in combination,[94,98–100, 103,105,108–111,114–119] vary in effectiveness in mediating postoperative analgesia in the immediate postoperative period, the evidence is weak or not significant for a salutary effect on the development of chronic postoperative pain syndromes.[92,97–99,112,118,120,121]

Evidence for Multimodal Pain Therapy

The consensus that postoperative pain is a multifactorial problem requiring a multimodal therapeutic plan is strongly supported by a number of clinical studies.[67,99,110,117,122–131] They show that multimodal therapy, in contrast to a single therapy, improves surgical outcome. Several outcome studies provide solid evidence for a multimodal approach to postoperative pain that includes pharmacotherapies directed at different sites of action as well as supportive or complementary measures supervised by an adequately resourced acute pain team.[132–135]

Evidence for "Acute Pain Teams"

The establishment of institutional pain services or "acute pain teams" is a major initiative to improve pain management in hospitalized patients.[136–142] Although some studies have questioned the effectiveness of acute pain teams, they have for the most part proved their worth.[50,143–145] However, considerable barriers challenge the establishment and/or effectiveness of acute pain teams.[144,146–150] A major impediment to their establishment is cost, as in a privatized system with limited reimbursement for their services.[147,148] The value of an acute pain service apart from its benefit for patient care also comes from the added benefit of reducing hospital costs by improving surgical outcome and facilitating patient recovery and early discharge.[145]

Evidence that the Establishment of Pain Standards Has Improved Patient Care

In 2000, as the primary agency for setting quality standards in the United States, the JCAHO proposed national goals and standards to address institutional deficiencies in the treatment of pain in hospitalized patients.[2] The proposal is based on the assumption that the development of effective pain management strategies will result in improved patient care.[143] However, surveys published in 2003 and 2004 suggest that despite improvements in pain management, a significant number of patients still experience moderate to severe pain during hospitalization.[12,50,146,149-151] The consensus is that although the management of pain in hospitalized patients has improved overall, much more work must be done with respect to patient education as well as the education of physicians and nurses to prioritize pain management objectives before further gains are observed.[12,152-154] This statement assumes that all staff members participating in the perioperative care of patients understand that relief of pain and suffering is a non-negotiable objective of care—i.e., pain management is not an adjuvant therapy but is integrated into the disease management plan.[155-157]

Recommendations

PATIENT-CENTERED MULTIMODAL THERAPY

The primary objective of postoperative pain management is to prevent and/or relieve pain and suffering as an integral component of surgical management. The perioperative pain management plan must be individualized to each patient's needs, wherein relief from pain and suffering due to both the patient's underlying disease and operative trauma hastens recovery and return to normal function.

A multimodal management plan should address the various mechanisms that may cause nociceptive stimuli and potentially unnecessary pain. The pain management plan must take into account preexisting painful conditions and must address fears, anxieties, and misunderstandings that will affect the patient's perception of pain, willingness to report pain states, and potential for somatic amplification.

INSTITUTIONAL COMMITMENT

Effective management of postoperative pain requires an institutional commitment with defined objectives of care in which all staff involved in patient care embrace pain relief as a primary objective in healing and recovery for all patients after surgery. Commensurate with this objective is the assignment of pain management as a priority. In order to ensure that all patients have access to appropriate pain measures, the institution is obligated to standardize management protocols throughout the organization and educate all healthcare personnel as to those practice standards. The overall establishment of institutional pain policies and staff education should be under the direction of a multidisciplinary pain management work group that involves pain specialists, anesthesiologists, surgeons, clinical nurse specialists, pharmacists, and house staff in developing policies, educating staff, and closely monitoring and implementing quality improvement measures (Fig. 10–1).

A key element of patient management is the establishment of acute pain management teams to direct and coordinate pain management plans in consultation with the primary treatment teams (Fig. 10–2). In view of the central importance of

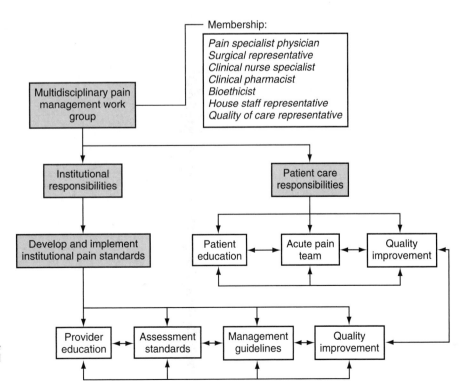

Figure 10–1 Suggested strategy for the development of institutional policies and procedures for "acute pain services."

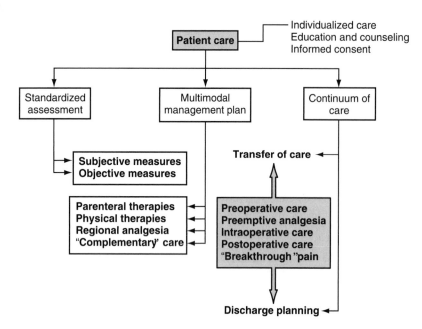

Figure 10–2 Integrated approach to perioperative pain management for surgical procedures.

effective pain management and the multiple "handoffs" that occur during a patient's hospitalization, a central task of the acute pain team is to ensure a continuum of care throughout a patient's hospitalization and discharge. The lack of systems that effectively manage the transition of a single patient through the seemingly disparate parts of the surgical journey (preoperative, perioperative, and postoperative periods) can be a significant barrier that will diminish effectiveness no matter the sophistication of pathways for measuring pain or treatment capabilities.

NATIONAL AGENDA

The realization of a national agenda to treat pain must start with a commitment to education in schools and other training institutions. Pain and its management must be part of the educational curriculums of nursing and medical schools, including graduate training programs. In addition, continuing medical and nursing education and recertification programs must ensure that qualified and licensed practitioners maintain their competence with respect to current practices in pain medicine. Notwithstanding these critically important steps, implementation of gains in systems and knowledge for pain management will require a cultural change in which medicine returns to its roots—curing when it can, but always caring for suffering. Current events suggest that if medicine does not meet its responsibilities for managing pain and suffering, it may well be forced to do so by regulators and legislators.

REFERENCES

1. Thomson H: A new law to improve pain management and end-of-life care: Learning how to treat patients in pain and near death must become a priority. West J Med 2001;174:161–162.
2. Phillips DM: JCAHO pain management standards are unveiled. Joint Commission on Accreditation of Healthcare Organizations. JAMA 2000; 284:428–429.
3. Acello B: Meeting JCAHO standards for pain control. Nursing 2000; 30:52–54.
4. Practice guidelines for acute pain management in the perioperative setting. A report by the American Society of Anesthesiologists Task Force on Pain Management, Acute Pain Section. Anesthesiology 1995;82:1071–1081.
5. Rich BA: Physicians' legal duty to relieve suffering. West J Med 2001; 175:151–152.
6. National Pharmaceutical Council, Inc: Pain: Current understanding of assessment, management, and treatments. Dec 1, 2001. Available at www.jcaho.org/news+room/health+care+issues/pain_mono_+npc.pdf
7. Practice guidelines for postanesthetic care: A report by the American Society of Anesthesiologists Task Force on Postanesthetic Care. Anesthesiology 2002;96:742–752.
8. Joint Commission on Accreditation of Healthcare Organizations: Joint Commission focuses on pain management. Aug 3, 1999. Available at www.jcaho.org/news+room/health+care+issues/jcaho+focus+on+pain+management.htm
9. Cousins MJ, Brennan F, Carr DB: Pain relief: A universal human right. Pain 2004;112:1–4.
10. Dolin SJ, Cashman JN, Bland JM: Effectiveness of acute postoperative pain management. I: Evidence from published data. Br J Anaesth 2002;89:409–423.
11. Svensson I, Sjostrom B, Haljamae H: Assessment of pain experiences after elective surgery. J Pain Symptom Manage 2000;20:193–201.
12. Apfelbaum JL, Chen C, Mehta SS, Gan TJ: Postoperative pain experience: Results from a national survey suggest postoperative pain continues to be undermanaged. Anesth Analg 2003;97:534–540.
13. Bruster S, Jarman B, Bosanquet N, et al: National survey of hospital patients. BMJ 1994;309:1542–1546.
14. Bostrom BM, Ramberg T, Davis BD, Fridlund B: Survey of post-operative patients' pain management. J Nurs Manag 1997;5:341–349.
15. McNeill JA, Sherwood GD, Starck PL, Thompson CJ: Assessing clinical outcomes: Patient satisfaction with pain management. J Pain Symptom Manage 1998;16:29–40.
16. Carroll KC, Atkins PJ, Herold GR, et al: Pain assessment and management in critically ill postoperative and trauma patients: A multisite study. Am J Crit Care 1999;8:105–117.
17. McNeill JA, Sherwood GD, Starck PL, Nieto B: Pain management outcomes for hospitalized Hispanic patients. Pain Manag Nurs 2001;2:25–36.
18. Blank FS, Mader TJ, Wolfe J, et al: Adequacy of pain assessment and pain relief and correlation of patient satisfaction in 68 ED fast-track patients. J Emerg Nurs 2001;27:327–334.
19. Corizzo CC, Baker MC, Henkelmann GC: Assessment of patient satisfaction with pain management in small community inpatient and outpatient settings. Oncol Nurs Forum 2000;27:1279–1286.
20. Jamison RN, Ross MJ, Hoopman P, et al: Assessment of postoperative pain management: Patient satisfaction and perceived helpfulness. Clin J Pain 1997;13:229–236.

21. Sherwood GD, McNeill JA, Starck PL, Disnard G: Changing acute pain management outcomes in surgical patients. AORN J 2003;77:374, 377–380, 384–390.

22. Yellen E, Davis GC: Patient satisfaction in ambulatory surgery. AORN J 2001;74:483–486, 489–494, 496–498.

23. Bauer KP, Dom PM, Ramirez AM, O'Flaherty JE: Preoperative intravenous midazolam: Benefits beyond anxiolysis. J Clin Anesth 2004;16:177–183.

24. Brander VA, Stulberg SD, Adams AD, et al: Predicting total knee replacement pain: A prospective, observational study. Clin Orthop 2003;(416):27–36.

25. Caumo W, Schmidt AP, Schneider CN, et al: Preoperative predictors of moderate to intense acute postoperative pain in patients undergoing abdominal surgery. Acta Anaesthesiol Scand 2002;46:1265–1271.

26. Daltroy LH, Morlino CI, Eaton HM, et al: Preoperative education for total hip and knee replacement patients. Arthritis Care Res 1998; 11:469–478.

27. Doering S, Katzlberger F, Rumpold G, et al: Videotape preparation of patients before hip replacement surgery reduces stress. Psychosom Med 2000;62:365–373.

28. Juhl IU, Christensen BV, Bulow HH, et al: Postoperative pain relief, from the patients' and the nurses' point of view. Acta Anaesthesiol Scand 1993;37:404–409.

29. Kain ZN, Sevarino F, Alexander GM, et al: Preoperative anxiety and postoperative pain in women undergoing hysterectomy: A repeated-measures design. J Psychosom Res 2000;49:417–422.

30. Kain ZN, Sevarino F, Pincus S, et al: Attenuation of the preoperative stress response with midazolam: Effects on postoperative outcomes. Anesthesiology 2000;93:141–147.

31. Kalkman CJ, Visser K, Moen J, et al: Preoperative prediction of severe postoperative pain. Pain 2003;105:415–423.

32. Karling M, Renstrom M, Ljungman G: Acute and postoperative pain in children: A Swedish nationwide survey. Acta Paediatr 2002;91: 660–666.

33. Lamontagne LL, Hepworth JT, Salisbury MH: Anxiety and postoperative pain in children who undergo major orthopedic surgery. Appl Nurs Res 2001;14:119–124.

34. McDonald S, Hetrick S, Green S: Pre-operative education for hip or knee replacement. Cochrane Database Syst Rev 2004;1:CD003526.

35. Messer B: Total joint replacement preadmission programs. Orthop Nurs 1998;17(Suppl):31–33.

36. Ozalp G, Sarioglu R, Tuncel G, et al: Preoperative emotional states in patients with breast cancer and postoperative pain. Acta Anaesthesiol Scand 2003;47:26–29.

37. Polomano RC, Heffner SM, Reck DL, et al: Evidence for opioid variability. Part 2: Psychosocial influences. Semin Perioper Nurs 2001;10:159–166.

38. Scott LE, Clum GA, Peoples JB: Preoperative predictors of postoperative pain. Pain 1983;15:283–293.

39. Sjoling M, Nordahl G, Olofsson N, Asplund K: The impact of preoperative information on state anxiety, postoperative pain and satisfaction with pain management. Patient Educ Couns 2003;51:169–176.

40. Winefield HR, Katsikitis M, Hart LM, Rounsefell BF: Postoperative pain experiences: Relevant patient and staff attitudes. J Psychosom Res 1990;34:543–552.

41. Bell ML, Reeves KA: Postoperative pain management in the non-Hispanic white and Mexican American older adult. Semin Perioper Nurs 1999;8:7–11.

42. Calvillo ER, Flaskerud JH: Evaluation of the pain response by Mexican American and Anglo American women and their nurses. J Adv Nurs 1993;18:451–459.

43. Dimmitt J: Rural Mexican-American and non-Hispanic white women: Effects of abuse on self-concept. J Cult Divers 1995;2:54–63.

44. Fenwick C, Stevens J: Post operative pain experiences of central Australian aboriginal women: What do we understand? Aust J Rural Health 2004;12:22–27.

45. Greer SM, Dalton JA, Carlson J, Youngblood R: Surgical patients' fear of addiction to pain medication: The effect of an educational program for clinicians. Clin J Pain 2001;17:157–164.

46. Bennett DS, Carr DB: Opiophobia as a barrier to the treatment of pain. J Pain Palliat Care Pharmacother 2002;16:105–109.

47. Beauregard L, Pomp A, Choiniere M: Severity and impact of pain after day-surgery. Can J Anaesth 1998;45:304–311.

48. Management approaches for improved patient outcomes. Orthop Nurs 2000;(19 Suppl):10–21.

49. Berge DJ, Dolin SJ, Williams AC, Harman R: Pre-operative and post-operative effect of a pain management programme prior to total hip replacement: A randomized controlled trial. Pain 2004;110:33–39.

50. Chung JW, Lui JC: Postoperative pain management: Study of patients' level of pain and satisfaction with health care providers' responsiveness to their reports of pain. Nurs Health Sci 2003;5:13–21.

51. Dalton JA, Blau W, Lindley C, et al: Changing acute pain management to improve patient outcomes: An educational approach. J Pain Symptom Manag 1999;17:277–287.

52. Dawkins S: Patient-controlled analgesia after coronary artery bypass grafting. Nurs Times 2003;99:30–31.

53. Devine EC, Bevsek SA, Brubakken K, et al: AHCPR clinical practice guideline on surgical pain management: Adoption and outcomes. Res Nurs Health 1999;22:119–130.

54. Gocen Z, Sen A, Unver B, et al: The effect of preoperative physiotherapy and education on the outcome of total hip replacement: A prospective randomized controlled trial. Clin Rehabil 2004;18:353–358.

55. Goldsmith DM, Safran C: Using the Web to reduce postoperative pain following ambulatory surgery. Proc AMIA Symp 1999;780–784.

56. Griffin MJ, Brennan L, McShane AJ: Preoperative education and outcome of patient controlled analgesia. Can J Anaesth 1998;45:943–948.

57. Harrington JT, Dopf CA, Chalgren CS: Implementing guidelines for interdisciplinary care of low back pain: A critical role for pre-appointment management of specialty referrals. Jt Comm J Qual Improv 2001;27:651–663.

58. LaMontagne LL, Hepworth JT, Cohen F, Salisbury MH: Cognitive-behavioral intervention effects on adolescents' anxiety and pain following spinal fusion surgery. Nurs Res 2003;52:183–190.

59. Ridge RA, Goodson AS: The relationship between multidisciplinary discharge outcomes and functional status after total hip replacement. Orthop Nurs 2000;19:71–82.

60. Shuldham CM, Fleming S, Goodman H: The impact of pre-operative education on recovery following coronary artery bypass surgery: A randomized controlled clinical trial. Eur Heart J 2002;23:666–674.

61. Teutsch C: Patient-doctor communication. Med Clin North Am 2003;87:1115–1145.

62. Watt-Watson J, Stevens B, Costello J, et al: Impact of preoperative education on pain management outcomes after coronary artery bypass graft surgery: A pilot. Can J Nurs Res 2000;31:41–56.

63. Watt-Watson J, Stevens B, Katz J, et al: Impact of preoperative education on pain outcomes after coronary artery bypass graft surgery. Pain 2004;109:73–85.

64. Nilsdotter AK, Petersson IF, Roos EM, Lohmander LS: Predictors of patient relevant outcome after total hip replacement for osteoarthritis: A prospective study. Ann Rheum Dis 2003;62:923–930.

65. Ostendorf M, Buskens E, van Stel H, et al: Waiting for total hip arthroplasty: Avoidable loss in quality time and preventable deterioration. J Arthroplasty 2004;19:302–309.

66. Bondy LR, Sims N, Schroeder DR, et al: The effect of anesthetic patient education on preoperative patient anxiety. Reg Anesth Pain Med 1999; 24:158–164.

67. Camu F, Beecher T, Recker DP, Verburg KM: Valdecoxib, a COX-2-specific inhibitor, is an efficacious, opioid-sparing analgesic in patients undergoing hip arthroplasty. Am J Ther 2002;9:43–51.

68. Giraudet-Le Quintrec JS, Coste J, Vastel L, et al: Positive effect of patient education for hip surgery: A randomized trial. Clin Orthop 2003;414:112–120.

69. Holtzman J, Saleh K, Kane R: Effect of baseline functional status and pain on outcomes of total hip arthroplasty. J Bone Joint Surg Am 2002; 84A:1942–1948.

70. Knutsson S, Engberg IB: An evaluation of patients' quality of life before, 6 weeks and 6 months after total hip replacement surgery. J Adv Nurs 1999;30:1349–1359.

71. Lilja Y, Ryden S, Fridlund B: Effects of extended preoperative information on perioperative stress: An anaesthetic nurse intervention for patients with breast cancer and total hip replacement. Intensive Crit Care Nurs 1998;14:276–282.

72. McGregor AH, Rylands H, Owen A, et al: Does preoperative hip rehabilitation advice improve recovery and patient satisfaction? J Arthroplasty 2004;19:464–468.

73. Meding JB, Anderson AR, Faris PM, et al: Is the preoperative radiograph useful in predicting the outcome of a total hip replacement? Clin Orthop 2000;376:156–160.

74. O'Connell T, Browne C, Corcoran R, Howell F: Quality of life following total hip replacement. Ir Med J 2000;93:108–110.

75. Scherak O, Kolarz G, Wottawa A, et al: [Effect of inpatient rehabilitation measures on patients with total hip endoprostheses—evaluation 15 months after operation. Acta Med Austriaca 1996;23:142–145.

76. Topol EJ: Failing the public health—rofecoxib, Merck, and the FDA. N Engl J Med 2004;351:1707–1709.

77. Lenzer J: US government agency to investigate FDA over rofecoxib. BMJ 2004;329:935.

78. Horton R: Vioxx, the implosion of Merck, and aftershocks at the FDA. Lancet 2004;364:1995–1996.

79. Couzin J: Drug safety: Withdrawal of Vioxx casts a shadow over COX-2 inhibitors. Science 2004;306:384–385.

80. Sibbald B: Rofecoxib (Vioxx) voluntarily withdrawn from market. CMAJ 2004;171:1027–1028.

81. Berenson A, Harris G, Meier B, Pollack AL: Despite warnings, drug giant took long path to Vioxx recall. NY Times, Nov 14, 2004:A1, A32.

82. Choi HK, Seeger JD, Kuntz KM: Effects of rofecoxib and naproxen on life expectancy among patients with rheumatoid arthritis: A decision analysis. Am J Med 2004;116:621–629.

83. Oakley G Jr: Lessons from the withdrawal of rofecoxib: Observational studies should not be forgotten. BMJ Dec 4 2004;329:1342.

84. Abenhaim L: Lessons from the withdrawal of rofecoxib: France has policy for overall assessment of public health impact of new drugs. BMJ 2004;329:1342.

85. Giaquinta D: Lessons learned after the withdrawal of rofecoxib. Manag Care Interface 2004;17:25–26, 46.

86. Dieppe PA, Ebrahim S, Martin RM, Juni P: Lessons from the withdrawal of rofecoxib. BMJ 2004;329:867–868.

87. Gallagher RM: Balancing risks and benefits in pain medicine: Wither Vioxx Pain Med 2004;5:329–330.

88. DeMaria AN: The fallout from Vioxx. J Am Coll Cardiol 2004;44:2080–2081.

89. Kelly DJ, Ahmad M, Brull SJ: Preemptive analgesia. I: Physiological pathways and pharmacological modalities. Can J Anaesth 2001;48:1000–1010.

90. Suzuki H: Recent topics in the management of pain: Development of the concept of preemptive analgesia. Cell Transplant 1995;(Suppl 1):S3–S6.

91. Wilder-Smith CH, Hill L, Dyer RA, et al: Postoperative sensitization and pain after cesarean delivery and the effects of single IM doses of tramadol and diclofenac alone and in combination. Anesth Analg 2003;97:526–533.

92. Halbert J, Crotty M, Cameron ID: Evidence for the optimal management of acute and chronic phantom pain: A systematic review. Clin J Pain 2002;18:84–92.

93. Redmond M, Florence B, Glass PS: Effective analgesic modalities for ambulatory patients. Anesthesiol Clin North Am 2003;21:329–346.

94. Subramaniam B, Subramaniam K, Pawar DK, Sennaraj B: Preoperative epidural ketamine in combination with morphine does not have a clinically relevant intra- and postoperative opioid-sparing effect. Anesth Analg 2001;93:1321–1326.

95. Joshi GP: Postoperative pain management. Int Anesthesiol Clin 1994;32:113–126.

96. Wright BD: Clinical pain management techniques for cats. Clin Tech Small Anim Pract 2002;17:151–157.

97. Gottschalk A, Smith DS, Jobes DR, et al: Preemptive epidural analgesia and recovery from radical prostatectomy: A randomized controlled trial. JAMA 1998;279:1076–1082.

98. Katz J, Cohen L: Preventive analgesia is associated with reduced pain disability 3 weeks but not 6 months after major gynecologic surgery by laparotomy. Anesthesiology 2004;101:169–174.

99. Rosaeg OP, Krepski B, Cicutti N, et al: Effect of preemptive multimodal analgesia for arthroscopic knee ligament repair. Reg Anesth Pain Med 2001;26:125–130.

100. Sekar C, Rajasekaran S, Kannan R, et al: Preemptive analgesia for postoperative pain relief in lumbosacral spine surgeries: A randomized controlled trial. Spine J 2004;4:261–264.

101. Horattas MC, Evans S, Sloan-Stakleff KD, et al: Does preoperative rofecoxib (Vioxx) decrease postoperative pain with laparoscopic cholecystectomy? Am J Surg 2004;188:271–276.

102. Akarsu T, Karaman S, Akercan F, et al: Preemptive meloxicam for postoperative pain relief after abdominal hysterectomy. Clin Exp Obstet Gynecol 2004;31:133–136.

103. Trampitsch E, Pipam W, Moertl M, et al: [Preemptive randomized, double-blind study with lornoxicam in gynecological surgery.] Schmerz 2003;17:4–10.

104. Settecase C, Bagilet D, Bertoletti F, Laudanno C: [Preoperative diclofenac does not reduce pain of laparoscopic cholecystectomy.] Rev Esp Anestesiol Reanim 2002;49:455–460.

105. Oztekin S, Hepaguslar H, Kar AA, et al: Preemptive diclofenac reduces morphine use after remifentanil-based anaesthesia for tonsillectomy. Paediatr Anaesth 2002;12:694–699.

106. Gilabert Morell A, Sanchez Perez C: [Effect of low-dose intravenous ketamine in postoperative analgesia for hysterectomy and adnexectomy]. Rev Esp Anestesiol Reanim 2002;49:247–253.

107. Giannoni C, White S, Enneking FK: Does dexamethasone with preemptive analgesia improve pediatric tonsillectomy pain? Otolaryngol Head Neck Surg 2002;126:307–315.

108. Kokki H, Salonen A: Comparison of pre- and postoperative administration of ketoprofen for analgesia after tonsillectomy in children. Paediatr Anaesth 2002;12:162–167.

109. Reuben SS, Bhopatkar S, Maciolek H, et al: The preemptive analgesic effect of rofecoxib after ambulatory arthroscopic knee surgery. Anesth Analg 2002;94:55–59.

110. Nagatsuka C, Ichinohe T, Kaneko Y: Preemptive effects of a combination of preoperative diclofenac, butorphanol, and lidocaine on postoperative pain management following orthognathic surgery. Anesth Prog 2000;47:119–124.

111. Norman PH, Daley MD, Lindsey RW: Preemptive analgesic effects of ketorolac in ankle fracture surgery. Anesthesiology 2001;94:599–603.

112. Cabell CA: Does ketorolac produce preemptive analgesic effects in laparoscopic ambulatory surgery patients? AANA J 2000;68:343–349.

113. Ko JC, Miyabiyashi T, Mandsager RE, et al: Renal effects of carprofen administered to healthy dogs anesthetized with propofol and isoflurane. J Am Vet Med Assoc 2000;217:346–349.

114. Zacharias M, Hunter KM, Baker AB: Effectiveness of preoperative analgesics on postoperative dental pain: A study. Anesth Prog 1996;43:92–96.

115. Likar R, Krumpholz R, Pipam W, et al: [Randomized, double-blind study with ketoprofen in gynecologic patients: Preemptive analgesia study following the Brevik-Stubhaug design.] Anaesthesist 1998;47:303–310.

116. Likar R, Krumpholz R, Mathiaschitz K, et al: [The preemptive action of ketoprofen: Randomized, double-blind study with gynecologic operations.] Anaesthesist 1997;46:186–190.

117. Rockemann MG, Seeling W, Bischof C, et al: Prophylactic use of epidural mepivacaine/morphine, systemic diclofenac, and metamizole reduces postoperative morphine consumption after major abdominal surgery. Anesthesiology 1996;84:1027–1034.

118. Katz J, Jackson M, Kavanagh BP, Sandler AN: Acute pain after thoracic surgery predicts long-term post-thoracotomy pain. Clin J Pain 1996;12:50–55.

119. Mezei M, Hahn O, Penzes I: [Preemptive analgesia—preoperative diclofenac sodium for postoperative analgesia in general surgery.] Magy Seb 2002;55:313–317.

120. Lakdja F, Dixmerias F, Bussieres E, et al: [Preventive analgesic effect of intraoperative administration of ibuprofen-arginine on postmastectomy pain syndrome.] Bull Cancer 1997;84:259–263.

121. Lambert A, Dashfield A, Cosgrove C, et al: Randomized prospective study comparing preoperative epidural and intraoperative perineural analgesia for the prevention of postoperative stump and phantom limb pain following major amputation. Reg Anesth Pain Med 2001;26:316–321.

122. Jin F, Chung F: Multimodal analgesia for postoperative pain control. J Clin Anesth 2001;13:524–539.

123. Paech MJ, Pavy TJ, Orlikowski CE, et al: Postcesarean analgesia with spinal morphine, clonidine, or their combination. Anesth Analg 2004;98:1460–1466.

124. Stephens J, Laskin B, Pashos C, et al: The burden of acute postoperative pain and the potential role of the COX-2-specific inhibitors. Rheumatology (Oxford) 2003;42(Suppl 3):iii40–iii52.

125. Schumann R, Shikora S, Weiss JM, et al: A comparison of multimodal perioperative analgesia to epidural pain management after gastric bypass surgery. Anesth Analg 2003;96:469–474.

126. Ochroch EA, Mardini IA, Gottschalk A: What is the role of NSAIDs in pre-emptive analgesia? Drugs 2003;63:2709–2723.

127. Bardiau FM, Taviaux NF, Albert A, et al: An intervention study to enhance postoperative pain management. Anesth Analg 2003;96:179–185.

128. Anderson AD, McNaught CE, MacFie J, et al: Randomized clinical trial of multimodal optimization and standard perioperative surgical care. Br J Surg 2003;90:1497–1504.

129. Issioui T, Klein KW, White PF, et al: Cost-efficacy of rofecoxib versus acetaminophen for preventing pain after ambulatory surgery. Anesthesiology 2002;97:931–937.

130. Doyle E, Bowler GM: Pre-emptive effect of multimodal analgesia in thoracic surgery. Br J Anaesth 1998;80:147–151.

131. Skinner HB: Multimodal acute pain management. Am J Orthop 2004;33(Suppl):5–9.

132. Skinner HB, Shintani EY: Results of a multimodal analgesic trial involving patients with total hip or total knee arthroplasty. Am J Orthop 2004;33:85–92.

133. Kamming D, Chung F, Williams D, et al: Pain management in ambulatory surgery. J Perianesth Nurs 2004;19:174–182.

134. Rosenberg J, Kehlet H: Does effective postoperative pain management influence surgical morbidity? Eur Surg Res 1999;31:133–137.

135. Baker AB: Analgesia for day surgery. Med J Aust 1992;156:274–280.

136. McDonnell A, Nicholl J, Read SM: Acute pain teams and the management of postoperative pain: A systematic review and meta-analysis. J Adv Nurs 2003;41:261–273.

137. McDonnell A, Nicholl J, Read SM: Acute pain teams in England: Current provision and their role in postoperative pain management. J Clin Nurs 2003;12:387–393.

138. Loughrey JP, Fitzpatrick G, Connolly J, Donnelly M: High dependency care: Impact of lack of facilities for high-risk surgical patients. Ir J Med Sci 2002;171:211–215.

139. Schafheutle EI, Cantrill JA, Noyce PR: Why is pain management suboptimal on surgical wards? J Adv Nurs 2001;33:728–737.

140. Rawal N, Allvin R: [Postoperative pain an unnecessary suffering: A model of "emergency pain relief" implemented in Orebro.] Lakartidningen 2001;98:1648–1654.

141. Rawal N: 10 years of acute pain services—achievements and challenges. Reg Anesth Pain Med 1999;24:68–73.

142. Chen PP, Ma M, Chan S, Oh TE: Incident reporting in acute pain management. Anaesthesia Aug 1998;53:730–735.

143. Stomberg MW, Wickstrom K, Joelsson H, et al: Postoperative pain management on surgical wards—do quality assurance strategies result in long-term effects on staff member attitudes and clinical outcomes? Pain Manag Nurs 2003;4:11–22.

144. Goldstein DH, VanDenKerkhof EG, Blaine WC: Acute pain management services have progressed, albeit insufficiently in Canadian academic hospitals. Can J Anaesth 2004;51:231–235.

145. Stadler M, Schlander M, Braeckman M, et al: A cost-utility and cost-effectiveness analysis of an acute pain service. J Clin Anesth 2004;16:159–167.

146. Powell AE, Davies HT, Bannister J, Macrae WA: Rhetoric and reality on acute pain services in the UK: A national postal questionnaire survey. Br J Anaesth 2004;92:689–693.

147. Joranson DE: Are health-care reimbursement policies a barrier to acute and cancer pain management? J Pain Symptom Manage 1994;9:244–253.

148. Pain management: Theological and ethical principles governing the use of pain relief for dying patients. Task Force on Pain Management, Catholic Health Association. Health Prog 1993;74:30–39, 65.

149. Jordan-Marsh M, Hubbard J, Watson R, et al: The social ecology of changing pain management: Do I have to cry? J Pediatr Nurs 2004;19:193–203.

150. Middleton C: Barriers to the provision of effective pain management. Nurs Times 2004;100:42–45.

151. Watt-Watson J, Chung F, Chan VW, McGillion M: Pain management following discharge after ambulatory same-day surgery. J Nurs Manag 2004;12:153–161.

152. Manias E, Bucknall T, Botti M: Assessment of patient pain in the postoperative context. West J Nurs Res 2004;26:751–769.

153. MacLellan KL: Postoperative pain: Strategy for improving patient experiences. J Adv Nurs 2004;46:179–185.

154. Idvall E: Quality of care in postoperative pain management: What is realistic in clinical practice? J Nurs Manag 2004;12:162–166.

155. Chavis SW, Duncan LH: Pain management—continuum of care for surgical patients. AORN J 2003;78(3):382–386, 389–399; quiz 400–401, 403–404.

156. Rawal N: Treating postoperative pain improves outcome. Minerva Anestesiol 2001;67(Suppl 1):200–205.

157. Krenzischek DA, Windle P, Mamaril M: A survey of current perianesthesia nursing practice for pain and comfort management. J Perianesth Nurs 2004;19:138–149.

11 Clinical Assessment of Postoperative Pain

GABRIELLA IOHOM

Clinical assessment of postoperative pain refers to the process of describing pain and its effect on function in sufficient detail to achieve the following goals:

1. To assist in diagnosis and to quantify postoperative pain.
2. To select appropriate therapy.
3. To evaluate the response to therapy.

The most common reason for the undertreatment of pain in U.S. hospitals is the failure of clinicians to assess pain and pain relief.[1] Ideally, pain assessment should involve a multidimensional approach. However, time and personnel constraints generally permit only unidimensional recordings in the postoperative period. Pain is assessed regularly (every 3 to 4 hours), at rest and on movement, and the scores are documented; this documentation makes pain the fifth vital sign. Protocol determines the maximum score above which further action is required to control pain.

A more comprehensive assessment of postoperative pain is sometimes required, involving history and examination. Pain history should reveal location, intensity, characteristics, and temporal aspects of pain as well as factors aggravating and relieving the pain, associated symptoms, and treatment to date.

The patient's self-report is the most reliable indicator of pain. Because pain is a subjective experience, it is the patient's perceptions and not those of the clinician that should be documented. Also, measures of pain intensity are not meant to compare one person's pain with another's; rather, they compare the intensity of one patient's pain at any given time with its intensity at another given time.[2]

The physical examination follows the history, although in urgent clinical situations there may be some overlap to save time. The patient usually gives both verbal and nonverbal clues to the severity of pain and the urgency of need for treatment. It may be appropriate to observe the patient's movement and his or her facial expression. The physical examination may exacerbate the patient's pain.[3]

During this examination, the clinician appraises the patient's general physical condition, with special attention to the site of pain. The clinician may also evaluate the effect of various physical factors (i.e., motion, deep breathing, changes in position) on the pain and/or performance measures of physical function (i.e., range of motion, ability to carry out activities of daily living).[4]

Several behavioral scales enable the clinician to assess pain in infants, children, elderly patients, and mentally impaired patients unable to communicate verbally about their pain through the evaluation of either physiologic responses (i.e., heart rate, blood pressure, oxygenation) or overt behaviors (i.e., cries, facial expressions, withdrawal behavior). The greater the number of distress signals, the higher the pain level. Although they provide an indirect assessment of pain, several distress scales have been validated for clinical use.

Postoperative pain management is a unique area of clinical practice. The occurrence of acute pain is largely predictable, and its intensity can be correlated with the operation site. Postoperative pain differs from other types of pain in that it is usually transient, with progressive improvement over a relatively short time. Typically, the affective component tends toward an anxiety state associated with diagnosis of the condition and fear of delay in provision of analgesic therapy by clinicians. The preoperative visit offers the clinician the opportunity to establish a positive relationship with patients and/or their families, to obtain a pain history, and to educate the patient about pain assessment and analgesic strategies. Postoperative pain assessment is centered on patient self-report except when patients are unable to communicate (behavior and/or vital signs are substituted). Pain is assessed at rest and during activity (i.e., moving, deep breathing, coughing) as follows: (1) at regular time intervals consistent with surgery type and pain severity, (2) with each new report of pain, and (3) at a suitable interval after each analgesic intervention (i.e., 30 minutes after parenteral drug therapy, and 1 hour after oral analgesics).[5] Measuring pain during function increases the sensitivity of measurements for clinical research. For example, the efficacy of two analgesic techniques may be similar when pain is measured in patients at rest but significantly different when dynamic pain measurements are taken, such as during breathing and coughing.[6]

Although the surgical wound is the most common and most obvious source of postoperative pain, there are many other potential sources and causes for postoperative pain. No assumptions should be made. The possibility of an alternative diagnosis or complication should always be considered when a patient demonstrated uncontrolled pain, unexpected pain, or a complex pain problem. There may be a new problem (e.g., compartment syndrome, peritonitis) or a concurrent one (e.g., angina). Alternatively, neuropathic pain may

No pain 0 1 2 3 4 5 6 7 8 9 10   Worst pain imaginable

Figure 11–1 Numerical rating scale (NRS).

be developing. This complication can develop within days of the original injury, can be difficult to treat, and may be more responsive if treatment is started at an early stage.[3]

Pain Measurement

Pain is a complex multidimensional symptom determined not only by tissue injury and nociception but also by previous pain experience, personal beliefs, motivation, environment, and so on. No satisfactory objective measurement of pain exists. Self-report is the most valid measure of the individual experience of pain.

Theoretically, postoperative pain should be evaluated in its multiple dimensions, such as intensity, location, emotional consequences, and semiological correlates. Scales developed to evaluate these dimensions are too complex for widespread and repetitive use in surgical patients, however. Only simple methods assessing pain intensity can be used in this clinical setting.[7]

Self-reported measurement tools can be classified as unidimensional or multidimensional according to the number of dimensions used.

UNIDIMENSIONAL TOOLS

Categorical Scales/Verbal Rating Scales/Verbal Descriptor Scales

The scale is the oldest form of pain measurement tool, in which the patient is asked to describe his or her current experience of pain by choosing from a list of adjectives that reflect gradations of pain intensity.[8] Such a scale may contain between two and seven words.

In its simplest form, it can be a choice of "yes" or "no" to questions such as "Are you in pain?" In clinical practice, a four-descriptor verbal rating scale (VRS) measuring pain intensity is commonly used, with the words *none, mild, moderate,* and *severe.*[3] The five-word scale consists of *mild, discomforting, distressing, horrible,* and *excruciating.*[9] Pain relief can also be measured in clinical practice using a five-descriptor scale consisting of *none, slight, moderate, good,* and *complete.*[3]

Disadvantages of this scale include the limited selection of descriptors, subjectivity to patient bias, and its noncontinuous nature, which requires nonparametric tests for statistical analyses. Nevertheless, a good correlation with the visual analogue scale (VAS) in the clinical setting of postoperative pain has been demonstrated.[10]

Numerical Rating Scales

Numerical rating scales (NRSs) are the simplest and most commonly used scales.[11] The numerical scale is most commonly 0 to 10, with 0 being "no pain" and 10 being "the worst pain imaginable." The patient picks (verbal version) or draws a circle around (written version, Fig. 11–1) the number that best describes the pain dimension, usually intensity.

Advantages of NRSs include simplicity, reproducibility, easy comprehensibility, and sensitivity to small changes in pain. Children as young as 5 years who are able to count and have some concept of numbers (i.e., that 8 is larger than 4) may use this scale.[9] Although claimed to be not necessarily linear, NRSs correlate well with the VAS.[12]

Visual Analogue Scales

The concept of quantifying subjective sensations (i.e., depression, anxiety, apprehension, well-being) by using VASs has long been employed by psychiatrists.[13,14] Huskisson[15,16] first presented the possibility[15] and later validated the VAS for pain intensity assessment. These are similar to the verbal NRSs, except that the patient marks on a measured line (of 10 cm/100 mm length), one end of which is labeled "no pain" and the other end "worst pain imaginable," where his or her pain falls (Fig. 11–2). The score is obtained by measuring the distance (mm) from the left end of the line. The anchoring text can influence the scores—i.e., higher VAS may be scored with "severe pain" rather than "unimaginable pain" defining the upper pain boundary. The line can be oriented vertically or horizontally without affecting the sensitivity of VAS.[17] Although more valid for research purposes, VASs are less commonly used in clinical practice because they are more time-consuming to administer than verbal scales.

DeLoach et al[18] have shown that the postoperative perceptual-cognitive impairment experienced by patients who have undergone anesthesia degrades the relationship of the VAS to the subjective pain experience, leading to an imprecision of ±20 mm for each measurement in this clinical setting.

The VAS has properties consistent with the linear scale, at least for patients with mild to moderate pain, and thus VAS scores can be treated as ratio data. This statement supports the notion that a change in the VAS score represents a relative change in the magnitude of pain sensation, and the use of parametric tests for analysis of VAS scores is appropriate.[19]

Picture Scales

Picture scales, like categorical rating scales, consist of a series of four to six faces depicting different expressions ranging from a happy, smiling face to a sad, teary face (Fig. 11–3). This scale may be extrapolated to the VAS by multiplying the chosen value by 2. It is perceived as being easier for patients to use than the NRS or VAS. The picture scale is useful in individuals with difficulty communicating (i.e., children as young as 3 years, the elderly, the mentally

No pain _____ Worst pain imaginable

Figure 11–2 Visual analogue scale (VAS).

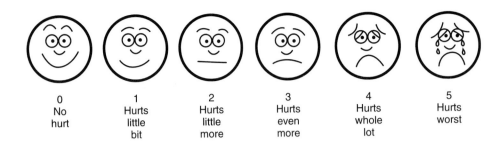

Figure 11-3 Faces Pain Scale. (From Wong DL, Hockenberry-Eaton M, Wilson D, et al: Wong's Essentials of Pediatric Nursing, 6th ed. St. Louis, Mosby, 2001, p 1301.)

impaired, individuals with limited language fluency or education).[9] Disadvantages of this approach include potentially distorted assessment (i.e., patients' tendency to point to the center of such a scale) and the need for instrumentation (i.e., printed form).

MULTIDIMENSIONAL TOOLS FOR RESEARCH PURPOSES

McGill Pain Questionnaire (MPQ)

The McGill Pain Questionnaire (MPQ) is one of the most extensively tested multidimensional scales in use.[20] This tool assesses pain in three dimensions (sensory, affective, and evaluative) on the basis of words that patients select from 20 sets of descriptors to characterize their pain (Fig. 11-4). The patient is instructed to select the words that best describe their pain. The following three indices are produced from this information:

- The Pain Rating Index (PRI). Each descriptor in each set has a rank value according to its implied intensity. The PRI is the sum total of the ranked values of each chosen descriptor. There are separate scores for each of the three dimensions as well as a miscellaneous subclass.
- The number of words chosen (NWC).
- The Present Pain Intensity Index (PPII). The patient is asked to complete a categorical Present Pain Intensity Scale (PPIS) using descriptors from "no pain" through "excruciating."

Initially developed for the general assessment of chronic pain, the MPQ has been validated for acute pain in general[21] and for postoperative pain in particular.[22]

Patients with acute pain tend to score higher in their use of sensory descriptors and lower with affective descriptors than patients with chronic pain.[21] The MPQ questionnaire is at least as sensitive to changes in postoperative pain after oral analgesics as the VRS and VAS.[22]

Short-Form McGill Pain Questionnaire

The short-form MPQ (SF-MPQ; Fig. 11-5) was developed for use in research when there is limited time to obtain information from patients and when more information is desired than that provided by intensity measures such as the VAS or the overall PPII.[23] The SF-MPQ takes about 2 to 5 minutes to complete, compared with 10 minutes for the longer form. The present pain intensity index is recorded as a number from 1 to 5, in which each number is associated with the following words: 1 mild, 2 discomforting, 3 distressing,

4 horrible, 5 excruciating. Both the VAS and the PPII provide data on pain intensity only and no data on the qualities of the pain. In the development of the SF-MPQ, the most commonly used set of words was chosen from the sensory and affective categories of the standard form. The words were divided into the two descriptive categories for sensory and affective components of pain. The most common sensory words are *throbbing, shooting, stabbing, sharp, cramping, gnawing, hot-burning, aching, heavy, tender,* and *splitting.* In the affective category, the most frequently used words are *tiring-exhausting, sickening, fearful,* and *cruel-punishing.* Each of the 15 descriptors is ranked by the patient on the following intensity scale: 0 = none, 1 = mild, 2 = moderate, and 3 = severe. The sensory and affective components can therefore be examined individually or as a total score.

The SF-MPQ has been shown to correlate well with the PRI of the longer form of the MPQ.[23] It has also been shown to be sensitive to clinical changes brought about by various interventions, postoperative analgesic drugs, and epidural agents used during labor.[23,24] Also, consistency has been demonstrated among young, middle-aged, and elderly patients in the ability to complete the questionnaire effectively.[25]

Quantitative Sensory Testing

Quantitative sensory testing (QST; Fig. 11-6) is a noninvasive form of somatosensory testing that provides information on the activity of the entire afferent pain pathway from the periphery (receptor) to the brain (supratentorium). Threshold and tolerance in response to a variety of painful stimuli are approximately normally distributed in the general population. Some objective measures of sensory and pain perception can be obtained through administration of standardized noxious stimuli and quantifying of pain responses under controlled laboratory conditions.[26] The modalities commonly used in testing are mechanical (i.e., static test with graded Von Frey hairs or dynamic tests of vibration sense) or thermal (using Peltier probes to alter skin temperature at specific rates). The subject is asked to report the threshold for sensory detection, the threshold for pain, the limit of pain tolerance, and the just-noticeable difference between stimuli. However, such testing can be time-consuming, requires considerable patient cooperation, and is still largely limited to use in research.

Several studies have examined preoperative experimental pain responses as predictors of postoperative pain. Among patients undergoing limb amputation, preamputation pressure pain thresholds were inversely correlated with postamputation stump pain and phantom pain.[27] Preoperative thermal QST responses predicted postoperative pain scores at rest

McGILL PAIN QUESTIONNAIRE

Patient's name _____ Date _____ Time _____ am/pm

PRI: S _____ A _____ E _____ M _____ PRI(T) _____ PPI _____
     (1–10)   (11–15)   (16)   (17–20)   (1–20)

Brief ___	Rhythmic ___	Continuous ___
Momentary ___	Periodic ___	Steady ___
Transient ___	Intermittent ___	Constant ___

1 Flickering ___
  Quivering ___
  Pulsing ___
  Throbbing ___
  Beating ___
  Pounding ___

2 Jumping ___
  Flashing ___
  Shooting ___

3 Pricking ___
  Boring ___
  Drilling ___
  Stabbing ___
  Lancinating ___

4 Sharp ___
  Cutting ___
  Lacerating ___

5 Pinching ___
  Pressing ___
  Gnawing ___
  Cramping ___
  Crushing ___

6 Tugging ___
  Pulling ___
  Wrenching ___

7 Hot ___
  Burning ___
  Scalding ___
  Searing ___

8 Tingling ___
  Itchy ___
  Smarting ___
  Stinging ___

9 Dull ___
  Sore ___
  Hurting ___
  Aching ___
  Heavy ___

10 Tender ___
  Taut ___
  Rasping ___
  Splitting ___

11 Tiring ___
  Exhausting ___

12 Sickening ___
  Suffocating ___

13 Fearful ___
  Frightful ___
  Terrifying ___

14 Punishing ___
  Gruelling ___
  Cruel ___
  Vicious ___
  Killing ___

15 Wretched ___
  Blinding ___

16 Annoying ___
  Troublesome ___
  Miserable ___
  Intense ___
  Unbearable ___

17 Spreading ___
  Radiating ___
  Penetrating ___
  Piercing ___

18 Tight ___
  Numb ___
  Drawing ___
  Squeezing ___
  Tearing ___

19 Cool ___
  Cold ___
  Freezing ___

20 Nagging ___
  Nauseating ___
  Agonizing ___
  Dreadful ___
  Torturing ___

PPI
0 No pain ___
1 Mild ___
2 Discomforting ___
3 Distressing ___
4 Horrible ___
5 Excruciating ___

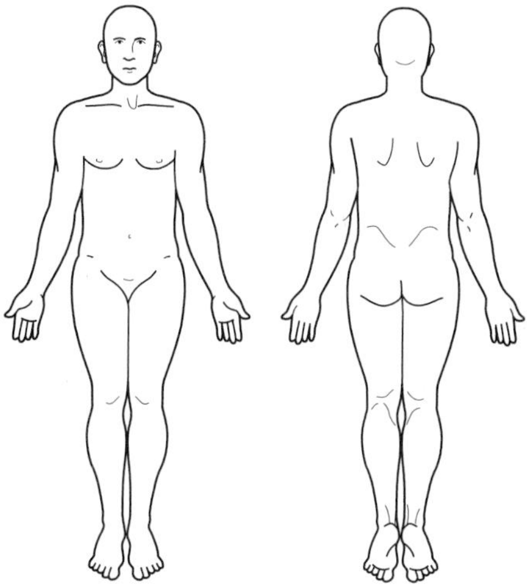

E = External
I = Internal

Comments:

Figure 11–4 McGill Pain Questionnaire. (Reprinted from Turk DC, Melzack R [eds]: Handbook of Pain Assessment. Copyright 1992, The Guilford Press, New York.)

Study #

Date:

Short-form McGill Pain Questionnaire:

I. Pain Rating Index (PRI):
    The words below describe average pain. Place a check mark (✓) in the column that represents the
    degree to which you feel that type of pain. Please limit yourself to a description of the pain in your
    pelvic area only.

		None		Mild		Moderate		Severe
	Throbbing	0	1		2		3	
	Shooting	0	1		2		3	
	Stabbing	0	1		2		3	
	Sharp	0	1		2		3	
	Cramping	0	1		2		3	
a	Gnawing	0	1		2		3	
	Hot-burning	0	1		2		3	
	Aching	0	1		2		3	
	Heavy	0	1		2		3	
	Tender	0	1		2		3	
	Splitting	0	1		2		3	
	Tiring-exhausting	0	1		2		3	
	Sickening	0	1		2		3	
b	Fearful	0	1		2		3	
	Punishing-cruel	0	1		2		3	

II. Present Pain Intensity (PPI)-Visual Analog Scale (VAS). Tick along scale below for pelvic pain:

No pain |————————————————————————————| Worst possible pain

III. Evaluative overall intensity of total pain experience. Please limit yourself to a description of the pain
    in your pelvic area only. Place a check mark (✓) in the appropriate column.

Evaluative		
0	No pain	
1	Mild	
2	Discomforting	
3	Distressing	
4	Horrible	
5	Excruciating	

IV. Scoring:

		Score
I-a	S-PRI (Sensory Pain Rating Index)	
I-b	A-PRI (Affective Pain Rating Index)	
I-a+b	T-PRI (Total Pain Rating Index)	
II	PPI-VAS (Present Pain Intensity-Visual Analog Scale)	
III	Evaluative overall intensity of total pain experience	

Figure 11–5 Short-form McGill Pain Questionnaire (SF-MPQ) for pelvic pain. (From www.med.umich.edu/obgyn/repro-endo/Lebovicresearch/PainSurvey.pdf/)

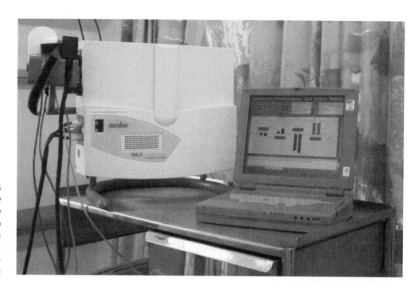

Figure 11–6   Quantitative Sensory Testing (QST). This picture shows the quantitative sensory testing machine with the thermode and patient response device, in the upper left of the photograph, connected to the laptop computer, which displays the results of testing. (From Heffernan A: Transcutaneous spinal electroanalgesia: Its effects in acute and chronic pain and healthy volunteers [Thesis]. Leicester, UK, Leicester University, 2002.)

and during activity in women undergoing cesarean section, explaining up to 54% of the variance in postsurgical pain.[28] In patients undergoing anterior cruciate ligament repair, preoperative ratings of an intense noxious thermal stimulus were strongly correlated with joint pain ratings for several weeks after surgery.[29] Preoperative cold pain tolerance predicted postoperative pain after laparoscopic cholecystectomy, even after data were controlled for neuroticism.[30] In summary, these findings identify suprathreshold experimental pain responses as important predictors of acute pain intensity after surgical procedures.[26]

Despite practical barriers to performing experimental pain evaluation in clinical settings, it is anticipated that QST will become an increasingly common pain assessment tool.[26]

Analgesic Requirements

Time to first request of analgesics and analgesic consumption are also used as measures of pain in clinical research. Patient-controlled analgesia (PCA) devices have been used in this respect. The assumption is that the dose of analgesia delivered by the device over a period of time gives a measure of pain intensity.[31] The numerical data generated are relatively easy to analyze. It has been suggested that the demand-to-delivery ratio may better reflect the patient's analgesic needs.[32] This measurement involves the use of a computerized PCA device and is influenced by factors other than pain intensity (i.e., dosing variables, side effects, psychological differences).

Summary Measures

In the research context, pain is typically assessed before the intervention and subsequently on multiple occasions afterwards. Ideally, the area under the time-analgesic effect curve is calculated. Summed pain intensity differences (SPID) or relief measures (total pain relief [TOTPAR]) indicate the cumulative response to the intervention. However, they do not impart information about the onset and peak of the analgesic effect. If these data are important, then time to maximum pain relief (or reduction in pain intensity) and

time for pain to return to baseline must also be measured; SPID and TOTPAR are then calculated with the following equations[33]:

$$SPID = \sum_{t=0-6}^{n} PID_t$$

$$TOTPAR = \sum_{t=0-6}^{n} PR_t$$

where, at the t assessment point ($t = 0, 1, 2, n$), P_t and PR_t are pain intensity and pain relief measured at that point, respectively; P_0 is pain intensity at $t = 0$; and PID_t is the pain intensity difference, calculated as ($P_0 - P_t$).

Conclusion

Repeated pain assessment is a fundamental tool for improving the quality of acute pain management. It is the performance of assessment, and not the measurement tool itself, that is important. The measurement must be a patient self-report when possible, because care providers tend to underestimate the patient's pain. As rehabilitation of function determines outcome after surgery, postoperative pain assessment should be performed both with the patient at rest and during relevant movement. Because patients have the right to appropriate pain management, pain assessment is no longer optional.

REFERENCES

1. Max MB, Payne R, Edwards WT, et al: Principles of Analgesic Use in the Treatment of Acute Pain and Cancer Pain, 4th ed. Glenview, IL, American Pain Society, 1999.
2. Slezak J, Hacobian A: The history and clinical examination. In Ballantyne J, Fishman SM, Abdi S (eds): The Massachusetts General Hospital Handbook of Pain Management, 2nd ed. Philadelphia, Lippincott Williams & Wilkins, 2002, pp 37–46.
3. Hobbs GJ, Hodgkinson V: Assessment, measurement, history and examination. In Rowbotham DJ, Macintyre P (eds): Acute Pain. London, Arnold, 2003, pp 93–111.

4. Loeser JD: Medical evaluation of the patient with pain. In Loeser JD, Butler SH, Chapman CR, et al (eds): Bonica's Management of Pain, 3rd ed. Baltimore, Lippincott Williams & Wilkins, 2001, pp 267–279.

5. McCaffery M, Pasero C: Assessment: Underlying complexities, misconceptions, and practical tools. In McCaffery M, Pasero C (eds): Pain Clinical Manual, 2nd ed. St. Louis, Mosby Inc, 1999, pp 35–102.

6. Dahl JB, Rosenberg J, Hansen BL, et al: Differential analgesic effects of low-dose epidural morphine and morphine-bupivacaine at rest and during mobilization after major abdominal surgery. Anesth Analg 1992;74:362–365.

7. Benhamou D: Evaluation de la douleur postoperatoire. Ann Fr Anesth Reanim 1998;17:555–572.

8. Keele KD: The pain chart. Lancet 1948;3:6–8.

9. LeBel AA: Assessment of pain. In Ballantyne J, Fishman SM, Abdi S (eds): The Massachusetts General Hospital Handbook of Pain Management, 2nd ed. Philadelphia, Lippincott Williams & Wilkins, 2002, pp 58–75.

10. Stubhaug A, Breivik H: Post-operative analgesic trials: Some important issues. Baillieres Clin Anaesthesiol 1995;9:555–584.

11. Price DD, Bush FM, Long S, Harkins W: A comparison of pain measurement characteristics of mechanical visual analogue and simple numerical rating scales. Pain 2004;56:217–226.

12. Murphy DF, McDonald A, Power C, et al: Measurement of pain: A comparison of the visual analogue with a non visual analogue scale. Clin J Pain 1988;3:197–199.

13. Aitken RCB: A growing edge of measurement of feelings. Proc Roy Soc Med 1969;62:989–993.

14. Clarke PRF, Spear FG: Reliability and sensitivity in the self-assessment of well-being [abstract]. Br J Psychol Soc 1964;17:55.

15. Huskisson EC: Measurement of pain. Lancet 1974;2:1127–1131.

16. Scott J, Huskisson EC: Graphic representation of pain. Pain 1976;2:175–184.

17. Brievik EK, Skoglund LA: Comparison of present pain intensity assessments on horizontally and vertically orientated visual analogue scales. Methods Find Exp Clin Pharmacol 1998;20:719–724.

18. DeLoach LJ, Higgins MS, Caplan AB, Stiff JL: The visual analog scale in the immediate postoperative period: Intrasubject variability and correlation with a numeric scale. Anesth Analg 1998;86:102–106.

19. Myles PS, Troedel S, Boquest M, Reeves M: The pain visual analog scale: Is it linear or nonlinear? Anesth Analg 1999;89:1517–1520.

20. Melzack R: The McGill Pain Questionnaire: Major properties and scoring methods. Pain 1975;1:277–299.

21. Reading AE: A comparison of the McGill pain questionnaire in chronic and acute pain. Pain 1982;13:185–192.

22. Jenkinson C, Carroll D, Egerton M, et al: Comparison of the sensitivity to change of long and short form pain measures. Quality Life Res 1995;4:353–357.

23. Melzack R: The short-form McGill Pain Questionnaire. Pain 1987;30:191–197.

24. Lowe NK, Walker SN, McCallum RC: Confirming the theoretical structure of the McGill pain questionnaire in acute clinical pain. Pain 1990;46:53–60.

25. Gagliese L, Melzack R: Age differences in the quality of chronic pain: A preliminary study. Pain Res Manage 1997;2:157–162.

26. Edwards R, Sarlani E, Wesselmann U, Fillingim RB: Quantitative assessment of experimental pain perception: Multiple domains of clinical relevance. Pain 2005;114:315–319.

27. Nikolajsen L, Ilkjaer S, Jensen TS: Relationship between mechanical sensitivity and postamputation pain: A prospective study. Eur J Pain 2000;4:327–334.

28. Granot M, Lowenstein L, Yarnitzky D, et al: Postcesarean section pain prediction by preoperative experimental pain assessment. Anesthesiology 2003;98:1422–1426.

29. Werner MU, Duun P, Kehlet H: Prediction of postoperative pain by preoperative nociceptive responses to heat stimulation. Anesthesiology 2004;100:115–119.

30. Bisgaard T, Klarskov B, Rosenberg J, Kehlet H: Characteristics and prediction of early pain after laparoscopic cholecystectomy. Pain 2001;90:261–269.

31. Lehmann KA: Patient-controlled intravenous analgesia for postoperative pain relief. In Max MB, Portenoy RK, Laska E (eds): The Design of Analgesic Clinical Trials. Advances in Pain Research and Therapy, vol 18. New York, Raven Press, 1991, pp 481–506.

32. McCoy EP, Furness G: Forum: Patient-controlled analgesia with and without background infusion. Analgesia assessed using the demand: delivery ratio. Anaesthesia 1993;48:256–265.

33. McQuay H, Moore A: An Evidence-Based Resource for Pain Relief. Oxford, Oxford Medical Publications, 1998, pp 14–18.

12 Prediction and Prevention of Acute Postoperative Pain: Moving Beyond Preemptive Analgesia

JOEL KATZ

Acute postoperative pain management has been dominated by an outdated concept of pain. Pain has been viewed as the end-product of a passive system that faithfully transmits a peripheral "pain signal" from receptor to a "pain center" in the brain.[1] This view has resulted in a strategy for managing postoperative pain that is inadequate, in part because it treats the patient only after the pain is well established. Patients arrive in the post-anesthesia care unit (PACU) after surgery, often in extreme pain, where they then receive multiple doses of opioids in an effort to bring the pain down to a tolerable level. However, basic science and clinical data show that brief, noxious inputs or frank injury due to C-fiber activation (e.g., cutting tissue, nerve, and bone) induces long-lasting changes in central neural function that persist well after the offending stimulus has been removed or the injury has healed.[2,3] This view of pain, involving a dynamic interplay between peripheral and central mechanisms, is inconsistent with the outdated notion that pain results from transmission of impulses along a straight-through pathway from the site of injury to the brain.[1]

The practice of treating pain only after it has become well entrenched is slowly being supplanted by a preventive approach that aims to block transmission of the primary afferent injury barrage before, during, and after surgery.[4-6] The idea behind this approach is not simply that it reduces nociception and stress during surgery—although these are obviously worthwhile goals. The hypothesis is that the transmission of noxious afferent input from the periphery (e.g., arising from preoperative pain, incision, noxious intraoperative events, postoperative inflammation, and ectopia) to the spinal cord induces a prolonged state of central neural sensitization or hyperexcitability that amplifies subsequent input from the wound, leading to heightened postoperative pain and a greater requirement for postoperative analgesics. By interrupting the transmission of the peripheral nociceptive barrage to the spinal cord at various points in time throughout the perioperative period, a preventive approach aims to block the induction of central sensitization, thereby reducing pain intensity and lowering analgesic requirements.

Targets of a Preventive Approach to Acute Pain Management

The perioperative period can be divided into three distinct phases: preoperative, intraoperative, and postoperative (Fig. 12–1). Specific factors within these phases contribute to the development of acute postoperative pain. The factors are as follows: (1) preoperative noxious inputs and pain, (2) C-fiber injury barrage arising from the cutting of skin, muscle, nerve and bone, wound retraction, and so on, and (3) postoperative peripheral nociceptive activity, including those arising from the inflammatory response, and ectopic neural activity in the case of postsurgical nerve injury. Each of these factors can contribute to peripheral and central sensitization, and each is a legitimate target for a preventive approach. The relative contributions of these three factors to acute postoperative pain depend on the surgical procedure, extent and nature of tissue damage, duration of surgery, timing of treatments relative to incision, pharmacokinetics of the agent(s) used preoperatively, presence or absence of additional analgesia intraoperatively, nature of postoperative analgesia, and a host of other variables. Minimizing the negative impact of as many of these factors in the three phases as possible increases the likelihood of preventing the induction and maintenance of peripheral and central sensitization. Preventing sensitization reduces pain and analgesic requirements.

Figure 12–1 depicts the eight possible treatment combinations of administering or not administering analgesics during the three perioperative phases (preoperative, intraoperative, and postoperative). The preoperative period encompasses interventions that begin days before surgery and includes those administered just minutes before the skin incision. The intraoperative period extends from interventions started immediately after incision to those initiated just prior to the end of surgery (i.e., skin closure). The postoperative period consists of interventions started immediately after the end of surgery and may extend for days thereafter.

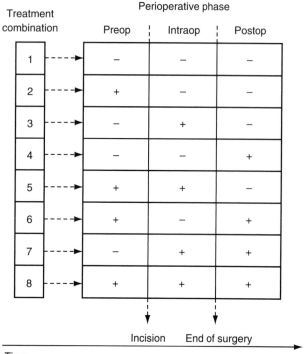

Figure 12–1 Schematic representation showing the administration (+) or nonadministration (–) of analgesic agents during the three perioperative phases of surgery—preoperative (preop), intraoperative (intraop), and postoperative (postop). The administration or nonadministration of analgesics during the three phases yields 8 different treatment combinations and 28 possible two-group study designs.

Within each phase there is potential for extensive variability in the timing of administration of analgesic agents. This potential is greatest in the preoperative and postoperative phases (e.g., ranging from days to minutes), but evidence shows that even within the intraoperative period there are considerable interstudy differences in timing of the postincisional intervention (e.g., ranging from minutes to hours).

Prediction of Pain

The ability to predict who will experience severe acute postoperative pain and who will go on to have chronic postsurgical pain is at the heart of efforts to understand the role played by the various factors within the three perioperative phases. One of the most robust findings to emerge from the postoperative pain and anesthesia literature is that current pain predicts future pain.[7–9] This appears to be true for all surgery types and regardless of time frame. Intense preoperative pain or preoperative pain of long duration is a risk factor for development of severe early acute postoperative pain,[10] for acute pain days[11–15] and weeks[16] after surgery, and for long-term postsurgical pain.[12,13,16–20] High preoperative pain ratings in response to the cold pressor task,[21] suprathreshold heat pain stimuli,[22] and a first-degree burn injury[23] also predict more intense acute postoperative pain days after surgery. Additionally, severe acute postoperative pain not only predicts pain after discharge[16,24] but also is a risk factor for development of chronic postsurgical pain.[25–30]

No other factor is as consistently related to the development of future pain problems as is current pain. Younger age,[10,16] female sex,[16] anxiety,[10,17] and various other psychological variables[7,31–34] predict postoperative pain in some studies, but not with the consistency or magnitude with which current pain predicts pain. What must be determined is the aspect of pain that is predictive. Is it something about the pain per se (e.g., intensity, quality, duration) or the individuals who report the pain (e.g., response bias, psychological vulnerability, genetic predisposition)? Will reducing surgery-induced sensitization alter the course of acute pain and lead to a lower incidence of long-term pain problems? What factors are responsible for the transition of acute postoperative pain to chronic, intractable, pathological pain? We do not have answers to these important questions, but one of the factors that have been linked to increased pain and analgesic consumption in the short and long term is the perioperative peripheral nociceptive injury barrage associated with surgery. The remainder of this chapter consists of an evidence-based presentation of the literature that examines the efficacy of preemptive and preventive interventions aimed at reducing surgically induced sensitization.

History of and Progress in Preemptive Analgesia

The idea that acute postoperative pain might be intensified by a state of central neural hyperexcitability induced during surgery was proposed first by Crile[35] and later by Wall,[36] who suggested that "preemptive preoperative analgesia" would block the induction of central neural sensitization brought about by the incision and, thus, reduce the intensity of acute postoperative pain. Since its introduction into the pain and anesthesia literatures, this concept has been refined, partly on the basis of confirmatory and contradictory evidence from clinical studies, new developments in basic science, and critical thought. The suggestion that surgical incision triggers central sensitization[36] has been expanded to include the sensitizing effects of preoperative noxious inputs and pain and of other noxious intraoperative stimuli, as well as the effects of postoperative peripheral and central inflammatory mediators and ectopic neural activity.

It is now well documented that general anesthesia may attenuate the transmission of afferent injury barrage from the periphery to the spinal cord and brain, but it does not block the transmission.[37] Moreover, systemic opioids may not provide a sufficiently dense blockade of spinal nociceptive neurons to prevent central sensitization.[38] The clinical significance of these findings for patients who receive general anesthesia during surgery is that although they are unconscious, the processes leading to sensitization of dorsal horn neurons are largely unaffected by general anesthesia or routine doses of opioids. This sets the stage for heightened postoperative pain and an increased requirement for analgesics.

Controversy and Confusion about Preemptive Analgesia

Debate over the appropriate definition of *preemptive analgesia*[5,39–45] has spawned a variety of different terms, including anoci-association,[46] preemptive preoperative analgesia,[36]

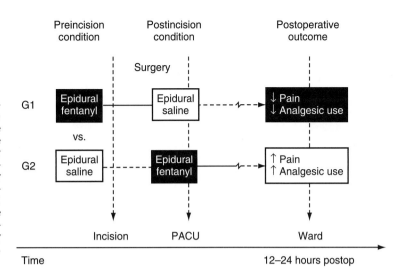

Figure 12–2 Experimental design and expected postoperative outcome for studies of preemptive analgesia in which a preincisional intervention is compared with the very same intervention initiated after incision but before the end of surgery. This design was used in the study by Katz et al,[52] in which the two groups of patients undergoing lateral thoracotomy received epidural fentanyl or saline before, and the other drug 15 minutes after, incision. Pain ratings in the group who received preincisional epidural fentanyl (G1) were significantly less intense 6 hours after surgery and morphine consumption was significantly lower between 12 and 24 hours after surgery than in the group who received preincisional saline (G2). PACU, post-anesthesia care unit.

preemptive analgesia,[47] preventive analgesia,[5,48] balanced periemptive analgesia,[49] broad versus narrow preemptive analgesia,[6] and protective analgesia.[50] Substantial confusion has developed about the benefits and meaning of *preemptive analgesia.*

Two general approaches have dominated the literature.[51] The classic study of *preemptive analgesia*[47] requires two groups of patients to receive identical analgesic treatment, one group before surgery and one group either after incision or after surgery (treatment combinations 2 versus 3 and 2 versus 4 in Fig. 12–1). The only difference between the two groups is the timing of administration of the pharmacological agent relative to incision, with one group receiving the target agent before surgery and the other group receiving it after incision (Fig. 12–2, the study by Katz et al[52]) or after surgery (Fig. 12–3, the study by Dierking et al[53]).

The constraint to include a postincision or postsurgical treatment group is methodologically appealing, because in the presence of a positive result, it provides a window of time within which the observed effect occurred and thus points to possible mechanisms underlying the effect. However, this view of preemptive analgesia is too restrictive

and narrow,[3,5,41] in part because we do not know the relative extent to which preoperative, intraoperative, and postoperative peripheral nociceptive inputs contribute to central sensitization and postoperative pain. The narrow conceptualization of preemptive analgesia in conjunction with the classic pre-/post-design assumes that the intraoperative nociceptive barrage contributes to postoperative pain to a greater extent than does the postoperative nociceptive barrage. However, the design does not allow for other equally plausible alternatives. For certain surgical procedures, central sensitization may be induced to an equal extent by incision and intraoperative trauma on the one hand (i.e., in the postsurgical treatment group) and postoperative inflammatory inputs and/or ectopia on the other (i.e., in the preoperative treatment group), leading to nonsignificant intergroup differences in pain and analgesic consumption.[4]

Two-group studies that fail to find significant differences in postoperative pain or analgesic consumption between groups treated either before or after incision or surgery are inherently flawed because of the absence of an appropriate control group (e.g., treatment combination 1, 8, or both

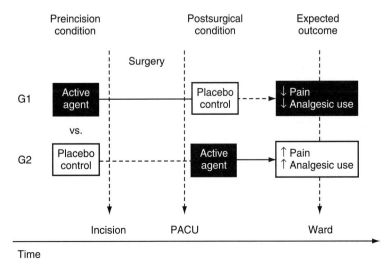

Figure 12–3 Experimental design and expected postoperative outcome for studies of preemptive analgesia in which a preincision intervention (G1) is compared with the very same intervention initiated after surgery (G2). Expected outcome is based on the hypothesis of classically defined preemptive analgesia, i.e., that the effects of intraoperative noxious inputs contribute to postoperative pain and analgesic use to a greater extent than postoperative noxious inputs. This design was used in the study by Dierking et al,[53] who compared a lidocaine inguinal field block administered 15 minutes before hernia repair with the same treatment administered immediately after surgery. Significant differences in pain or analgesic use were not found between the presurgical and postsurgical treatment groups, raising the possibility that a preventive effect went undetected owing to lack of a control group (see Figs. 12–4 and 12–5). PACU, post-anesthesia care unit.

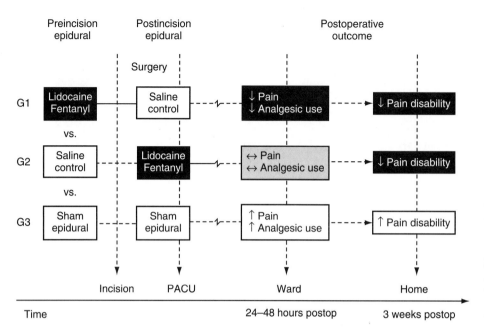

Figure 12–4 Experimental design used by Katz et al[54,55] to address the design flaw inherent in two-group studies of preemptive analgesia (see Fig. 12–2). In women undergoing abdominal gynecological surgery by laparotomy, preincisional (G1) but not postincisional (G2) administration of epidural lidocaine and fentanyl was associated with a significantly lower rate of morphine use, lower cumulative morphine consumption, and reduced hyperalgesia compared with a sham epidural condition (G3).[54] Three-week follow-up showed that pain disability ratings were significantly lower in the two groups that received the epidural than in the standard treatment group.[55] Results highlight the importance of including a standard treatment control group to avoid the problems of interpretation that arise when two-group studies of preemptive analgesia (preincision versus postincision) fail to find the anticipated effects. PACU, post-anesthesia care unit; postop, after surgery.

in Fig. 12–1). The negative results may point to the relative efficacy of postincisional or postsurgical blockade in reducing central sensitization and not to the inefficacy of preoperative blockade (for examples, see Figs. 12–4 and 12–5, which depict studies Katz et al[54,55] and Gordon et al[56]). Later studies have highlighted the critical importance of a standard treatment control group.[54,55] Inclusion of such a group has made it possible to demonstrate reductions in acute postoperative pain and morphine consumption[54] as well as pain disability 3 weeks after surgery[55] that would have gone undetected in studies using classic two-group design. Other reports have demonstrated that for certain types of surgery,

blocking the peripheral nociceptive barrage in the hours after surgery decreases pain at later periods, whereas blocking the intraoperative nociceptive barrage does not (Fig. 12–5).[56] The near-exclusive focus in the literature on this narrow view of preemptive analgesia has had the unintended effect of diverting attention away from certain clinically significant findings because they do not conform to what has become the accepted definition of preemptive analgesia.[4]

A more encompassing approach, *preventive analgesia*,[4,5] has evolved with the aim of minimizing sensitization induced by noxious perioperative stimuli, including those arising

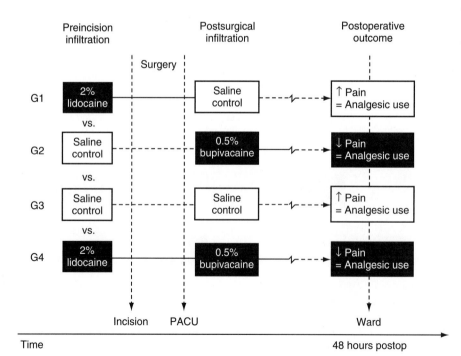

Figure 12–5 Experimental design used by Gordon et al[56] to assess the relative effects on late postoperative pain of blocking, or not blocking, noxious intraoperative and/or postoperative inputs. Patients were randomly assigned in a double-blind manner to receive a local anesthetic (lidocaine or bupivacaine) or saline before and/or at the end of surgery for third molar extraction. Preventive analgesia is demonstrated by the finding that 48 hours after surgery, pain intensity was significantly less in the groups whose postoperative pain was blocked by bupivacaine (G2, G4) than in the group receiving preoperative administration of lidocaine (G1) or the saline control group (G3). The results suggest that for third molar extraction surgery, the peripheral nociceptive barrage in the hours after surgery contributes to a greater extent to central sensitization and late postoperative pain than the intraoperative nociceptive barrage, because local anesthetic blockade after surgery was more efficacious than preoperative blockade. PACU, post-anesthesia care unit; postop, after surgery.

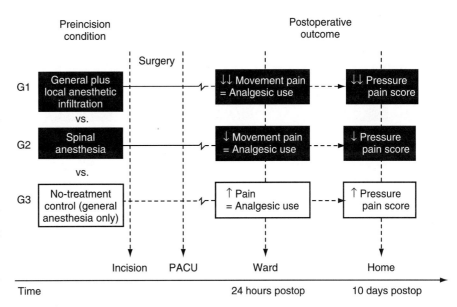

Figure 12–6 Experimental design comparing two different preoperative interventions with a no-treatment control condition. This design was used by Tverskoy et al[57] in the very first prospective study of preventive analgesia. Patients undergoing inguinal herniorrhaphy were randomly assigned to receive one of three types of anesthesia: general plus local anesthetic infiltration (G1), spinal anesthesia (G2), or general anesthesia only (G3). Although anesthesia (infiltration or spinal) significantly decreased movement-associated pain intensity at 24 hours after surgery compared with control, the infiltration group reported the least pain overall. This pattern of pain scores was still apparent 10 days after surgery in response to mechanical pressure applied to the wound. PACU, post-anesthesia care unit; postop, after surgery.

preoperatively, intraoperatively, and postoperatively. A preventive analgesic effect is demonstrated when postoperative pain and/or analgesic consumption is reduced relative to another treatment and/or a placebo treatment or no treatment as long as the effect is observed at a point in time that exceeds the clinical duration of action of the target agent (e.g., treatment combination 1 versus 2, and treatment combination 1 versus 5 in Fig. 12–1). The requirement that the reduced pain and/or analgesic consumption be observed after the duration of action of the target agent ensures that the preventive effect is not simply an analgesic effect. Such a design, however, does not provide information about the factors underlying the effect or the time frame within which the effect occurred, owing to the absence of a post-treatment condition. Figs. 12–6 and 12–7 illustrate studies by Tverskoy et al[57] and Reuben et al,[58] respectively, who used these designs.

Demonstration of a preventive effect does not require that an intervention be initiated before surgery; the treatment may occur during the procedure (e.g., treatment combination

1 versus 3 in Fig. 12–1) or even after surgery (e.g., treatment combination 1 versus 4 in Fig. 12–1). For example, a preventive effect is present if postoperative administration of a target analgesic agent, but not of a placebo, results in less postoperative pain or lower analgesic consumption after the effects of the target agent have worn off. (For a case in point, see Fig. 12–8, which depicts a study by Reuben et al.[59]) The focus of preventive analgesia is not on the relative timing of anesthetic interventions but on attenuating the effect of noxious perioperative stimuli that both induce peripheral and central sensitization and increase postoperative pain intensity and analgesic requirements.

Synopsis of Literature

Evidence-based reviews of randomized double-blind studies reported in the literature on preemptive analgesia[4,48,50,60,61] and preventive analgesia[4,48,62] suggest that clinically significant benefits are associated with both approaches to postoperative

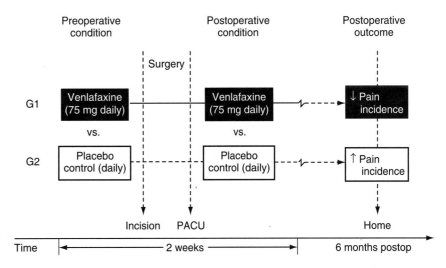

Figure 12–7 Experimental design comparing a preoperative plus postsurgical intervention with a placebo-controlled condition. Preventive analgesia is demonstrated if the preoperative plus postsurgical intervention condition shows less pain and/or analgesic consumption than the placebo control group beyond the clinical duration of action of the target analgesic. This design was used by Reuben et al,[58] who randomly assigned women to receive venlafaxine (75 mg daily) or placebo (daily) for a 2-week period beginning the night before radical mastectomy. Six-month follow-up showed that the incidence of chest wall pain, arm pain, and axilla pain was significantly lower in the venlafaxine group than in the placebo group. PACU, post-anesthesia care unit; postop, after surgery.

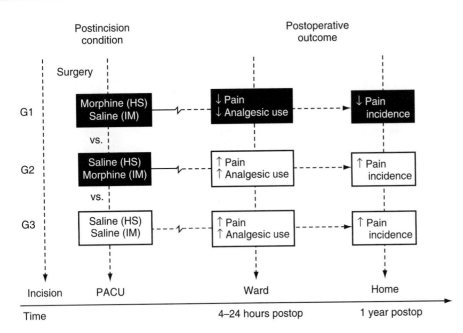

Figure 12–8 Experimental design comparing a postincision analgesic intervention with a placebo or no-treatment control condition. Preventive analgesia is demonstrated if the postincision condition shows less pain and/or analgesic consumption than the control group in the time beyond the clinical duration of action of the target analgesic. This design was used by Reuben et al,[59] who showed that morphine, but not saline, administered into the iliac bone graft harvest site (HS) during cervical spinal fusion surgery (G1) reduced short-term pain and analgesic consumption as well as the incidence of chronic donor site pain 1 year after surgery compared with a group that received intramuscular (IM) morphine (G2) and a placebo control group that received saline (G3). The study illustrates that preventive analgesia can be achieved even when the analgesic intervention is started *after* incision and bone graft harvest (i.e., in the context of an unchecked peripheral nociceptive injury barrage). PACU, post-anesthesia care unit; postop; after surgery.

pain prevention, although the positive evidence is more abundant for the latter than the former. The more equivocal results for preemptive analgesia likely reflect the fact that intraoperative and postoperative noxious inputs contribute to central sensitization, thus diminishing the magnitude of the effect when preoperatively and postoperatively treated groups are compared.

Katz[4] and Katz and McCartney[48] evaluated 175 randomized, double-blind, controlled trials of preventive and preemptive analgesia using the definitions provided previously. The reviews spanned the period from December 1987 through April 2002. The investigators concluded that throughout the classes of agents reviewed, the proportion of significant preventive analgesic effects was significantly greater than what one would expect by chance alone (Table 12–1). Local anesthetic administration before tonsillectomy[63–67] or inguinal hernia repair[57,68–71] appears to produce clinically significant reductions in postoperative pain beyond the duration of action of the local anesthetic.

Results of studies that examined the timing of administration of opioids, with or without local anesthetics, were less conclusive, possibly because of the competing processes associated with acute opioid tolerance[72–74] and opioid-induced hyperalgesia.[75–77] In general, opioid-induced reductions in pain and analgesic consumption associated with preemptive or preventive effects were small.

There appears to be little evidence that the timing of administration of nonsteroidal anti-inflammatory drugs (NSAIDs)

| TABLE 12–1 | Summary of Studies of Preemptive and Preventive Analgesia According to Target Agent Administered* |

Agent(s)	No. of Studies	Preemptive Effects (%)		Preventive Effects (%)		Opposite Effects (%)	Total No. Effects (%)
		Positive	Negative	Positive	Negative		
Local anesthetics*	65	8 (10.7)	16. (21.3)	27 (36.0)	18 (24.0)	6 (8.0)	75 (100)
Opioids	25	7 (25.0)	5 (17.9)	10 (35.7)	3 (10.7)	3 (10.7)	28 (100)
NSAIDs	25	3 (11.5)	12 (46.2)	1 (3.8)	8 (30.8)	2 (7.7)	26 (100)
NMDA antagonists	31	5 (13.2)	6 (15.8)	19 (50.0)	7 (18.4)	1 (2.6)	38 (100)
Clonidine	2	0 (0.0)	0 (0.0)	2 (100.0)	0 (0.0)	0 (0.0)	2 (100)
Local anesthetics and opioids	21	4 (17.4)	5 (21.7)	7 (30.4)	6 (26.1)	1 (4.3)	23 (100)
Multimodal	6	2 (25.0)	0 (0.0)	2 (25.0)	3 (37.5)	1 (12.5)	8 (100)
Total†	175	29 (14.5)	44 (22.0)	68 (34.0)	45 (22.5)	14 (7.0)	200 (100)

*$P = .05$ for the number of positive preventive effects by Fisher exact test.

†$P = .01$ for the number of positive preventive effects by chi-square test. The total number of effects exceeds the number of studies because some studies were designed to evaluate both preemptive and preventive effects. See text for definition of *preemptive effects* and *preventive effects*.

NMDA, N-methyl-D-aspartate; NSAIDs, nonsteroidal anti-inflammatory drugs.

Combined data from Katz J: Timing of treatment and pre-emptive analgesia. In Rice A, Warfield C, Justins D, et al: Clinical Pain Management: Acute Volume. London, Arnold, 2003, pp 113–162; and Katz J, McCartney CJL: Current status of pre-emptive analgesia. Curr Opin Anaesthesiol 2002;15:435–441.

produces preemptive or preventive effects.[4,48] This conclusion is consistent with results of the meta-analysis by Moiniche et al[50] but conflicts with the results of the later meta-analyses conducted by Ong et al[61] and Dahl and Moiniche.[60] Ong et al[61] report an effect size of 0.39 for the preemptive administration of NSAIDs, and Dahl and Moiniche[60] report that 6 of the 8 later studies demonstrated less pain after presurgical than after postsurgical administration of NSAIDs. The discrepancy may, in large part, be explained by the different time frames over which the reviews were conducted. Both Ong et al[61] and Dahl and Moiniche[60] report that since 2001 there has been an increase in the number of significant studies of preemptive analgesia using NSAIDs, whereas the reviews by Katz[4,48] extended only to April 2002.

In view of the higher risk of cardiovascular thrombotic events associated with the cyclooxyegnase-2 (Cox-2) inhibitor rofecoxib,[78,79] and notwithstanding the potential importance of this class of NSAID for the prevention of pain,[80] it is important to point out that only one of the studies evaluating the efficacy of NSAIDs used a Cox-2 inhibitor.[81]

Reviews by Katz[4] and Katz and McCartney[48] reported significant benefits associated with the preventive use of the N-methyl-D-aspartate (NMDA) antagonists ketamine and dextromethorphan. Together, the two reviews indicate that 73% of the 26 preventive effects evaluated resulted in significantly lower pain intensity and/or reduced analgesic requirements (see Table 12–1). These conclusions were bolstered by the qualitative systematic review by McCartney et al,[62] who used a more conservative test in evaluating the preventive analgesic effects of several NMDA receptor antagonists. The relevant outcomes were a reduction in pain, analgesic consumption, or both in studies that provided these measures at a point in time that exceeded five half-lives of the NMDA receptor antagonist under examination. Forty articles met the inclusion criteria (24 ketamine, 12 dextromethorphan, and 4 magnesium). The evidence in favor of preventive analgesia was strongest in the case of dextromethorphan and ketamine, with 67% and 58% of studies, respectively, demonstrating a reduction in pain, analgesic consumption, or both beyond the clinical duration of action of the drug concerned. The four reports on magnesium did not provide evidence of preventive analgesia. The meta-analyses indicate that NMDA receptor antagonists showed no evidence of a preemptive effect,[50,60,61] a finding consistent with basic science data showing that these agents are equally effective at preventing and reversing central sensitization.[82]

Given the small number of studies of multimodal analgesia and the relatively large variability in the routes of administration, agents, timing, and patient populations, there were insufficient data to generate a reliable conclusion on the efficacy of the timing of combined administration of local anesthetics, opioids, and NSAIDs.[4]

Conclusions

Preoperative pain intensity is a risk factor for development of severe acute postoperative pain as well as long-term postsurgical pain. Severity of acute postoperative pain predicts pain after discharge and is also a risk factor for chronic postsurgical pain. These findings have fueled preventive and preemptive efforts to reduce acute pain intensity and long-term pain problems by blocking noxious perioperative inputs.

The evidence points to a significantly greater proportion of preventive analgesia studies than preemptive analgesia studies with positive results (see Table 12–1). The nature of the designs differ considerably among the 175 clinical trials (200 effects) evaluated,[4,48] but it appears that in general there is a benefit in terms of reduced pain and/or analgesic consumption that extends beyond the duration of action of the target drug. The preponderance of evidence for preventive analgesia is understandable when one considers that both preincisional and postincisional (or postsurgical) noxious inputs contribute to postoperative sensitization.[4] The most likely conclusion is that for a certain proportion of studies of preemptive analgesia, the postincision or postsurgical administration condition is as beneficial in reducing central sensitization as the preoperative condition, but these benefits go undetected when the comparison is made between the two groups. The lack of a control group in studies of preemptive analgesia is a serious limitation that confounds interpretation of the results and has contributed to the premature and erroneous conclusion that there is no clinical benefit to preoperative nociceptive blockade.

The continued use of incomplete designs that consist of preincisional and postincisional or postsurgical conditions without a standard treatment group or a complete blockade condition will hinder progress in our understanding of the benefits of preemptive analgesia. Adhering to the narrow definition of preemptive analgesia currently accepted by many in the field will perpetuate problems of interpretation and will not lead to the evolution and progress that are needed to move us beyond the current state of confusion. Inclusion of appropriate control conditions is essential if we are to advance our knowledge about the factors that contribute to acute postoperative pain and enhance our ability to detect clinical benefits associated with blockade of noxious perioperative inputs. Future work should focus on maximizing the prevention of surgically induced sensitization by ensuring as complete a blockade as possible of nociceptive transmission throughout the three phases of the perioperative period.

Given the prominent role of psychosocial factors in chronic pain[83] and the recommendations for assessment of core measures and domains in clinical trials,[84,85] relevant psychological, emotional, and physical variables should be added to those routinely assessed before and after surgery. Assessment of additional domains of functioning may help shed light on the predictors of severe acute postoperative pain, the processes involved in recovery from surgery, and the risk factors for development of chronic postsurgical pain.

Acknowledgments

Joel Katz is supported by a Canada Research Chair in Health Psychology.

REFERENCES

1. Melzack R, Wall PD: The Challenge of Pain, 2nd ed. New York, Basic Books, 1988.
2. Woolf CJ, Salter MW: Neuronal plasticity: Increasing the gain in pain. Science 2000;288:1765–1769.

3. Coderre TJ, Katz J, Vaccarino AL, Melzack R: Contribution of central neuroplasticity to pathological pain: Review of clinical and experimental evidence. Pain 1993;52:259–285.
4. Katz J: Timing of treatment and pre-emptive analgesia. In Rice A, Warfield C, Justins D, et al (eds): Clinical Pain Management: Acute Volume. London, Arnold, 2003, pp 113–162.
5. Kissin I: Preemptive analgesia: Terminology and clinical relevance. Anesth Analg 1994;79:809.
6. Kissin I: Preemptive analgesia. Anesthesiology 2000;93:1138–1143.
7. Perkins FM, Kehlet H: Chronic pain as an outcome of surgery: A review of predictive factors. Anesthesiology 2000;93:1123–1133.
8. Katz J: Pain begets pain—predictors of long-term phantom limb pain and post-thoracotomy pain. Pain Forum 1997;6:140–144.
9. Dworkin RH: Which individuals with acute pain are most likely to develop a chronic pain syndrome? Pain Forum 1997;6:127–136.
10. Kalkman CJ, Visser K, Moen J, et al: Preoperative prediction of severe postoperative pain. Pain 2003;105:415–423.
11. Tasmuth T, Blomqvist C, Kalso E: Chronic post-treatment symptoms in patients with breast cancer operated in different surgical units. Eur J Surg Oncol 1999;25:38–43.
12. Jensen TS, Krebs B, Nielsen J, Rasmussen P: Immediate and long-term phantom limb pain in amputees: Incidence, clinical characteristics and relationship to pre-amputation limb pain. Pain 1985;21:267–278.
13. Nikolajsen L, Ilkjaer S, Kroner K, et al: The influence of preamputation pain on postamputation stump and phantom pain. Pain 1997;72:393–405.
14. Caumo W, Schmidt AP, Schneider CN, et al: Preoperative predictors of moderate to intense acute postoperative pain in patients undergoing abdominal surgery. Acta Anaesthesiol Scand 2002;46:1265–1271.
15. Scott LE, Clum GA, Peoples JB: Preoperative predictors of postoperative pain. Pain 1983;15:283–293.
16. Thomas T, Robinson C, Champion D, et al: Prediction and assessment of the severity of post-operative pain and of satisfaction with management. Pain 1998;75:177–185.
17. Harden RN, Bruehl S, Stanos S, et al: Prospective examination of pain-related and psychological predictors of CRPS-like phenomena following total knee arthroplasty: A preliminary study. Pain 2003;106:393–400.
18. Brander VA, Stulberg SD, Adams AD, et al: Predicting total knee replacement pain: A prospective, observational study. Clin Orthop 2003;416:27–36.
19. Liem MS, van Duyn EB, van der Graaf Y, van Vroonhoven TJ: Recurrences after conventional anterior and laparoscopic inguinal hernia repair: A randomized comparison. Ann Surg 2003;237:136–141.
20. Poobalan AS, Bruce J, King PM, et al: Chronic pain and quality of life following open inguinal hernia repair. Br J Surg 2001;88:1122–1126.
21. Bisgaard T, Klarskov B, Rosenberg J, Kehlet H: Characteristics and prediction of early pain after laparoscopic cholecystectomy. Pain 2001;90:261–269.
22. Granot M, Lowenstein L, Yarnitsky D, et al: Postcesarean section pain prediction by preoperative experimental pain assessment. Anesthesiology 2003;98:1422–1426.
23. Werner MU, Duun P, Kehlet H: Prediction of postoperative pain by preoperative nociceptive responses to heat stimulation. Anesthesiology 2004;100:115–119.
24. Beauregard L, Pomp A, Choiniere M: Severity and impact of pain after day-surgery. Can J Anaesth 1998;45:304–311.
25. Lau H, Patil NG, Yuen WK, Lee F: Prevalence and severity of chronic groin pain after endoscopic totally extraperitoneal inguinal hernioplasty. Surg Endosc 2003;17:1620–1623.
26. Callesen T, Bech K, Kehlet H: Prospective study of chronic pain after groin hernia repair. Br J Surg 1999;86:1528–1531.
27. Katz J, Jackson M, Kavanagh BP, Sandler AN: Acute pain after thoracic surgery predicts long-term post-thoracotomy pain. Clin J Pain 1996;12:50–55.
28. Hayes C, Browne S, Lantry G, Burstal R: Neuropathic pain in the acute pain service: A prospective survey. Acute Pain 2002;4:45–48.
29. Senturk M, Ozcan PE, Talu GK, et al: The effects of three different analgesia techniques on long-term postthoracotomy pain. Anesth Analg 2002;94:11–15.
30. Tasmuth T, Kataja M, Blomqvist C, et al: Treatment-related factors predisposing to chronic pain in patients with breast cancer—a multivariate approach. Acta Oncol 1997;36:625–630.
31. Jorgensen T, Teglbjerg JS, Wille-Jorgensen P, et al: Persisting pain after cholecystectomy: A prospective investigation. Scand J Gastroenterol 1991;26:124–128.
32. Borly L, Anderson IB, Bardram L, et al: Preoperative prediction model of outcome after cholecystectomy for symptomatic gallstones. Scand J Gastroenterol 1999;34:1144–1152.
33. Cohen L, Fouladi RT, Katz J: Preoperative coping strategies and distress predict postoperative pain and analgesic consumption in women undergoing abdominal gynecologic surgery. J Psychosom Res 2005;58:201–209.
34. Hanley MA, Jensen MP, Ehde DM, et al: Psychosocial predictors of long-term adjustment to lower-limb amputation and phantom limb pain. Disabil Rehabil 2004;26:882–893.
35. Katz J: George Washington Crile, anoci-association, and pre-emptive analgesia. Pain 1993;53:243–245.
36. Wall PD: The prevention of post-operative pain. Pain 1988;33:289–290.
37. Rundshagen I, Kochs E, Schulte am Esch J: Surgical stimulation increases median nerve somatosensory evoked responses during isoflurane-nitrous oxide anaesthesia. Br J Anaesth 1995;75:598–602.
38. Abram SE, Yaksh TL: Morphine, but not inhalation anesthesia, blocks post-injury facilitation: The role of preemptive suppression of afferent transmission. Anesthesiology 1993;78:713–721.
39. Taylor BK, Brennan TJ: Preemptive analgesia: Moving beyond conventional strategies and confusing terminology. J Pain 2000;1:77–84.
40. Futter M: Preventive not pre-emptive analgesia with piroxicam. Can J Anaesth 1997;44:101–102.
41. Katz J: Pre-emptive analgesia: Evidence, current status and future directions. Eur J Anaesthesiol Suppl 1995;10:8–13.
42. Kissin I: Preemptive analgesia: Why its effect is not always obvious. Anesthesiology 1996;84:1015–1019.
43. Yaksh TL, Abram SE: Preemptive analgesia: A popular misnomer, but a clinically relevant truth? APS J 1993;2:116–121.
44. Penning JP: Pre-emptive analgesia: What does it mean to the clinical anaesthetist? Can J Anaesth 1996;43:97–101.
45. Dionne R: Preemptive vs preventive analgesia: Which approach improves clinical outcomes? Compend Contin Educ Dent 2000;21:48,51–54,56.
46. Crile GW: The kinetic theory of shock and its prevention through anoci-association (shockless operation). Lancet 1913;185:7–16.
47. McQuay HJ: Pre-emptive analgesia. Br J Anaesth 1992;69:1–3.
48. Katz J, McCartney CJL: Current status of pre-emptive analgesia. Curr Opin Anaesth 2002;15:435–441.
49. Amantea B, Gemelli A, Migliorini F, Tocci R: Preemptive analgesia or balanced periemptive analgesia? Minerva Anestesiol 1999;65:19–37.
50. Moiniche S, Kehlet H, Dahl JB: A qualitative and quantitative systematic review of preemptive analgesia for postoperative pain relief: The role of timing of analgesia. Anesthesiology 2002;96:725–741.
51. Kissin I: Preemptive analgesia at the crossroad. Anesth Analg 2005;100:754–756.
52. Katz J, Kavanagh BP, Sandler AN, et al: Preemptive analgesia: Clinical evidence of neuroplasticity contributing to postoperative pain. Anesthesiology 1992;77:439–446.
53. Dierking GW, Dahl JB, Kanstrup J, et al: Effect of pre- vs postoperative inguinal field block on postoperative pain after herniorrhaphy. Br J Anaesth 1992;68:344–348.
54. Katz J, Cohen L, Schmid R, et al: Postoperative morphine use and hyperalgesia are reduced by preoperative but not intraoperative epidural analgesia: Implications for preemptive analgesia and the prevention of central sensitization. Anesthesiology 2003;98:1449–1460.
55. Katz J, Cohen L: Preventive analgesia is associated with reduced pain disability 3 weeks but not 6 months after major gynecologic surgery by laparotomy. Anesthesiology 2004;101:169–174.
56. Gordon SM, Brahim JS, Dubner R, et al: Attenuation of pain in a randomized trial by suppression of peripheral nociceptive activity in the immediate postoperative period. Anesth Analg 2002;95:1351–1357.
57. Tverskoy M, Cozacov C, Ayache M, et al: Postoperative pain after inguinal herniorrhaphy with different types of anesthesia. Anesth Analg 1990;70:29–35.
58. Reuben SS, Makari-Judson G, Lurie SD: Evaluation of efficacy of the perioperative administration of venlafaxine XR in the prevention of postmastectomy pain syndrome. J Pain Symptom Manage 2004;27:133–139.

59. Reuben SS, Vieira P, Faruqi S, et al: Local administration of morphine for analgesia after iliac bone graft harvest. Anesthesiology 2001;95: 390–394.
60. Dahl JB, Moiniche S: Pre-emptive analgesia. Br Med Bull 2004;71:13–25.
61. Ong KS, Lirk P, Seymour RA, Jenkins BJ: The efficacy of preemptive analgesia for acute postoperative pain management: A meta-analysis. Anesth Analg in press.
62. McCartney CJ, Sinha A, Katz J: A qualitative systematic review of the role of N-methyl-D-aspartate receptor antagonists in preventive analgesia. Anesth Analg 2004;98:1385–1400.
63. Agren K, Engquist S, Danneman A, Feychting B: Local versus general anaesthesia in tonsillectomy. Clin Otolaryngol 1989;14:97–100.
64. Jebeles JA, Reilly JS, Gutierrez JF, et al: The effect of pre-incisional infiltration of tonsils with bupivacaine on the pain following tonsillectomy under general anesthesia. Pain 1991;47:305–308.
65. Jebeles JA, Reilly JS, Gutierrez JF, et al: Tonsillectomy and adenoidectomy pain reduction by local bupivacaine infiltration in children. Int J Pediatr Otorhinolaryngol 1993;25:149–154.
66. Molliex S, Haond P, Baylot D, et al: Effect of pre- vs postoperative tonsillar infiltration with local anesthetics on postoperative pain after tonsillectomy. Acta Anaesthesiol Scand 1996;40:1210–1215.
67. Johansen M, Harbo G, Illum P: Preincisional infiltration with bupivacaine in tonsillectomy. Arch Otolaryngol Head Neck Surg 1996; 122:261–263.
68. Sinclair R, Cassuto J, Hogstrom S, et al: Topical anesthesia with lidocaine aerosol in the control of postoperative pain. Anesthesiology 1988;68: 895–901.
69. McLoughlin J, Kelley CJ: Study of the effectiveness of bupivacaine infiltration of the ilioinguinal nerve at the time of hernia repair for post-operative pain relief. Br J Clin Pract 1989;43:281–283.
70. Teasdale C, McCrum AM, Williams NB, Horton RE: A randomised controlled trial to compare local with general anaesthesia for short-stay inguinal hernia repair. Ann R Coll Surg Engl 1982;64:238–242.
71. Fischer S, Troidl H, MacLean AA, et al: Prospective double-blind randomised study of a new regimen of pre-emptive analgesia for inguinal hernia repair: Evaluation of postoperative pain course. Eur J Surg 2000;166:545–551.
72. Kissin I, Bright CA, Bradley EL Jr: The effect of ketamine on opioid-induced acute tolerance: Can it explain reduction of opioid consumption with ketamine-opioid analgesic combinations? Anesth Analg 2000;91: 1483–1488.
73. Li X, Angst MS, Clark JD: Opioid-induced hyperalgesia and incisional pain. Anesth Analg 2001;93:204–209.
74. Vinik HR, Kissin I: Rapid development of tolerance to analgesia during remifentanil infusion in humans. Anesth Analg 1998;86:1307–1311.
75. Celerier E, Laulin J, Larcher A, et al: Evidence for opiate-activated NMDA processes masking opiate analgesia in rats. Brain Res 1999;847: 18–25.
76. Celerier E, Rivat C, Jun Y, et al: Long-lasting hyperalgesia induced by fentanyl in rats: Preventive effect of ketamine. Anesthesiology 2000;92: 465–472.
77. Crain SM, Shen KF: Antagonists of excitatory opioid receptor functions enhance morphine's analgesic potency and attenuate opioid tolerance/dependence liability. Pain 2000;84:121–131.
78. Topol EJ: Rofecoxib, Merck, and the FDA. N Engl J Med 2004;351: 2877–2878.
79. Bombardier C, Laine L, Reicin A, et al: Comparison of upper gastrointestinal toxicity of rofecoxib and naproxen in patients with rheumatoid arthritis. VIGOR Study Group. N Engl J Med 2000;343:1520–1528.
80. Samad TA, Sapirstein A, Woolf CJ: Prostanoids and pain: Unraveling mechanisms and revealing therapeutic targets. Trends Mol Med 2002; 8:390–396.
81. Reuben SS, Bhopatkar S, Maciolek H, et al: The preemptive analgesic effect of rofecoxib after ambulatory arthroscopic knee surgery. Anesth Analg 2002;94:55–59.
82. Woolf CJ, Thompson SW: The induction and maintenance of central sensitization is dependent on N-methyl-D-aspartic acid receptor activation: Implications for the treatment of post-injury pain hypersensitivity states. Pain 1991;44:293–299.
83. Turk DC: Cognitive-behavioral approach to the treatment of chronic pain patients. Reg Anesth Pain Med 2003;28:573–579.
84. Dworkin RH, Turk DC, Farrar JT, et al: Core outcome measures for chronic pain clinical trials: IMMPACT recommendations. Pain 2005; 113:9–19.
85. Turk DC, Dworkin RH, Allen RR, et al: Core outcome domains for chronic pain clinical trials: IMMPACT recommendations. Pain 2003; 106:337–345.

13 Acute Pain Services

NARINDER RAWAL

Pain relief after surgery continues to be a major medical challenge. Improvement in perioperative analgesia not only is desirable for humanitarian reasons but also is essential for its potential to reduce postoperative morbidity[1–4] and mortality.[2] Unrelieved postoperative pain may delay discharge and recovery and may prevent a patient from participating in rehabilitation programs, resulting in a poor outcome. Studies now show that undertreatment of pain continues despite the availability of drugs for its effective management. It is generally accepted that the solution to the problem of inadequate pain relief lies not so much in development of new analgesic drugs or technologies as in development of appropriate organizations to make use of existing expertise.[5]

Although several editorials in the late 1970s advocated the introduction of an analgesia team to supervise and administer pain relief and to take responsibility for teaching and training in postoperative pain management, almost a decade passed before specialized in-hospital postoperative pain services emerged. Various medical and healthcare organizations have recommended a widespread introduction of *acute pain service* (APS).[6–12] Furthermore, provision of an APS is currently a prerequisite for accreditation for training by the Royal College of Anaesthetists and the Australian and New Zealand College of Anaesthetists.[13]

Prevalence of Acute Pain Services

The Joint Colleges of Surgery and Anaesthesia Working Party Report in the United Kingdom recommended that a multidisciplinary team including specialist-nursing staff should run APSs. They further recommended that the services should assume day-to-day responsibility for the management of postoperative pain, in-service training for nursing and medical staff, and research and audit.[7] Similar recommendations have been made by national expert committees from Australia,[6] the United States,[8,10] Germany,[9] Sweden,[11] and again in an updated form by the American Society of Anesthesiologists (ASA) Task Force.[12] In the United Kingdom, two national surveys were conducted to determine the extent to which the recommendations of the Working Party Report had been implemented.[14,15] There appeared to be a large variation in what was thought to constitute an APS, and some hospitals had only some of the elements recommended by the Working Party Report.[14,15] Table 13–1 shows the prevalence of APSs in Europe, North America, Australia, and New Zealand.[14–27]

Claims about the number of APSs in different countries, however, do not mean much in the absence of established standards.[25] Many hospitals considered their services adequate for their needs even though they had only some components of an APS.[12] Furthermore, the numbers do not give any indication as to the nature of service provided, the staffing and facilities of the service, the training and competence of those running the APS, or the effectiveness of the APS. For example, a recent Canadian survey showed that the percentage of academic hospitals with an APS had risen from 53% in 1993 to 92%. However, the number of APSs staffed only by anesthesiologists had decreased from 36% to 22% owing to growing clinical demands and lower numbers of anesthesiologists. Only 44% of centers had a designated group of APS physicians, and nurses were represented in only 55%. Additionally, only 29% of centers reported having an ongoing prospective data collection system. The survey investigators commented that no information was obtained about management of acute pain in patients who were not followed by the APS, which is the vast majority of postoperative patients.[26] In common with others performing similar surveys,[27,28] the Canadian investigators concluded with a call for a national consensus to produce standards with defined criteria on the basis of which the performance of APSs can be evaluated and compared with national audits.

The Structure of Acute Pain Services

The main organizational model for managing postoperative pain has been the APS, largely catalyzed by developments in the United States[21] and gradually introduced in the United Kingdom during the 1990s after the landmark report *Pain after Surgery*.[7] Yet the implementation of APSs since 1990 has been piecemeal and haphazard, with successive reports up to the late 1990s providing evidence of continuing variation within and between hospitals in the structure and function.[27]

Although there is a consensus that one of the major functions of an APS is to ensure safe and effective delivery of the newer types of postoperative analgesic techniques, such as patient-controlled analgesia (PCA) and epidural analgesia, many hospitals without an APS may also provide these services.[29] It is important to differentiate between the advantages of the analgesic techniques themselves and the advantages conferred by the greater specialist supervision and education provided by the dedicated staff of an APS.

In spite of the increased numbers of APSs, evidence still indicates that some face financial problems and may provide a "token" service only. Currently there is little work exploring the clinical efficacy and cost-effectiveness of APSs. McDonnell et al[29] concluded that although the findings of their study indicated that APSs are associated with a number of initiatives

TABLE 13–1	National Surveys of the Prevalence of Acute Pain Services*		
Study	**Region/Country**	**Survey Year**	**Prevalence**
Zimmerman & Stewart[16]	Canada	1991	24/47 (53%)[†]
Goucke & Owe[17]	Australia, New Zealand	1992/1993	37/111 (33%)
Rawal & Allvin[18]	Europe	1993	37/105 (34%)
Davies[19]	United Kingdom	1994	77/221 (35%)[†]
Windsor et al[15]	United Kingdom	1994[‡]	151/354 (43%)
		1990	10/358 (3%)
Merry et al[20]	New Zealand	1994	12/62 (19%)
Merry et al[20]	New Zealand	1996	17/22[§]
Harmer & Davies[14]	United Kingdom	1995[‖]	97/221 (44%)[†]
Ready[21¶]	United States	1995	236/324 (73%)
Warfield & Kahn[22]	United States	1995	126/300 (42%)
Neugebauer et al[23]	Germany	1997	390/1000 (39%)
Stamer et al[24]	Germany	1999	161/446 (36%)
O'Higgins & Tuckey[25]	United Kingdom	2000[‖]	>49%**
Goldstein et al[26]	Canada	2004	50/62 (93%)[†]
Powell et al[27]	United Kingdom	2004	270/325 (83%)

*Formal "acute pain service" assumes provision of staff and funding.
[†]Only university affiliated.
[‡]Survey was conducted in 1994 and contained a retrospective analysis of 1990 data.
[§]This part of the survey included only 22 publicly funded Crown Health Enterprises with ≥ 150 beds.
[‖]Year of survey not stated.
[¶]Letter.
**A total of 118 of 240 Anaesthetic College tutors confirmed the presence of an acute pain team to review epidural analgesia on the wards.
Adapted from Werner MU, Søholm L, Rotbøll-Nielsen P, Kehlet H: Does an acute pain service improve postoperative outcome? Anesth Analg 2002; 95:1361–1372.

seen as hallmarks of good postoperative pain management, they did not explore the impact of APSs on patient outcomes.

Requirements of an Acute Pain Service

Stamer et al[24] reviewed the literature on APSs and concluded that in spite of guidelines, most APSs worldwide did not meet basic quality criteria, which were defined as follows:

- Regular assessment and documentation of pain scores at least once a day
- Written protocols for pain management
- Personnel assignment for APSs
- Policies for postoperative pain management during nights and weekends

Although each institution has different requirements for its APS and modifications of published models will be necessary to accommodate local conditions, the main components of an APS should be as follows[29]:

1. Designated personnel responsible for 24-hour APSs; in small hospitals, one or two people may be adequate.
2. Regular pain assessment at rest and during movement, maintaining of pain scores below a predetermined threshold level, and documentation ("making pain visible"), with appropriate scales for children and patients with cognitive impairment.
3. Active cooperation with surgeons and ward nurses for development of protocols and critical pathways to achieve preset goals for postoperative mobilization and rehabilitation.
4. Ongoing teaching programs for ward nurses on the provision of safe and cost-effective analgesic techniques.

5. Patient education about pain monitoring and treatment options, goals, benefits, and adverse effects.
6. Regular audit of the cost-effectiveness of analgesic techniques on surgical wards and of patient satisfaction among inpatients and outpatients.

Does an Acute Pain Service Improve Outcome?

It is believed that the introduction of APSs has led to an increase in the use of specialized pain relief methods, such as epidural and perineural analgesic technique and PCA on surgical wards. Implementation of these methods may represent real advances in improving patient well-being and in reducing postoperative morbidity.[12,13] Evaluation of safety aspects is an important objective of an APS, but the role of an APS in preventing and reducing these events has not been established. This lack is unfortunate, because implementation and supervision of epidural analgesia and PCA are important objectives of any APS.

One study reported a decrease in the incidence of lower respiratory tract infection from 1.3% to 0.4% after the introduction of an APS.[30] Tsui et al[31] investigated patients with esophageal carcinoma undergoing esophagectomy. The patients either were supervised by an APS (n = 299) or received conventional treatment in a non-APS setting (n = 279). In the APS group, patients received opioid-based postoperative epidural or systemic-infusion analgesia, and in the non-APS group, patients received intermittent intramuscular morphine injections. A significantly lower incidence of pulmonary and cardiac complications and shorter hospital stay were reported for patients in the APS group.[31] However, some studies have not found any reduction of hospital stay in patients supervised by APSs.[13,32,33]

In a 2002 literature review, Werner et al[13] studied APS and outcome in 44 audits and 4 clinical trials containing outcome data from 84,097 postoperative patients. The researchers concluded that implementation of an APS was associated with a significant diminution in pain ratings. The overall incidence of serious postoperative respiratory depression (requiring naloxone reversal) was 0% to 1.7% with intravenous morphine infusion, 0.1% to 2.2% with PCA, 0.1% to 1.0% with spinal opioids, and 0% to 0.5% with a mixture of local anesthetic and opioid given epidurally, confirming the general belief that opioids given by any route are associated with a very low but similar risk of respiratory depression.[13] This finding is echoed by a report from the ASA Task Force that supports the use of epidural anesthesia, PCA, and regional techniques by anesthesiologists when appropriate and feasible. The literature indicates that adverse effects are no more common with these three analgesic techniques than with other, less effective techniques.[12] Werner et al[13] also reported that the introduction of an APS might have been associated with less postoperative nausea and vomiting and less urinary retention. However, they could not draw clear conclusions about the side effects of analgesic modalities, patient satisfaction, or postoperative morbidity because of a large variability in the studies regarding APS function and the services provided.[13] Hospital administrators may be more likely to invest in an APS if they are persuaded that it would achieve measurable improvements in patient outcomes at an affordable cost.

Are Acute Pain Services Cost-Effective?

Cost-benefit analyses that include complications, adverse effects, and outcome measures are necessary to justify the need for APSs, and no such studies have been conducted. Cost-benefit analyses of postoperative pain management must consider the costs of analgesic drugs, devices, and nursing and physician time; the duration of stay in the intensive care unit (ICU), post-anesthesia care unit (PACU), and/or surgical ward; and postoperative morbidity.[13]

Brodner et al[34] have shown that the introduction of a multimodal analgesia program with improved pain relief, stress reduction, and early extubation decreased the number of patients who required an ICU stay in the immediate postoperative period after major surgery. Because of an earlier discharge from the high-dependency areas, a net savings of approximately $43 (U.S.) per patient was achieved.[34] Several other researchers have advocated for a low-cost nurse-based, anesthesiologist-supervised model[5,35–37] as an alternative to the more expensive multidisciplinary APS.[38–41] Cost analyses of acute pain management are impeded by the lack of a well-defined baseline and outcome assessments. There is no valid method to assign financial cost to differing levels of analgesia, and the effect of perioperative regional analgesia on economic outcomes has not been adequately examined.[13] Currently, there is no evidence that a physician-based multidisciplinary APS is better or more cost-effective than a specialist nurse–based, anesthesiologist-supervised APS. Although cost-benefit

studies are difficult to perform, there is a great need for such studies.

How to Implement an Acute Pain Service

The first step in initiating a pain management program is to organize an interdisciplinary team of interested and motivated individuals who represent diverse professional skills and approaches to patient care.

EDUCATION

One of the most basic, yet essential, activities of a pain management program is to develop and implement educational programs for patients and healthcare providers. For patients, the educational process should begin at the time of the preoperative evaluation. Content should include the importance of adequate pain control, the commitment of hospital staff to provide effective pain control, the various options available to manage postoperative pain, practical information about how to report pain intensity (e.g., visual analogue scale [VAS] or numerical scale), and how to participate in the pain management plan when techniques such as PCA and regional analgesia are used.[5,41,42]

DEFINING MAXIMUM ACCEPTABLE PAIN SCORES AND "MAKING PAIN VISIBLE"

In the absence of formal, documented pain assessment, many medical and nursing staff continue to believe that patients who do not report pain do not feel pain. It is therefore essential that a maximum acceptable pain score be defined and that pain intensity be routinely documented before and after treatment. Documentation also provides data for audit and facilitates review and improvement of care. Traditionally, patients have assumed that pain after surgery is inevitable; they are unlikely to be aware of the standard of care they can expect to receive and the potential benefits of effective pain relief. Quality assurance measures can no longer be ignored; patients should be informed that their pain will be maintained at or below a predefined threshold level (generally 3 on a 10-grade VAS) and that pain scores in excess of the threshold will trigger interventions to reduce pain.[41] "Analgesic gaps" are common during the transition from epidural analgesia or PCA to oral analgesic therapy. The quality improvement activities of a dedicated APS may reduce such gaps and enhance patient comfort.

DEVELOPMENT OF A SPECIALIST PAIN NURSE–BASED ACUTE PAIN SERVICE

It is becoming increasingly clear that simpler and less expensive models must be developed if the aim is to improve the quality of postoperative analgesia for all patients (including outpatient surgery patients) who undergo surgery. At Örebro University Hospital, our specialist pain nurse–based, anesthesiologist-supervised model is founded on the concept that postoperative pain relief can be greatly improved by provision of in-service training for surgical nursing staff,

TABLE 13–2	Organization of Acute Pain Services at Örebro University Hospital, Örebro, Sweden*
Healthcare Member "Pain Representatives"	**Responsibility**
Director of acute pain service	Responsible for coordinating hospital-wide acute pain services and in-service teaching
Section anesthesiologist	Responsible for preoperative, perioperative, and postoperative care (including postoperative pain) for his/her surgical section
"Pain representative" ward surgeon	Formally responsible for pain management for his/her surgical ward
	Helps in integration of analgesia routines into clinical pathways for individual surgical procedures
"Pain representative" day nurse and "pain representative" night nurse	Responsible for implementation of pain management guidelines and monitoring routines on the ward†
Acute pain nurse (specialist pain nurse)	Daily rounds of all surgical wards
	Data collection (EDA, PCA, peripheral nerve blocks) for annual audits
	"Troubleshooting" of technical problems (PCA, EDA)
	Referral of problem patients to section anesthesiologist (link between surgical ward and anesthesiologist)
	"Bedside" teaching of ward nurses

*This organization benefits about 16,000 patients a year (visual analogue score ≤3); it has been functioning satisfactorily since 1991. Cost per patient is about US $3 (excluding drug and equipment costs).

†Patients are treated on the basis of standard orders and protocols developed jointly by chiefs of anesthesiology, surgery, and nursing sections. Pain representatives meet every 3 months to discuss and implement improvements in surgical ward pain management routines.

EDA, epidural analgesia; PCA, patient-controlled analgesia.

optimal use of systemic opioids, and use of regional analgesia techniques and PCA in selected patients.[5] Regular recording of each patient's pain intensity by VAS score every 3 hours and recording of treatment efficacy on the vital sign chart is the cornerstone of this model. This assessment includes pain at rest and during movement and also before and after an intervention. A VAS score above 3 is promptly treated.

Surgeon and ward nurse participation is crucial in this organization. A specialist pain nurse or "acute pain nurse" (APN) makes daily rounds of all surgery departments; the APN's duties are described in Table 13–2. In this organization the treatment of individual patients is based on standard orders and protocols developed jointly by the section anesthesiologist, surgeon, and ward nurse. This arrangement gives ward nurses the flexibility to administer the analgesics when necessary. The section anesthesiologist has the overall responsibility for preoperative, perioperative, and postoperative anesthesia care of the section's patients, including postoperative pain management. The section anesthesiologist selects the patients for special pain therapies such as PCA and epidural or peripheral nerve blocks on the basis of the departmental policy mandating use of the "acute pain analgesic ladder."

During regular working hours, this anesthesiologist is available for consultation or any emergency; at other times, the anesthesiologist on call has the same function. Postoperative pain management can be improved by a team approach, as shown in Table 13–3.

The "pain representatives" from each surgical ward meet regularly with anesthesiologist and APN to discuss improvements based on annual audit data. In the organization described here, the only additional cost is that of two APNs. At our hospital, about 16,000 surgical procedures are performed each year; our low-cost organization (about US $3 per patient, excluding drug and equipment costs) is designed to benefit all of these patients. Regular audits have confirmed that the aims of our APS are achieved in more than 90% of patients. The number of times anesthesiologists are consulted or called has fallen over the years; currently it is in the range of one or two consultations a week. However, our latest audit showed the need for a more detailed comparison of pain relief during nighttime than in daytime.

The general principles for this organizational model have been accepted and recommended for Swedish hospitals by the Swedish Medical Association.[11] The choice of

TABLE 13–3	How Can Postoperative Pain Management Be Improved?
On wards	"Make pain visible" (regular assessment, documentation)
	Allow ward nurses to treat pain based on standardized protocols
Surgeon	Preset goals for postoperative mobilization and rehabilitation
Anesthesiologists	Selection of evidence-based analgesic techniques, teaching, supervision of acute pain nurses (APNs)
APN	Bedside teaching of ward nurses; "troubleshooting" epidural analgesia, patient-controlled analgesia, peripheral nerve block, etc.; regular audit of acute pain service
Hospital administration	Hospital-wide pain management policy

medication, dose, route, and duration of therapy should be individualized.[12]

Bardiau et al[43] described the process of implementing an APS based on our model in a Belgian general hospital of 1005 beds, of which 240 are on surgical wards. The process was divided into eight stages over a 3-year period. This program anticipated an improvement in postoperative pain relief for all surgical inpatients and the maintenance of this service over time. First, a pain management committee (PMC) was formed, comprising anesthesiologists, surgeons, pharmacists, and nurses. The second month, a survey of nurses' attitudes toward and knowledge of postoperative care was conducted by means of an anonymous 35-item questionnaire. The third month, a 10-cm VAS device was introduced for routine assessment of pain intensity. Then, for a 6-month period, a baseline survey (survey I) was designed to analyze current practices of pain treatment.

After that 6-month survey, a specialist nurse–based, anesthesiologist-supervised APS model was set up based on APNs and pain representatives. Standardized treatment protocols, regular assessments of pain intensity by VAS every 4 hours, recording of treatment efficacy, and APNs are the bases of this model. The PMC developed a clinical pathway to create an optimal regimen of postoperative pain management. Three months later, a second survey (survey II) of 671 patients was conducted to assess the effect of APS implementation. Finally, a third confirmation survey (survey III) of 2383 patients was conducted to investigate whether the initial improvements had been maintained.

The survey of nurses identified a lack of knowledge and skills among nurses in assessing and managing pain effectively because of the absence of nursing guidelines and pain treatment protocols. Pain relief improved significantly after the implementation of the APS. Paracetamol consumption rose significantly. The rate of administration of nonsteroidal anti-inflammatory drugs increased from 20% in survey I to 64% and 99% in surveys II and III, respectively. Morphine consumption decreased slightly. The researchers in this study concluded that standardization of pain treatment and nursing practice and also regular feedback about performance are essential factors in improvement of pain management. Organizing teams of surgeons, anesthesiologists, and nurses is necessary for this improvement. Cost-benefit analyses are now needed to further substantiate these results.[43]

Problems with United States–Style Acute Pain Services

Most major institutions in the United States have anesthesiologist-based APSs. The comprehensive pain management teams usually consist of staff anesthesiologists, resident anesthesiologists, specially trained nurses, pharmacists, and physical therapists. Sometimes biomedical and infusion pump dispensing personnel are included. Secretarial and billing personnel are also a part of a United States–style APS. Patients under the care of APSs are visited and assessed regularly by members of the team.

Anesthesiologist-based APS organization models usually provide "high-tech" pain management services, and most APSs in the United States are essentially epidural analgesia and PCA services only. A good APS organization should provide optimal pain management for every patient who undergoes surgery, including children and patients undergoing surgery on an ambulatory basis. The costs of United States–style APSs are very high and are being increasingly questioned by healthcare payers. In many institutions, PCA management has been taken over by surgeons. A downsizing of many APSs is taking place in the United States, with further reductions predicted.

There is a clear need for new APS models that provide effective pain relief for all surgical patients. The Joint Commission on Accreditation of Healthcare Organizations (JCAHO), an independent not-for-profit organization that sets healthcare standards in the United States, recognizes this need. Accreditation of healthcare facilities in the United States is determined, in part, by how they adhere to the JCAHO standards of pain assessment and care. Healthcare facilities must recognize that patients have the right to assessment and management of their pain. JCAHO standards require that hospitals assess, treat, and document patients' pain, guarantee the competence of their staff in pain assessment and management, and educate patients and families about effective pain management. Hospitals must also consider the needs of ambulatory surgery patients for information and guidelines about pain management after discharge from the hospital.[41]

Upgrading the Role of Ward Nurses

Nurses on surgical wards are responsible for assessing every patient's pain intensity, administering prescribed analgesic treatments, and monitoring their efficacy and adverse effects as well as the extent of regional block. Studies have demonstrated the key role that nurses have in improving the efficacy of analgesic regimens.[5,14,43,44] Clinical nurse specialists or APNs with particular training in pain management are increasingly being appointed as parts of an acute pain team. They can educate nurses, give necessary support, and help initiate and supervise analgesia. They also facilitate collaboration among surgeons, anesthesiologists, and nurses on surgical wards.

The nursing role must be upgraded if postoperative pain management is to improve on surgical wards. In many countries and institutions, ward nurses are not allowed to inject opioids in intravenous IV lines or epidural catheters, but they are expected to call APS physicians every time PCA and epidural doses need adjustment. This latter requirement is time-consuming, unrealistic, cost-ineffective, and unnecessary. Such restrictions for ward nurses seem strange in view of the growing trends toward patient self-treatment. Outside hospitals, diabetic children are allowed to self-administer injections of potentially dangerous doses of insulin, and cancer patients are allowed to self-administer epidural and intrathecal drugs for pain relief. Uses of home ventilators, home dialysis, home PCA devices, and opioids for noncancer pain are increasingly accepted. Notably, in many hospitals, midwives are allowed to "top up" epidural catheters for labor pain, but ward nurses are not allowed to do the same for postoperative pain.

There is convincing evidence from many countries and institutions that with appropriate teaching and training, ward nurses are able to dose-titrate, monitor, and manage analgesic modalities such as PCAs and epidurals on surgical wards. Nurse education is widely recognized as an important priority in pain management.[5,14,41–43] At our institution, ward nurses have been allowed to give intravenous opioid titrated bolus doses, set up PCA pumps, administer drugs in epidural catheters, and reduce or increase drug delivery (within prescribed limits) with PCA and epidural techniques. The nurses were not allowed to perform such tasks at the time of implementation of the APS in 1991. Regular teaching and daily visits by APNs have resulted in effective and safe pain relief, confirmed by annual audit data.

Role of the Surgeon

Although all guidelines emphasize the importance of a multidisciplinary APS as a tool to improve postoperative pain relief, no distinctions have been made in the literature among the roles of individual members of the multidisciplinary team. The role of the surgeon is far more important than, say, that of the pharmacist; indeed, it would be no exaggeration to say that an APS without surgeon cooperation is doomed to fail. Surgeon participation is important for the following reasons: (1) development of protocols for all analgesic techniques, with consideration of the fact that a majority of surgical patients do not need epidural or PCA techniques for effective analgesia, (2) development of clinical pathways to achieve preset goals for postoperative mobilization and rehabilitation that can be expected to reduce hospital stay, (3) strategies for pain management after outpatient surgery (which accounts for up to 70% of the surgical population and is rising), and (4) improved ward nurse compliance for implementation of APS goals, including frequent pain assessment and documentation.[41]

Audits and Continuous Quality Improvement

Regular audits of APSs are necessary to assess quality of pain management and to confirm that the techniques such as epidural analgesia, PCA, and peripheral blocks are cost-effective. Such audits show the problems with the techniques that must be addressed and the changes that must be made before the next audit.

Taverner[44] reported in 2003 that an audit was carried out in the Northern and Yorkshire region of the United Kingdom to assess postoperative pain management outcomes. All patients in the region undergoing surgery for a range of procedures over a 2-week period were included in the study. Sixteen hospitals were involved in the audit, ranging from the large teaching hospitals with 5500 beds to smaller district general hospitals with fewer than 400 beds. Pain scores were measured in the recovery room at 24 hours and at 7 days postoperatively, at rest and during movement. Data on the modalities of pain management were also collected. The results showed that a large percentage of patients reported unacceptable levels of pain despite changes in practice and the development of acute pain management teams. Sites with pain management teams did not provide better pain management for postoperative patients.[44] Such results emphasize the need

for regular audits to address the problems of APSs and to justify their costs.

One of the most important activities of a pain management program is to provide ongoing review of institutional policies and practices regarding pain control and the mechanisms to deal with problems as they arise. The members of the program should meet regularly to provide formal feedback and opportunities for further improvement. Such meetings are important as a forum for assessment of the efficiency of the APS, to highlight practical problems, and to find solutions to less well-functioning aspects of the APS.[42] In general, the literature on audits is very limited.

Future Perspectives

The aims of APS treatment have expanded to embrace not merely a reduction of pain intensity but also the promotion of comfort and rehabilitation. The widening of objectives, together with the insidious elevation of standards and expectations, has placed a burden on an old order that is often ill-equipped to serve the new ambitions of anesthesiologists.[45] Evidence that standards are improving can be found in the way that pain is assessed. As pain control has improved, its evaluation has become more demanding. Although the goal of management remains a reduction in pain intensity, it is no longer sufficient to measure efficacy at rest; measurements must also be made during mobilization and during coughing in patients who have undergone abdominal and thoracic surgery.

APSs have a leading educational role that no one else can assume. With success on the educational front, other healthcare providers might be incorporated into the team. Expanding the multidisciplinary approach could extend the role of APSs to all matters pertaining to patient rehabilitation. Such enlargement of the role might have the double benefit of improving overall patient care and persuading hospital managers that APSs are worthy of support.[45]

In the United Kingdom there has been debate about the future direction of APSs. Suggested developments include integration with other pain services (chronic and palliative care), alignment with critical care outreach teams,[46] and the development of comprehensive postoperative rehabilitation programs.[16] Central to concerns about out-of-hours care is the debate about whether the key role of APSs is to provide a hands-on, direct patient care service or, instead, to serve as a resource for education and training, and for the promotion of good practice. Powell et al[27] speculate that if an APS is well resourced and able to stimulate the kinds of widespread organizational and attitudinal changes required to overcome barriers to good pain management, it may not matter whether the APS itself is a daytime service, because good practice should continue throughout the 24-hour period.[27] However, combined with the evidence that many patients perceive pain at night as more severe,[47] the current "office hours" model of APSs, which covers only about 50 hours of the 168 hours in a week, would seem destined to leave many patients in pain.[27]

The key role of the APS is not to provide a hands-on, direct patient care service but to serve as a resource for education and training as well as for promotion of good practice based on algorithms and protocols that have been developed jointly by anesthesiologists, surgeons, and nurses. These protocols must be integrated into predefined clinical pathways for each surgical procedure. Regular audits will show whether the goals of an APS are being achieved.[41]

It has been proposed by some that APSs should be integrated with other pain services (chronic pain, palliative care). This will work only if an anesthesiologist on the team is responsible only for APS, because the practical issues related to management of postoperative pain and chronic pain are entirely different. The APS anesthesiologist should be involved with the preoperative, perioperative, and postoperative phases, including administering anesthesia and training others in the administration of regional anesthesia. Not all chronic pain services are run by anesthesiologists; even when they are, the anesthesiologists are rarely involved with delivery of anesthesia services. Thus, such anesthesiologists are not familiar with the day-to-day practical issues of postoperative pain management on surgical wards. Therefore it is unclear whether the problems of postoperative pain can be solved by the development of a more comprehensive service.[27] In our institution the organization of the APS is separate from that of chronic pain management. There is good cooperation between the two teams for patients with chronic pain who undergo surgery, patients with drug problems, and patients with postoperative complications for which long-term pain relief may be necessary. For organizational purposes, the hand-off time is 7 days; that is, after the 7th postoperative day, the chronic pain team takes over the management of postoperative pain.

Web-based, surgical procedure–specific guidelines and recommendations are now available, to take advantage of the versatile information management inherent in a web-based format that makes the information readily available.[48,49] The role of an APS is to integrate appropriate evidence-based analgesic techniques into clinical pathways for each surgical procedure. Surgical procedure–specific postoperative pain management recommendations can be expected to provide better outcome results than the "one size fits all" routines of the past. Fundamental changes to practice patterns require clear recommendations based on clinical evidence.

PROSPECT[50] (from *procedure-specific postoperative pain management*) is a web-based program that provides evidence-based arguments for each analgesic and anesthetic intervention and operative technique used in a particular procedure, allowing the clinician to make informed treatment decisions. The evidence is derived from systematic reviews of the literature using the Cochrane protocol, transferable evidence from comparable procedures, and current clinical practice. Procedure-specific analgesic strategies differ from those of previously published acute pain guidelines, which presented the range of postoperative pain control methods without making recommendations for specific techniques to control pain after certain operations. An important feature of PROSPECT is the role of surgical interventions in postoperative pain and outcome. Recommendations for laparoscopic cholecystectomy and primary total hip replacement are currently available on the PROSPECT website, and the PROSPECT Working Group of anesthesiologists and surgeons is currently reviewing hysterectomy, colonic resection, herniorrhaphy, and thoracotomy.[51,52] Initiatives such as PROSPECT, together with a greater awareness of procedure-specific analgesic requirements, support appropriate and targeted use of the growing range of drugs and modalities available to treat postoperative pain.

Rosenquist et al,[48] in conjunction with the U.S. Veterans Health Affairs (VHA) Office of Quality and Performance, used a standardized rating of the evidence gleaned from comprehensive electronic searches to develop an interactive electronic and traditional "paper" guideline with a preoperative and postoperative algorithm. They constructed a table listing a menu of analgesic choices organized by specific operation. Preferences for particular analgesic techniques and classes of medications were identified. The guideline may be reviewed at the VHA's website.[53] In contrast to this website, the PROSPECT website provides updated references and all available evidence about analgesic and surgical interventions, allowing the user to make his/her own decisions to accept or modify recommendations made by the PROSPECT consensus group. Such modifications may be necessary because of issues related to costs, availability of drugs, therapy traditions, and regulatory issues.

Summary

Freedom from postoperative pain is a central concern of surgical patients, and alleviation of pain may contribute considerably to better clinical outcomes. However, despite long-standing recognition, undertreatment of postoperative pain continues to be a major problem internationally. It is clear from the literature that the introduction of APSs has increased the awareness that postoperative pain techniques contribute to patients' well-being.

It has become increasingly evident that an organized team of dedicated physicians and nurses is a fundamental prerequisite for a well-functioning acute postoperative pain management program in surgical wards. Although randomized comparative literature is not available, preoperative/postoperative studies support the efficacy of an APS for reducing pain and suggest that adverse effects are also less.[12] The number of hospitals running an APS using advanced techniques such as catheters for regional anesthesia and PCA has been growing. At the same time there is usually no national consensus on the optimal structure or responsibilities that an APS should adopt. Therefore, there is an obvious need to produce national standards with defined criteria on the basis of which the performance of APSs at individual hospitals can be evaluated and comparisons with national audits can be made. Web-based, surgical procedure–specific initiatives such as PROSPECT, which provide evidence-based recommendations and allow the clinician to select appropriate drugs and modalities, could become a part of APS protocols in the future.

Selection of an appropriate organizational structure may be as important to the success of the APS as the choice of treatment modalities. Currently there is no consensus about the standards for staffing and facilities and what constitutes a good APS. It is important to recognize that quality improvement initiatives must be specifically tailored to the local environment, because no single approach is guaranteed to be successful in all settings. The integration of effective analgesia into general surgical care should be mandatory to improve outcome and depends on close cooperation between the surgeon and anesthesiologist. APSs will also have to document their value and demonstrate justification of allotted resources and expertise.

Acknowledgment

The author wishes to acknowledge the excellent secretarial assistance of Marianne Welamsson.

REFERENCES

1. Ballantyne JC, Carr DB, deFerranti S, et al: The comparative effects of postoperative analgesic therapies on pulmonary outcome: Cumulative meta-analyses of randomised, controlled trials. Anesth Analg 1998; 86:598–612.
2. Rodgers A, Walker N, Schug S, et al: Reduction of postoperative mortality and morbidity with epidural or spinal anaesthesia: Results from overview of randomised trials. BMJ 2000;321:1493.
3. Kehlet H, Holte K: Effect of postoperative analgesia reduces on surgical outcome. Br J Anaesth 2001;87:62–72.
4. Beattie WS, Badner NH, Choi P: Epidural analgesia reduces postoperative myocardial infarction: A meta-analysis. Anesth Analg 2001;93:853–858.
5. Rawal N, Berggren L: Organization of acute pain services—a low cost model. Pain 1994;57:117–123.
6. National Health & Medical Research Council of Australia: Acute Pain Management Scientific Evidence. Canberra, Australia, Ausinfo, 1999.
7. Royal College of Surgeons and College of Anaesthetists Working Party on Pain after Surgery: Pain after Surgery. London, Royal College of Surgeons, 1990.
8. US Department of Health and Human Services, Agency for Health Care Policy and Research: Acute Pain Management: Operative and Medical Procedures and Trauma. (Publication No. 92-0032.) Rockville, Md, AHCPR Publications, 1992.
9. Wulf H, Neugebauer E, Maier C: Die behandlung akuter perioperativer und posttraumatischer schmerzen: Empfehlungen einer interdisziplinaeren expertenkommission. New York, G Thieme, 1997.
10. Joint Commission on Accreditation of Healthcare Organizations: 1992 Hospital Accreditation Standards. Oakbrook Terrace, Ill, JCAHO, 2001.
11. Behandling av postoperativ smärta, riktlinjer och kvalitetsindikatorer [Treatment of postoperative pain, guidelines, and quality indicators]. Svenska Läkaresällskapet [Swedish Medical Association], Förlagshuset Gothia AB, Stockholm, 2001. Available at www.gothia.nu/
12. Practice guidelines for acute pain management in the perioperative setting: An updated report by American Society of Anesthesiologists Task Force on Acute Pain Management. Anesthesiology 2004;100: 1573–1581.
13. Werner MU, Søholm L, Rotbøll-Nielsen P, Kehlet H: Does an acute pain service improve postoperative outcome? Anesth Analg 2002;95: 1361–1372.
14. Harmer M, Davies KA: The effect of education, assessment and a standardised prescription on postoperative pain management: The value of clinical audit in the establishment of acute pain services. Anaesthesia 1998;53:424–430.
15. Windsor AM, Glynn CJ, Mason DG: National provision of acute pain services. Anaesthesia 1996;51:228–231.
16. Zimmerman DL, Stewart J: Postoperative pain management and acute pain service activity in Canada. Can J Anaesth 1993;40:568–575.
17. Goucke CR, Owe H: Acute pain management in Australia and New Zealand. Anaesth Intensive Care 1995;23:715–717.
18. Rawal N, Allvin R: Acute pain services in Europe: A 17-nation survey of 105 hospitals. The EuroPain Acute Pain Working Party. Eur J Anaesthesiol 1998;15:354–363.
19. Davies K: Findings of a national survey of acute pain services. Nurs Times 1996;92:31–33.
20. Merry A, Jugde MA, Ready B: Acute pain services in New Zealand hospitals: A survey. N Z Med J 1997;110:233–235.
21. Ready LB: How many acute pain services are there in the United States, and who is managing patient-controlled analgesia [letter]? Anesthesiology 1995;82:322.

22. Warfield CA, Kahn CH: Acute pain management: Programs in US hospitals and experiences and attitudes among US adults. Anesthesiology 1995;83:1090–1094.
23. Neugebauer E, Hempel K, Sauerland S, et al: [The status of perioperative pain therapy in Germany: Results of a representative, anonymous survey of 1,000 surgical clinics. Pain Study Group.] Chirurg 1998;69: 461–466.
24. Stamer UM, Mpasios N, Stuber F, Maier C: A survey of acute pain services in Germany and a discussion of international survey data. Reg Anesth Pain Med 2002;27:125–131.
25. O'Higgins, Tuckey JP: Thoracic epidural anaesthesia and analgesia: United Kingdom practice. Acta Anaesthesiol Scand 2000;44: 1087–1092.
26. Goldstein DH, Van Den Kerkhof EG, Blaine WC: Acute pain management services have progressed albeit insufficiently in Canadian academic hospitals. Can J Anesth 2004;51:231–235.
27. Powell AE, Davies HTO, Bannister J, Macrae WA: Rhetoric and reality on acute pain services in the UK: A national postal questionnaire survey. Br J Anaesth 2004;92:689–693.
28. Reference deleted.
29. McDonnell A, Nicholl J, Read S: Acute pain teams in England: Current provision and their role in postoperative pain management. J Clin Nurs 2003;12:387–393.
30. Wheatley RG, Madej TH, Jackson IJ, Hunter D: The first year's experience of an acute pain service. Br J Anaesth 1991;67:353–359.
31. Tsui SL, Law S, Fok M, et al: Postoperative analgesia reduces mortality and morbidity after esophagectomy. Am J Surg 1997;173:472–478.
32. Lempa M, Gerards P, Koch G, et al: Efficacy of an acute pain service: A controlled comparative study of hospitals. Langenbecks Arch Chir Suppl Kongressbd 1998;115:673–676.
33. Rose DK, Cohen MM, Yee DA: Changing the practice of pain management. Anesth Analg 1997;84:764–772.
34. Brodner G, Mertes N, Buerkle H, et al: Acute pain management: Analysis, implications and consequences after prospective experience with 6349 surgical patients. Eur J Anaesthesiol 2000;17:566–575.
35. Coleman SA, Booker-Milburn J: Audit of postoperative pain control: Influence of a dedicated acute pain nurse. Anaesthesia 1996;51: 1093–1096.
36. Mackintosh C, Bowles S: Evaluation of a nurse-led acute pain service: Can clinical nurse specialists make a difference? J Adv Nurse 1997; 25:30–37.
37. Bardiau FM, Braeckman MM, Seidel L, et al: Effectiveness of an acute pain service inception in a general hospital. J Clin Anesth 1999;11: 583–589.
38. Stacey BR, Rudy TE, Nelhaus D: Management of patient-controlled analgesia: A comparison of primary surgeons and a dedicated pain service. Anesth Analg 1997;85:130–134.
39. Mackey DC, Ebener MK, Howe BL: Patient-controlled analgesia and the acute pain service in the United States: Health-Care Financing Administration policy is impeding optimal patient-controlled analgesia management [letter; comment]. Anesthesiology 1995;83: 433–434.
40. Ready LB: Organization and operation of an acute pain service. In Ashburn MA, Fine PG, Stanley TH (eds): Pain Management and Anesthesiology. Dordrecht, The Netherlands, Kluwer Academic, 1998, pp 125–135.
41. Rawal N: Acute Pain Services revisited: Good from far, far from good [editorial]? Reg Anesth Pain Med 2002;27:117–121.
42. Blau WS, Dalton AB, Lindley C: Organization of hospital-based acute pain management programs. Southern Med J 1999;92:465–471.
43. Bardiau FM, Taviaux NF, Albert A, et al: An intervention study to enhance postoperative pain management. Anest Analg 2003;96: 179–185.
44. Taverner T: A regional pain management audit. Nurs Times 2003; 99:34–37.
45. Bonnet F: Postoperative pain management: A continuing struggle. ESA Newsletter 2004;17:8–9.
46. Counsell DJ: The acute pain service: A model for outreach critical care. Anaesthesia 2001;56:925–926.
47. Closs S, Briggs M, Everitt VE: Implementation of research findings to reduce postoperative pain at night. Int J Nurs Stud 1999;36:21–31.
48. Rosenquist RW, Rosenberg J: Postoperative pain guidelines. Reg Anesth Pain Med 2003;28:279–288. Available at www.oqp.med.va.gov/cpg/cpg.htm/

49. Rowlingson JC, Rawal N: Postoperative pain guidelines: Targeted to the site of surgery. Reg Anesth Pain Med 2003;28:265–267.
50. PROSPECT: Procedure-specific pain management. Available at www.postoppain.org/
51. Rawal N, McCloy RF, PROSPECT Working Group: Incisional and intraperitoneal local anaesthetics in laparoscopic cholecystectomy and abdominal hysterectomy: A systematic review. Reg Anesth Pain Med 2004;29:A307.
52. Fischer B, Camu F, PROSPECT Working Group: Comparative benefits of epidural analgesia following hysterectomy and colonic resection. Reg Anesth Pain Med 2004;29:A309.
53. U.S. Veterans Health Affairs, Office of Quality and Performance: Clinical Practice Guidelines: Postoperative Pain. Available at www.oqp.med.va.gov/cpg/PAIN/PAIN_base.htm/

14 Applied Clinical Pharmacology of Opioids

DAMIAN MURPHY

Opioid drugs are among the most commonly used analgesics in clinical practice. Their pharmacological effects were known to the ancient Sumerians and have been cited in the literature of many cultures. The word *opium* itself is derived from the Greek name for "juice," appropriately so because the drug is obtained from the juice of the poppy *Papaver somniferum*. Opium itself contains more than 20 distinct alkaloids. Serturner first isolated morphine in 1803; other derivatives of opium quickly followed and became established in medical practice. The term *opioid* refers to all substances, natural and synthetic, that have morphine-like properties.

The reason for the widespread use of opioids as analgesics in most countries is their easy availability, low cost, and effectiveness in providing relief.[1] However, a survey performed more than 30 years ago revealed that most patients received inadequate dosing because of a poor understanding of the intensity of pain, overestimation of the duration of action of the opioids, and the fear of abuse.[2] Progress since then has not been rapid; at present, even with the accessibility and widespread use of opioids in postoperative pain management, more than 60% of patients still experience moderate to severe pain after surgery.[3]

This chapter aims to outline the basic pharmacology of opioids with particular reference to their clinical use in the perioperative period. The main characteristics of individual opioids used in the perioperative period are addressed elsewhere.

Mechanisms of Action of Opioid Analgesics

Opioid analgesics used in clinical practice produce their pharmacological effects by binding to specific membrane receptors identified as opioid receptors (ORs). These receptors, together with putative peptide transmitters (endogenous opioid peptides [EOPs]), form the endogenous opioid system (EOS), which among other functions physiologically modulates nociceptive transmission in mammals.[4]

THE ENDOGENOUS OPIOID SYSTEM

Naturally occurring EOPs are synthesized from protein precursor molecules and include endorphins, dynorphins, and enkephalins. Among other locations, EOPs are present in the central and peripheral nervous systems, cardiovascular and gastrointestinal systems, and immune cells.[4] Although EOPs appear to function as neurotransmitters or modulators of sensory transmission, their precise physiological roles remain poorly understood. Other endogenous ligands (endomorphins) with a high selectivity for the μ opioid receptor were first identified in 1997.[5] Both endomorphin-1 and endomorphin-2 are peptides of only four amino acids. Their specific role is under investigation, but it is clear that they are involved in nociceptive modulation in mammals.[6]

OPIOID RECEPTORS: CENTRAL AND PERIPHERAL LOCALIZATION

The importance of the EOS in pain and analgesia was established approximately 30 years ago, and the distribution of the μ opioid receptor (MOR or OP_3), κ opioid receptor (KOR or OP_2), and δ opioid receptor (DOR or OP_1) in the central nervous system is well known.[7] A fourth receptor that is highly homologous with the traditional OR has been described and is designated ORL-1 (opioid receptor–like-1) or OP_4; nociceptin/orphanin-FQ has been characterized as the endogenous ligand for the ORL-1 and shown to share a high sequence homology with dynorphin.[8] This system is involved in several physiological processes, including central modulation of pain, but is not implicated in respiratory depression.[9] Experimentally, the activation of ORL-1 by agonists induces spinal analgesia and supraspinal hyperalgesia; thus, the potential for pain reduction by the activation of the ORL-1 receptor will not be established until more selective pharmacological research is performed. Nociceptin receptor antagonists are candidate antidepressants and analgesics.

MORs are abundant in the cortex, amygdala, hippocampus, thalamus, mesencephalon, pons, medulla, and spinal cord. KORs are similarly distributed but are also found in the hypothalamus. DORs are not as widespread but are present throughout the telencephalon and the spinal cord. Opioid receptors have also been identified in peripheral tissues, and when administered locally, opioids have been shown to have analgesic effects in humans.[10] The main advantage of the peripheral administration of opioids is the absence of centrally mediated side effects, in particular respiratory depression. However, the clinical efficacy of opioids when administered by different peripheral routes or at different sites remains controversial.[11]

Opioid receptors were initially classified according to their pharmacological effects when activated by opioid agonists or blocked by antagonists. On the basis of the pharmacological studies, subtypes for each one of the ORs have been described. For the MOR, the two major subtypes seem to mediate analgesia (MOR-1) and respiratory depression (MOR-2).[4] Unfortunately, we still lack clinically available opioids specific to the MOR-1 receptor. Their advent will be a major advance in pain management.

Activation of the three main ORs by agonists induces analgesia (Table 14–1), which is associated with other pharmacological effects. Interestingly, binding of opioid agonists to the KORs induces dysphoria and diuresis but not respiratory depression.

Opioid receptors belong to the family of G-protein–coupled receptors, and they signal via a second messenger (cyclic adenosine monophosphate) and ion channels. Activation of opioid receptors decreases calcium entry into the cell, which in turn reduces the release of presynaptic excitatory neurotransmitters (e.g., substance P). Potassium efflux is promoted, resulting in hyperpolarization and a decrease in synaptic transmission. Opioids may modulate inhibition of gamma-aminobutyric acid (GABA)–ergic transmission in spinal circuits. This disinhibitory action of opioids has been postulated to enhance the modulation of nociceptive transmission induced by the descending inhibitory pathways.

Opioid analgesics exert their effects by activating one or more of the three conventional opioid receptors (MOR, DOR, KOR), which at present have been characterized through the use of pharmacological methods (bioassays, stereospecific binding) and cloning. A full understanding of the mechanisms involved in opioid analgesia is still unclear[12] because (1) the different drugs may act as agonists in one species and antagonists in another, (2) it is difficult to find opioids (agonists and antagonists) that are receptor specific, (3) opioids may interact with more than one site on the receptor protein and induce conformational changes, and (4) the receptors undergo dimerization to form complexes (such as MOR/MOR,

TABLE 14–2	Opioid Analgesics Commonly Used in the Perioperative Period
Agonist	Morphine
	Fentanyl
	Alfentanil
	Sufentanil
	Pethidine
	Oxycodone
	Diamorphine
	Remifentanil
Partial agonist	Buprenorphine
Agonist antagonist	Butorphanol
	Pentazocine
Antagonist	Naloxone
	Naltrexone

DOR/KOR, and MOR/DOR). The pharmacological profiles of these complexes are poorly understood.[13]

CLASSIFICATION OF OPIOID ANALGESICS

Clinically used opioids are usually classified according to their affinity and efficacy for the different opioid receptors. They are also categorized as weak or strong according to the intensity of pain they suppress (Table 14–2).

Pharmacokinetics of Opioids

Pharmacokinetic parameters involving the processes of absorption, distribution, metabolism, and excretion of the opioids and their formulations are central to our understanding of their clinical usage. In general, opioids are well absorbed when given by all routes of administration. The absorption profile is of growing importance owing to the numerous routes of administration available (transdermal, spinal, buccal-transmucosal, nasal, inhalational, parenteral, oral, and rectal) and to the higher number of sustained-release oral formulation offered.

Distribution of the drug from the blood to the different tissues and compartments, including skeletal muscle and fat, depends on lipid solubility and pKa. Lipid solubility and level of ionization at physiological pH affect the rate of transmembrane passage and binding to the receptors. All opioid drugs have similar molecular weights but relatively large differences in lipid solubility and pKa (the lower the pKa, the larger the nonionized portion at physiological pH). The nonionized forms have far greater membrane permeability than the ionized, and thus alfentanil (pKa 6.5) has a more rapid onset of action than other opioids, which in general have pKa values between 8 and 9.[13] Lipid solubility is commonly determined by measurement of the oil/water partition coefficient (Table 14–3). This value varies quite a bit for the opioid compounds (morphine 1.4, sufentanil 1.778). The higher the value of the coefficient, the greater the lipophilicity. Drugs with high lipid solubility have an early onset of action because of the rapid passage from plasma to the active sites.[14]

TABLE 14–1	Activation of the Different Opioid Receptors (ORs) by Agonists
Receptor Type	**Effect**
μ (MOR)	Supraspinal, spinal, and peripheral analgesia
	Respiratory depression
	Gastrointestinal: ileus, constipation, nausea, emesis
	Pruritus, urinary retention
	Cardiovascular depression
	Tolerance/dependence
	Sedation, euphoria
	Miosis
κ (KOR)	Spinal analgesia
	Dysphoria
	Sedation
	Diuresis
δ (DOR)	MOR receptor modulation
	Spinal/supraspinal analgesia

TABLE 14-3	Physiochemical Characteristics of Opioids			
Opioid	Molecular Weight (kDa)	pKa	Percentage Ionization*	O/W Partition Coefficient†
Morphine	285	7.9	76	1.4
Fentanyl	336	8.4	91	813
Alfentanil	416	6.5	11	128
Sufentanil	386	8.0	80	1778
Pethidine	247	8.5	76	39

*Percentage ionization indicates the % of the opioid that is in the ionized form at a pH of 7.4.

†Oil/water partition coefficient represents the n-octanol/water partition coefficient at a pH of 7.4. The higher the value, the greater the agent's lipid solubility; lower values correspond to hydrophilic opioids.

Modified from Gourlay G: Clinical Pharmacology of opioids in the treatment of pain. In Giamberardino MA (ed): Pain 2002—An Updated Review: Refresher Course Syllabus, 10th World Congress on Pain. Seattle, IASP Press, 2002, pp 381–394.

Most opioids have similar elimination half-lives, which are directly related to the volumes of distribution (Vd) and inversely related to the clearance (Cl). Drugs with large Vd, such as fentanyl, have longer elimination half-lives, whereas the rapid clearance and small Vd of remifentanil is responsible for its very short half-life.[15] However, because the opioids are widely distributed through the body, the sole comparison of their half-lives does not predict the duration of effect of different drugs.[14]

A more useful measure is the context-sensitive half-time, which is the time required, after discontinuation of an intravenous infusion, for the drug concentration in the central compartment to decrease by 50%. When an infusion is interrupted, the drug present in the peripheral compartment is redistributed back into the central compartment, thus prolonging the half-time.[16] There is no clear correlation between plasma levels of opioids and clinical analgesia that

has practical value.[17] In clinical practice, opioid plasma levels are almost exclusively used in relation to toxicity .

The liver is the main site of metabolism of most opioids. Because hepatic clearance of many opioids is high, liver blood flow is one of the major determinants of the rate of metabolism. Minor biotransformation may occur in the organ of the body that interfaces with the opioid (e.g., gut, lung), but this statement cannot be applied to all opioids or routes; for example, fentanyl is not metabolized during transdermal absorption in the skin.[18] Opioids in general undergo phase I or phase II reactions in the liver, and the resultant metabolites can have pharmacological activity (Table 14–4).

ANALGESIC EFFICACY OF OPIOID METABOLITES

Morphine is mainly metabolized by conjugation with glucuronic acid, to form morphine-3-glucuronide (M3G) and morphine-6-glucuronide (M6G), and by a minor route via demethylation, to produce normorphine. M6G, the major metabolite in humans, has been shown to be 10 to 20 times more potent than morphine when given by the intrathecal route in rats.[19] The analgesic effects of M6G in humans are still unclear because data from different studies show conflicting results.

Using an experimental pain model in healthy volunteers, Lotsch et al[20] found that the intravenous infusion of low doses of M6G did not induce analgesia in comparison with morphine and placebo.[20] In another study in a postoperative pain model, patients were randomly assigned to receive intravenous morphine (0.15 mg/kg), placebo, or M6G (0.1 mg/kg) at skin closure. Analgesic requirements were significantly greater in the M6G and placebo groups during the first 24 postoperative hours.[21] In contrast, other human volunteer studies in which analgesia was assessed using either a submaximal ischemic pain model[22] or electrical stimulation[23] suggest an analgesic effect of M6G when given in doses of 3.3 to 5 mg per 70 kg. Overall, M6G may have potential as an analgesic, but its usefulness in clinical practice has yet to be demonstrated.

TABLE 14-4	Opioid Pharmacokinetics and Metabolites						
Opioid	Half-life	Equipotent IV Dose (mg/kg)	Equipotent PO Dose (mg/kg)	Clearance (mL/min/kg)	Duration (hr)	Oral Bioavailability (%)	Active Metabolites
Morphine	2–4 hr	0.1	0.3–0.5	15	3–5	10–50	M6G
Fentanyl	1.7 (α) min	0.001	0.001–0.015 transmucosal	13	0.75–1	Transdermal, 90	None
Pethidine	3–4 hr	1	1.5–2	12	2–3	30–60	Norpethidine
Alfentanil	1.4 (α) min	0.05	N/A	6	0.5		None
Sufentanil	1.4 (α) min	0.0001	N/A	12.7	1		None
Codeine	3 hr	1.2	2		4–6	60–90	Morphine
Oxycodone	2–6 hr	N/A	0.1		4–6	40–130	Oxymorphone
Remifentanil	5 min independent of infusion time	0.05–2µg/kg/hr	N/A	40	Depends on infusion	N/A	Nitric oxide

IV, intravenous; M6G, morphine-6-glucuronide; N/A, not applicable; PO, oral.

M3G has no affinity for the MOR receptor and may be responsible for some of the excitatory effects seen after high doses of morphine, such as myoclonus, convulsions, and hyperalgesia.

Cytochrome P450 2D6 is responsible for the metabolism of codeine into morphine, and 10% of white persons lack the ability to perform this conversion (poor metabolizers). Patients who are poor metabolizers may show absence of analgesia after administration of codeine in analgesic doses.[24]

The metabolites of fentanyl are considered to be inactive, but the metabolites of pethidine (i.e., norpethidine), although lacking clinical analgesic effect, can accumulate with repeated dosing or prolonged infusion (especially in the elderly and in patients with renal impairment) and thereby have neuroexcitatory effects.[25]

FACTORS THAT INFLUENCE OPIOID PHARMACOKINETICS

The main factors that affect the pharmacokinetics of opioids and may have clinical consequences are age, sex, systemic disease, obesity, and plasma protein concentration or binding.

Age

Predictably, the extremes of age are when most variations are noted and have important clinical sequelae. In neonates the following factors may alter the duration and effects of opioids: (1) an immature cytochrome P450 system, (2) a decreased renal clearance (leading to a prolonged half-life), and (3) an immature blood-brain barrier, which may result in higher opioid concentrations in the brain. Seizures have been reported in newborn infants at doses considered acceptable for other age groups.[26] Consequently, the administration of opioids to neonates requires careful control of dosage and continuous assessment of the effects. Several studies have found intravenous morphine infusions (20 μg/kg/hr) to be effective in the management of postoperative pain in children between 3 months and 14 years of age.[27]

In a prospective randomized double-blind study, van Dijk et al[28] reported that administration of continuous or intermittent intravenous morphine in infants up to 1 year who had undergone major thoracic surgery was effective. Differences in pain intensity and morphine requirements were most prominent between neonates and infants 1 to 6 months old; neonates had lower pain scores, whereas infants 1 to 6 months old had higher pain responses and required higher doses of morphine.

Older patients exhibit a greater sensitivity to opioids, a fact that seems to be related to their lower clearance and reduced volume of distribution compared with younger patients. These differences would result in higher morphine concentration per a given dose, so caution is advised in the use of opioids in this population.[29]

Sex

A review of animal and human literature suggested that opioids produce more effective analgesia in males than in females.[30] In a pain model using transcutaneous electrical stimulation in healthy volunteers, however, Sarton et al[31] were able to demonstrate that the efficacy of intravenous morphine (0.1 mg/kg bolus followed by an infusion of 0.03 mg/kg for 1 hour) was higher in females, even though the onset and offset of the analgesic effects were later than in males. More controlled studies are necessary to clarify possible dosing requirement differences between the sexes.

Liver and Renal Disease

Most metabolites originating from opioids that are metabolized by the liver are excreted via the kidney. Renal impairment does not seem to alter the pharmacokinetics of an opioid after bolus administration, but the potential exists for accumulation of active metabolites with continuous infusion, causing an increase in the pharmacological effects. In this situation, M6G or norpethidine, rather than the parent compounds morphine or pethidine, respectively, are likely to accumulate.[32] Although the pharmacokinetics of buprenorphine, alfentanil, sufentanil, and remifentanil change little in patients with renal failure, the continuous administration of fentanyl can lead to prolonged sedation. Because of its ultra-short half-life, remifentanil would seem the logical choice in patients with renal failure.

The use of opioids in patients with liver disease does not appear to cause major clinical problems when used in the recommended doses for pain relief.[33] However, animal studies have demonstrated increases in morphine half-life and of the pharmacological effects in animals without liver function.[34]

In humans, conflicting results have been generated; one study found lower morphine plasma clearance rates and longer half-life in cirrhotic patients than in healthy controls,[35] but in another study performed in children undergoing liver transplantation, no changes in opioid pharmacokinetics could be demonstrated.[36] The pharmacokinetics of single doses of fentanyl and sufentanil are not affected in liver and renal failure; however, continuous infusion of fentanyl may result in accumulation and a prolonged effect.[37] Plasma clearance and elimination of alfentanil are reduced in patients with liver failure, so this agent's clinical use cannot be recommended.[38] Remifentanil would appear to be the opioid of choice in patients with liver or renal failure.

Obesity

Obesity is defined as an excessive amount of body fat or adipose tissue in relation to lean body mass. The body mass index (BMI) is commonly used to identify obesity, and individuals with a BMI higher than 30 are traditionally considered obese.[39] Obese people have larger absolute lean body masses than non-obese individuals of the same age, sex, and height. The current knowledge of the influence of obesity on drug pharmacokinetics is limited, but it seems reasonable that drugs with a narrow therapeutic index should be given cautiously to obese patients.

The pharmacokinetics of remifentanil, a lipophilic opioid, was studied in 24 patients undergoing elective surgery, 12 of whom had a lean body mass of 62 ± 14 kg and total body weight of 113 ± 17 kg and 12 of whom were of normal weight. The results suggest that dosing to ideal body weight for remifentanil could be adequate in morbidly obese patients.[40]

Furthermore, a detailed study suggests that actual body weight overestimates fentanyl dose requirements in obese patients undergoing surgery[41]; therefore, dosing should be tailored to ideal body weight.

Plasma Protein Binding

The concentration of plasma proteins, especially α_1-acid glycoprotein (AAG), is decreased in various situations, especially after trauma or surgery and in chronic inflammatory disorders and cancer. Because most opioids are bound to these proteins, patients with reduced AAG may exhibit greater sensitivity to the opioid as a result of higher plasma concentrations of the free drug.

Routes of Administration

INTRAVENOUS

Opioids are well absorbed by all routes. In general, with the intravenous route there is little difference in onset times among the opioids commonly used in clinical practice (2–5 minutes). The intravenous route is easier to titrate than oral and intramuscular routes. Pain relief has been shown to be similar with intravenous infusion and intermittent boluses after major surgery in children.[28]

INTRAMUSCULAR

The lipophilicity of the drug is a determining factor for rate of onset after intramuscular administration. Intramuscular administration can provide good analgesia if the doses and dosing intervals are correctly customized to the individual patient. However, the systemic absorption after intramuscular morphine in the immediate postoperative period may be variable because of factors such as hypothermia, hypovolemia, and peripheral vasoconstriction.[42] This finding, together with the pain induced by repeated intramuscular injections, precludes the routine use of intramuscular administration in the perioperative period.

ORAL

In most standard oral formulations of opioids, onset of analgesia takes approximately 1 hour. The oral bioavailability displays significant variability, with almost 0 for fentanyl and between 10% and 50% for morphine (see Table 14–4). The influence of food, especially high-fat meals, on morphine absorption has been described; oral morphine absorption is slower in the fed state than in the fasting state. Not enough data are available on the effect on other opioids.[43]

In the management of postoperative pain, oral opioids can be useful, depending on the type of surgery. In a review from the Cochrane Database,[44] a single dose of oral dihydrocodeine (30 mg) was ineffective for acute postoperative pain after various types of surgery. However, data from pooled studies in a second review suggested that a single dose of oxycodone (from 5 mg upward) with or without paracetamol provided greater analgesia than placebo. On the basis of these results, the researchers suggested that the combination

is as efficacious as intramuscular morphine plus a nonsteroidal anti-inflammatory drug (NSAID) but had a higher incidence of adverse effects.[45] Perioperative oral opioids seem useful for mild to moderate pain but appear to be limited by side effects.

BUCCAL-TRANSMUCOSAL

Drugs given by the buccal-transmucosal route enter the systemic circulation via the mucosa of the mouth and bypass hepatic first-pass metabolism. Factors that influence absorption include pKa, lipid solubility, molecular weight, rate of diffusion, and the pH of the mouth.[46] Fentanyl is used in a unique formulation that allows direct absorption through the oral mucosa and also the gut, via swallowed saliva. It is used as a "lollipop stick," although this term is being actively discouraged.[47] The inability to deliver high doses limits the clinical usefulness of this route in the acute postoperative period.

TRANSDERMAL

At present, transdermal administration allows delivery of drugs in two forms, conventional (passive) and iontophoresis (active).

Conventional

Drugs that have low molecular weight and high lipophilicity and are nonionized are able to penetrate the dermal layers and avoid first-pass metabolism. Relevant factors in drug delivery after the application of an opioid patch (transdermal delivery system [TDS]) include permeability of the stratum corneum, skin temperature, placement site, integrity of the skin, and patient age and ethnicity. Transdermal fentanyl and buprenorphine are at present the two most commonly used TDS opioids in the management of chronic pain. Once a system is applied, the drug is released at a constant rate and accumulates within the skin layers over 12 to 16 hours. This accumulation behaves as a secondary reservoir, and constant blood levels of the drug are maintained for approximately 3 days.[48] The apparent terminal half-life of fentanyl is 15 to 24 hours, so there will still be significant drug available to reach the circulation after removal of the patch.

The use of a TDS in the postoperative period is discouraged because there is considerable risk of respiratory depression when supplemental analgesia is administered[49] or when pain subsides.

Iontophoresis

Iontophoresis was designed to overcome the stratum corneum barrier to drug absorption. The application of an electric field allows the charged component of a drug to pass through the skin. A study performed in more than 600 patients with postoperative pain shows that 40 µg of fentanyl delivered over a period of 10 minutes in a patient-controlled manner is similar in analgesic efficacy to a standard morphine intravenous patient-controlled analgesia (PCA) device.[50] However, this system is limited by the fixed dosing that can be delivered and may not as yet be suitable for patients at the extremes of age.

INTRANASAL ADMINISTRATION

The intranasal route offers the advantages of ease of administration, rapid onset, and patient control. At present it is used in the management of breakthrough pain. Presystemic hepatic metabolism is bypassed, leading to a relative potency similar to that with intravenous administration. However, drug absorption may be variable compared with conventional routes. The best agents to be administered intranasally are those with low molecular weight and high lipid solubility. Several opioids have been used in this manner, including fentanyl, sufentanil, pethidine, diamorphine, and butorphanol. Only intranasal fentanyl, pethidine, and butorphanol have been evaluated for postoperative pain. The mean onset time of these agents ranges from 12 to 22 minutes, and the time to peak effect from 24 to 60 minutes, showing considerable individual variation in pharmacokinetics and clinical outcome.[51]

Although nasally administered opioids have potential use in ambulatory or hospitalized patients and patients with chronic pain, the production of better formulations and devices is needed.

RECTAL

Rectal administration is not commonly used in the postoperative period, because the absorption of drugs from the rectum is exceedingly variable and depends (among other factors) on the formulation used. Absorption occurs by diffusion into the systemic and portal circulations, thus limiting the level of first-pass metabolism. In general, doses used for rectal administration are similar to those for oral administration.

SUBCUTANEOUS

For subcutaneous administration, water-soluble drugs are more rapidly absorbed. Subcutaneous morphine was found to be similar to intramuscular morphine in an elderly postoperative population.[52] Limitations to its use include the presence of an edematous state, hypotension, and poor peripheral circulation.

SPINAL ROUTE: EPIDURAL AND INTRATHECAL

Opioid receptors located in the dorsal horn of the spinal cord are not confined to the superficial layers but are also present in the substantia gelatinosa, implying that spinally administered opioids must diffuse into the deep layers of the spinal cord in order to induce analgesia. Diffusion depends on molecular weight, concentration gradient, ionic-to-nonionic ratio, and, most important, lipid solubility. Several studies have documented the use of either epidural or intrathecal opioids for postoperative pain, with morphine and fentanyl being the most common in Europe.[53]

When an opioid is injected directly into the cerebrospinal fluid (CSF), only small doses are required because there are no additional anatomical barriers, and uptake by the vascular system is slow. However, when drugs are administered epidurally they must cross the dura matter to reach the spinal cord and subsequently bind to the opioid receptors.[54] Systemic absorption of the drugs administered epidurally is rapid, and for lipophilic agents the plasma concentrations achieved are similar to those after intramuscular injection.

In a pig model using a microdialysis technique, which enabled continuous sampling of opioid concentrations in the epidural and intrathecal spaces, Bernards et al[55] showed that there is a strong correlation between lipid solubility of a drug and (1) the time spent in the epidural space and (2) the terminal elimination half-life (i.e., the more lipid-soluble the drug, the greater its half-life).

Morphine was the first and is probably the most commonly used spinal opioid. It produces long-lasting analgesia but has side effects via redistribution by rostral spread to the brain, the most serious being respiratory depression. Most opioids available in clinical practice have been administered via the intrathecal route in search of the "ideal opioid," which would induce effective analgesia with minimal side effects. The ideal intrathecal opioid would have rapid distribution from the CSF to the spinal cord, a slow clearance, and moderate or no rostral distribution.

The efficacy and duration of intrathecal analgesia vary significantly for different opioids. In clinical practice, the major differences are related to duration of action, rostral spread, and relative potency compared with intravenous administration. These factors are influenced by the lipophilicity of the drug (the more lipid-soluble drugs are taken up into the spinal cord faster than hydrosoluble drugs; see Table 14–3), affinity for the opioid receptors, intrinsic activity, and drug removal via the systemic circulation.

The hydrophilic opioids, such as morphine, are slowly removed from the CSF, leading to rostral spread of relatively high concentrations of the drug. In animal studies, morphine is more potent when delivered intrathecally than intravenously, in contrast to fentanyl, which is only slightly more potent when delivered intrathecally.[56] Lipophilic drugs such as fentanyl move from the CSF rapidly to the lipid rich tissues of the spinal cord, with a rapid onset of analgesia in a more segmental fashion. It is unclear what role metabolism plays in the termination of the effects of neuraxially administered opioids.

The exact site of action of lipophilic agents administered epidurally is uncertain, because plasma levels of these drugs, analgesia, and side effects are similar for both epidural and intravenous administrations.[55] A few studies suggest a spinal site of action for the lipophilic agents.[57,58] A small study using 10 volunteers investigated the analgesic effects of epidural fentanyl when administered either as a single bolus or by infusion. The data suggest that the epidural bolus induced analgesia via a spinal mechanism, whereas fentanyl given by infusion produced its analgesic effect through uptake into the general circulation and redistribution.[59] Nonetheless, it is likely that for the lipophilic compounds, analgesia is mediated mainly via systemic uptake into the circulation, although they also spread rostrally in the CSF and can induce serious complications.[60]

Opioid-Induced Adverse Effects

The goal of opioid administration is effective analgesia, which is generally obtained by careful titration. Opioids have little or no use outside this realm in clinical practice. Systemically administered conventional opioids have both central and peripheral effects, a fact that is related to the wide distribution of opioid receptors throughout the body. In general, beneficial effects (analgesia) and adverse effects occur simultaneously, although the incidence and severity may vary according to the opioid, dose, route, and patient. The main adverse effects on the different systems are briefly reviewed here.

RESPIRATORY DEPRESSION

The true incidence of clinically significant respiratory depression is unknown, but an estimation of the risk of severe respiratory depression from therapeutic doses of opioids, regardless of the route of administration, is less than 1%.[61] However, no definite evidence is available about the incidence of respiratory depression for the various opioids, dosing regimens, and routes of administration, or for the concomitant use of neuraxial and parenteral opioids (with or without sedatives).

Opioids in general decrease minute ventilation by diminishing both respiratory rate and tidal volume. The major effect is a decrease in responsiveness of the respiratory center in the medulla to carbon dioxide tension. Thus, after opioid administration, the carbon dioxide curve is shifted to the right and its slope is reduced. A decrease in respiratory rate is a late and therefore not useful sign of opioid-induced respiratory depression, and indeed, patients may be awake yet apneic after the intravenous administration of rapid-acting opioids.[62]

Opioids also inhibit the respiratory response to hypoxia. The relative influences of intrathecal versus intravenous morphine on the ventilatory response to sustained isocapnic hypoxia has been studied in volunteers.[63] The study showed that the depression of the ventilatory response to hypoxia after intrathecal morphine was similar in magnitude to an equianalgesic dose of intravenous morphine; however, for the intrathecal route, the response lasted longer (up to 12 hours), suggesting that opioids affect ventilation via central mechanisms.

Opioid-induced respiratory depression is mediated by activation of MORs, a fact demonstrated in animal studies using MOR-knockout mice; these animals displayed absence of respiratory depression as well as no spinal/supraspinal antinociception after the administration of systemic morphine.[64] Thus, in the absence of pain, opioid-mediated analgesia and respiratory depression are difficult to separate. However, opioids given to volunteers behave differently from those given to patients in pain. It has been postulated that the respiratory center receives nociceptive input, which could attenuate the opioid-induced respiratory depression.[65] In acute pain states, opioids must be titrated for analgesia, and concern about opioid respiratory depression should not hinder the appropriate use of opioids in the postoperative patient. The titration, dose, and timing of administration must be considered to minimize risks to the patient.[66]

The management of opioid-induced respiratory depression depends on its severity and involves careful titration with intravenous naloxone (100 to 400 μg) and, if necessary, a naloxone infusion, because this agent's half-life is significantly shorter than that of most opioids (see Chapter 15).

PRURITUS

Opioids such as morphine and fentanyl may induce local transitory pruritus after intravenous administration related to histamine release. Pruritus is also a common adverse effect of neuraxial opioid administration, occurring with variable incidence according to the population studied. The precise mechanism of neuraxial opioid–induced pruritus is unclear. Several mechanisms have been postulated, such as abnormal skin sensitivity related to opioid administration, the presence of an itch center, and the activation of specific neurons in the dorsal horn of the spinal cord.[67] The treatment of neuraxial opioid–induced pruritus remains a challenge. Many pharmacological therapies—antihistamines, 5-hydroxytriptamine receptor antagonists, opioid antagonists, propofol, NSAIDs, and droperidol—have been evaluated. Drugs that do not reverse analgesia or induce profound sedation should be favored. Intravenous ondansetron, 2 to 4 mg, is among the most effective treatments for neuraxial opioid–induced pruritus in various patient populations,[68] including children.[69]

GASTROINTESTINAL EFFECTS

Opioids delay gastric emptying, increase small and large bowel transit times, and inhibit fluid secretion and permeability. Ileus/constipation is a predictable consequence of opioid therapy. Several physiological factors may inhibit or promote gastric emptying. Thus, stimulation of the sympathetic nervous system and pain, delay gastric emptying. Opioids decrease secretion of hydrochloric acid and increase antral tone. Delayed gastric emptying has several important sequelae, including slow absorption of orally administered drugs or nutrients, nausea, and increased risk of aspiration.[70] Smooth muscle tone increases throughout the small and large intestines, and biliary and pancreatic secretions are diminished.

Although oral and parenteral routes are the major culprits in opioid delay of gastrointestinal motility, several studies in volunteers have demonstrated that opioids administered epidurally or intrathecally also delay gastric emptying.[71] In a study in which neuraxial analgesia was provided with local anesthetic alone in patients undergoing laparotomy and compared with systemic or epidural opioid techniques, there was a more rapid return to gastrointestinal function in the local anesthetic group.[72]

The mechanism by which epidural opioids delay gastric emptying is unclear because the relative contributions of local and systemic effects are not entirely established. In the postoperative period, ileus is multifactorial, and opioid administration plays an important role.[73] Opioid receptors are constitutively expressed throughout the gut, and opioid-induced inhibition of gastrointestinal function occurs as a consequence of binding of the opioid to MORs located in the gut as well as in the central nervous system. The proportion of central versus peripheral MORs that is affected seems to be dose related. Opioid-induced delay in gastric emptying and gastrointestinal transit in humans can be partially reversed with a peripheral opioid antagonist, methylnaltrexone, suggesting a predominantly peripheral mechanism of action.[74,75] The use of the novel peripherally acting MOR antagonist alvimopan, which has limited ability to cross the blood-brain barrier, has been shown to accelerate gastrointestinal recovery and shorten time to hospital discharge compared with placebo in patients undergoing major bowel or radical hysterectomy procedures.[76]

Therapeutic doses of opioids cause a rise in biliary tract pressure, owing to either spasm or contraction of the sphincter of Oddi, that can persist for up to 12 hours. The effects of opioids on the sphincter are complex, and the clinical symptoms can be attenuated by the administration of low doses of naloxone or nitroglycerin.[77]

There is no good evidence to suggest that equianalgesic doses of pethidine offer any advantage over other opioids for the treatment of biliary or renal colic.

URINARY EFFECTS

Opioids increase the tone and amplitude of contraction of the ureter and bladder, but the response in humans is variable. Although the mechanism is not clearly understood, the endogenous opioid system seems to play a role in the physiological control of bladder function via modulation of the parasympathetic outflow at the level of the sacral spinal cord.[78]

Urinary retention after neuraxial administration of opioids is variable but tends to be higher than after intravenous or intramuscular administration of equivalent doses, suggesting that the underlying mechanism after neuraxial administration is not related to the systemic absorption of the drug.[79] In a human study, epidural morphine caused detrusor muscle relaxation within 15 minutes that persisted for hours and was reversible by naloxone; other opioids studied in this setting suggest that intrathecal lipophilic opioids may have less of an effect on time to voluntary voiding.[80]

Other factors that could delay voiding in the postoperative period include the volume status of the patient, type and anatomical location of surgery, and factors that promote antidiuretic hormome activation.[81]

NAUSEA AND VOMITING

Postoperative nausea and vomiting (PONV) are common and troublesome events after surgery. Although they are multifactorial, intraoperative and postoperative administration of opioids seems to play an important role. However, the extent by which these effects are mediated by opioid receptors located at the chemoreceptor trigger zone (CRTZ) and related centers in the medulla is unclear at present.[82,83] The route of opioid administration does not alter PONV, because its incidence after intrathecal or epidural administration of opioids is similar to that after intravenous administration.[84] However, cephalad migration of the opioid after spinal administration would seem a likely mechanism. Other relevant factors involved in promoting PONV are pain, hypotension, type of surgery, movement, gastric distention, delayed gastric emptying, and sex (more common in females).

CARDIOVASCULAR EFFECTS

In the supine individual, analgesic doses of opioids have minimal effects on blood pressure, heart rate, and rhythm. Hypotension may occur upon rising from the supine position. Other effects are seen in patients with coronary artery disease, in whom therapeutic doses of opioids may cause a decrease in oxygen consumption, cardiac work, left ventricular pressure, and diastolic pressure.[85] Hypotension due to histamine release may be observed after morphine administration,[86]

and opioids in general induce vasodilatation of peripheral arterioles and veins. Thus, intravenous administration of opioids should be used with caution in patients with hypovolemia. Fentanyl and other short-acting opioids can cause bradycardia when used alone or in conjunction with vagal stimulation procedures (i.e., laryngoscopy).

Partial agonists and mixed agonist-antagonist compounds are rarely used in the acute perioperative period and are not addressed in this chapter.

Summary

The pharmacology of opioids is complex, given the individual variability of the responses and factors that may affect their pharmacokinetics and pharmacodynamics. Morphine is still the standard by which all other drugs are measured, although most strong opioids have similar analgesic efficacy. The presence of pain alters the pharmacology of opioids; as a result, opioids must be titrated against pain on the basis of pain intensity and the clinical condition of the patient. The most common reason for inadequate pain relief with opioids is fear of adverse effects. However, concern about respiratory depression should not restrain the rational and appropriate use of opioids. The titration, size of the dose, timing, and rescue dosing must be optimized for the individual patient to provide good perioperative analgesia.

REFERENCES

1. Arner S, Bolund C, Rane A, et al: Narcotic analgesics in the treatment of cancer and postoperative pain. Acta Anaesthesiol Scand 1982; 26(Suppl 74):1–78.
2. Marks RM, Sacher EJ: Under treatment of medical inpatients with narcotic analgesics. Ann Intern Med 1973;78:173–181.
3. Apfelbaum JL, Chen C, Matha SS, et al: Postoperative pain experience results from a national pain survey suggest postoperative pain continues to be undermanaged. Anesth Analg 2003;97:534–550.
4. Vaccarino AL, Kastin AJ: Endogenous opiates. Peptides 2000;21: 1975–2034.
5. Zadina JE, Hackler L, Ge LJ, Kastin AJ: A potent and selective endogenous agonist for the mu-opiate receptor. Nature 1997;386:499–502.
6. Horvath G: Endomorphin-1 and endomorphin-2: Pharmacology of the selective endogenous mu-opioid receptor agonists. Pharmacol Ther 2000;88:437–463.
7. Mansour A, Khachaturian H, Lewis ME, et al: Anatomy of CNS opioid receptors. Trends Neurosci 1988;11:308–314.
8. Darland T, Heinricher MM, Grandy DK: Orphanin FQ/nociceptin: A role in pain and analgesia, but so much more. Trends Neurosci 1998; 21:215–221.
9. Calo G, Guerrini R, Rizzi A, et al: Pharmacology of nociceptin and its receptor: A novel therapeutic target. Br J Pharmacol 2000;129: 1261–1283.
10. Stein C, Yassouridis A: Peripheral morphine analgesia. Pain 1997;71: 119–121.
11. Picard PR, Tramer MR, McQuay HJ, Moore RA: Analgesic efficacy of peripheral opioids (all except intra-articular): A qualitative systematic review of randomised controlled trials. Pain 1997;72:309–318.
12. Kosterlitz HW, Paterson SJ: Opioid receptors and mechanism of opioid analgesia. In Benedetti C, Chapman CR, Giron G (eds): Advances in Pain Research and Therapy, vol 14. New York, Raven Press, 1989, pp 37–43.
13. Levac, BAR, O'Dowd BF, George SR: Oligomerization of opioid receptors: Generation of novel signalling units. Curr Opin Pharmacol 2002; 2:76–81.
14. Bovill JG: Pharmacokinetics of opioids. In Bowdle TA, Hortia A, Kharasch ED (eds): The Pharmacological Basis of Anaesthesiology. New York, Churchill Livingstone, 1994, pp 37–81.

15. Thompson JP, Rowbotham DJ: Remifentanil: An opioid for the 21st century. Br J Anaesth 1996;76;341–343.
16. Hughes MA, Glass PSA, Jacobs JR: Context sensitive half time in a multicompartment model for intravenous anaesthetic drugs. Anesthesiology 1992;76:334–341.
17. Dalhstrom B, Tamsen A, Paalzow L, et al: Patient controlled analgesic therapy. Part IV: Pharmacokinetic and analgesic plasma concentrations of morphine. Clin Pharmacokinet 1982;7:266–279.
18. Gourlay GK: Treatment of cancer pain with transdermal fentanyl. Lancet Oncol 2001;2:165–172.
19. Sullivan AF, McQuay HJ, Baily D, et al: The spinal antinociceptive actions of morphine metabolites morphine 6 glucuronide and normorphine in the rat. Brain Res 1989;482:219–224.
20. Lotsch J, Kobal G, Stockmann, et al: Lack of analgesic activity of morphine-6-glucuronide intravenous administration in healthy volunteers. Anesthesiology 1997;87:1348–1358.
21. Motamed C, Mazoit X, Ghanouchi K, et al: Pre-emptive intravenous morphine-6-glucuronide is ineffective for postoperative pain relief. Anesthesiology 2000;92:355–360.
22. Buetler TM, Wilder-Smith OGH, Aebi S, et al: Analgesic actions of i.v. morphine-6-glucuronide in healthy volunteers. Br J Anaesth 2000;84: 97–99.
23. Penson RT, Joel SP, Bakhshi K, et al: Randomised placebo controlled trial of the activity of the morphine glucuronides. Clin Pharmacol Ther 2000;68:667–676.
24. Desmeules J, Gascon MP, Dayer P, Magistris M: Impact of environmental and genetic factors on codeine analgesia. Eur J Clin Pharmacol 1991; 41:23–26.
25. Danziger LH, Martin SJ, Blum RA: Central nervous system toxicity associated with meperidine use in hepatic disease. Pharmacotherapy 1994;14:235–238.
26. Koren G, Butt W, Pape K, et al: Morphine induced seizures in newborn infants. Vet Hum Toxicol 1985;27:519–520.
27. Lynn Am, Opheim KE, Tyler DC: Morphine infusions after paediatric cardiac surgery. Crit Care Med 1984;12:863–866.
28. van Dijk M, Bouwmeester NJ, Duivenvoorden HJ, et al: Efficacy of continuous versus intermittent morphine administration after major surgery in 0–3 year old infants: A double-blind randomised controlled trial. Pain 2002;98:305–313.
29. Kaiko RF, Walssenstein SL, Rogers AG, et al: Narcotics in the elderly. Medi Clin North Am 1982;66:1079–1089.
30. Keat B, Sarton E, Dahan A: Gender differences in opioid mediated analgesia: Animal and human studies. Anesthesiology 2000;93: 539–547.
31. Sarton E, Olofsen E, Den Hartigh J, et al: Sex differences in morphine analgesia: An experimental study in healthy volunteers Anesthesiology 2000;93:670–675.
32. Angst MS, Buhrer M, Lotsch J: Insidious intoxication after morphine treatment in renal failure: Delayed onset of morphine-6-glucuronide action. Anesthesiology 2000;92;1473–1476.
33. Patwardhan RV, Johnson RF, Hoyumpa A, et al: Normal metabolism of morphine in cirrhosis. 1981;81:1006–1011.
34. Greene NM, Hug CC: Pharmacokinetics. In Kitaha LM, Collins JG (eds): Narcotic Analgesics in Anesthesiology. Baltimore, Williams & Wilkins, 1982, pp 1–41.
35. Hasselstrom J, Eriksson LS, Person A, et al: The metabolism and bioavailability of morphine in patients with liver cirrhosis. Eur J Pharmacol 1990;29:289–297.
36. Davis JP, Stiller RL, Cook DR, et al: Effects of cholestatic hepatic disease and chronic renal failure on alfentanil pharmacokinetics in children. Anesth Analg 1989;68:579–583.
37. Davies G, Kingswood C, Street M: Pharmacokinetics of opioids in renal dysfunction. Clin Pharmacokinet 1996;31:410–422.
38. Hohne C, Donaubauer B, Kaisers U: Opioids during anaesthesia in liver and renal failure. Anaesthesist 2004;53:291–303.
39. National Institutes of Health: Clinical guidelines on the identification, evaluation, and treatment of overweight and obesity in adults. Bethesda, Md, Department of Health and Human Services, National Institutes of Health, National Heart, Lung, and Blood Institute, 1998.
40. Egan TD, Huizinga B, Gupta SK, et al: Remifentanil pharmacokinetics in obese versus lean patients. Anesthesiology 1998;89:562–573.
41. Shibutani K, Inchiosa MA, Sawada K, et al: Accuracy of pharmacokinetic models for predicting fentanyl concentrations in lean and obese surgical patients: Deviation of dosing weight. Anesthesiology 2004; 101:603–613.
42. Forrest J: Pharmacology of opioids. In Acute Pain Path... Treatment. Ontario, Canada, Manticore, 1998, pp 77–9...
43. Kaiko RF: The effect of food intake on the pharmac... sustained-release morphine sulphate capsules. Clin The... 296–303.
44. Edwards JE, Moore RA, McQuay HJ: Single dose dihydrocodeine... acute postoperative pain. Cochrane Database Syst Rev 2000;(4):CD002760.
45. Edwards JE, Moore RA, McQuay HJ: Single dose oxycodone and oxycodone plus paracetamol (acetaminophen) for acute postoperative pain. Cochrane Database Syst Rev 2000;(4):CD002763.
46. Ripamonti C, Bruera E: Rectal, buccal and sublingual narcotics for the management of cancer pain. J Palliative Care 1991;7:30–35.
47. Schechter NL, Weisman SJ, Rosenblum M, et al: The use of oral transmucosal fentanyl citrate for painful procedures in children. Paediatrics 1995;95:335–339.
48. Varel JR, Shafter SL, Hwang SS, et al: Absorption characteristics of transdermally applied fentanyl. Anesthesiology 1989;70:928–934.
49. Sandler AN, Baxter AD, Katz J: A double blind patient controlled trial of transdermal fentanyl after abdominal hysterectomy. Anesthesiology 1994;81:1169–1180.
50. Viscusi E, Reyonlds L, Chung F, et al: Patient controlled transdermal fentanyl HCl vs intravenous morphine pump for postoperative pain. JAMA 2004;291:1293.
51. Dale O, Hjortkjaer R, Kharasch ED: Nasal administration of opioids for pain management in adults. Acta Anesthesiol Scand 2002;46:759–770.
52. Semple TJ, Upton RN, Macintyre PE, et al: Morphine blood concentrations in elderly postoperative patients following administration via an indwelling subcutaneous cannula. Anaesthesia 1997;52:318–323.
53. Rawal N, Alllvin RL: Epidural and intrathecal opioids for postoperative pain in Europe—a 17 nation questionnaire study of selective hospitals. Euro Pain Study Group on Acute Pain. Acta Anaesthesiol Scand 1996; 40:1119–1126.
54. Nordberg G: Pharmacokinetic aspects of spinal morphine analgesia. Acta Anesthesiol Scand Suppl 1984;79:1–38.
55. Bernards CM, Shen DD, Sterling ES, et al: Epidural cerebrospinal fluid and plasma pharmacokinetics of epidural opioids. Part 1: Difference among opioids. Anesthesiology 2003;99:455–465.
56. Abram SE, Mampilly GA, Milsavljevic D: Assessment of the potency and intrinsic activity of systemic versus intrathecal opioids in the rat. Anesthesiology 1997;87:127–134.
57. D'Angelo R, Gerachner JC, Eisenach J, et al: Epidural fentanyl produces labor analgesia by a spinal mechanism. Anesthesiology 1998;88: 1519–1523.
58. Salomaki TE, Latinen JO, Nuutinen LS: A randomised double blind comparison of epidural versus intravenous infusion for analgesia after thoracotomy by rostral spread. Anesthesiology 1991;75:790–795.
59. Ginosar Y, Riley ET, Angst MS: The site of action of epidural fentanyl in humans: The difference between infusion and bolus administration. Anesth Analg 2003;97:1428–1438.
60. Eisenach JC: Lipid soluble opioids do move in cerebrospinal fluid. Reg Anesth Pain Med 2001;26:296–297.
61. Rygnestad T, Borchgrevink PC, Eide E: Postoperative epidural infusion of morphine and bupivacaine is safe on surgical wards: Organisation of the treatment, effects and side effects of 2000 consecutive patients. Acta Anesthesiol Scand 1997;41:868–876.
62. Babenco HD, Conard PF, Gross JB: The pharmacodynamic effect of a remifentanil bolus on ventilatory control. Anesthesiology 2000;92: 393–398.
63. Bailey PL, Lu JK, Pace NL, et al: Effects of intrathecal morphine on the ventilatory response to hypoxia. N Engl J Med 2000;343:1228–1234.
64. Dahan M, Sarto E, Teppema L, et al: Anaesthetic potency and influence of morphine and sevoflurane on respiration in mu opioid receptor knockout mice. Anesthesiology 2001;94:824–832.
65. Borgbjerg FM, Nielsen K, Franks J: Experimental pain stimulates respiration and attenuates morphine-induced respiratory depression: A controlled study in human volunteers. Pain 1996;64:123–128.
66. Hopf HW, Weitz S: Postoperative pain management. Arch Surg 1994; 129:128–132.
67. Szarvas S, Harmon D, Murphy D: Neuraxial opioid-induced pruritus: A review. J Clin Anesth 2003;15:234–239.
68. Borgeat A, Stirnemann HR: Ondansetron is effective to treat spinal or epidural morphine-induced pruritus. Anesthesiology 1999;90:432–436.
69. Arai L, Stayer S, Schwartz R, Dorsey A: The use of ondansetron to treat pruritus associated with intrathecal morphine in two paediatric patients. Paediatr Anesth 1996;6:337–339.

70. Nimmo WS: The effects of anaesthesia on gastric motility and emptying. Br J Anaesth 1984;56:29–36.
71. Thoren T, Wattwil M: The effects on gastric emptying on thoracic epidural analgesia with morphine or bupivacaine. Anesth Analg 1988;67:687–694.
72. Jorgensen H, Wetterslev J, Moiniche S, Dahl JB: Epidural local anaesthetics versus opioid-based analgesic regimens on postoperative gastrointestinal paralysis, PONV and pain after abdominal surgery. Cochrane Database Syst Rev 2000;(4):CD001893.
73. Luckey A, Livingston E, Tache Y: Mechanism and treatment of postoperative ileus. Arch Surg 2003;128:206–214.
74. Murphy D, Sutton JA, Prescott LF, Murphy MB: Opioid induced changes in gastric emptying: A peripheral mechanism in man. Anesthesiology 1997;87:765–770.
75. Yuan CS, Foss JF: Oral methylnaltrexone for opioid-induced constipation. JAMA 2000;284:1383–1384.
76. Wolff BG, Michelassi F, Tood M, et al: Alvimopan, a novel peripheral acting μ opioid antagonist. Ann Surg 2004;240:728–735.
77. Isenhower HL, Muller BA: Selection of narcotic analgesic for pain associated with pancreatitis. Am J Health Syst Pharm 1998;55:480–486.
78. Malinovsky LM, Le Normand L, LePage JY, et al: The urodynamic effects of intravenous opioids and ketoprofen in humans. Anesth Analg 1998;87:456–461.
79. Peterson TK, Husted SE, Rybo L, et al: Urinary retention during i.m. and extradural morphine analgesia. Br J Anaesth 1982;54:1175–1178.
80. Lui S, Chiu AA, Carpenter RL, et al: Fentanyl prolongs lidocaine spinal anaesthesia without prolonging recovery. Anesth Analg 1995;80:730–734.
81. Rawal N, Mollefors KM, Axelsson K, et al: An experimental study of urodynamic effects of epidural morphine and naloxone reversal. Anesth Analg 1983;62:641–647.
82. Andrews PLR: Physiology of nausea and vomiting. Br J Anaesth 1992;69:2S–19S.
83. Hornby PJ: Central neurocircuitry associated with emesis. Am J Med 2001;111(Suppl 8A):106S–112S.
84. Correll DJ, Viscusi ER, Grunwald Z, Moore JH Jr: Epidural analgesia compared with intravenous morphine patient-controlled analgesia: Postoperative outcome measures after mastectomy with immediate TRAM flap breast reconstruction. Reg Anesth Pain Med 2001;26:444–449.
85. Estafanous F (ed): Opioids in Anaesthesia II. London, Butterworth-Heinemann, 1990, pp 93–109.
86. Rosow CE, Moss J, Philbin DM, et al: Histamine release during morphine and fentanyl anaesthesia. Anesthesiology 1982;56:93–96.

15 Use of Opioid Analgesics in the Perioperative Period

COLIN J. L. McCARTNEY • AHTSHAM NIAZI

The primary role of the anesthetist is the management of pain, and opioid analgesics have been commonly used since the beginning of the specialty to achieve this aim. Opioid analgesics remain the mainstay of management for moderate to severe postoperative pain, and despite the development of new opioids, morphine remains the "gold standard" against which all other opioids are compared. However, each opioid may have advantages in certain clinical situations and also when given by specific routes. In acute pain management, opioids are usually prescribed within the confines of a multimodal analgesic regimen[1] that includes the administration of nonsteroidal anti-inflammatory drugs (NSAIDs), acetaminophen, local anesthetic techniques, and other analgesic adjuvants. Such regimens both improve pain control and decrease opioid consumption, leading to reduction in opioid-related adverse effects.

The International Association for the Study of Pain (IASP) defines *pain* as "An unpleasant sensory and emotional experience associated with actual or potential tissue damage, or described in terms of such damage."[2] Postsurgical pain is typically nociceptive and is caused by tissue damage and the inflammatory response that occurs in response to trauma. This type of pain commonly responds well to opioid treatment. Occasionally postsurgical pain can be neuropathic, especially if direct peripheral nerve or central nervous system (CNS) injury has occurred. Neuropathic pain is usually described as a shooting (electric shock) or burning pain and, unlike nociceptive pain, was traditionally thought to respond poorly to opioid analgesics. This concept has now been challenged, however, and a number of studies have demonstrated benefit from the use of opioids in patients with neuropathic pain.[3,4]

This chapter examines the available evidence for the analgesic benefit of administration of opioids in the perioperative period. Advantages and disadvantages of particular opioids given by each route of administration are examined. Newer techniques, such as the use of controlled-release oral opioids and opioid administration in the periphery, are also discussed.

Methodology

The literature was reviewed systematically from 1966 to December 2004 by a search of the Medline database using the following terms: opioid, morphine, fentanyl, hydromorphone, oxycodone, diamorphine, oral, intravenous, epidural, intrathecal, transcutaneous, peripheral, intra-articular, and controlled-release. The Cochrane database and the Oxford Pain Internet Site were also searched for relevant material. Randomized and double-blind studies with a relevant assessment of pain were predominantly included. Other relevant studies have been incorporated to answer specific questions in the absence of higher-quality evidence; where necessary, their inclusion has been indicated in the text.

The data for the use of opioids via intravenous, intramuscular, and oral routes for acute pain management are presented as Number Needed to Treat (NNT) and as Number Needed to Harm (NNH). The data for the use of opioids by other routes has been presented as percentages and frequencies. The NNT, which is used as a measure to compare treatment outcomes of two interventions, is the reciprocal of the absolute risk reduction compared with placebo for that treatment.[5] In the case of a hypothetical tramadol study—in which risk of severe pain decreased from 0.30 without tramadol to 0.05 with tramadol, for an absolute risk reduction of 0.25 (0.3 − 0.05)—the NNT would be 1 ÷ 0.25, or 4.

In clinical terms, an NNT of 4 means that one would have to treat four patients with tramadol to prevent pain from occurring in one patient. However, few studies demonstrate 100% reduction in pain with a single treatment; for that reason, it is easier to calculate the NNT for a 50% reduction in pain. The concept encompassed in the NNT can also be calculated and expressed for adverse events; this is known as the number needed to harm (NNH). The use of NNT is limited, in that it usually refers to the effect of a single-dose intervention at one point in time and may not accurately represent the temporal quality of effect. It is a useful tool, however, for demonstrating the relative effectiveness of different treatments.

Intravenous Opioid Therapy

Box 15–1 summarizes this discussion.

MORPHINE

Morphine remains the gold standard opioid analgesic, with a 10-mg intramuscular dose having an NNT of 2.9 for 50% pain relief.[6] Unfortunately, data needed to calculate the NNT for intravenous morphine are not available. It is generally accepted in modern acute pain practice, however, that the repeated painful injections of the intramuscular route are

Morphine remains the gold standard for intravenous opioid analgesia when pain is moderate to severe; hydromorphone in equianalgesic doses is a good alternative.

Short-acting opioids may be useful in patients undergoing outpatient surgery because of their effective pain relief and lower incidence of nausea and vomiting.

Tramadol, owing to its efficacy in mild to moderate postoperative pain and low incidence of serious side effects, has a "user-friendly" profile.

Meperidine (pethidine) has no advantages over morphine or other opioids, and many disadvantages.

undesirable and that the intravenous route should be used whenever possible.[7] The many studies comparing analgesic and side effect profiles of other opioids with morphine are detailed in the following sections.

MEPERIDINE

At present, systemic meperidine is not recommended in the management of postoperative pain owing to a significant potential for adverse effects (tachycardia, hypertension, accumulation of neurotoxic metabolites) and its lack of advantages over other strong opioids, such as morphine and hydromorphone.[8]

For patients with intolerance or allergy to other opioids, meperidine does provide analgesia in doses of at least 100 mg (NNT 2.9 for 70-kg individual)[9] but has a shorter duration of action (2–3 hours) than morphine. Using dosing intervals of 4 hours will therefore provide windows of inadequate analgesia. Meperidine has no clinical advantages over other opioids in patients with biliary or renal colic.[8] Prolonged administration in the postoperative period has several disadvantages, including potential for accumulation of the metabolite normeperidine, which has two to three times the neurotoxic potential of the parent compound (causing seizures) and has a plasma half-life of 14 to 48 hours. Meperidine is the opioid that most frequently causes delirium in the elderly, especially with the use of patient-controlled analgesia (PCA) devices.[8] Fatal drug interactions between meperidine and the monoamine oxidase inhibitors have been reported.[8] Overall, meperidine is a poor choice of parenteral opioid because of its short duration of action, anticholinergic effects, and potential for neurotoxicity. This is confirmed by the NNH for meperidine, 2.9, whereas that for morphine is 9.1.[9] Patients who have postoperative pain and morphine intolerance or allergy may benefit more from the use of an agent with less potential for adverse effects, such as intravenous hydromorphone.

HYDROMORPHONE

Hydromorphone is a semisynthetic derivative of morphine. The parenteral dose equivalence is approximately 2 mg hydromorphone to 10 mg morphine in a 70-kg patient; that is, hydromorphone is about five times more potent than morphine.[10] When given by the intravenous route, hydromorphone has a rapid onset (within 5 minutes), a short time to peak effect (10–20 minutes), and a relatively short half-life

(3–4 hours).[11] The major metabolite of hydromorphone (hydromorphone 3-glucuronide) does not have analgesic activity, although it is neuroexcitatory in rats[12] and may accumulate in patients with renal impairment.[13] Intravenous hydromorphone is purported to produce fewer adverse effects in elderly patients and patients with renal impairment, although there are no randomized studies to support this statement. Rapp et al[14] randomly assigned 61 patients aged 18 to 65 years who were undergoing lower abdominal or pelvic surgery to receive equipotent doses of intravenous PCA-administered hydromorphone or morphine. Analgesia was equivalent in the two groups, but interestingly, patients in the morphine group suffered less cognitive impairment. No randomized blinded studies comparing hydromorphone and other opioid analgesics in postoperative patients with renal impairment have been performed.

FENTANYL

Fentanyl was one of a series of opioids synthesized by Janssen Pharmaceutica in the 1950s and 1960s in an effort to produce opioid analgesics with greater analgesic activity and potency and fewer adverse effects than morphine and meperidine. Fentanyl, or N-(1-phenethyl-4-piperidyl) propionanilide, is structurally related to meperidine.[15] Fentanyl is 80 to 100 times more potent than morphine when given by the parenteral route; thus, 100 μg fentanyl is equivalent to 10 mg morphine. Because the onset of analgesia occurs sooner with fentanyl than with morphine when administered intravenously,[15] boluses of fentanyl, 0.25 to 0.5 μg/kg, are commonly administered in the post–anesthesia care unit (PACU) for analgesia immediately after patients' recovery from anesthesia. Time to peak effect of fentanyl (5 minutes) allows for repeated boluses every 5 minutes, facilitating titration to achieve adequate pain control. Fentanyl can be used in PCA devices or continuous infusion to provide postoperative analgesia.[15]

TRAMADOL

Tramadol is an atypical centrally acting opioid and a synthetic 4-phenyl-piperidine analogue of codeine. Tramadol possesses a low affinity for the μ, κ, and δ opioid receptors,[16] and intravenous tramadol in a dose of 50 to 150 mg is equivalent to intravenous morphine 5 to 15 mg for a 70-kg patient.[17] Tramadol is also a useful analgesic for mild to moderate pain.

Tramadol is well tolerated for short-term use, with dizziness, nausea, sedation, dry mouth, and sweating being its principal adverse effects. Respiratory depression is uncommon.[16] Tramadol may induce seizures, especially when used in the presence of proconvulsive drugs (such as monoamine oxidase inhibitors, tricyclic antidepressants, and selective serotonin uptake inhibitors) and in epileptic patients, and should be used with caution in patients with head injury.[17]

PARENTERAL OPIOIDS IN AMBULATORY SURGERY

The main reasons for failure to achieve discharge criteria after ambulatory surgery (outpatient surgery) continue to be pain and nausea.[18] Claxton et al,[19] examining the use of either intravenous morphine or fentanyl for pain control after ambulatory surgery in 58 patients, found that although morphine provided better quality and duration of pain relief, a greater number of patients given morphine suffered nausea and vomiting at home (59% versus 24%; $P = .01$). Another large multicenter study compared intravenous remifentanil with fentanyl in 2438 patients (1496 outpatients and 942 inpatients) 18 years or older and studied the hemodynamic effects of surgery as well as the recovery profile. The study found that patients given remifentanil had fewer hemodynamic changes and were discharged home earlier than patients who received fentanyl.[20]

Other short-acting opioids, such as alfentanil and sufentanil, have been compared with fentanyl to determine the incidence of postoperative nausea and vomiting in ambulatory patients who have undergone anesthesia. When equipotent doses of fentanyl, alfentanil, and sufentanil were studied in 274 patients, alfentanil was shown to have the lowest incidence of postoperative nausea and vomiting.[21] Therefore, shorter-acting opioid analgesics may be more appropriate for patients undergoing ambulatory surgery because of fewer adverse effects, especially when used in a multimodal analgesic regimen.

Oral Opioid Therapy

Box 15–2 summarizes this discussion.

IMMEDIATE-RELEASE PREPARATIONS

The opioid analgesics morphine, hydromorphone, oxycodone, dextropropoxyphene, dihydrocodeine, codeine, and tramadol are all commonly used in oral form and are available as immediate-release (IR) preparations (Table 15–1).

Both codeine and dextropropoxyphene (60–65 mg) were found to be poor analgesics, with NNTs of 16.7 and 7.7, respectively.[22,23] Dihydrocodeine has also shown similar poor efficacy when used individually. It compares poorly with a drug such as ibuprofen, which has an NNT of 2.4.[24] However, tramadol is an effective sole analgesic, a 100-mg dose having an NNT of 4.6 and NNHs of 11 for dizziness and 7 to 8 for nausea.[22] Oxycodone, 5 mg, demonstrated no difference from placebo; raising the dose to 15 mg provided effective analgesia for patients after abdominal and gynecological surgery[25] (NNT 2.4), although with significant drowsiness

| BOX 15–2 | ORAL OPIOIDS |

All oral opioids should be prescribed when possible within a multimodal analgesic regimen including acetaminophen, NSAIDS, and, where necessary, other adjuvants.
Transition from intravenous to oral opioid therapy can be performed with the use of a CR opioid, with intermittent on-demand doses of IR opioid every 2 hours as required.
Greater attention should be given to the conversion of opioids from one route of administration to another to prevent underdosing and overdosing.
Compound analgesics such as acetaminophen with oxycodone or codeine are useful for mild to moderate pain.

(NNH 3.3). The NNTs for oral opioids are compared in Table 15–2.

Codeine is a prodrug that must be metabolized to morphine in the liver by cytochrome P450 2D6 (CYP2D6) to have an analgesic effect.[26] Seven percent to 10% of the population does not express functional CYP2D6, and such patients will not obtain analgesic benefit from codeine. Because most of the adverse effects of codeine (sedation, dizziness, dysphoria, nausea, and pruritus) are mediated by both the prodrug (codeine) and the active metabolite (morphine), this group of patients will experience no analgesia but will instead suffer adverse effects.[26]

Commonly used doses of IR preparations in the opioid-naive 70-kg patient are morphine 5 to 10 mg, oxycodone 5 to 10 mg, and hydromorphone 1 to 2 mg.

CONTROLLED-RELEASE OPIOIDS

Several opioids (morphine, hydromorphone, oxycodone, codeine, and tramadol) are available as controlled-release (CR) oral preparations, which significantly extends plasma half-life, allowing patients to remain pain free for greater periods.[25,27] These drugs are commonly administered on a fixed-dose schedule every 8 to 12 hours. Fentanyl is also available as a transdermal patch, which is changed every 72 hours. CR preparations are useful for patients requiring or likely to require frequent dosages (>4 doses daily) of IR opioids.

In patients tolerating oral intake, CR preparations can be combined with intravenous or oral IR opioids. The starting dose of a CR opioid in such patients should be calculated according to the last 24-hour intake of intravenous or IR preparation. The intravenous consumption of opioid is converted to the oral equivalent (morphine, oxycodone, or hydromorphone). The patient can then be given 50% to 75% of the total daily opioid requirement in the CR preparation in two or three divided doses,[28] which can be titrated to achieve good pain control with either intravenous or oral IR opioids. If the patient is taking oral IR opioids, the total daily opioid dose can be calculated and, once again, 50% to 75% of the total dose is administered in the CR preparation in two or three divided doses per day, with the balance administered, as required, in the IR preparation. After the CR opioid is initiated, the dose can be titrated up or down according to analgesic effect, opioid-related adverse effects, and requirement for further IR opioid.

A number of studies examining the benefit of adding CR opioids to conventional pain regimens have demonstrated significant benefits, including improved pain control, reduced overall (CR + IR) opioid requirements, and fewer opioid-related adverse effects.[25,29–33] However, care is warranted in the unrestricted use of CR opioids in opioid-naive patients, in whom serious respiratory adverse effects have been reported after the use of transdermal fentanyl.[34,35] Perioperative analgesia in the opioid-tolerant patient lies outside the scope of this chapter.

COMPOUND OPIOID ANALGESICS

Tramadol, codeine, and oxycodone, which are available as compound analgesics combined with acetaminophen and/or

TABLE 15–1	Equianalgesic Doses for Commonly Used Opioid Analgesics in the Perioperative Period for 70-kg Individual					
Drug	Oral	Intravenous/ Intramuscular	Patient-Controlled Analgesia (bolus)	Epidural (bolus)	Intrathecal	Comments
Morphine	10–30 mg every 2–3 hr	10–15 mg every 3–4 hr	1–2 mg	1–4 mg	100–300 μg	Gold standard for moderate to severe pain Active metabolites accumulate in renal impairment
Codeine	30–60 mg every 4 hr	15–60 mg every 4 hr	No PCA; IM use only	Not available	Not available	Use in mild to moderate pain Common in fixed-dose oral preparations Not converted to morphine in 10% of the population
Hydromorphone	2–3 mg	2–3 mg every 4 h	0.2–0.4 mg	0.5–1 mg	100–200 μg	Higher oral bioavailability Fewer adverse effects when given in epidural or intrathecal space than with other opioids
Diacetylmorphine (diamorphine)	N/A	5–10 mg	0.5–1 mg	2–3 mg[98]	200–300 μg [99]	
Fentanyl	N/A	20–50-μg boluses every 5 min up to 150 μg for postoperative pain in post–anesthesia care unit	20–50 μg	50–100-μg bolus	12.5–25-μg bolus	Transdermal not recommended With epidural or intrathecal route, risk of early respiratory depression
Oxycodone	10–20 mg	N/A		Not available	Not available	Controlled-release preparation available
Tramadol	50–150 mg every 4–6 hr	50–100 mg every 4–6 hr	20 mg	Not recommended	Not recommended	Sustained-release preparation available
Meperidine (pethidine)	100–300 mg every 3 hr	100 mg*	10 mg	Not recommended	Not recommended	Poor oral bioavailability Toxic metabolite: normeperidine

*Limit total dose to 1000 mg in the first 24 hr and then 600 mg/day thereafter. Reduce doses in the elderly or in those with renal impairment.
IM, intramuscular; PCA, patient-controlled anesthesia.

acetylsalicylic acid, are commonly used for both inpatient and outpatient surgery as soon as the patient is tolerating oral fluids.

The compound analgesic agents are effective in mild to moderate pain, as can be seen by their corresponding NNTs: The NNT for aspirin 650 mg plus codeine 60 mg is 5.3[22]; that for acetaminophen plus codeine 60 mg is 2.2[36]; that for acetaminophen plus dextropropoxyphene is 4.4[37]; and that for acetaminophen plus tramadol is 2.7.[38] Oxycodone 5 mg combined with acetaminophen 325 mg was found to be as effective (NNT 2.5) as 15 mg oxycodone, with no increase in adverse effects over placebo. Raising the dose of either oxycodone (10 mg) or acetaminophen (500 or 1000 mg) produced no better analgesia but increased the incidence of adverse effects such as drowsiness, dizziness, nausea, and vomiting (NNH 2.1 for drowsiness to 8.4 for vomiting) (see Table 15–2).[39]

The use of compound analgesics may be limited by the maximum daily dose of aspirin or acetaminophen. Therefore, in acute mild to moderate pain, it is useful to

TABLE 15–2	Number Needed to Treat (NNT) for At Least 50% Pain Control for Commonly Used Oral Opioids and Compound Analgesics

Drug and Dosage	NNT (50% pain relief)
Codeine 60 mg	16.7
Dextropropoxyphene 65 mg	7.7
Tramadol 100 mg	4.6
Acetaminophen 1000 mg/650 mg + codeine 60 mg	2.2/4.2
Oxycodone 5 mg + acetaminophen 325 mg	2.5
Acetaminophen 1000 mg + dextropropoxyphene 65 mg	4.4
Aspirin 650 mg + codeine 60 mg	5.3
Acetaminophen 1000 mg/650 mg	3.8/4.6

administer acetaminophen individually on a fixed-dose basis (650–1000 mg every 6 hours) and to combine it with the required doses of an oral opioid to control pain.

Spinal Opioid Therapy

The first reports in humans of intrathecal and epidural administration of opioids appeared in 1979.[40,41] Since that time, almost every opioid has been administered by the spinal route. In general, spinally administered opioids produce effective analgesia with lower doses than required for the intravenous route, since injection takes place close to the sites of action (spinal cord). The use of spinally administered opioids has the potential to produce greater morbidity than seen with opioids given by more conventional routes.[42] Nevertheless, the significant benefits produced by this route of administration support the use of spinal opioids in the perioperative period.

EPIDURAL OPIOID ADMINISTRATION

Box 15–3 summarizes this discussion.

Benefits of Epidural Opioids

The advantage of epidural opioids is that they produce analgesia without motor or sympathetic blockade.[43] When compared with the conventional intramuscular route, the

BOX 15–3	EPIDURAL OPIOIDS

Lipophilic epidural opioids (fentanyl, sufentanil) act primarily by systemic redistribution.
Hydrophilic epidural opioids (morphine, diamorphine, hydromorphone) induce analgesia at spinal sites of action.
Epidural morphine provides effective and sustained analgesia and is effective when administered at levels below the surgical dermatome.

epidural route was shown to be associated with significantly earlier recovery of peak flow rates, fewer pulmonary complications (atelectasis and parenchymal infiltrates), and a shorter hospital stay in patients undergoing thoracic and upper abdominal surgery.[44] In high-risk patients undergoing major abdominal, thoracic, or vascular surgery and receiving epidural block and postoperative epidural local anesthetics and/or opioids, there was decreased postoperative morbidity and mortality, as well as improved outcome (shorter hospital stays and lower costs), than in patients receiving general anesthesia and postoperative parenteral opioids.[44] Patient-controlled epidural analgesia (PCEA) using opioids in patients with peripheral vascular disease who were undergoing aortic bypass surgery was associated with significantly fewer thrombotic, infectious, and cardiovascular complications.[44] In high-risk patients undergoing major surgery, epidural analgesia using local anesthetics and/or opioids is the method of choice and is also cost-effective.[44]

Which Opioid Produces the Greatest Spinal Analgesic Benefit?

When administered as sole analgesic agents by the epidural route, lipophilic opioids such as fentanyl, sufentanil, and alfentanil are redistributed into the blood stream and epidural fat[44,45] and have a predominantly systemic analgesic effect. An epidural bolus of fentanyl would appear to have a (limited) spinal effect and therefore may be more beneficial than the same dose given intravenously for short-term (<1 hour) rescue analgesia.[46] Hydrophilic drugs are less bound to epidural fat and less absorbed into the systemic circulation, and opioids such as morphine[47] and hydromorphone[48] produce superior or equivalent analgesia at lower doses when given in the epidural space than when given intravenously. Table 15–3 indicates the likelihood of specific opioids' producing spinal cord–mediated analgesia.

Data from the literature indicate that the best choice of opioid for epidural infusion is hydromorphone, which

TABLE 15–3	Likelihood of Individual Opioids to Produce Spinal-Mediated Analgesia in the Management of Postoperative Pain

| | Route of Administration | |
Opioid	Epidural Administration	Intrathecal Administration
Morphine	High	High
Hydromorphone	High	High
Diamorphine	High	High
Alfentanil	Negligible	Unknown
Fentanyl	Low	Moderate
Sufentanil	Negligible	Moderate
Meperidine*	Unknown	Unknown

*Difficult to ascertain spinal selectivity of this agent because of local anesthetic effect.

Modified from Bernards CM: Understanding the physiology and pharmacology of epidural and intrathecal opioids. Best Pract Res Clin Anaesthesiol 2002;16:489–505.

balances good pain control and fewer adverse effects than morphine.[49-51] However, epidural morphine has the advantage of prolonged duration of action,[52] and a single dose of 2 to 4 mg can produce analgesia for at least 12 hours. Morphine and hydromorphone provide a similar quality of analgesia,[49] but hydromorphone appears to have a faster onset and shorter duration of action.[53]

In one study comparing morphine with hydromorphone as an epidural infusion, morphine caused pruritus four times more often.[49] For nausea and vomiting, the incidence ranges between 17% and 34% with morphine,[54] coinciding with the rostral spread of morphine that usually occurs after 4 to 6 hours.[55]

Level of Administration—Does It Matter?

A number of investigators have questioned whether the level of administration (i.e., lumbar versus thoracic) would alter rostral spread of opioids and, consequently, their efficacy and toxicity. Several studies demonstrate no difference in analgesia between the two approaches using lipophilic opioid infusions (fentanyl, buprenorphine), a fact that could be related to systemic absorption and supraspinal analgesia. However, Grant et al,[56] randomly assigning 20 patients undergoing thoracotomy to receive either lumbar or thoracic epidural morphine, demonstrated no difference in pain scores or adverse effects but greater opioid consumption in the lumbar group. This study provides limited evidence that an epidural hydrophilic opioid such as morphine can provide analgesic benefit even if injected distant from the dermatomal level of surgery.

Epidural Opioids and Local Anesthetics

Studies evaluating postoperative pain have shown a significant improvement of analgesic efficacy when local anesthetics are combined with spinal hydrophilic opioids.[57,58] This approach has provided effective analgesia while decreasing the required dose of each drug, with a consequent reduction in adverse effects. Adding an epidural lipophilic opioid such as fentanyl or sufentanil to local anesthetic infusions for postoperative pain, however, provides no benefit over the local

anesthetics alone while raising the risk of opioid-related adverse effects.[59-61] Suggested dose regimens for bolus and infusion are listed in Table 15–4.

INTRATHECAL OPIOIDS

All intrathecal opioids have spinally mediated mechanisms of action, although larger doses of lipophilic opioids are required to produce effective analgesia owing to systemic absorption (Box 15–4). This feature is demonstrated by the potency of morphine and fentanyl when administered either by the intravenous or the intrathecal route. Although the potency ratio of intravenous fentanyl to morphine is approximately 100:1, the intrathecal ratio is more like 8:1 (i.e., 25 µg of fentanyl is required to produce the same analgesic effect as 200 µg of morphine). Duration of action is also considerably different, with the effects of morphine lasting for up to 24 hours but those of fentanyl lasting only 2 to 3 hours. The binding of hydrophilic opioids to supraspinal receptors due to rostral spread in the cerebrospinal fluid (CSF) induces analgesia, which occurs at the same time as the spinally mediated effect is decreasing.[45] Intrathecal opioids allow a reduction in the dose of local anesthetic, thereby decreasing motor block, a fact that is especially relevant in outpatient surgery.[62]

The use of intrathecal hydrophilic opioids such as morphine (0.1 to 0.4 mg) provides effective, prolonged analgesia. Rathmell et al[63] compared placebo with 0.1, 0.2, and 0.3 mg of intrathecal morphine in 120 patients after total hip and knee arthroplasty. Intrathecal morphine provided up to 24 hours of analgesia, with the 0.2-mg and 0.3-mg doses being most effective. Incidence of nausea was significantly higher in the 0.3-mg group, and all patients receiving morphine had significant pruritus that required treatment. Because total hip arthroplasty is associated with shorter duration or intensity of postoperative pain than total knee replacement, a smaller dose of intrathecal opioid may be adequate, especially in the elderly.[64]

Intrathecal diamorphine (0.2 mg) also induces prolonged analgesia and produces less pruritus and drowsiness than morphine.[65] The characteristics of hydromorphone are similar to those of diamorphine. Drakeford et al[66] compared the effects of adding hydromorphone 0.14 mg, morphine 0.5 mg,

TABLE 15–4	Suggested Epidural Opioid Regimens in a 70-kg Patient*			
Drug	Solution	Single-Bolus Dose	Basal Infusion	Patient-Controlled Epidural Analgesia Bolus
Hydromorphone	0.015–0.03 mg/mL	0.2–1 mg	0.15–0.3 mg/hr	0.15–0.3 mg every 10 to 20 min
Hydromorphone 0.015–0.03 mg/mL + bupivacaine 0.0625–0.125%	N/A	N/A	5–10 mL/hr	2–4 mL every 15 to 20 min
Fentanyl	5–10 µg/mL	25–50 µg	50–100 µg/hr	10–15 µg every 10 to15 min
Fentanyl 2–4 µg/mL + bupivacaine 0.0625–0.125%	Not available	Not available	5–10 mL/hr	2–4 mL every 15 to 20 min
Morphine	0.1 mg/mL	2–4 mg	0.5–0.8 mg/hr	0.2–0.3 mg every 10 to 15 min
Sufentanil	1 µg/mL	2.5–5 µg	5–10 µg/hr	2–4 µg every 5 to 10 min

*Doses administered through a thoracic or lumbar epidural catheter.
Modified from de Leon-Casasola OA, Lema MJ: Potoperative epidural opioid analgesia: What are the choices? Anesth Analg 1996;83:867–875.

BOX 15–4   INTRATHECAL OPIOIDS

Lipophilic intrathecal opioids (fentanyl, sufentanil) provide analgesia by both spinal and systemic mechanisms. Low-dose intrathecal opioids allow a reduction in the dose of local anesthetic with a consequent decrease in motor block.

Hydrophilic opioids (morphine, diamorphine, hydromorphone) act predominantly at spinal sites and induce slow onset of analgesia and adverse effects.

Intrathecal morphine (100–200 μg) provides effective analgesia after pelvic and lower limb surgery but induces more adverse effects than intrathecal diamorphine (200 μg).

BOX 15–5   FACTORS INCREASING THE RISK OF RESPIRATORY DEPRESSION AFTER SPINAL OPIOIDS

- Increasing age
- Concomitant use of parenteral opioids or sedatives
- High doses of opioid
- Repeated bolus doses
- Coexisting respiratory disease or American Society of Anesthesiologists (ASA) risk score >3
- Thoracic or prolonged surgery

Data from references 65 and 77.

or placebo to spinal tetracaine anesthesia for total hip and knee arthroplasty; they observed an improved duration and quality of analgesia for the two opioids compared with placebo, with no difference in effect or adverse events.

SPINAL OPIOIDS AND RESPIRATORY DEPRESSION

The administration of spinal opioids (epidural or intrathecal) is associated with a number of adverse effects (Table 15–5), the clinically most significant of which is respiratory depression.[67] Respiratory depression after spinal opioids is dose dependent; other predictive factors, however, are concomitant use of parenteral opioids or sedatives, and elderly patients appear to be especially vulnerable (Box 15–5). The incidence of respiratory depression requiring medical intervention after conventional doses of intrathecal or epidural opioids is the same as that after intramuscular or intravenous opioid therapy (0.1%–1%).[68,69]

Respiratory depression tends to fall into two patterns, early and delayed. Early respiratory depression usually occurs within 2 hours of administration of spinal opioids and therefore is diagnosed and managed in the operating room or recovery room. The effect is usually associated with the lipophilic opioids and is mainly related to systemic absorption, because blood concentration is proportional to level of respiratory depression.[70,71] Most reports of respiratory depression are associated with large doses of epidural fentanyl and sufentanil;

this complication is uncommon after intrathecal administration, especially of lower doses.[69]

Delayed respiratory depression characteristically occurs 6 to 12 hours after the administration of a hydrophilic opioid and occurs slowly but progressively (as opposed to the sudden and rapid early respiratory depression).[72] Onset of respiratory depression roughly corresponds with the rate of CSF flow from the thoracolumbar spinal level to the brainstem.[45] Most reports have been associated with the administration of epidural or intrathecal morphine[73-76]; however, it would be possible to induce delayed respiratory depression when infusing large doses of a lipophilic opioid. Clinically relevant respiratory depression has not been reported more than 24 hours after the last injection of intrathecal or epidural morphine, and large series suggest that it is extremely uncommon after 12 hours.[74]

Monitoring and detection of respiratory depression after epidural or intrathecal administration of opioids requires suitable levels of supervision by nursing staff and appropriate risk awareness. Controversy exists regarding the appropriate type and duration of monitoring. Respiratory monitors such as pulse oximetry and capnography have been tried but are unreliable because of an excessive rate of false alarms.[77] Extensive experience suggests that monitoring of respiratory rate and sedation on an hourly basis for the first 24 hours is sufficient to detect onset of respiratory depression.[77] Patients receiving continuous opioid infusions should continue to be monitored every 4 hours until cessation of treatment, and those with several risk factors may benefit from supplemental oxygen and observation in a high-dependency environment for the first 24 hours. Excessive sedation appears to be a good clinical indicator of respiratory depression, especially when associated with a reduction in respiratory rate below 10 breaths/minute.[77-79]

Opioid-induced respiratory depression is readily reversed with intravenous naloxone. Care is required to avoid complete antagonism of analgesia, and the naloxone dose should be titrated in 0.1-mg increments. Repeated dosing or infusion is usually necessary, because naloxone has a duration of action of 35 to 45 minutes,[80] significantly shorter than that of most spinal opioids. Infusion rates in the range of 2 to 5 μg/kg/hr have been found to provide reversal of respiratory effects without antagonizing analgesia.[81] Availability of an anesthesiologist is of vital importance when opioid-related respiratory depression occurs.

Box 15–6 summarizes this discussion.

TABLE 15–5   Common Adverse Effects of Intrathecal and Epidural Opioids[105-107]

Adverse Effect	Incidence (%)
Pruritus	11–44[48]
Nausea and vomiting	17–34[53]
Urinary retention	33–50[105]
Respiratory depression	0.1–1*
Mental status changes: sedation, drowsiness	—

*Equivalent to the risk of respiratory depression following administration of intramuscular or intravenous opioids.

SPINAL OPIOIDS AND RESPIRATORY DEPRESSION

Spinal opioids produce respiratory depression in 0.1% to 1% of patients, and the incidence is similar to that for opioids administered by other parenteral routes.

Lipophilic opioids may produce early and rapid onset (<2 hr) respiratory depression primarily through systemic absorption. The condition is usually associated with high doses of epidural lipophilic opioids.

Hydrophilic opioids may produce delayed or slow-onset (>2 hr) respiratory depression owing to rostral spread in the CSF. It usually occurs between 6 and 12 hours but can take place up to 24 hours after administration.

All patients who receive spinal opioids in the perioperative period should be monitored in a suitable environment with the support of a readily available anesthesiologist.

TABLE 15–6 Outcomes of 15 Studies Examining the Effect of Perineural Opioids (Excluding Tramadol and Buprenorphine)

Overall outcomes	8 supportive
	7 negative
Systemic control outcomes*	6 systemic control:
	4 supportive
	2 negative
	9 no systemic control:
	4 supportive
	5 negative

*Three group studies included an active group (local anesthetic + opioid and intravenous saline), a placebo control group (local anesthetic alone + intravenous saline), and a systemic opioid control group (local anesthetic alone + intravenous opioid).

Use of Opioids for Peripherally Mediated Analgesia

During inflammation, opioid receptors and endogenous opioids are expressed in peripheral sensory fibers and immune cells.[82,83] Numerous studies have evaluated the effects of opioids applied to peripheral nerves or to the intra-articular space. Although many studies claim an analgesic benefit of peripherally applied opioids, fewer studies use a control group with a systemically administered opioid for comparison. Without this control, it is impossible to infer whether the peripheral opioid is having a true peripheral effect or in fact is being carried by the circulation to the CNS to induce analgesia. True peripherally mediated opioid analgesia may be beneficial if it is associated with fewer adverse effects: if the analgesia is mediated centrally, then there is no clear benefit.

PERINEURONAL OPIOIDS

Opioid receptors identified on primary afferent fibers are transported from the dorsal root ganglion to the site of inflammation; however, while undergoing axonal transport, these receptors are not easily reached for interaction with agonists. This may explain the reason that two systematic reviews published in 1997 and 2000[84,85] found little evidence for the benefit of adding opioids to local anesthetics in peripheral nerve blocks. An updated summary of studies examining perineuronal administration of opioids (excluding buprenorphine and tramadol) shows that analgesic benefit remains equivocal (Table 15–6).[86–90] In addition, Choyce and Peng[91] reviewed the use of opioids in intravenous regional anesthesia and came to similar disappointing conclusions. Two opioids that have shown analgesic efficacy when administered perineuronally are buprenorphine and tramadol. Candido et al,[92] adding 0.3 mg buprenorphine to a combination of mepivacaine and tetracaine in axillary blocks, found an almost 100% increase in the duration of analgesia in comparison with the administration of an axillary block plus the same dose of intramuscular buprenorphine. This report supports findings of two earlier studies that examined buprenorphine without a systemic control group.[93,94]

Kapral et al[95] used tramadol 100 mg as an adjuvant to mepivacaine in axillary brachial plexus block. They randomly assigned 60 patients to three groups; the first group received mepivacaine 1% with 2 mL saline, the second group received mepivacaine 1% with 100 mg tramadol, and the third group received mepivacaine 1% with 2 mL saline and 100 mg tramadol intravenously. These researchers found a greater duration of motor and sensory block in the axillary tramadol group that significantly ($P < .01$) outlasted that in both the intravenous and placebo groups. Robaux et al[96] subsequently performed a dose-response study with placebo, and 40, 100, and 200 mg tramadol added to a fixed dose of mepivacaine 1.5% in axillary block; they found that the 200-mg dose provided the best analgesia with no increase in adverse effects. However, these investigators did not compare the effects with those of intravenous tramadol.

INTRA-ARTICULAR OPIOIDS AND OTHER PERIPHERAL ROUTES OF ADMINISTRATION

Opioid agonists administered into inflamed tissue bind to opioid receptors on sensory terminals and induce analgesia.[97] In humans, opioid analgesia is obtained after intra-articular (IA) administration in the presence of preexisting inflammation. In 1997, Kalso et al[98] systematically examined the role of IA opioids and established that there is evidence for a prolonged benefit from IA morphine, without significant adverse effects, at doses of 1 to 5 mg. However, a dose-response relationship could not be established. Later articles support this finding and show the benefit of IA morphine,[99,100] tramadol,[101] buprenorphine,[102] and sufentanil.[103]

A study by Reuben et al[104] investigated the use of morphine (5 mg) injected into the iliac crest bone graft donor site during cervical spine fusion surgery. Morphine significantly reduced both the rate of acute pain and the incidence of development of chronic pain (assessed 1 year after surgery) compared with intramuscular morphine and placebo (5% versus 37% and 33%, respectively).

Box 15–7 summarizes this discussion.

BOX 15–7	**PERIPHERAL OPIOIDS**

Morphine in doses up to 5 mg provides significant analgesia when injected intra-articularly but requires preexisting peripheral inflammation.

Morphine 5 mg injected into the donor site during bone graft harvest may reduce acute and chronic bone graft pain.

Tramadol 200 mg or buprenorphine 0.3 mg enhances local anesthetic effect during peripheral nerve blocks.

Summary

Opioid analgesics remain an integral part of the postoperative pain control regimen in all but the most minor surgery.

Morphine remains the best opioid for intravenous use, whereas agents such as oxycodone have pharmacokinetic advantages for the oral route.

Spinal opioids produce significant analgesia in the postoperative period as long as the ratio of benefit compared with risk is observed. Spinal diamorphine or hydromorphone appears to have greatest benefit with fewest adverse effects.

Use of opioids in peripheral sites can produce significant analgesia with lower risk of central adverse effects. Generally, the benefit of perineuronal application of opioids has not been observed, but tramadol and buprenorphine produce peripherally mediated analgesia when used in addition to local anesthetic for peripheral nerve block. Morphine has been demonstrated to produce analgesia in the intra-articular space.

The analgesic benefits of opioids can be enhanced, and their adverse effects minimized, through use as part of a multimodal analgesic regimen that includes the use of acetaminophen, NSAIDs, and, where necessary, other adjuvants, such as N-methyl-D-aspartate receptor antagonists, α_2 agonists, and anticonvulsant agents.

REFERENCES

1. Kehlet H, Dahl JB: The value of "multimodal" or "balanced analgesia" in postoperative pain treatment. Anesth Analg 1993;77:1048–1056.
2. Pain terms: A list with definitions and notes on usage. Recommended by the IASP Subcommmitee on Taxonomy. Pain 1979;6:249–252.
3. Kalso E, Edwards JE, Moore RA, et al: Opioids in chronic non-cancer pain: Systematic review of efficacy and safety. Pain 2004;112:372–380.
4. Watson CP, Watt-Watson JH, Chipman ML: Chronic noncancer pain and the long term utility of opioids. Pain Res Manag 2004;9:19–24.
5. Cook RJ, Sackett DL: The number needed to treat: A clinically useful measure of treatment effect. BMJ 1995;310:452–454.
6. McQuay HJ, Carroll D, Moore RA: Injected morphine in postoperative pain: A quantitative systematic review. J Pain Symptom Manage 1999;17:164–174.
7. Bollish SJ, Collins CL, Kirking DM, et al: Efficacy of patient-controlled versus conventional analgesia for postoperative pain. Clin Pharm 1985;4:48–52.
8. Latta KS, Ginsberg B, Barkin RL: Meperidine: A critical review. Am J Ther 2002;9:53–68.
9. Smith LA, Carroll D, Edwards JE, et al: Single-dose ketorolac and pethidine in acute postoperative pain: Systematic review with meta-analysis. Br J Anaesth 2000;84:48–58.
10. Lawlor P, Turner K, Hanson J, et al: Dose ratio between morphine and hydromorphone in patients with cancer pain: A retrospective study. Pain 1997;72:79–85.
11. Coda BA, O'Sullivan B, Donaldson G, et al: Comparative efficacy of patient-controlled administration of morphine, hydromorphone, or sufentanil for the treatment of oral mucositis pain following bone marrow transplantation. Pain 1997;72:333–346.
12. Wright AW, Mather LE, Smith MT: Hydromorphone-3-glucuronide: A more potent neuro-excitant than its structural analogue, morphine-3-glucuronide. Life Sci 2001;69:409–420.
13. Dean M: Opioids in renal failure and dialysis patients. J Pain Symptom Manage 2004;28:497–504.
14. Rapp SE, Egan KJ, Ross BK, et al: A multidimensional comparison of morphine and hydromorphone patient-controlled analgesia. Anesth Analg 1996;82:1043–1048.
15. Peng, PW, Sandler H, Alan NA: Review of the use of fentanyl analgesia in the management of acute pain in adults. Anesthesiology 1999;90:576–599.
16. Shipton EA: Tramadol—present and future. Anaesth Intensive Care 2000;28:363–374.
17. Lee CR, McTavish D, Sorkin EM: Tramadol: A preliminary review of its pharmacodynamic and pharmacokinetic properties, and therapeutical potential in acute and chronic pain states. Drugs 1993;46:313–340.
18. Chung F, Mezei G: Factors contributing to a prolonged stay after ambulatory surgery. Anesth Analg 1999;89:1352–1359.
19. Claxton AR, McGuire G, Chung F, et al: Evaluation of morphine versus fentanyl for postoperative analgesia after ambulatory surgical procedures. Anesth Analg 1997;84:509–514.
20. Twersky RS, Jamerson B, Warner DS, et al: Hemodynamics and emergence profile of remifentanil versus fentanyl prospectively compared in a large population of surgical patients J Clin Anesth 2001;13:407–416.
21. Langevin S, Lessard MR, Trepanier CA, et al: Alfentanil causes less postoperative nausea and vomiting than equipotent doses of fentanyl or sufentanil in outpatients. Anesthesiology 1999;6:1666–1673.
22. Moore RA, McQuay HJ: Single-patient data meta-analysis of 3453 postoperative patients: Oral tramadol versus placebo, codeine and combination analgesics. Pain 1997;69:287–294.
23. Collins SL, Edwards JE, Moore RA, et al: Single-dose dextropropoxyphene in post-operative pain: A quantitative systematic review. Eur J Clin Pharmacol 1998;54:107–112.
24. Collins SL, Moore RA, McQuay HJ, et al: Oral ibuprofen and diclofenac in post-operative pain: A quantitative systematic review. Eur J Pain 1998;2:285–291.
25. Sunshine A, Olson NZ, Colon A, et al: Analgesic efficacy of controlled-release oxycodone in postoperative pain. J Clin Pharmacol 1996;36:595–603.
26. Cleary J, Mikus G, Somogyi A, et al: The influence of pharmacogenetics on opioid analgesia: Studies with codeine and oxycodone in the Sprague-Dawley/Dark Agouti rat model. J Pharmacol Exp Ther 1994;271:1528–1534.
27. Hale ME, Fleischmann R, Salzman R, et al: Efficacy and safety of controlled-release versus immediate-release oxycodone: Randomized, double-blind evaluation in patients with chronic back pain. Clin J Pain 1999;15:179–183.
28. Ginsberg B, Sinatra RS, Adler LJ, et al: Conversion to oral controlled-release oxycodone from intravenous opioid analgesic in the postoperative setting. Pain Med 2003;4:31–38.
29. Bourke M, Hayes A, Doyle M, et al: A comparison of regularly administered sustained release oral morphine with intramuscular morphine for control of postoperative pain. Anesth Analg 2000;90:427–430.
30. Cheville A, Chen A, Oster G, et al: A randomized trial of controlled-release oxycodone during inpatient rehabilitation following unilateral total knee arthroplasty. J Bone Joint Surg Am 2001;83A:572–576.
31. Kampe S, Warm M, Kaufmann J, et al: Clinical efficacy of controlled-release oxycodone 20 mg administered on a 12-h dosing schedule on the management of postoperative pain after breast surgery for cancer. Curr Med Res Opin 2004;20:199–202.
32. Kaufmann J, Yesiloglu S, Patermann B, et al: Controlled-release oxycodone is better tolerated than intravenous tramadol/metamizol for postoperative analgesia after retinal surgery. Curr Eye Res 2004;28:271–275.
33. Reuben SS, Connelly NR, Maciolek H: Postoperative analgesia with controlled-release oxycodone for outpatient anterior cruciate ligament surgery. Anesth Analg 1999;88:1286–1291.
34. Sandler A: Transdermal fentanyl: Acute analgesic clinical studies. J Pain Symptom Manage 1992;7:S27–S35.

35. Sandler AN, Baxter AD, Katz J, et al: A double-blind, placebo-controlled trial of transdermal fentanyl after abdominal hysterectomy: Analgesic, respiratory, and pharmacokinetic effects. Anesthesiology 1994;81:1169–1180.

36. Smith LA, Moore RA, McQuay HJ, et al: Using evidence from different sources: An example using paracetamol 1000 mg plus codeine 60 mg. BMC Med Res Methodol 2001;1:1.

37. Collins SL, Edwards JE, Moore RA, et al: Single-dose dextropropoxyphene in post-operative pain: A quantitative systematic review. Eur J Clin Pharmacol 1998;54:107–112.

38. Edwards JE, McQuay HJ, Moore RA: Combination analgesic efficacy: Individual patient data meta-analysis of single-dose oral tramadol plus acetaminophen in acute postoperative pain. J Pain Symptom Manage 2002;23:121–130.

39. Edwards JE, Moore RA, McQuay HJ: Single dose oxycodone and oxycodone plus paracetamol (acetaminophen) for acute postoperative pain. Cochrane Database Syst Rev 2000;4:CD002763.

40. Behar M, Magora F, Olshwang D, et al: Epidural morphine in treatment of pain. Lancet 1979;1(8115):527–529.

41. Wang JK, Nauss LA, Thomas JE: Pain relief by intrathecally applied morphine in man. Anesthesiology 1979;50:149–151.

42. Morgan M: The rational use of intrathecal and extradural opioids. Br J Anaesth 1989;63:165–188.

43. de Leon-Casasola OA, Lema MJ: Postoperative epidural opioid analgesia: What are the choices? Anesth Analg 1996;83:867–875.

44. Rawal N: Opioids and non opioids' efficacy, safety and cost benefit. Pain Reviews 1996;3:31–62.

45. Bernards CM: Understanding the physiology and pharmacology of epidural and intrathecal opioids. Best Pract Res Clin Anaesthesiol 2002;16:489–505.

46. Ginosar Y, Riley ET, Angst MS: The site of action of epidural fentanyl in humans: The difference between infusion and bolus administration. Anesth Analg 2003;97:1428–1438.

47. Kilbride MJ, Senagore AJ, Mazier WP, et al: Epidural analgesia. Surg Gynecol Obstet 1992;174:137–140.

48. Liu S, Carpenter RL, Mulroy MF, et al: Intravenous versus epidural administration of hydromorphone: Effects on analgesia and recovery after radical retropubic prostatectomy. Anesthesiology 1995;82:682–688.

49. Chaplan SR, Duncan SR, Brodsky JB, et al: Morphine and hydromorphone epidural analgesia: A prospective, randomized comparison. Anesthesiology 1992;77:1090–1094.

50. Goodarzi M: Comparison of epidural morphine, hydromorphone and fentanyl for postoperative pain control in children undergoing orthopaedic surgery. Paediatr Anaesth 1999;9:419–422.

51. Halpern SH, Arellano R, Preston R, et al: Epidural morphine vs hydromorphone in post-caesarean section patients. Can J Anaesth 1996;43:595–598.

52. Celleno D, Capogna G, Sebastiani M, et al: Epidural analgesia during and after cesarean delivery: Comparison of five opioids. Reg Anesth 1991;16:79–83.

53. Brose WG, Tanelian DL, Brodsky JB, et al: CSF and blood pharmacokinetics of hydromorphone and morphine following lumbar epidural administration. Pain 1991;45:11–15.

54. Rauck RL: Epidural and spinal narcotics. American Society of Anesthesiologists' Annual Refresher Course Lectures 1991;274:1–7.

55. Tawfik MO: Mode of action of intraspinal opioids. Pain Rev 1994;1:275–294.

56. Grant GJ, Zakowski M, Ramanathan S, et al: Thoracic versus lumbar administration of epidural morphine for postoperative analgesia after thoracotomy. Reg Anesth 1993;18:351–355.

57. Crews JC, Hord AH, Denson DD, et al: Comparison of the analgesic efficacy of 0.25% levobupivacaine combined with 0.005% morphine, 0.25% levobupivacaine alone, or 0.005% morphine alone for the management of postoperative pain in patients undergoing major abdominal surgery. Anesth Analg 1999;89:1504–1509.

58. Dahl JB, Rosenberg J, Hansen BL, et al: Differential analgesic effects of low-dose epidural morphine and morphine-bupivacaine at rest and during mobilization after major abdominal surgery. Anesth Analg 1992;74:362–365.

59. Berti M, Casati A, Fanelli G, et al: 0.2% ropivacaine with or without fentanyl for patient-controlled epidural analgesia after major abdominal surgery: A double-blind study. J Clin Anesth 2000;12:292–297.

60. Finucane BT, Ganapathy S, Carli F, et al: Prolonged epidural infusions of ropivacaine (2 mg/mL) after colonic surgery: The impact of adding fentanyl. Anesth Analg 2001;92:1276–1285.

61. Scott DA, Blake D, Buckland M, et al: A comparison of epidural ropivacaine infusion alone and in combination with 1, 2, and 4 microg/mL fentanyl for seventy-two hours of postoperative analgesia after major abdominal surgery. Anesth Analg 1999;88:857–864.

62. Ben David B, Solomon E, Levin H, et al: Intrathecal fentanyl with small-dose dilute bupivacaine: Better anesthesia without prolonging recovery. Anesth Analg 1997;85:560–565.

63. Rathmell JP, Pino CA, Taylor R, et al: Intrathecal morphine for postoperative analgesia: A randomized, controlled, dose-ranging study after hip and knee arthroplasty. Anesth Analg 2003;97:1452–1457.

64. Murphy PM, Stack D, Kinirons B, et al: Optimizing the dose of intrathecal morphine in older patients undergoing hip arthroplasty. Anesth Analg 2003;97:1709–1715.

65. Husaini SW, Russell IF: Intrathecal diamorphine compared with morphine for postoperative analgesia after caesarean section under spinal anaesthesia. Br J Anaesth 1998;81:135–139.

66. Drakeford MK, Pettine KA, Brookshire L, et al: Spinal narcotics for postoperative analgesia in total joint arthroplasty: A prospective study. J Bone Joint Surg Am 1991;73:424–428.

67. Chaney MA: Side effects of intrathecal and epidural opioids. Can J Anaesth 1995;42:891–903.

68. Leon-Casasola OA, Parker B, Lema MJ, et al: Postoperative epidural bupivacaine-morphine therapy: Experience with 4,227 surgical cancer patients. Anesthesiology 1994;81:368–375.

69. Rygnestad T, Borchgrevink PC, Eide E: Postoperative epidural infusion of morphine and bupivacaine is safe on surgical wards: Organisation of the treatment, effects and side-effects in 2000 consecutive patients. Acta Anaesthesiol Scand 1997;41:868–876.

70. Koren G, Sandler AN, Klein J, et al: Relationship between the pharmacokinetics and the analgesic and respiratory pharmacodynamics of epidural sufentanil. Clin Pharmacol Ther 1989;46:458–462.

71. Whiting WC, Sandler AN, Lau LC, et al: Analgesic and respiratory effects of epidural sufentanil in patients following thoracotomy. Anesthesiology 1988;69:36–43.

72. Stenseth R, Sellevold O, Breivik H: Epidural morphine for postoperative pain: Experience with 1085 patients. Acta Anaesthesiol Scand 1985;29:148–156.

73. Gustafsson LL, Schildt B, Jacobsen K: Adverse effects of extradural and intrathecal opiates: Report of a nationwide survey in Sweden. Br J Anaesth 1982;54:479–486.

74. Rawal N, Arner S, Gustafsson LL, et al: Present state of extradural and intrathecal opioid analgesia in Sweden: A nationwide follow-up survey. Br J Anaesth 1987;59:791–799.

75. Krenn H, Jellinek H, Haumer H, et al: Naloxone-resistant respiratory depression and neurological eye symptoms after intrathecal morphine. Anesth Analg 2000;91:432–433.

76. Neustein SM, Cottone TM: Prolonged respiratory depression after intrathecal morphine. J Cardiothorac Vasc Anesth 2003;17:230–231.

77. Mulroy MF: Monitoring opioids. Reg Anesth 1996;21(Suppl):89–93.

78. Etches RC, Sandler AN, Daley MD: Respiratory depression and spinal opioids. Can J Anaesth 1989;36:165–185.

79. Ready LB, Loper KA, Nessly M, et al: Postoperative epidural morphine is safe on surgical wards. Anesthesiology 1991;75:452–456.

80. Stoelting RK: Opioid antagonists. In Pharmacology and Physiology in Anesthetic Practice, 3rd ed. Philadelphia, Lippincott Williams & Wilkins, 1999, pp 106–107.

81. Rawal N, Schott U, Dahlstrom B, et al: Influence of naloxone infusion on analgesia and respiratory depression following epidural morphine. Anesthesiology 1986;64:194–201.

82. Brack A, Rittner HL, Machelska H, et al: Control of inflammatory pain by chemokine-mediated recruitment of opioid-containing polymorphonuclear cells. Pain 2004;112:229–238.

83. Likar R, Mousa SA, Philippitsch G, et al: Increased numbers of opioid expressing inflammatory cells do not affect intra-articular morphine analgesia. Br J Anaesth 2004;93:375–380.

84. Murphy DB, McCartney CJ, Chan VW: Novel analgesic adjuncts for brachial plexus block: A systematic review. Anesth Analg 2000;90:1122–1128.

85. Picard PR, Tramer MR, McQuay HJ, et al: Analgesic efficacy of peripheral opioids (all except intra-articular): A qualitative systematic review of randomised controlled trials. Pain 1997;72:309–318.

86. Reuben SS, Connelly NR, Maciolek H: Postoperative analgesia with controlled-release oxycodone for outpatient anterior cruciate ligament surgery. Anesth Analg 1999;88:1286–1291.

87. Fanelli G, Casati A, Magistris L, et al: Fentanyl does not improve the nerve block characteristics of axillary brachial plexus anaesthesia performed with ropivacaine. Acta Anaesthesiol Scand 2001;45:590–594.

88. Karakaya D, Buyukgoz F, Baris S, et al: Addition of fentanyl to bupivacaine prolongs anesthesia and analgesia in axillary brachial plexus block. Reg Anesth Pain Med 2001;26:434–438.

89. Likar R, Koppert W, Blatnig H, et al: Efficacy of peripheral morphine analgesia in inflamed, non-inflamed and perineural tissue of dental surgery patients. J Pain Symptom Manage 2001;21:330–337.

90. Nishikawa K, Kanaya N, Nakayama M, et al: Fentanyl improves analgesia but prolongs the onset of axillary brachial plexus block by peripheral mechanism. Anesth Analg 2000;91:384–387.

91. Choyce A, Peng P: A systematic review of adjuncts for intravenous regional anesthesia for surgical procedures. Can J Anaesth 2002;49:32–45.

92. Candido KD, Winnie AP, Ghaleb AH, et al: Buprenorphine added to the local anesthetic for axillary brachial plexus block prolongs postoperative analgesia. Reg Anesth Pain Med 2002;27:162–167.

93. Candido KD, Franco CD, Khan MA, et al: Buprenorphine added to the local anesthetic for brachial plexus block to provide postoperative analgesia in outpatients. Reg Anesth Pain Med 2001;26:352–356.

94. Viel EJ, Eledjam JJ, De La Coussaye JE, et al: Brachial plexus block with opioids for postoperative pain relief: Comparison between buprenorphine and morphine. Reg Anesth 1989;14:274–278.

95. Kapral S, Gollmann G, Waltl B, et al: Tramadol added to mepivacaine prolongs the duration of an axillary brachial plexus blockade. Anesth Analg 1999;88:853–856.

96. Robaux S, Blunt C, Viel E, et al: Tramadol added to 1.5% mepivacaine for axillary brachial plexus block improves postoperative analgesia dose-dependently. Anesth Analg 2004;98:1172–1177.

97. Mousa SA, Zhang Q, Sitte N, et al: β-endorphin-containing memory-cells and mu-opioid receptors undergo transport to peripheral inflamed tissue. J Neuroimmunol 2001;115:71–78.

98. Kalso E, Tramer MR, Carroll D, et al: Pain relief from intra-articular morphine after knee surgery: A qualitative systematic review. Pain 1997;71:127–134.

99. Brandsson S, Karlsson J, Morberg P, et al: Intraarticular morphine after arthroscopic ACL reconstruction: A double-blind placebo-controlled study of 40 patients. Acta Orthop Scand 2000;71:280–285.

100. Rasmussen S, Larsen AS, Thomsen ST, et al: Intra-articular glucocorticoid, bupivacaine and morphine reduces pain, inflammatory response and convalescence after arthroscopic meniscectomy. Pain 1998;78:131–134.

101. Alagol A, Calpur OU, Kaya G, et al: The use of intraarticular tramadol for postoperative analgesia after arthroscopic knee surgery: A comparison of different intraarticular and intravenous doses. Knee Surg Sports Traumatol Arthrosc 2004;12:184–188.

102. Varrassi G, Marinangeli F, Ciccozzi A, et al: Intra-articular buprenorphine after knee arthroscopy: A randomised, prospective, double-blind study. Acta Anaesthesiol Scand 1999;43:51–55.

103. Vranken JH, Vissers KC, de Jongh R, et al: Intraarticular sufentanil administration facilitates recovery after day-case knee arthroscopy. Anesth Analg 2001;92:625–628.

104. Reuben SS, Vieira P, Faruqi S, et al: Local administration of morphine for analgesia after iliac bone graft harvest. Anesthesiology 2001;95:390–394.

105. Petersen TK, Husted SE, Rybro L, et al: Urinary retention during i.m. and extradural morphine analgesia. Br J Anaesth 1982;54:1175–1178.

106. Leon-Casasola OA, Parker B, Lema MJ, et al: Postoperative epidural bupivacaine-morphine therapy. Experience with 4,227 surgical cancer patients. Anesthesiology 1994;81:368–375.

107. Rygnestad T, Borchgrevink PC, Eide E: Postoperative epidural infusion of morphine and bupivacaine is safe on surgical wards: Organisation of the treatment, effects and side-effects in 2000 consecutive patients. Acta Anaesthesiol Scand 1997;41:868–876.

16 Patient-Controlled Analgesia

JEREMY N. CASHMAN

Patient-controlled analgesia (PCA) was first developed as a research tool to more accurately quantify patients' analgesic requirements.[1] At about the same time, concerns about the ineffective relief of postoperative pain had prompted an exploration of more effective routes and methods of administration of opioid analgesic drugs, including PCA.[2] One of the earliest PCA devices was a mechanical spring-loaded clamp on the tubing of an intravenous infusion–giving set that the patient squeezed to allow free flow from a bag containing meperidine (pethidine).[3] As the patient became sedated, his or her grip on the clamp relaxed and the flow stopped. However, it took the development of apparatus that incorporated an infusion pump with a timing device and patient interface in the form of a demand button before PCA became an accepted technique. The Cardiff Palliator was the first commercially available PCA device when it was introduced into clinical practice in the United Kingdom in 1976.[4] Since then, PCA machines have become more and more refined, with sophisticated computer-controlled pumps, enhanced levels of security, and data output capacity. However, "low-tech" disposable elastomeric devices have also been developed.[5]

PCA is now widely accepted for postoperative pain relief, commonly administered under the supervision of an acute pain service. In 1995, two thirds of European hospitals were using PCA for postoperative pain relief,[6] and the figure is likely to be much higher now. In a prospective multisite study conducted in 23 hospitals in the United States and published in 1999, Miaskowski et al[7] reported that of 2824 patients cared for by an acute pain service, three quarters received PCA. These investigators observed that anesthesia-based acute pain services were associated with an improved quality of postoperative pain management, a lower incidence of side effects, higher patient satisfaction scores, and earlier discharge from the hospital (level III evidence); see Box 16–1).[7]

Basic Principles

PCA involves the on-demand, intermittent self-administration of a predetermined dose of analgesic drug (usually an opioid) by a patient. Nurse-controlled, parent-controlled, and spouse-controlled methods of analgesia have all been described. The most common route of administration is intravenous, but subcutaneous, epidural, and intranasal routes can also be used. PCA takes advantage of the phenomenon that with opioids, analgesia occurs at lower doses than does sedation. PCA is based on the concept of a simple feedback loop in which the perception of pain by the patient triggers a demand

for a dose of analgesic. Inadequate relief of pain triggers further demands, but if pain relief is satisfactory, no further demands are made until such time as pain returns. However, subsequent demands for analgesia may be influenced by the patient's experience of drug-induced side effects, such as nausea, vomiting, hallucinations, and itching which, if extreme may result in the patient's not making any further demands.

PHARMACOKINETICS AND PHARMACODYNAMICS

There is considerable variability in opioid pharmacokinetics and pharmacodynamics. Together with a narrow therapeutic index, the variability requires titration of dose to effect in patients. Thus, in one study, the minimum effective analgesic concentration (MEAC) of meperidine (pethidine) varied threefold in postoperative patients (level III evidence).[8] The theoretical basis of PCA is that the patient will titrate the delivery of opioid to achieve plasma concentrations of drug consistent with good analgesia and minimal side effects.[1] All of the commonly used opioids have kinetic and dynamic properties that make them suitable for use in PCA.[9] Table 16–1 summarizes the pharmacokinetic variables for the opioids used in PCA.

There are no major differences in efficacy of the different opioids used for PCA (level II evidence).[10] Morphine is most commonly used in PCA, but fentanyl may be preferred in patients with renal impairment because of its lack of active metabolites. In contrast, meperidine is probably best avoided owing to the potential for normeperidine toxicity.

ROUTES OF ADMINISTRATION

Traditionally, PCA is administered by the intravenous route, but the subcutaneous, epidural, and intranasal routes can also be used. Employing the subcutaneous rather than

BOX 16–1	LEVELS OF EVIDENCE

Level I—Evidence from systematic reviews ± meta-analysis.
Level II—Evidence from one or more randomized controlled trials.
Level III—Evidence from nonrandomized controlled trials, cohort (audit) studies, or case-controlled studies.
Level IV—Expert opinion, descriptive studies, or reports of expert committees.

TABLE 16–1	Pharmacokinetic Variables for Opioid Analgesics Used in Patient-Controlled Analgesia		
	Volume of Distribution (L/kg)	Clearance (mL/min/kg)	Elimination Half-life (hr)
Alfentanil	0.8	6.0	1.6
Fentanyl	4.0	13.0	3.5
Hydromorphone	4.1	22.0	3.1
Meperidine	4.0	12.0	4.0
Morphine	3.5	15.0	3.0
Oxycodone	2.6	9.7	3.7
Tramadol	2.9	6.0	7.0

intravenous route for PCA necessitates the use of a more concentrated solution of opioid (see later). Apart from a higher opioid use for subcutaneous administration, the two routes provide comparable analgesia with no difference in the incidence of nausea and vomiting (level II evidence).[11,12] Patient-controlled epidural analgesia (PCEA) is becoming increasingly popular,[13] although some have argued that the higher cost and greater complexity of the technique are not justified.[14] A low-rate background infusion (up to 30% of the maximum hourly bolus dose) linked to an extended lockout period (up to 30 minutes) is usually employed. Lipid-soluble opioids such as fentanyl, diamorphine, and butorphanol have been successfully administered by metered-dose intranasal spray (level III evidence).[15] The system is simple but has limited options for varying the dose of analgesic or for monitoring.

Dosing Parameters

BOLUS DOSE

The *bolus dose* is the amount of medication administered by the PCA pump when the patient presses the button. The size of the bolus influences the success of PCA: Too small, and analgesia will be inadequate; too big, and side effects will be excessive. The optimal bolus dose is the dose that provides satisfactory analgesia without excessive side effects; for morphine, the optimal dose is 1 mg, but patients can partially compensate by increasing their demand rate if this dose proves to be too small (level II evidence).[16] The size of the bolus

dose may need to be adjusted according to the patient's subsequent pain scores. It has been suggested that the rapid change in blood morphine concentration associated with PCA bolus delivery may contribute to side effects such as nausea and vomiting. However, prolonging the duration of bolus delivery to a brief infusion does not decrease the side effects (level II evidence).[17]

LOCKOUT INTERVAL

The *lockout interval* is the time after delivery of a bolus dose during which no further drug will be delivered by the PCA device. The lockout interval should be sufficiently long to allow the patient to gauge whether the pain has been adequately relieved. The length of the lockout interval is influenced by the drug used, the size of the bolus dose, and the route of administration. Conventionally, lockout intervals between 5 and 10 minutes have been used, but the few studies that have investigated the influence of lockout interval have not shown any difference (level II evidence).[18,19] Recommended bolus doses and lockout intervals for various opioid analgesics are shown in Tables 16–2 and 16–3.

LOADING DOSE

The *loading dose* is the initial dose of analgesic needed to establish analgesia. The loading dose varies enormously among patients but does seem to correlate with subsequent analgesic consumption. Therefore, the size of the loading dose and pain scores during the first 30 minutes may be valuable for predicting individual pain management (level II evidence).[20]

BACKGROUND INFUSION

A *background infusion* is an infusion of analgesic at a constant rate that can be supplemented by bolus dosing. Intuitively, it might be expected that a background infusion would improve the quality of pain relief in adults. However, background infusions actually increase the amount of opioid delivered and raise the risk of side effects without significantly improving analgesia or sleep profile (level II evidence).[21–24] Background infusions also raise the risk of respiratory depression and are therefore not recommended for routine use in adults. However, background infusions may be reasonable in some patients. For instance, in the patient who is already receiving opioids and who is likely to have some opioid tolerance, a background infusion can be used to replace the patient's maintenance

TABLE 16–2	Guidelines for Bolus Dose, Lockout Interval, and Background Infusion Rate for Opioid Analgesics Used in Intravenous Patient-Controlled Analgesia			
	Drug Concentration (mg/mL)	Bolus Dose (mg)	Lockout Interval (min)	Background Infusion Rate (mg/hr)*
Fentanyl	0.01	0.01–0.02	5–10	0.02–0.1
Hydromorphone	0.2	0.1–0.5	5–10	0.2–0.5
Meperidine	10	5–15	5–12	5–40
Morphine	1	0.5–3.0	5–12	1–10
Oxymorphone	0.25	0.2–0.4	8–10	0.1–1.0

*The routine use of background infusions with PCA is NOT recommended (see text).

TABLE 16–3	Guidelines for Bolus Dose and Lockout Interval for Opioid Analgesics Used in Subcutaneous Patient-Controlled Analgesia		
	Drug Concentration (mg/mL)	Bolus Dose (mg)	Lockout Interval (min)
Hydromorphone	1.0	0.2	15
Morphine	5.0	1.0	10
Oxymorphone	1.5	0.3	10

dose of opioid (level IV evidence).[25] If a patient receiving a background infusion does not demand a bolus dose, the background infusion rate is too high.[21]

In contrast, background infusions are beneficial in children (level II evidence),[26] although there is some doubt as to the ideal rate of infusion. Thus, PCA in combination with a very-low-dose background infusion rate of morphine (4 µg/kg/hr) is associated with a better sleep pattern, less hypoxia, and less nausea and vomiting than PCA with either no background infusion or with a background infusion rate of 10 µg/kg/min (level II evidence).[27] Other studies have found the addition of slightly higher background infusion rates of morphine, up to16 µg/kg/hr, to result in better analgesia without any increase in side effects (level II evidence).[26–28] An even higher background infusion rate of morphine, 20 µg/kg/hr, was not found to improve analgesia but was associated with a greater incidence of hypoxemia, excessive sedation, nausea, and vomiting than associated with a PCA-only regimen (level II evidence).[29]

DOSE LIMIT

The *dose limit* is the maximum number of doses the patient can receive over a given period, irrespective of the number of demands made. There is no real evidence that limiting the dose improves the safety of PCA.

INJECTION/ATTEMPTS

Injection/attempts—more commonly recorded as attempts/ injections or demand:delivery—is the number of successful doses of analgesic the patient has received compared with the total number of times the patient has demanded a dose. It can be used to "profile" the adequacy of analgesia[30]; a demand:delivery ratio of greater than 3:1 suggests either an inadequate pump program (usually the lockout interval is too long) or poor patient understanding.

Management

PATIENT SELECTION AND EDUCATION

PCA can be used for the treatment of acute postoperative pain in adults and in children as young as 5 years, in trauma, in obstetrics, in acute medical diseases such as sickle cell crisis, and in malignant pain. Box 16–2 outlines some of the

indications for and contraindications to using PCA. Some patients worry about overdose, addiction, lack of personal contact with nurses, and machine dysfunction. Preoperative counseling in the use of PCA is helpful in reducing not only these fears but also PCA opioid consumption and, hence, the severity of side effects (level II evidence).[31–33]

STAFF EDUCATION AND CONDUCT OF PCA

Effective use of PCA requires adequate maintenance of equipment, appropriate protocols, and standardized monitoring records. For PCA to be used safely, all staff involved in the assessment and treatment process should be well educated in its uses and dangers. Indeed, the benefits of PCA can be negated by a lack of knowledge in both patients and ward staff (level IV evidence).[34]

Monitoring of the effectiveness, safety, and side effects is obviously important. Frequent evaluation of the patient should include pain scores (at rest and on movement), sedation scores, respiratory rate, opioid consumption (attempts/injections), any side effects and their severity, and any PCA pump program changes. PCA should be continued until regular oral analgesia has been established for the patient. In addition, it may be helpful to set a threshold below which opioid consumption must fall before discontinuation of PCA is considered.

Efficacy

ANALGESIA

PCA with opioids provides significantly better analgesia than opioids administered by conventional techniques of administration (level I evidence).[35–37] However, overall opioid consumption is not significantly different (level I evidence).[35,36] Although it is associated with lower pain scores and better pain relief scores than intramuscular analgesia, PCA is not as effective as epidural analgesia (level I evidence).[37]

PATIENT SATISFACTION

Patients appear to expect some pain after surgery, and patient satisfaction with PCA remains higher than with conventional techniques of administration (level I evidence),[35,36] even when PCA does not provide perfect analgesia (level II evidence).[38–40] Furthermore, patients who have experienced traditional intramuscular analgesia and PCA express an overwhelming preference for PCA (level IV evidence).[41] Satisfaction is significantly correlated with a sense of control over pain relief rather than the intensity of the pain itself.[32,42] Patients are apparently satisfied by the fact that their care providers are attempting to provide pain relief even if the results are not always successful, as judged from postoperative pain scores. An alternative possibility is that patients may report higher satisfaction for fear of offending those providing their postoperative care.

Safety

RESPIRATORY DEPRESSION

A number of criteria have been used to define *respiratory depression,* including respiratory rate, percutaneous oxygen saturation, arterial blood gas analysis, and the need to administer respiratory stimulants. Of these, respiratory rate is the most commonly used. A Europe-wide survey of acute pain services found that respiratory rate was routinely measured in 81% of hospitals, whereas oxygen saturation was measured in only 41% (level IV evidence).[43] A respiratory rate of less than 10 breaths/minute and an oxygen saturation value of less than 90% are most commonly used to define respiratory depression. PCA provides for better ventilation than conventional routes of opioid administration (level I evidence).[35] The incidence of respiratory depression with PCA, as indicated by a low respiratory rate, is 1.2%; the incidence of arterial desaturation, although higher, is still less than with intramuscular opioid analgesia (level I evidence).[44]

HEMODYNAMIC DEPRESSION

Morphine administration via both PCA and intramuscular analgesia, as well as via epidural analgesia, can result in a reduction in blood pressure (hypotension). However, hypotension may be the result of factors other than the analgesic technique. *Hypotension* has been defined in a number of ways: a decrease in systolic blood pressure greater than 20% to 30% of a stable preoperative value, absolute values of systolic blood pressure less than 80 to 100 mm Hg, and systolic/diastolic blood pressures less than 90/60 mm Hg. The incidence of hypotension with PCA, at less than 1%, is lower than with both intramuscular and epidural analgesia techniques (level I evidence).[44]

Tolerability

NAUSEA AND VOMITING

A large number of surveys have considered the incidence of nausea and vomiting associated with PCA. The overall incidence would seem to be in the region of 20% (level I evidence).[45,46] A number of strategies have been employed to reduce the incidence of postoperative nausea and vomiting (PONV), including adding an antiemetic to the PCA infusate. Promethazine, cyclizine, droperidol, ondansetron, and granisetron have all been tried. However, the only antiemetic that is effective with PCA is droperidol (level I evidence).[47] The optimal dose is 0.05 mg droperidol per 1 mg morphine (level I evidence).[48] However, the practice of adding an antiemetic to the PCA infusate is not popular; only 30 of every 100 patients so treated would obtain benefit (level I evidence),[47] and conversely, 70 of every 100 patients would be exposed to the potential adverse effects of droperidol.

SEDATION

Sedation occurs frequently in the postoperative period, not just in association with PCA. However, excessive sedation associated with PCA may indicate impending respiratory depression.[41] In a Europe-wide survey, sedation was routinely assessed by 82% of acute pain services (level IV evidence).[43] In another large review, the incidence of excessive sedation associated with PCA was 5%, but the reviewers made no attempt to correlate sedation with respiratory depression (level I evidence).[46] Other psychological effects associated with PCA are nightmares, hallucinations, and panic attacks.

PRURITUS

Pruritus is a relatively common side effect, affecting 14% of patients receiving PCA (level I evidence).[46] It varies in severity, can be difficult to manage, and may be resistant to conventional treatment such as antihistamines. Opioid antagonists such as naloxone and naltrexone, as well as nalbuphine and droperidol, are effective in preventing pruritus (level I evidence).[49]

URINARY RETENTION

There is conflicting evidence relating to the influence of PCA on urinary retention. One large review observed that the incidence of urinary retention was six times greater with PCA than with intramuscular analgesia (level III evidence).[45] Another review, however, found the incidences of urinary retention to be very similar for PCA and intramuscular analgesia (level I evidence).[46]

BOWEL FUNCTION

Information on the influence of PCA on bowel function is also conflicting. An equal number of studies report that the risk of prolonged postoperative ileus is increased by PCA as show no difference. Nevertheless, the use of PCA by patients to alleviate gas pain is likely to prolong recovery of bowel motility after abdominal surgery.

Hazards

Current PCA pumps are highly sophisticated and reliable, and medication mishaps are rare. In one study, mishaps occurred in 1.2% of PCA usage, of which 52% were due to operator errors, 36% were equipment-related, and 12% were adverse drug effects.[50] Operator errors include programming errors, problems with PCA machine setup, and inappropriate patient selection or patient-related errors. Mechanical problems with PCA technology, when they occur, can be classified as due to overdelivery, underdelivery, or siphoning. Box 16–3 summarizes the hazards associated with PCA.

In early PCA machines, static electricity discharge could result in corruption of the software used to control the syringe driver mechanism. This is no longer a problem. In addition, the routine use of antireflux valves prevents retrograde flow of opioid in the intravenous line, while siphoning is prevented by correct loading of the syringe into the PCA machine and checking for cracks in the syringe/reservoir chamber.

Finally, one study observed that use of PCA was significantly associated with an increase in in-hospital postoperative wound infection after abdominal surgery. The mechanism was unclear, and there were a number of confounding variables (level IV evidence).[51]

REPLACEMENT OF PUMPS

To prevent mechanical problems, PCA pumps should be maintained regularly. An estimate of the likely length of life of the pump (commonly 8 years) should be made, and the pump carefully inspected when the estimated time has elapsed.[52] The U.K. Department of Health's Medicines and Healthcare Products Regulatory Agency (MHRA) has issued guidelines that set out the criteria for when to replace an infusion pump (which should also apply to replacement of PCA pumps); these criteria are given in Box 16–4.

DEATHS ASSOCIATED WITH PATIENT-CONTROLLED ANALGESIA

Fortunately, deaths associated with PCA are extremely rare. PCA-associated death is predominantly the result of drug

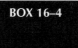

BOX 16–3	HAZARDS ASSOCIATED WITH PATIENT-CONTROLLED ANALGESIA

Wrong drug
Misprogramming of pump
False trigger
Drug accumulation
Pump malfunction
Underdelivery, overdelivery, siphoning
Defective delivery system
Retrograde flow
Poor medical judgment
Inappropriate patient selection
Anaphylaxis
Extraordinary sensitivity to opioid
Reprogramming of pump with criminal intent

BOX 16–4	CRITERIA FOR DECIDING WHEN TO REPLACE A PATIENT-CONTROLLED ANALGESIA PUMP[52]

Levels of wear and damage beyond economic repair
Chronic unreliability
Obsolescence
Spare parts no longer available
More cost-effective or clinically effective pumps available

overdose, whether due to a programming error or pump malfunction, but there are often other contributory factors, such as hypovolemia.[53–55] According to one report, 5 deaths associated with the use of one particular PCA device occurred over the course of 12 years and 22 million patients, all of which were due to programming errors.[54] The authors of this report estimated that the probability of mortality from a programming error was very similar to the likelihood of death from a general anesthetic (1:300,000). It is also important to point out that these figures relate to one specific PCA pump that had a software configuration whereby the default drug concentration setting could result in administration of an excessive dose; the software configuration has now been updated.

Summary

The following statements about PCA are supported by level I evidence:
- Opioids delivered by PCA will provide better pain relief than opioids administered by conventional techniques.
- Patient satisfaction with PCA is higher than that with conventional techniques of analgesia.
- The incidence of respiratory depression for PCA with opioids is lower than with intramuscular opioid analgesia.
- The incidence of hypotension for PCA with opioids is lower than with intramuscular opioid analgesia.
- Droperidol is effective against PCA-induced emesis by opioids.

The next statements are supported by level II evidence:
- Intravenous PCA and subcutaneous PCA provide comparable analgesia.
- Low-dose background infusions are beneficial in children.
- Adding an antiemetic to the PCA infusate will benefit 30 patients out of every 100.

REFERENCES

1. Sechzer PH: Objective measurement of pain. Anesthesiology 1968; 29:209–210.
2. Harmer M, Rosen M, Vickers MD: Patient-controlled analgesia: Proceedings of the First International Workshop on Patient-Controlled Analgesia. Oxford, Blackwell Scientific Publications, 1985.
3. Scott JS: Obstetric analgesia: A consideration of labor pain on a patient-controlled technique for its relief with meperidine. Am J Obstet Gynecol 1970;106:959–978.
4. Evans JM, McCarthy JP, Rosen M, Hogg MIJ: Apparatus for patient-controlled administration of intravenous narcotics during labour. Lancet 1976;1(7949):17–18.

5. Sawaki Y, Parker RK, White PF: Patient and nurse evaluation of patient-controlled analgesia delivery systems for postoperative pain management. J Pain Symptom Manag 1992;7:443–453.

6. Rawal N: Post-operative Pain Management: Into the 21st Century. EuroPain Opinion Leader Meeting Report. Paris, European Society of Anaesthesiology, 1995.

7. Miaskowski C, Crews J, Ready LB, et al: Anesthesia based pain services improve the quality of postoperative pain management. Pain 1999;80:23–29.

8. Austin KL, Stapleton JV, Mather LE: Relationship between blood meperidine concentration and analgesic responses: A preliminary report. Anesthesiology 1980;53:460–466.

9. Upton RN, Semple TJ, Macintyre PE: Pharmacokinetic optimisation of opioid treatment in acute pain therapy. Clin Pharmacokinet 1997;33:225–244.

10. Woodhouse A, Ward M, Mather L: Inter-subject variability in post-operative patient-controlled analgesia (PCA): Is the patient equally satisfied with morphine, pethidine and fentanyl? Pain 1999;80:545–553.

11. Dawson L, Brockbank K, Carr EC, Barrett RF: Improving patients' post-operative sleep: A randomised control study comparing subcutaneous with intravenous patient-controlled analgesia. J Adv Nurs 1999;30:875–881.

12. Urquhart ML, Klapp K, White PF: Patient-controlled analgesia: A comparison of intravenous versus subcutaneous hydromorphone. Anesthesiology 1989;69:428–432.

13. Wigfull J, Welchew E: Survey of 1057 patients receiving postoperative patient-controlled epidural analgesia. Anaesthesia 2001;56:471–476.

14. Ammar AD: Postoperative epidural analgesia following abdominal aortic surgery: Do the benefits justify the costs? Ann Vasc Surg 1988;12:359–363.

15. Toussaint S, Maidl J, Schwagmeier R, Striebel HW: Patient-controlled intranasal analgesia: Effective alternative to intravenous PCA for postoperative pain relief. Can J Anaesth 2000;47:299–302.

16. Owen H, Plummer JL, Armstrong I, et al: Variables of patient-controlled analgesia. 1: Bolus size. Anaesthesia 1989;44:7–10.

17. Woodhouse A, Mather LE: The effect of duration of dose delivery with patient-controlled analgesia on the incidence of nausea and vomiting after hysterectomy. Br J Clin Pharmacol 1998;45:57–62.

18. Ginsberg B, Gil KM, Muir M, et al: The influence of lockout intervals and drug selection on patient-controlled analgesia following gynecological surgery. Pain 1995;62:95–100.

19. Badner NH, Doyle JA, Smith MH, Herrick IA: Effect of varying intravenous patient-controlled analgesia dose and lockout interval while maintaining a constant hourly maximum dose. J Clin Anesth 1996;8:382–385.

20. Stamer UM, Grond S, Maier C: Responders and non-responders to post-operative pain treatment: The loading dose predicts analgesic needs. Eur J Anaesthesiol 1999;16:103–110.

21. Owen H, Szekely SM, Plummer JL, et al: Variables of patient-controlled analgesia. 2: Concurrent infusion. Anaesthesia 1989;44:11–13.

22. Parker RK, Holtmann B, White PF: Effect of nighttime opioid infusion with PCA therapy on patient comfort and analgesic requirements after abdominal hysterectomy. Anesthesiology 1992;76:362–367.

23. Owen H, Plummer J: Patient-controlled analgesia: Current concepts in acute pain management. CNS Drugs 1997;8:203–218.

24. Sidebotham D, Dijkhuizen MR, Schug SA: The safety and utilization of patient-controlled analgesia. J Pain Symptom Manag 1997;14:202–209.

25. Macintyre P, Ready LB: Acute pain management: A practical guide. London, WB Saunders, 1996.

26. Berde CB, Lehn BM, Yee JD, et al: Patient controlled analgesia in children and adolescents: A randomized, prospective comparison with intramuscular administration of morphine for post-operative analgesia. J Pediatr 1991;118:460–466.

27. Doyle E, Harper I, Morton NS: PCA with low dose background infusions after lower abdominal surgery in children. Br J Anaesth 1993;71:818–822.

28. Gaukroger PB, Tomkins DP, van der Walt JH: Patient controlled analgesia in children. Anaesth Intensive Care 1989;17:264–268.

29. Doyle E, Robinson D, Morton NS: Comparison of PCA with and without a background infusion after lower abdominal surgery in children. Br J Anaesth 1993;71:670–673.

30. McCoy EP, Furness G, Wright PM: Patient-controlled analgesia with and without background infusion: Analgesia assessed using the demand:delivery ratio. Anaesthesia 1993;48:256–260.

31. Kluger MT, Owen H: Patients' expectations of patient-controlled analgesia. Anaesthesia 1990;45:1072–1074.

32. Chumbley GM, Hall G, Salmon P: Patient-controlled analgesia: An assessment by 200 patients. Anaesthesia 1998;53:216–221.

33. Lam KK, Chan MT, Chen PP, Kee WD: Structured preoperative patient education for patient-controlled analgesia. J Clin Anesth 2001;13:465–469.

34. Coleman SA, Booker-Milburn J: Audit of postoperative pain control: Influence of a dedicated pain nurse. Anaesthesia 1997;51:1093–1096.

35. Ballantyne JC, Carr DB, Chalmers TC, et al: Postoperative patient-controlled analgesia: Meta-analysis of initial randomised control trials. J Clin Anesth 1993;5:182–193.

36. Walder B, Schafer M, Heinzi I, Tramer MR: Efficacy and safety of patient-controlled opioid analgesia for postoperative pain. Acta Anaesthesiol Scand 2001;45:795–804.

37. Dolin SJ, Cashman JN, Bland JM: Effectiveness of acute postoperative pain management. I: Evidence from published data. Br J Anaesth 2002;89:409–424.

38. McArdle CS: Continuous and patient controlled infusions. In Doyle E (ed): International Symposium on Pain Control. (Royal Society of Medicine International Congress and Symposium Series No. 123.) London, Royal Society of Medicine, 1986, pp 17–22.

39. Wheatley RG, Madej TH, Jackson IJ, Hunter D: The first year's experience of an Acute Pain service. Br J Anaesth 1991;67:353–359.

40. Donovan B: Patient attitudes to postoperative pain relief. Anaesth Intensive Care 1983;11:125–128.

41. Ready LB: Patient-controlled analgesia—does it provide more than comfort? Can J Anaesth 1990;37:719–721.

42. Pellino TA, Ward SE: Perceived control mediates the relationship between pain severity and patient satisfaction. J Pain Symptom Manag 1998;15:110–116.

43. Rawal N, Allvin R: Epidural and intrathecal opioids for postoperative pain management in Europe—a 17-nation questionnaire study of selected hospitals. Euro Pain Study Group on Acute Pain. Acta Anaesthesiol Scand 1996;40:1119–1126.

44. Cashman JN, Dolin SJ: Respiratory and haemodynamic effects of acute postoperative pain management: Evidence from published data. Br J Anaesth 2004;93:212–223.

45. Werner MU, Soholm L, Rotboll-Nielsen P, Kehlet H: Does an acute pain service improve postoperative outcome? Anesth Analg 2002;95:1361–1372.

46. Dolin SJ, Cashman JN: Tolerability of acute postoperative pain management: Nausea, vomiting, sedation, pruritus and urinary retention. Evidence from published data. Br J Anaesth 2005;95:584–591.

47. Tramer MR, Walder B: Efficacy and adverse effects of prophylactic antiemetics during patient-controlled analgesia therapy: A quantitative systematic review. Anesth Analg 1999;88:1354–1361.

48. Culebres X, Corpatuaux JB, Gaggero G, Tramer M: The antiemetic efficacy of droperidol added to morphine patient-controlled analgesia: A randomised, controlled, multicenter dose-finding study. Anesth Analg 2003;97:816–821.

49. Kjelberg F, Tramer MR: Pharmacological control of opioid-induced pruritus: A quantitative systematic review of randomised trials. Eur J Anaesthesiol 2001;18:346–357.

50. Oswalt KE, Shrewsbury P, Stanton-Hicks M: The incidence of medication mishaps in 3,299 PCA patients. Pain 1990;5(Suppl):S152.

51. Horn SD, Wright HL, Couperus JJ, et al: Association between patient-controlled analgesia pump use and postoperative surgical site infection in intestinal surgery patients. Surg Infect 2002;3:109–118.

52. Medicines and Healthcare Products Regulatory Agency: Bulletin DB2003(02)—Infusion Systems. Available at www.mhra.gov.uk/home/idcplg?IdcService=SS_GET_PAGE&nodeId=233

53. Grey TC, Sweeney ES: Patient-controlled analgesia [letter]. JAMA 1988;259:2240.

54. Doyle DJ, Vicente KJ: Electrical short circuit as a possible cause of death in patients on PCA machines: Report on an opiate overdose and a possible preventive remedy. Anesthesiology 2001;94:940.

55. Vicente KJ, Kada-Bekhaled K, Hillel G, et al: Programming errors contribute to death from patient-controlled analgesia: Case report and estimate of probability. Can J Anaesth 2003;50:328–332.

Regional and Peripheral Techniques

BRIAN KINIRONS • DOMINIC HARMON

Regional anesthesia has enjoyed a revival of interest and usage. It can provide excellent analgesia in the awake patient. New drugs, improvement in equipment design, and the introduction of imaging techniques have improved the quality and safety of regional anesthesia. Continuous infusion techniques allow the rate of administration to be titrated and facilitate adjustment of drug concentrations and combinations. Patient-controlled regional anesthesia at home is a major advance in this field.

Regional anesthesia has long been perceived as having a role in the high-risk surgical patient.[1] Minimizing the area of anesthesia in patients with decreased cardiorespiratory reserve is potentially advantageous. Use of regional anesthesia avoids the complications associated with general anesthesia. In this chapter, four specific questions regarding regional techniques and postoperative pain management are discussed, and the available evidence to answer them is examined.

Is There Evidence that Spinal Anesthesia Decreases Morbidity and Mortality Compared with General Anesthesia in the High-Risk Patient?

To examine this question, let us choose a clearly defined surgical group—patients receiving anesthesia for hip fracture surgery. Hip fracture is a common condition. It has been estimated that as many as 6.3 million patients worldwide may have presented with this condition by 2050.[2] This estimate has significant resource implications for any healthcare system.

Patients with hip fracture commonly present with significant coexisting cardiorespiratory disease, and for them, significant mortality and morbidity may be associated with surgery. Twenty percent of all patients will die within the first year after surgery.[3] Of those who survive, one in four will require a higher level of long-term care, and a significant number will experience difficulty with activities of daily living.[4] Morbidity includes infection, venous thrombosis, pneumonia, pulmonary embolism, myocardial ischemia or infarction, cerebrovascular accident, and pressure sores.

EVIDENCE

The controversy as to whether regional anesthesia has advantages over general anesthesia in reducing mortality and morbidity is not new. As far back as 1933, Nygaard[1] demonstrated fewer complications with spinal anesthesia than with open drop ether anesthesia.

Methodological flaws and inadequate power have limited interpretation of available data. It has been estimated that using 30-day mortality as an outcome measure, assuming a mortality rate of 4.8% and an ability to detect a 25% difference, would require a study population of 13,000 to 14,000 patients. This may explain why some meta-analyses may have been unable to demonstrate an improvement in mortality after regional anesthesia.

The first reported meta-analysis comparing general anesthesia with regional anesthesia for hip fracture was performed by Sorenson and Pace[5] in 1992. This meta-analysis compared regional anesthesia to general anesthesia in 13 randomized controlled trials of patients undergoing surgical repair of fractured neck of femur ($N=2000$). Outcome measures were mortality at 1 month, the incidence of venous thrombosis, and blood loss. Although this meta-analysis showed no difference in mortality between the two groups at 1 month, patients who received general anesthesia were four times more likely to experience deep vein thrombosis (DVT). Limitations in this meta-analysis included inadvertent duplication of patients from several studies and the fact that most patients did not receive any DVT prophylaxis.

Urwin et al[6] subsequently performed a similar meta-analysis, reviewing 15 randomized controlled trials involving 2162 patients. Outcome measures were mortality at 1 month, incidence of DVT, blood loss, incidence of hypotension, myocardial infarction, congestive cardiac failure, urinary retention, vomiting, pneumonia, postoperative hypoxemia, confusion, and renal failure. In contrast to Sorenson and Pace,[5] Urwin et al found a lower 1-month mortality in the regional anesthesia group than in the general anesthesia group (49/766 versus 76/812, respectively; odds ratio [OR] 0.68, 95% confidence interval [CI] 0.49–0.97). The data reviewed showed a reduction in the incidence of DVT in the regional anesthesia group (30% versus 47%). The regional anesthesia group also had a significantly lower incidence of fatal pulmonary embolism. Other than a shorter operation time, general anesthesia had no advantage over regional anesthesia.

A retrospective analysis by O'Hara et al[7] reviewed outcomes in all patients undergoing surgical repair for fractured hip between 1983 and 1993 ($N = 9425$) at 20 U.S. hospitals. Primary outcome measures were 7-day and 1-month mortality. Secondary outcome measures included congestive heart failure, myocardial infarction, nosocomial pneumonia, and altered cognitive function. The investigators concluded that there was no association between the choice of anesthetic technique and morbidity or mortality.[7] They also suggested that coexisting disease and American Society of Anesthesiologists Physical Status (ASA-PS) classification may be more important in determining outcome. Limitations of this study include the fact the study was nonrandomized, was observational, and depended on medical record review and, therefore, on the accurate recording of perioperative problems.

Rodgers et al[8] reviewed all studies in which patients were randomly assigned to receive central neuraxial blockade or not. Outcomes measured were mortality, DVT, pneumonia, respiratory depression, myocardial infarction, renal failure, and pulmonary embolism. Although the study population was not exclusive to orthopedic surgery, the overall mortality was one third lower in the group who received a central neuraxial block (OR 0.68, 95% CI 0.49–0.96). This reduction in mortality was not affected by the type of surgery or whether patients received either epidural or spinal anesthesia. Mortality reduction occurred irrespective of whether the regional technique was continued postoperatively. Rodgers et al[8] demonstrated a reduction in rates of DVT, postoperative pneumonia, renal failure, myocardial infarction, bleeding complications, and respiratory depression in the central neuraxial anesthesia group.

Although earlier reviews of anesthesia for hip fracture surgery in the Cochrane Database showed a reduction in early mortality in the regional anesthesia group,[9] a later review has questioned the statistical significance of this outcome.[8] Patients in the regional anesthesia group, however, did have a lower rate of postoperative confusion.

CONCLUSION

There is currently insufficient data to make definitive statements regarding the outcome benefits of regional anesthesia in this surgical population. Further large, multicenter studies will be required to answer this question. What is clear from the evidence is that the use of neuraxial blockade decreases the incidence of venous thrombosis in patients undergoing surgical repair of hip fracture. Although the results from the studies by Urwin et al[6] and Rodgers et al[8] would suggest that the use of regional anesthesia decreases mortality at 1 month, the Cochrane Database System Review is less emphatic about the reduction in mortality afforded by regional anesthesia. There is certainly no evidence to suggest that there is a difference in mortality rates between the two anesthesia techniques at 1 year. On the basis of available evidence, best practice guidelines consistently advocate the use of regional anesthesia in this surgical population.[11–13] Because central neuraxial blockade has been proven to consistently decrease the incidence of venous thrombosis in this at-risk group, advocating the use of this blockade in the management of patients undergoing surgical repair of hip fracture would seem reasonable.

Is There Evidence to Recommend the Use of Pharmacological Adjuncts in Peripheral Nerve Blockade?

Pharmacological adjuncts have been used in combination with local anesthetic solutions in the belief that a synergistic effect is produced. These agents may have local anesthetic effects themselves or may have potential targets in the peripheral nerve. The desired clinical effect is to improve not only the duration but also the quality of peripheral nerve blockade. Evidence for the efficacy of alkalinization and the addition of adrenaline to local anesthetic solutions is not discussed. The use of other adjuncts is more recent, and evidence regarding these agents must be clarified. Such agents are opioids, clonidine, neostigmine, and tramadol.

EVIDENCE

Opioids

A meta-analysis examining efficacy of opioids as adjuncts in peripheral nerve blockade was reported by Picard et al.[14] Of the 26 studies examined, 10 showed an improvement in efficacy of intraoperative or postoperative blockade. In no study was this statistically significant improvement considered to be clinically relevant. The investigators further stated that trials of poorer quality were more likely to report greater efficacy with opioids. They concluded that there was no evidence to support the addition of opioids to peripheral nerve blockade.

Murphy et al[15] performed a systematic review of the addition of novel adjuncts for brachial plexus block. The adjuncts studied were opioids, clonidine, tramadol, and neostigmine. Their survey exposed current limitations in the available literature due to either poor study design (lack of a systemic opioid control group) or lack of adequate power. With respect to the use of opioid adjuncts, they stated that studies with a systemic opioid control group were less likely to demonstrate an analgesic benefit than those without one. They concluded that there is insufficient evidence to support the use of opioids as adjuncts for brachial plexus block. Their conclusions support the findings previously reported by Picard et al.[14] On the basis of these reviews, there is insufficient evidence to support the adjunctive use of opioids for plexus blockade.

Clonidine

Alpha-2 receptors are found in brainstem nuclei, spinal cord, and primary afferent neurons, suggesting that clonidine has both peripheral and central effects.[16] Although the exact mechanism of action of clonidine is unknown, multiple hypotheses have been suggested. Clonidine may modify the composition of the local anesthetic, may alter its pharmacokinetic properties, or may have a direct drug effect on the nerve.[17] Clonidine is also known to diminish sympathetic output.[18]

Multiple studies have demonstrated that clonidine administered centrally or peripherally prolongs the duration of anesthesia and analgesia and intensifies the block associated with local anesthetic agents (without increasing the duration of motor blockade).[17,19] Murphy et al,[15] in their systematic review, reported that the addition of clonidine prolonged analgesia of brachial plexus blockade in five of the six studies in their review. They concluded that the addition of up to 150 μg of clonidine prolonged analgesia without increasing side effects. Thus, there is evidence to support the adjunctive use of clonidine for plexus blockade (Table 17–1).[20–27]

Neostigmine

Intrathecal administration of neostigmine has an analgesic effect,[28] thought to be due to greater release of gamma-aminobutyric acid in the dorsal horn.[29] There are limited data concerning the use of neostigmine as an adjunct for peripheral plexus anesthesia. Bone et al[26] added neostigmine to mepivacaine in brachial plexus blockade. Patients who received neostigmine required less analgesia in the first 24 hours after surgery. In contrast, Bouaziz et al[27] reported that neostigmine did not prolong sensory blockade associated with axillary blocks. Furthermore, the incidence of nausea and/or vomiting was significantly higher in the groups that received neostigmine than in the control group. The researchers further postulated that in studies in which neostigmine had a therapeutic effect, the effect may have been due to local administration of the agent at the surgical site.[27] Currently, there is insufficient evidence to recommend the addition of neostigmine as an adjunct for peripheral nerve blockade (see Table 17–1).

Tramadol

Tramadol has both peripheral and central effects.[30] It is a weak μ receptor agonist,[31] prevents synaptic reuptake of noradrenaline, and enhances serotonin release.[32] These neurotransmitters are important in the descending pathways that modulate pain.[33] Tramadol has also been postulated to have a local anesthetic effect.[34] The reversal of analgesia by α_2 antagonists[35] would suggest that tramadol causes indirect activation of the postsynaptic α_2 receptors. The first study assessing the efficacy of tramadol as an adjunct in the brachial

plexus blockade was reported by Kapral et al.[36] These investigators demonstrated that the addition of 100 mg of tramadol to 40 mL of 1% mepivacaine significantly prolonged the duration of brachial plexus blockade.[30] By including a group in which tramadol was administered systemically, and demonstrating no difference in block duration between systemic and control groups, Kapral et al[36] were able to hypothesize that the effect of tramadol was locally mediated at the peripheral nerve. This local anesthetic effect has been supported by results of an elegant animal study.[37] Robaux et al[38] described a dose-response study using 40, 100, or 200 mg of tramadol added to 40 mL of 1% mepivacaine in brachial plexus blockade. They reported a dose-dependent reduction in postoperative analgesic requirements when tramadol was included.[38] Mannion et al,[39] however, were not able to demonstrate a better analgesic effect for adjunctive use of tramadol, 0.5 mg/kg, in psoas blocks. The current data concerning the use of tramadol as an adjunct for plexus anesthesia are limited (Table 17–2), and further studies are required before definitive recommendations can be made.

Is There Evidence to Recommend the Use of Regional Anesthesia to Decrease Postoperative Cognitive Dysfunction?

A large international multicenter trial involving approximately 1200 patients older than 60 years noted that postoperative cognitive dysfunction (POCD) was present in 25.8% of patients 1 week after surgery and in 9.9% of patients 3 months after surgery (versus 3.4% at 1 week and 2.8% at 3 months for nonsurgical control subjects).[40] The presence of POCD is an independent predictor of long-term outcome.[41] Postoperative delirium is independently associated with higher mortality, major morbidity, longer hospital stay, and higher rates of discharge to rehabilitative facilities.[41]

The general etiology of POCD is unclear; however, a multifactorial model is supported by available studies.[42,43] Elderly patients[44] and patients with poor preoperative cognitive[44–46] or functional[47] status are generally at higher risk for POCD. Certain surgical procedures are associated with higher rates of POCD. Patients undergoing cardiac surgery with cardiopulmonary bypass[48] or thoracic or aortic aneurysm procedures are at higher risk for POCD.[43] Particular subgroups of patients

TABLE 17–1	Studies Using Clonidine and Neostigmine as Adjuncts to Brachial Plexus Blocks				
Study	**Technique**	**Adjunct**		**Systemic Control?**	**Result**
Eledjam et al[20]	Supraclavicular	Clonidine, 150 μg		No	Prolonged analgesia
Singelyn et al[21]	Axillary	Clonidine, 150 μg		Yes	Prolonged analgesia
Gaumann et al[22]	Axillary	Clonidine, 150 μg		No	No difference
Buttner et al[23]	Axillary	Clonidine, 120 and 240 μg		No	Prolonged analgesia
Singelyn et al[24]	Axillary	Clonidine, 0.1–0.5 μg/kg		No	Prolonged analgesia
Bernard & Macaire[25]	Axillary	Clonidine, 30, 90, and 300 μg		No	Prolonged analgesia
Iskandar et al[17]	Midhumeral	Clonidine, 50 μg		No	Prolonged analgesia
Erlacher et al[19]	Axillary	Clonidine, 150 μg		No	Prolonged analgesia
Bone et al[26]	Axillary	Neostigmine, 500 μg		No	Improved analgesia
Bouaziz et al[27]	Axillary	Neostigmine, 500 μg		Yes	No difference

TABLE 17–2	Studies Using Tramadol as Adjunct to Plexus Blocks			
Study	Technique	Tramadol Dose	Systemic Control?	Result
Kapral et al[36]	Axillary	100 mg	Yes	Prolonged analgesia
Robaux et al[38]	Axillary	40, 100, or 200 mg	No	Prolonged analgesia
Mannion et al[39]	Psoas	1.5 mg/kg	Yes	No difference

are at higher risk for POCD. The overall incidence of POCD in elderly orthopedic surgery patients may be as high as 7.5% to 17.5%[49]; however, patients with hip fractures have a much higher incidence (28%–50%).[47,50] The overall contribution of intraoperative factors to the development of POCD is unclear.[51] A longer duration of anesthesia is associated with a higher incidence of POCD.[52] The administration of certain drugs has been independently associated with development of POCD, especially postoperative delirium. The use of psychoactive medications, such as anticholinergic drugs,[44] meperidine,[43] and benzodiazepines,[43] is significantly associated with development of POCD.[43,53] In other studies, opioids other than meperidine and anticholinergic agents have not been associated with delirium.[54] The presence of postoperative infections and respiratory complications is also associated with the development of POCD.[40]

Although many of the strongest risk factors for POCD may be those that cannot be altered (i.e., increasing age, preexisting cognitive impairment, and severity of coexisting illness), it does appear that other factors, such as poorly controlled pain and presence of respiratory complications, may be associated with a higher incidence of POCD. A possible therapeutic option is the use of perioperative epidural analgesia (with a local anesthetic–based regimen) in a multimodal approach. This type of intervention may attenuate known risk factors for POCD, such as lowering the incidence of respiratory complications,[55] providing better postoperative pain control,[56] and improving patient-oriented outcomes (e.g., sleep)[57] that may contribute to POCD or postoperative delirium.[58]

EVIDENCE

In a systematic review by Wu et al[59] of 19 trials, 18 did not demonstrate a difference in cognitive function between intraoperative general anesthesia and regional anesthesia. It is possible that a relatively brief unimodal intervention, such as intraoperative neuraxial anesthesia, might have only a small impact on a complex perioperative complication such as POCD, which has a multifactorial etiology. Unlike the beneficial effects seen with other organ systems, intraoperative neuraxial anesthesia does not confer any apparent direct physiological benefit on cognitive function and, because of its limited duration of action, may be unable to provide adequate postoperative pain control, which has been shown to be a factor in the development of POCD.[60]

Study-Design Issues

Study-design concerns may contribute to ambiguity in the interpretation of currently available studies. Almost all of the trials comparing the effects of intraoperative neuraxial

anesthesia and general anesthesia have allowed the routine use of benzodiazepines in the perioperative period, which is significantly associated with development of POCD.[43]

Another area of potential concern is the general lack of control of postoperative analgesia in currently available trials. The effect of postoperative analgesia on mental function has not been rigorously investigated, and it is recognized that higher levels of postoperative pain are associated with a higher rate of POCD (especially delirium).[60] Thus, control of postoperative pain may theoretically influence the incidence of POCD, which typically peaks within the first 3 postoperative days.[39] Furthermore, different analgesic regimens may potentially have different effects on postoperative cognitive function; certain types of analgesic regimens (e.g., epidural analgesia with a local anesthetic–based solution) not only provide better pain control than systemic opioids[56] but also avoid the systemic side effects of opioids, which may be associated with development of POCD.[43] Finally, like almost all "regional versus general" anesthesia trials, none of the randomized controlled trials was blinded, leading to the possibility of bias.[57]

Future studies in this area will allow correlation of the level of cognitive impairment (as assessed by appropriate neuropsychological testing) with a clinically relevant drop in cognitive function.[61] Peripheral nerve blockade is a component of regional anesthesia practice. Its role in diminishing postoperative cognitive dysfunction in those at risk must also be examined in future studies.

Is There Evidence to Recommend the Use of Regional Anesthesia Techniques to Decrease Postoperative Pulmonary Complications?

In assessing the impact of regional anesthesia techniques on postoperative pulmonary complications, one must consider the following two questions:
1. Does the choice of postoperative analgesic therapy affect pulmonary outcome?
2. Is more effective postoperative pain control associated with a reduction in postoperative pulmonary morbidity?

ETIOLOGY OF LUNG DYSFUNCTION

Pulmonary complications after surgery are common and may be associated with significant morbidity and mortality (Fig. 17–1), especially after upper abdominal and thoracic procedures. The pathophysiology of postoperative pulmonary dysfunction is multifactorial and is due not only to the effects

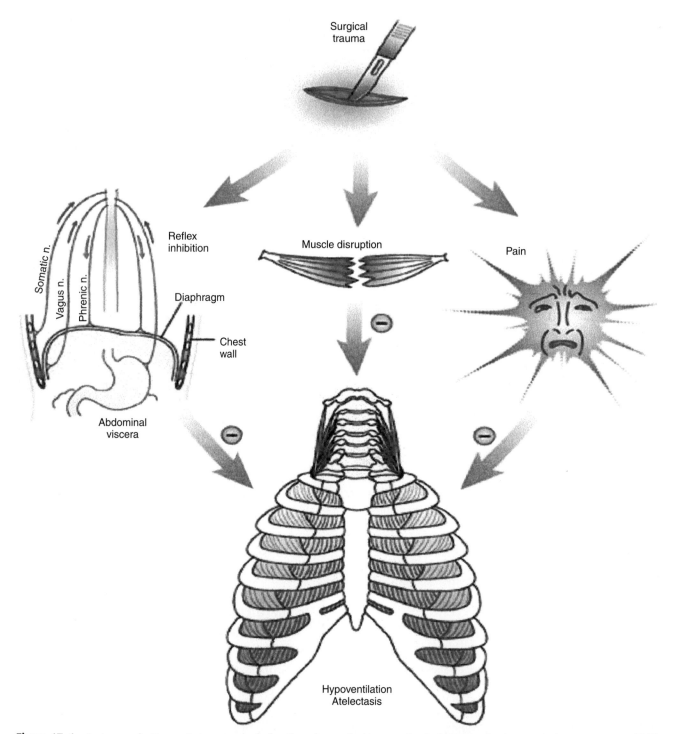

Figure 17–1 Factors producing respiratory muscle dysfunction after surgical trauma. Surgical trauma stimulates central nervous system (CNS) reflexes mediated by both visceral and somatic nerves; these reflexes produce reflex inhibition of the phrenic and other nerves innervating respiratory muscle. Mechanical disruption of respiratory muscles impairs their efficiency, and pain produces voluntary limitation of respiratory motion. These factors all tend to reduce lung volumes and can produce hypoventilation and atelectasis. (From Warner DO: Preventing postoperative pulmonary complications: The role of the anaesthesiologist. Anesthesiology 2000;92:1467–1472.)

of the surgical trauma but also to the anesthesia itself. General anesthesia is associated with respiratory depression, a reduction in both functional residual capacity and vital capacity. Surgical trauma may exacerbate this reduction with a muscle-splitting incision, which causes functional impairment of the respiratory muscle group. Inadequate postoperative analgesia may limit the patient's ability to breathe deeply or to cough, thus predisposing to atelectasis, pneumonia, and subsequent respiratory failure. Visceral surgery may cause phrenic nerve impairment and hence diaphragmatic dysfunction. Associated ventilation/perfusion mismatch results in hypoxemia, which may impair both cognitive function and wound healing.[62,63]

EVIDENCE

Interpretation of the evidence is limited by multiple factors. Difficulties include the heterogenicity of the study populations, different epidural techniques and infusion regimens, the lack of uniformity of block levels, and a variable definition of what constitutes a respiratory complication. Furthermore, bias and small sample sizes make definitive conclusions difficult.

One of the largest studies assessing the effects of epidural analgesia was reported by Jayr et al.[63] They studied 153 patients undergoing upper abdominal surgery. After performance of a standardized general anesthetic technique, patients were randomly assigned to receive either subcutaneous morphine or epidural bupivacaine and morphine postoperatively. Pulmonary outcome measures included arterial partial pressure of oxygen (PaO_2), pulmonary function tests, and chest radiographs. Although patients in the epidural group had significantly less pain, the incidences of pulmonary complications were similar in the two groups.[63]

Ballantyne et al[64] performed a meta-analysis of the effect of seven different analgesic therapies on pulmonary outcome. They compared epidural opioids, epidural local anesthetics, epidural opioids with local anesthetic, intercostal nerve block, intrapleural infusion of local anesthetic, thoracic versus lumbar epidural, and wound infiltration versus no wound infiltration. Measures of pulmonary outcome were forced expiratory volume in 1 second (FEV_1), forced vital capacity (FVC), vital capacity (VC), peak expiratory flow rate (PEFR), PaO_2, atelectasis, and pneumonia. Epidural opioids, epidural local anesthetics, and the combination of the two decreased the incidence of atelectasis, pulmonary infection, and pulmonary complications compared with systemic opioids. There was a higher PaO_2 in the epidural local anesthetic group. The addition of opioids in the epidural space improved analgesia but failed to demonstrate an improvement in pulmonary measurements (FEV_1 and FVC). Intercostal nerve block, wound infiltration, and intrapleural local anesthetic infusion were not associated with improved pulmonary outcome. No benefit was associated with thoracic epidural catheter placement. Although this meta-analysis supports the use of epidural analgesia, these findings suggest that better pain control is not always associated with an improvement in conventional measures of pulmonary function.

In a later systematic review, Rodgers et al[65] performed a meta-analysis assessing reduction of postoperative morbidity and mortality associated with central neuraxial blockade. They demonstrated a significant reduction in mortality and morbidity in all operations, and they showed that in patients who received central neuraxial blockade, postoperative pneumonia was less likely.[65] These investigators also stated that there is some evidence to support that the proportional reduction in pneumonia was associated with thoracic epidural anesthesia. Respiratory depression was reduced by 59% in patients who were randomly assigned to receive central neuraxial blockade. This reduction was independent of whether the patient received a concomitant general anesthetic. The findings of Rodgers et al[65] would support the use of epidural analgesia as recommended by the Ballantyne meta-analysis.[64]

Kehlet and Holte[66] studied the effect of postoperative analgesia on surgical outcome. Their findings support the use of epidural local anesthetics or local anesthetics and opioid mixtures to reduce postoperative pulmonary morbidity after major abdominal surgery.

In summary, there is sufficient evidence to support the use of epidural analgesia in an effort to decrease postoperative pulmonary complications.

REFERENCES

1. Nygaard KK: Routine spinal anaesthesia in provincial hospital: With comparative study of postoperative complications following spinal and general ether anesthesia. Acta Chir Scand 1936;78:379–446.
2. Melton LJ. Hip fractures: A world-wide problem of today and tomorrow. Bone 1993;14(Suppl 1):S1–S8.
3. Schurch M-A, Rizzoli R, Mermillod B, et al: A prospective study on the socio-economic aspects of fracture of the proximal femur. J Bone Miner Res 1996;11:1935–1942.
4. Hochberg MC, Williamson J, Skinner EA, et al: The prevalence and impact of self-reported hip fracture in elderly community-dwelling women: The women's Health and Aging Study. Osteoporos Int 1998;8:385–389.
5. Sorenson RM, Pace NL: Anaesthetic techniques during surgical repair of femoral neck fractures: A meta-analysis. Anesthesiology 1992;77:1095–1104.
6. Urwin SC, Parker MJ, Griffiths R: General versus regional anaesthesia for hip fracture surgery: A meta-analysis of randomized trials [erratum in Br J Anaesth 2002;88:619]. Br J Anaesth 2000;84:450–455.
7. O'Hara DA, Duff A, Berlin JA, et al: The effect of anesthetic technique on postoperative operative outcomes in hip fracture repair. Anesthesiology 2000;92:947–957.
8. Rodgers A, Walker N, Schug S, et al: Reduction in postoperative mortality and morbidity with epidural or spinal anaesthesia: Results from overview of randomised trials. BMJ 2000;231:1493–1497.
9. Parker MJ, Urwin SC, Handoll HH, Griffiths R: General versus spinal/epidural anaesthesia for hip fracture in adults. Cochrane Database Syst Rev 2000;2:CD000521.
10. Parker MJ, Handoll HH, Griffiths R: Anaesthesia for hip fracture surgery in adults. Cochrane Database Syst Rev 2004;4:CD000521.
11. Gillespie WJ: Extracts from "clinical evidence": Hip fracture. BMJ 2001;322:968–975.
12. March LM, Chamberlain AC, Cameron ID, et al: How best to fix a broken hip. Fractured Neck of Femur Health Outcomes Project Team. Med J Aust 1999;170:489–494.
13. Chilov MN, Cameron ID, March LM: Evidence-based guidelines for fixing broken hip: An update. Med J Aust 2003:179:489–493.
14. Picard PR, Tramer MR, McQuay HJ, Moore RA: Analgesic efficacy of peripheral opioids (all except intra-articular): A qualitative systematic review of randomised controlled trials. Pain 1997;72:309–318.
15. Murphy DB, McCarthy CJ, Chan VW: Novel analgesic adjuncts for brachial plexus block: A systemic review. Anesth Analg 2000;90:1122–1128.
16. Elliott JA, Smith HS. α_2-Agonists. In Smith HS (ed): Drugs for Pain. Philadelphia, Hanley & Belfus, 2003, pp 191–200.
17. Iskandar H, Guillaume E, Dixmerias F, et al: The enhancement of sensory blockade by clonidine selectively added to mepivacaine after midhumeral block. Anesth Analg 2001;93:771–775.
18. Eisenach JC, Tong C: Site of hemodynamic effects of intrathecal α_2-adenergic agonists. Anesthesiology 1991;74:766–771.
19. Erlacher W, Schusching C, Koinig H, et al: Clonidine as adjunct for mepivacaine, ropivacaine and bupivacaine in axillary, perivascular brachial plexus block. Can J Anaesth 2001;48:522–525.
20. Eledjam JJ, Viel E, Charavel P, du Caliar J: Brachial plexus block with bupivacaine: Effects of added alpha-adrenergic agonists. Comparison between clonidine and epinephrine. Can J Anaesth 1991;38:870–875.
21. Singelyn FJ, Dangoisse M, Bartholomee S, Gouverneur JM: Adding clonidine to mepivacaine prolongs the duration of anesthesia and analgesia after axillary brachial plexus block. Reg Anesth 1992;17:148–150.
22. Gaumann D, Forster A, Griessen M, et al: Comparison between clonidine and epinephrine admixture to lidocaine in brachial plexus block. Anesth Analg 1992;75:69–74.
23. Buttner J, Ott B, Klose R: Der einflub von clonidinzusatz zu mepivacain. Anaesthesist 1992;41:548–554.

24. Singelyn FJ, Gouverneur JM, Robert A: A minimum dose of clonidine added to mepivacaine prolongs the duration of anesthesia and analgesia after axillary brachial plexus block. Anesth Analg 1996;83: 1046–1050.

25. Bernard JM, Macaire P: Dose-range effects of clonidine added to lidocaine for brachial plexus block. Anesthesiology 1997;87:277–284.

26. Bone HG, Van Aken H, Booke M, et al: Enhancement of axillary brachial block anaesthesia by coadministration of neostigmine. Anesth Analg 1999;24:405–410.

27. Bouaziz H, Paqueron X, Bur ML, et al: No enhancement of sensory and motor blockade by neostigmine added to mepivacaine axillary plexus block. Anesthesiology 1999;91:78–84.

28. Hood DD, Eisenach JC, Tuttle R: Phase 1 safety assessment of intrathecal neostigmine methylsulphate in humans. Anesthesiology 1995;82: 331–343.

29. Cohen SP, Abdi S: Clinical applications of spinal analgesia. In Smith HS (ed): Drugs for Pain. Philadelphia, Hanley & Belfus, 2003, pp 339–351.

30. Smith HS: Miscellaneous analgesic agents. In Smith HS (ed): Drugs for Pain. Philadelphia, Hanley & Belfus, 2003, pp 271–287.

31. Collart L, Luthy C, Dayer P: Partial inhibition of tramadol antinociceptive effect by naloxone in man. Br J Clin Pharmacol 1993;35:73P.

32. Raffa RB, Friderichs E, Reimann E, et al: Opioid and nonopioid components independently contribute to the mechanism of action of tramadol, an "atypical" opioid analgesic. J Pharmacol Exp Ther 1992; 260:275–285.

33. Iosifescu DV, Alpert JE, Fava M: Antidepressants: Basic mechanisms and pharmacology. In Smith HS (ed): Drugs for Pain. Philadelphia, Hanley & Belfus, 2003, pp 215–222.

34. Mert T, Gunes Y, Guven M, et al: Comparison of nerve conduction blocks by an opioid and a local anesthetic. Eur J Pharmacol 2002; 439:77–81.

35. Desmeules JA, Piguet V, Collart L, Dayer P: Contribution of monoaminergic modulation to the analgesic effect of tramadol. Br J Clin Pharmacol 1996;41:7–12.

36. Kapral S, Gollman G, Waltl B, et al: Tramadol added to mepivacaine prolongs the duration of axillary brachial plexus blockade. Anesth Analg 1999;88:853–856.

37. Tsai YC, Chang PJ, Jou IM: Direct tramadol application on sciatic nerve inhibits spinal somatosensory evoked potentials in rats. Anesth Analg 2001;92:1547–1551.

38. Robaux S, Blunt C, Viel E, et al: Tramadol added to 1.5% mepivacaine for axillary brachial plexus block improves postoperative analgesia dose dependently. Anesth Analg 2004;98:1172–1177.

39. Mannion S, O'Callaghan S, Murphy DB, Shorten GD: Tramadol as adjunct to psoas compartment block with levobupivacaine 0.5%: A randomized double-blinded study. Br J Anaesth 2005;94:352–356.

40. Moller JT, Cluitmans P, Rasmussen LS, et al: Long-term postoperative cognitive dysfunction in the elderly ISPOCD1 study: ISPOCD investigators. International Study of Post-Operative Cognitive Dysfunction. Lancet 1998;351:857–861.

41. Inuoye SK, Schlesinger MJ, Lydon TJ: Delirium: A symptom of how hospital care is failing older persons and a window to improve quality of hospital care. Am J Med 1999;106:565–573.

42. Inouye SK, Charpentier PA: Precipitating factors for delirium in hospitalized elderly persons: Predictive model and interrelationship with baseline vulnerability. JAMA 1996;275:852–857.

43. Marcantonio ER, Juarez G, Goldman L, et al: The relationship of postoperative delirium with psychoactive medications. JAMA 1994;272: 1518–1522.

44. Dyer CB, Ashton CM, Teasdale TA: Postoperative delirium: A review of 80 primary data-collection studies. Arch Intern Med 1995;155: 461–465.

45. Litaker D, Locala J, Franco K, et al: Preoperative risk factors for postoperative delirium. Gen Hosp Psychiatry 2001;23:84–89.

46. Ancelin ML, de Roquefeuil G, Ledesert B, et al: Exposure to anaesthetic agents, cognitive functioning and depressive symptomatology in the elderly. Br J Psychiatry 2001;178:360–366.

47. Zakriya KJ, Christmas C, Wenz JF Sr, et al: Preoperative factors associated with postoperative change in confusion assessment method score in hip fracture patients. Anesth Analg 2002;94:1628–1632.

48. Arrowsmith JE, Grocott HP, Reves JG, Newman MF: Central nervous system complications of cardiac surgery. Br J Anaesth 2000;84: 378–393.

49. Fisher BW, Flowerdew G: A simple model for predicting postoperative delirium in older patients undergoing elective orthopedic surgery. J Am Geriatr Soc 1995;43:175–178.

50. Marcantonio ER, Flacker JM, Wright RJ, Resnick NM: Reducing delirium after hip fracture: A randomized trial. J Am Geriatr Soc 2001;49: 516–522.

51. Marcantonio ER, Lee G, Orav JE, et al: The association of intraoperative factors with the development of postoperative delirium. Am J Med 1998;105:380–384.

52. Goldstein MZ, Young BL, Fogel BS, Benedict RH: Occurrence and predictors of short-term mental and functional changes in older adults undergoing elective surgery under general anaesthesia. Am J Geriatr Psychiatry 1998;6:42–52.

53. Berggren D, Gustafson Y, Eriksson B, et al: Postoperative confusion after anesthesia in elderly patients with femoral neck fractures. Anesth Analg 1987;66:497–504.

54. Schor JD, Levkoff SE, Lipsitz LA, et al: Risk factors for delirium in hospitalized elderly. JAMA 1992;267:827–831.

55. Ballantyne JC, Carr DB, deFerranti S, et al: The comparative effects of postoperative analgesic therapies on pulmonary outcome: Cumulative meta-analyses of randomized, controlled trials. Anesth Analg 1998; 86:598–612.

56. Dolin SJ, Cashman JN, Bland JM: Effectiveness of acute postoperative pain management. I: Evidence from published data. Br J Anaesth 2002;89:409–423.

57. Wu CL, Fleisher LA: Outcomes research in regional anesthesia and analgesia. Anesth Analg 2000;91:1232–1242.

58. Hanania M, Kitain E: Melatonin for treatment and prevention of postoperative delirium. Anesth Analg 2002;94:338–339.

59. Wu CL, Hsu W, Richman JM, Raja SN: Postoperative cognitive function as an outcome of regional anesthesia and analgesia. Reg Anesth Pain Med 2004;29:257–268.

60. Lynch EP, Lazor MA, Gellis JE, et al: The impact of postoperative pain on the development of postoperative delirium. Anesth Analg 1998; 86:781–785.

61. Flacker JM, Marcantonio ER: Delirium in the elderly: Optimal management. Drugs Aging 1998;13:119–130.

62. Warner DO: Preventing postoperative pulmonary complications: The role of the anaesthesiologist. Anesthesiology 2000;92:1467–1472.

63. Jayr C, Thomas H, Rey A, et al: Postoperative pulmonary complications: Epidural analgesia using bupivacaine and opioids versus parenteral opioids. Anesthesiology 1993;78:666–676.

64. Ballantyne JC, Carr DB, deFerranti S, et al: The comparative effect of postoperative analgesic therapies on pulmonary outcome: Cumulated meta-analyses of randomized controlled trials. Anesth Analg 1998; 86:598–612.

65. Rodgers A, Natalie W, Schug S, et al: Reduction of postoperative mortality and morbidity with epidural or spinal anaesthesia: Results from overview of randomised trials. BMJ 2000;321:1493–1497.

66. Kehlet H, Holte K: Effect of postoperative analgesia on surgical outcome. Br J Anaesth 2001;87:62–72.

18 Nonsteroidal Anti-inflammatory Drugs in Postoperative Pain

JAMES HELSTROM • CARL E. ROSOW

Nonsteroidal anti-inflammatory drugs (NSAIDs) are the most commonly prescribed analgesic medications in the world. In addition to providing good relief of acute and chronic pain, NSAIDS have potent anti-inflammatory effects. The analgesic effects are dose related, but limited, so NSAIDs are often used perioperatively as supplements to opioid analgesics or regional anesthesia. The fact that these drugs do not cause respiratory depression or ileus gives them distinct advantages over opioids, although side effects such as bleeding and renal dysfunction may occasionally cause problems.

The clinical literature on NSAIDs is immense, so this chapter focuses on NSAID pharmacology as it pertains to perioperative pain. The first section briefly reviews NSAID pharmacology, cyclooxygenase isoforms, and the available drugs. The second section presents the evidence regarding NSAID efficacy in various types of postsurgical pain. The last section covers NSAID toxicity, which is often the deciding factor in the clinical decision to use these drugs. Unfortunately, many studies of NSAID toxicity are directed at the problems of long-term administration, and it is often unclear whether the data are relevant to brief use of these agents in the perioperative period. Concerns about cardiovascular risks associated with the use of selective cyclooxygenase-2 (Cox-2) inhibitors led to the removal of rofecoxib and valdecoxib from the U.S. market, a story that is still unfolding. For consistency, we use the term *NSAID* to refer to nonselective cyclooxygenase inhibitors (or all inhibitors, without regard to selectivity). The term *coxib* refers specifically to a drug with high selectivity for the Cox-2 isoform.

Pharmacology of NSAIDS

CYCLOOXYGENASE-1 AND CYCLOOXYGENASE-2

NSAIDs reversibly inhibit cyclooxygenase (prostaglandin endoperoxide synthase), the enzyme mediating production of prostaglandins (PGs) and thromboxane A_2 (TXA_2). The substrate for cyclooxygenase is arachidonic acid, a fatty acid derived from cell membrane phospholipids through the action of phospholipase A_2. Arachidonic acid also serves as the starting material for 5-lipoyxgenase (5-LO), the initial step in the production of the leukotriene family of inflammatory mediators. Prostaglandins are autocrines, mediating physiological functions in a variety of tissues, such as maintenance of the gastric mucosal barrier, regulation of renal blood flow, and regulation of endothelial tone. TXA_2 promotes platelet aggregation. Additionally, prostaglandins play an integral part in inflammatory and nociceptive processes, acting to produce localized swelling and sensitization of nociceptors.[1] There are three cyclooxygenase isoenzymes, although information on the third is still incomplete and not universally acknowledged. Cox-1 and Cox-2 are products of genes on different chromosomes, with different tissue localization, substrate specificities, and functions. Cox-1 provides constitutive PG synthesis for the homeostatic processes mentioned previously. Cox-2 is not normally present in many tissues (the central nervous system [CNS] and kidney are exceptions), but it is inducible by inflammation, fever, pain, and a wide variety of cytokines. Cox-3 may mediate the central analgesic effects of acetaminophen and appears to be an alternative protein product of the gene for Cox-1. The constitutive versus inducible distinction between Cox-1 and Cox-2 is undoubtedly an oversimplification, because there is evidence for Cox-2's homeostatic roles and for Cox-1's upregulation in inflammation.

MECHANISM OF ACTION

Cyclooxygenase inhibition offers a simple, but incomplete, explanation for the analgesic, anti-inflammatory, and toxic effects of NSAIDs. Prostaglandin E_2 (PGE_2) is generated at sites of tissue injury and sensitizes peripheral afferent nociceptors to the actions of bradykinin, substance P, and other pain mediators.[2] This gives rise to a state of hyperalgesia, in which the magnitude of the response to subsequent stimulation is increased and/or the threshold for stimulation is decreased.[3] NSAID treatment does not elevate the normal pain threshold but normalizes the hyperalgesic response after tissue injury, an effect largely attributed to reduction of peripheral PGs. NSAIDs inhibit a variety of non–PG-associated inflammatory processes as well, such as superoxide production in neutrophils[4] and mononuclear cell phospholipase C activity.[5] Interestingly, the anti-inflammatory, analgesic, and cyclooxygenase-inhibitory effects of NSAIDs are not well correlated, as described here:

- Analgesic doses of aspirin (650 mg taken orally every 3 to 4 hours) inhibit PG synthesis in kidney and platelets but do not suppress inflammation.[6]
- Diclofenac and etodolac are stronger inhibitors of peripheral PG synthesis than aspirin, yet neither demonstrates superior analgesic efficacy in dental patients undergoing third molar extraction.[7] Conversely, naproxen and azapropazone are weaker inhibitors of PG synthesis but stronger analgesics in this model.
- Microdialysis catheters implanted after third molar removal demonstrated that ketorolac can produce analgesia in a dose that does not reduce tissue PGE_2 concentrations.[8]

Brain and spinal cord PGs involved in the hyperalgesic response are both constitutive and inducible.[9] Prostaglandins have been isolated from spinal cord preparations,[10,11] and PGE_2 administered intrathecally provokes hyperalgesia.[12] Repetitive stimulation or treatment with cytokines causes hyperalgesia with a concomitant upregulation of spinal Cox-2 messenger RNA (mRNA).[13,14] Intrathecal administration of NSAIDs or coxibs blocks the hyperalgesia, but Cox-1–specific inhibitors have no effect.[15] This suggests that Cox-2 may play a dominant role in central sensitization.[16]

GENERAL PROPERTIES OF NSAIDS

This discussion does not review the properties of individual drugs, because this information is readily available in standard pharmacology textbooks. NSAIDs are a chemically heterogeneous group with many common features. Generally, the choice of drug depends on pharmacokinetics (including available dosage forms) and selectivity for Cox-1 or Cox-2. The NSAIDs most useful in perioperative pain vary widely in potency but tend to have shorter half-lives and therefore more rapid onset and more rapid approach to steady-state concentrations after repeated doses (Table 18–1). Long-acting NSAIDs (e.g., piroxicam, with a half-life of 57 hours) are more advantageous in chronic pain states, in which a

longer dose interval may improve compliance. NSAIDs with parenteral formulations (e.g., ketorolac) are obviously useful in the acute surgical setting. Most NSAIDs have excellent oral bioavailability and are cleared by hepatic metabolism. The majority of NSAIDs are highly protein bound, and for some of them (e.g., aspirin), protein binding may become saturated within the clinical dose range—meaning that an increase in dose may lead to a higher free drug concentration.[17,18] The majority of NSAIDs are weakly acidic, and they are largely ionized at physiological pH. Because intracellular pH is relatively alkaline compared with the extracellular inflammatory milieu, intracellular ion trapping can occur and facilitate NSAID entry into cells.[17] Nonselective NSAIDs are surprisingly variable in their relative amounts of Cox-1 and Cox-2 inhibition, and they affect PG synthesis differently in various compartments within the body.[19]

Clinical Efficacy in Postoperative Pain

GENERAL CONSIDERATIONS

Oral and parenteral NSAIDs are effective postoperative analgesics in most types of surgery. Virtually all have been compared with placebo through the use of the classic model of third molar extraction. In this mild to moderate pain model, the NSAID is used alone when local anesthesia wears off, and the results are usually expressed directly as changes in pain scores. In more severe pain states, NSAIDs are combined with opioids, and the magnitude of "opioid-sparing" is more likely to be the measurement.

A word of caution is necessary regarding the design and interpretation of opioid-sparing studies. In these studies, an opioid is typically titrated to make the patient comfortable and then is stopped until the patient requests more analgesia. The NSAID or comparator is given, and demand intravenous (IV) opioid dosing from a patient-controlled analgesia (PCA) device is used to maintain acceptable analgesia. The problem with these studies can be seen in Figure 18–1. Opioids have steep concentration–response curves, meaning that the

TABLE 18–1	NSAID Half-lives and Plasma Concentrations of NSAIDs at Usual Therapeutic Doses	
Drug	**Half-life (hr)**	**Concentration (μM)[*]**
Naproxen	14	1.3
Ibuprofen	2	38–111
Fenoprofen	3	89.5
Ketoprofen	2	9.4
Indomethacin	4	1.4
Sulindac	7[†]	14.6[‡]
Diclofenac	1	6.1
Ketorolac	5	8.0

[*]Data from Cryer B, Feldman M: Cyclooxygenase-1 and cyclooxygenase-2 selectivity of widely used nonsteroidal anti-inflammatory drugs. Am J Med 1998;104:413–421.

[†]Half-life of parent drug.

[‡]Concentration of active sulfide metabolite.

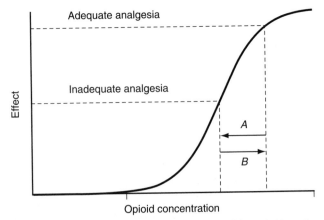

Figure 18–1 NSAID effect may be exaggerated by opioid-sparing analgesic protocols (see text for details). The small decrement in opioid plasma concentration necessary to move from adequate to inadequate analgesia is represented by *A*, and the comparably small increase necessary to restore adequate analgesia is represented by *B*.

difference between adequate and inadequate pain relief may represent a very small decrement in opioid concentration (*A* in Fig. 18–1). It follows that a relatively modest change in opioid effect (due to *potentiation* by an NSAID) may be sufficient to restore adequate pain relief (*B* in Fig. 18–1). The result is an apparently large analgesic effect from the NSAID, but much of it is actually due to the opioid. Opioid-sparing studies have been used to support misleading claims that various NSAIDs are similar in efficacy to morphine in moderate to severe postoperative pain. (See also the Addendum on page 176.)

The following sections describe the literature on NSAID use for acute pain in a variety of clinical settings. The discussion of analgesic efficacy is limited to surgical procedures that have been reasonably well-studied—that is, a sufficient number of randomized controlled trials (RCTs) have been performed to permit recommendations for clinical practice. The strength of evidence is categorized by the following criteria[20]:

Level A—Recommendations are based on good and consistent scientific evidence.

Level B—Recommendations are based on limited or inconsistent scientific evidence.

Level C—Recommendations are based primarily on consensus viewpoint or expert opinion.

THORACIC SURGERY

Posterolateral thoracotomy is among the most debilitating procedures, typically involving a skin incision that begins in the second or third thoracic dermatome and extends anteriorly to cross many additional dermatomes. Postoperative discomfort from the incision and rib shingling accompanies tidal breathing, pulmonary toilet, and movement. Typically, two large thoracic drains are placed at the conclusion of the procedure, one of which extends superiorly into the posterior thoracic gutter and may cause pleuritic pain, even with a successful epidural block.[21] In addition, thoracotomy often produces severe ipsilateral shoulder pain that results from reflection of pericardial and diaphragmatic pleura, which is referred via phrenic afferents.[22] In one series of 1200 postoperative patients, those undergoing posterolateral thoracotomy most often required additional analgesia in the immediate postoperative period.[23]

BOX 18–1	NSAIDS IN THORACIC SURGERY

NSAIDs are associated with an opioid-sparing effect and a modest improvement in pain after thoracotomy (level B evidence); however, the efficacy is no greater than that which can be achieved with opioid alone (level A evidence). Studies that add NSAIDs to thoracic epidural analgesia demonstrate little further benefit. Too few patients have been assessed for one to conclude that NSAID therapy (and decreased opioid) improves pulmonary function. One study showed that a Cox-2 preferential inhibitor, nimesulide, lowered morphine requirements after thoracotomy. NSAIDs reduce opioid consumption in video-assisted thoracoscopic surgery but do not increase analgesic effect or improve pulmonary function (level B evidence). Insufficient data are available about NSAID treatment of ipsilateral shoulder pain.

Because thoracotomy is associated with such severe postoperative pain, NSAIDs are not considered for use alone (Box 18–1). Diclofenac, indomethacin, ketorolac, piroxicam, and tenoxicam have all been studied in small RCTs as part of multimodal approaches that include opioids and/or regional anesthesia (Table 18–2). The endpoints are generally visual analogue scale (VAS) scores for incisional pain, amount of opioid consumed, and indices of pulmonary function. No NSAIDs have been studied for treatment of ipsilateral shoulder pain that accompanies thoracotomy. Results of these trials can be summarized as follows:

• Diclofenac[24,25] and indomethacin[26,27] have been found to reduce post-thoracotomy opioid use and VAS pain scores. Continuous intravenous infusion of diclofenac added to intercostal nerve blocks (T3–T7) lowered morphine consumption by 60% and 76% during the first and second postoperative days, respectively, and significantly reduced shoulder pain at 20 and 24 hours after surgery.

• Intramuscular ketorolac diminished the need for analgesic rescue (i.e., additional analgesic needed to treat acute pain) when added to a combination of intercostal nerve blocks and intramuscular (IM) papaveretum; no differences in opioid consumption or pain scores were

TABLE 18–2	Efficacy of NSAIDs in Thoracotomy					
Study	**Number of Patients**	**NSAID**	**Regional Block**	**↓ Pain**	**↓ Opioid**	**RCT**
Perttunen et al[24]	30	Diclofenac	Intercostal	Yes	Yes	Yes
Rhodes et al[25]	44	Diclofenac	Intercostal	Yes	Yes	Yes
Murphy & Medley[26]	50	Indomethacin		Yes*	Yes*	No
Pavy et al[27]	60	Indomethacin		Yes	Yes	Yes
Power et al[28]	75	Ketorolac	Intercostal	No	No	Yes
Merry et al[31]	20	Tenoxicam		No	Yes	Yes
Merry et al[32]	45	Tenoxicam	Intercostal, epidural	Yes	No	Yes
Bigler et al[33]	28	Piroxicam	Epidural	No	No	Yes
Singh et al[29]	62	Ketorolac	Epidural	Yes	Yes	Yes
Carretta et al[240]	30	Ketorolac		No	Yes	Yes

*Historical controls.
RCT, randomized controlled trial.

noted, however.[28] The requirement for patient-controlled epidural hydromorphone was reduced to the same extent by intravenous ketorolac and the addition of bupivacaine to the epidural mixture.[29] In this study, postoperative peak expiratory flow rates were significantly greater in the ketorolac group, although still decreased from baseline. One study showed that pretreatment with ketorolac and morphine produced identical analgesic effects during chest tube removal.[30]

- Addition of IV or oral tenoxicam[31,32] or piroxicam[33] to thoracic epidural anesthesia decreased pain at rest but did not improve pain with coughing or pulmonary function.

Video-assisted thoracoscopic surgery (VATS) is a common procedure for lung biopsies and small parenchymal resections. It is less invasive and produces more limited tissue damage than thoracotomy. Although there is no universal agreement on the analgesic benefits of endoscopic surgery, VATS appears to cause less postoperative pain than thoracotomy, as measured by need for intercostal or epidural block and opioid rescue.[34] A single trial assessed the efficacy of a 48-hour continuous infusion of diclofenac or ketorolac in 30 patients after VATS.[35] Cumulative morphine consumption was reduced by equivalent amounts in both NSAID groups relative to placebo; no differences in VAS scores or pulmonary function were found.

Evidence also suggests a role for central Cox-2 in mediating post-thoracotomy pain. In one study, cerebrospinal fluid from 30 thoracotomy patients was evaluated for 6-keto-$PGF_{1\alpha}$, the principal metabolite of PGE_2. Levels of the metabolite rose fourfold after surgery—a change that was suppressed by nimesulide, a Cox-2 preferential inhibitor. Pain scores and morphine requirements were each lower in the nimesulide arm of the study.[36]

GYNECOLOGICAL LAPAROSCOPY

Laparoscopic surgery is probably associated with less pain,[37,38] earlier discharge from the hospital,[39] and reduced overall morbidity[40] than the corresponding procedures performed with laparotomy. Reviews, however, now suggest that the advantage is not as consistent or as large as originally thought.[41] Pain after laparoscopic procedures can be related to the incision or abdominal distention or it can be referred to the shoulder, and it follows a variable course. Important factors are the volume of residual gas, pressure created by the pneumoperitoneum, and the rate of insufflation. Distention can cause pain through tearing of blood vessels, traction of nerves, and release of inflammatory mediators. Intraperitoneal acidosis, from either accumulation of carbonic acid or tissue ischemia, may contribute as well.[42] Postlaparoscopy shoulder pain is similar to that experienced after thoracotomy and reflects diaphragmatic irritation that is referred via phrenic afferents. Shoulder pain accompanies 35% to 63% of laparoscopic procedures and has been reported to be the predominant type of pain on the second postoperative day, whereas visceral pain dominates within the initial 24 hours.[43]

Gynecological laparoscopic procedures are diagnostic or involve the fallopian tubes or ovaries. Tubal ligation, the most common operation, can be accomplished by several methods, with clip sterilization producing less postoperative

discomfort.[44] The magnitude of visceral pain after tubal or ovarian manipulation may be influenced by local PG release. The concentration of $PGF_{2\alpha}$ in the fallopian tube is approximately 10 times higher than that in plasma, and the ovarian follicle contains both PGE_2 and $PGF_{2\alpha}$ in significant amounts.[45] Laparoscopic manipulation of the oviduct and ovary may therefore result in PG release, so one might predict that this type of pain would be particularly responsive to NSAID treatment.

Surprisingly, NSAIDs are inconsistently effective in these settings (Box 18–2). There have been numerous trials, but they differ in surgical approach, timing of NSAID administration, and scheduling of pain assessment, as summarized here:

- Ketorolac has been most commonly studied, with seven prospective trials and more than 350 patients (Table 18–3). Green et al[46] investigated parenteral ketorolac in comparison with placebo administered 30 minutes before the end of surgery in 126 patients undergoing diagnostic laparoscopy or tubal ligation. Pain scores at recovery room admission, fentanyl requirements for breakthrough pain, and time to ambulation and recovery room discharge were all significantly reduced by ketorolac in patients undergoing diagnostic laparoscopy but not in those undergoing tubal ligation. Shapiro and Duffy[47] also failed to find opioid-sparing or pain reduction with use of ketorolac in 40 women having tubal ligation. DeLucia and White[48] reported that preoperative intramuscular ketorolac decreased postoperative pain and fentanyl use in unspecified laparoscopic procedures. A subsequent trial by Pandit et al[49] produced the opposite result for a nearly identical population. Finally, Campbell et al[50] studied the use of 24- to 36-hour subcutaneous infusion of ketorolac or placebo in 72 women after laparoscopic surgery. Fentanyl and codeine use was significantly greater in the placebo group, and a trend toward improved pain scores was noted in the ketorolac group; interestingly, pain scores were equivalent for patients experiencing diagnostic laparoscopy and tubal ligation.
- Naproxen,[51,52,53] diclofenac,[54,55] and tenoxicam[56,57] have not been consistently better than placebo in relation to level of postoperative pain or need for opiate rescue.

BOX 18–2	NSAIDS IN GYNECOLOGICAL LAPAROSCOPY

In gynecological laparoscopic surgery, perioperative NSAIDs produce a modest improvement in postoperative pain scores and a small decrease in the need for analgesic rescue relative to placebo (level B evidence). By themselves, NSAIDs are less effective than longer-acting opioids (level A evidence). Efficacy may be higher in diagnostic laparoscopy (level B evidence). Ketorolac is the best-studied NSAID, and the majority of data suggest a benefit relative to placebo (level B evidence); no trend is evident regarding the timing of ketorolac administration and its relationship to postoperative pain or opioid rescue (level B evidence). With the exception of a piroxicam patch (level B evidence), NSAIDs have not been effective in postlaparoscopy shoulder pain.

TABLE 18–3	Efficacy of Ketorolac in Gynecological Laparoscopy				
Study	Number of Patients	Comparator	↓ Pain	↓ Opioid	RCT
Ng et al[59]	36	Parecoxib	Yes	No	Yes
Campbell et al[50]	72	Placebo	No	Yes	Yes
DeLucia & White[48]	76	Placebo	Yes	Yes	Yes*
Green et al[46]	80	Placebo	Yes	Yes	Yes
Shapiro & Duffy[47]	40	Placebo	No	No	Yes
Pandit et al[49]	54	Placebo	No	No	Yes*
Prados & Blaylock[241]	57	Placebo	No	No	Yes*

*Abstract.
RCT, randomized controlled trial.

- Celecoxib and parecoxib have each been investigated in a single prospective study. Celecoxib demonstrated no benefit over placebo in reducing wound pain or analgesic requirements.[58] Parecoxib was less effective than ketorolac in women undergoing tubal ligation, but no placebo arm was included in the study.[59]
- Prospective comparisons of NSAIDS with opiates have been largely equivocal or unfavorable. For tubal ligation pain, NSAIDs were less effective than morphine,[60] oxycodone,[61] and tramadol[62] in the immediate postoperative period. One study, however, found that ketorolac and meperidine were equally effective.[63] Patients receiving preoperative ibuprofen were more comfortable later in the recovery period than those treated with intraoperative fentanyl,[64] although the timing of the fentanyl dose suggests that the agent may have worn off. Tenoxicam was less efficacious than intraperitoneal bupivacaine or intravenous fentanyl in individuals undergoing minor laparoscopic procedures.[65]

A few studies have examined the effect of NSAID treatment on postlaparoscopy shoulder pain. Edwards et al[55] found no difference between diclofenac and placebo in treating shoulder pain after diagnostic laparoscopy or tubal ligation. Shoulder pain was unchanged in indomethacin-treated patients[66] and greater in naproxen-treated[53] patients despite global reductions in pain scores. Celecoxib produced a significant reduction in postlaparoscopy shoulder pain, but overall pain scores and analgesic requirements were indistinguishable from those in individuals receiving placebo.[58] A piroxicam patch was more effective than bilateral suprascapular blocks in reducing pain and analgesic requirements 6 and 12 hours after outpatient (ambulatory) laparoscopy.[67]

LAPAROSCOPIC CHOLECYSTECTOMY

As stated previously, the benefits of the laparoscopic approach for postoperative pain are not universally acknowledged, although some studies find less pain and better pulmonary function after laparoscopy than after the open procedure.[68] Nonselective NSAIDs and coxibs have been extensively investigated for postcholecystectomy pain, with much more consistent benefit than seen in gynecological procedures (Box 18–3). Perioperative ketorolac,[69,70] diclofenac,[71] indomethacin,[72] rofecoxib,[73] and a parecoxib/valdecoxib[74] combination regimen have all been shown to

be more effective than placebo at reducing postoperative pain and/or analgesic requirements (see Table 18–4). Lane et al[70] studied intramuscular administration of ketorolac (before and after the procedure) in 125 patients and found that its activity compared favorably with that of meperidine. Liu et al[75] investigated the effects of ketorolac pretreatment on postoperative analgesia and ventilation. Pain and several indices of pulmonary function were significantly improved in the ketorolac group. Intraperitoneal (IP) instillation of a lidocaine/tenoxicam mixture was superior to IP lidocaine plus IV tenoxicam with respect to both pain and analgesic consumption.[76] Preoperative IV parecoxib and a 4-day course of postoperative oral valdecoxib was investigated in 193 patients and found to reduce both morphine consumption and opioid-related symptoms.[74] Rofecoxib premedication reduced the number of patients requiring opioid after discharge from the post–anesthesia care unit (PACU) but made no difference in times to hospital discharge.[73]

NONLAPAROSCOPIC GYNECOLOGICAL SURGERY

NSAIDs have been evaluated as treatment for discomfort associated with nonlaparoscopic gynecological procedures, including hysteroscopy, endometrial biopsy, hysterectomy, and dilation and curettage (Box 18–4). Pain is the most common reason for failure to complete diagnostic hysteroscopy with endometrial biopsy.[77] Painful aspects of the procedure include cervical dilation and penetration, uterine expansion, and endometrial biopsy. It has been suggested that the discomfort of hysteroscopy may in part be related to PG-mediated uterine contractions,[78] indicating possible efficacy for NSAIDs during this procedure.

BOX 18–3	NSAIDS IN LAPAROSCOPIC CHOLCYSTECTOMY

NSAIDs consistently reduce pain and analgesia requirements after laparoscopic cholecystectomy (level A evidence). No benefit is proven for postoperative pulmonary function. Coxibs require more study, although parecoxib/valdecoxib reduced postoperative pain and opioid use (level B evidence).

TABLE 18–4	Efficacy of NSAIDs in Laparoscopic Cholecystectomy					
Study	Number of Patients	NSAID	Comparator	↓ Pain	↓ Opioid	RCT
Forse et al[72]	52	Indomethacin (I)	Ketorolac (K)	Yes (I = K)	Yes (I = K)	Yes
Fredman et al[69]	60	Diclofenac (D)	Ketorolac	Yes (D = K)	Yes (D = K)	Yes
Wilson et al[71]	55	Diclofenac	Placebo	Yes	No	Yes
Yeh et al[242]	88	Tenoxicam	Placebo	No	No	Yes
Elhakim et al[76]	90	Tenoxicam (intraperitoneal)	Placebo	Yes	Yes	Yes
Munro et al[243]	37	Tenoxicam	Placebo	No	Yes	Yes
Lane et al[70]	125	Ketorolac	Placebo	Yes	Yes	Yes
Liu et al[75]	60	Ketorolac	Placebo	Yes	Yes	Yes
Horattas et al[73]	116	Rofecoxib	Placebo	Yes	Yes	Yes
Gan et al[74]	193	Parecoxib + valdecoxib	Placebo	Yes	Yes	Yes

RCT, randomized controlled trial.

Whereas NSAIDs are not effective in treating pain during hysteroscopy, they may be useful afterward. Preoperative administration of mefenamic acid[78] or diclofenac[79] did not reduce pain associated with cervical or uterine manipulation, although recovery room discomfort was reduced with mefenamic acid. Oral dexketoprofen pretreatment was less effective than intracervical mepivacaine injection at reducing pain during or after the procedure.[80] Naproxen[53] given preoperatively reduced posthysteroscopy/postlaparoscopy pain in 60 women undergoing infertility assessment.

Data from other gynecological procedures have generally confirmed the results for hysteroscopy. Ketorolac was not an adequate substitute for fentanyl during propofol–nitrous oxide general anesthesia for dilation and curettage, cone biopsy, and vulvar laser surgery,[81] and combining ketorolac with fentanyl did not reduce recovery times or postoperative side effects. Oral flurbiprofen, by itself, was inferior to intramuscular morphine for moderate to severe pain after hysterectomy, laparotomy, and cesarean section.[82] After tenoxicam pretreatment, patients self-administered significantly fewer epidural boluses of a bupivacaine/fentanyl mixture after major gynecological procedures.[83] Postoperative administration of parecoxib was associated with significantly decreased morphine PCA use during the first 24 hours.[84]

OBSTETRICAL PROCEDURES

Obstetrical indications for NSAID use include treatment of pain accompanying episiotomy, postpartum vaginal tears, cesarean section, and uterine cramping (Box 18–5).

Episiotomy and uterine cramping have been well studied as models of analgesic efficacy and have shown excellent sensitivity for detecting differences among peripherally and centrally acting analgesics.[85] Episiotomy pain and uterine cramps probably represent qualitatively different pain states, because aspirin is effective in both but codeine is ineffective for uterine cramping.[86] Efficacy for both types of pain is desirable in postpartum pain. Results of other studies can be summarized as follows:

- Naproxen has demonstrated superiority over codeine and placebo in postpartum uterine pain that includes cramping.[87]
- Sunshine et al[88,89] compared ketoprofen and indoprofen with aspirin and placebo in two studies of parturients with moderate to severe postepisiotomy, cramping, or cesarean section pain. Both ketoprofen and indoprofen were significantly better than placebo, and ketoprofen gave faster and significantly longer pain relief than aspirin.
- Ibuprofen alone and in combination with codeine was effective in a study of mixed gynecological procedures, including use for postepisiotomy pain.[90]

NSAIDs are consistently effective in reducing post–cesarean section pain and uterine cramping as well as lowering postoperative opioid consumption. Table 18–5 lists trials of NSAIDs in cesarean section using general or regional anesthesia with or without a neuraxial opiate.

BOX 18–4	NSAIDS IN NONLAPAROSCOPIC GYNECOLOGICAL SURGERY

NSAIDs were ineffective when used intraoperatively during diagnostic hysteroscopy but were more effective after the procedure (level B evidence). NSAIDs and parecoxib were effective after open gynecological procedures when combined with opioids and/or epidural analgesia (level B evidence).

BOX 18–5	NSAIDS FOR OBSTETRICAL PROCEDURES

NSAIDs reduce pain after vaginal delivery, episiotomy, and cesarean section (level B evidence); NSAIDs also appear to provide relief from postcesarean uterine cramps (level B evidence). NSAIDs should not be routinely administered prior to cesarean section because they may induce premature closure of the fetal ductus arteriosus (level C evidence). NSAIDs do not accumulate in breast milk during typical perioperative therapy (level B evidence).

TABLE 18–5	Efficacy of NSAIDs in Cesarean Section						
Study	Number of Patients	NSAID	Comparator(s)	Anesthesia	↓ Pain	↓ Opioid	RCT
Rorarius et al[244]	90	Diclofenac	Ketoprofen & placebo	Any	Yes	Yes	Yes
Elhakim et al[245]	50	Tenoxicam	Placebo	GA	Yes	Yes	Yes
Bush et al[246]	50	Diclofenac	Placebo	GA	Yes	Yes	Yes
Pavy et al[247]	50	Ketorolac	Placebo	Any	No	Yes	Yes
Lowder et al[248]	44	Ketorolac	Placebo	Any	Yes	Yes	Yes
Wilder-Smith et al[249]	120	Diclofenac	Tramadol & placebo	Spinal	Yes	Yes	Yes
Olofsson et al[250]	50	Diclofenac	Placebo	Spinal	Yes	Yes	Yes
Lim et al[251]	48	Diclofenac	Placebo	Any	No	Yes	Yes
Dennis et al[252]	50	Diclofenac	Placebo	Spinal	No	Yes	Yes
Cardoso et al[253]	120	Diclofenac q8h	Diclofenac PRN	Spinal	q8h >PRN*	Yes	Yes
Sun et al[254]	120	Diclofenac	Placebo	Epidural	No	No	Yes

*Diclofenac administered at regular 8-hr intervals (q8h) was more effective than diclofenac dosed as needed (PRN).
RCT, randomized controlled trial.

The use of NSAIDs before or after delivery may produce a number of unwanted effects. The tocolytic effect and platelet inhibition may cause excessive bleeding, and maternal-to-fetal transfer may affect the fetal ductus arteriosus. The tocolytic dose appears to be lower than that causing premature ductal closure.[91] Administration of indomethacin was demonstrated to inhibit premature labor without evidence of premature ductal closure.[92] NSAIDs do not accumulate to any appreciable extent in breast milk and are not thought to represent a hazard to the infants of breast-feeding mothers.[93]

ORTHOPEDIC SURGERY

NSAID treatment has been extensively studied for a variety of orthopedic procedures, including joint replacement, arthroscopy, and spinal surgery (Box 18–6). Apart from the considerable tissue trauma that may accompany them, many procedures involve the manipulation of tissues in which a substantial amount of inflammation already exists. Unlike in other clinical situations, patients presenting for orthopedic surgery have commonly been treated with NSAIDs preoperatively, so the presence of residual analgesia or toxicity can be incorrectly attributed to perioperative therapy. Efficacy has been demonstrated with oral, rectal, intravenous, and intra-articular NSAID preparations. They have been used in conjunction with general, spinal, and epidural anesthesia, but almost no information is available on their use to supplement regional blocks.

Arthroscopy

In aggregate, the data show that NSAIDs are active in postarthroscopy pain (Table 18–6); these findings can be summarized as follows:

- Code et al[94] randomly assigned 66 patients to receive preoperative naproxen or placebo. Postoperative pain was decreased during hospitalization and 24 hours after discharge in the NSAID group, and a reduction in postdischarge analgesic use was also noted.
- Ogilvie-Harris et al[95] studied individuals undergoing arthroscopic meniscectomy who were randomly assigned to receive either naproxen or placebo. Naproxen treatment was associated with significantly less pain at rest and with movement, reduced analgesic use, and less synovitis and effusion than placebo.
- Several studies have compared preoperative and postoperative NSAID treatment, with conflicting results. Three studies of diclofenac concluded that timing did not seem to influence pain relief before discharge.[96-98] A 60-patient study of rofecoxib found that preoperative treatment was better than postoperative treatment with respect to time to first opioid use, 24-hour analgesic consumption, and pain with movement.[99] The difference may be related to pharmacokinetics, because diclofenac (half-life 1 hour) reaches peak steady-state concentrations much faster than rofecoxib (half-life 17 hours).
- Comparisons of diclofenac with ketorolac[100] and of ketoprofen with dexketoprofen[101] demonstrated equivalence between these nonselective NSAIDs; diclofenac was superior to indomethacin with respect to pain relief and analgesic requirements.[102]

BOX 18–6	NSAIDS IN ORTHOPEDIC SURGERY

NSAIDs are consistently effective analgesics for pain after arthroscopic surgery (level A evidence), and timing of administration does not influence analgesia with the short-acting NSAID diclofenac. Most direct comparisons show that various NSAIDs have similar efficacy and are equivalent or superior to oral opioids (level A evidence). In spine surgery and in total joint arthroplasties, NSAIDs are effective in lowering pain scores and decreasing opioid requirements (level A evidence). There are insufficient data to demonstrate efficacy for coxibs in spine surgery, but these agents are effective in total joint arthroplasty (level B evidence).

| TABLE 18–6 | Efficacy of NSAIDs in Arthroscopy |

Study	Number of Patients	NSAID	Comparator(s)	↓ Pain	↓ Opioid	RCT
Dahl et al[105]	61	Ibuprofen	Acetaminophen	Yes	Yes	Yes
Reuben et al[99]	60	Rofecoxib	Placebo	Yes	Yes	Yes
Rautoma et al[255]	200	Diclofenac	Placebo	Yes	No	Yes
Hoe-Hansen & Norlin[256]	41	Ketoprofen	Placebo	Yes	Yes	Yes
Code et al[94]	66	Naproxen	Placebo	Yes	Yes	Yes
Sandin et al[97]	64	Diclofenac	Placebo	Yes	No	Yes
Nelson et al[96]	67	Diclofenac	Placebo	Yes	Yes	Yes
Rasmussen et al[257]	120	Naproxen	Placebo	Yes	No	Yes
Smith et al[258]	60	Ketorolac	Placebo	No	No	Yes
Arviddson & Eriksson[259]	40	Piroxicam	Placebo	Yes	N/A	Yes
Ogilvie-Harris et al[95]	139	Naproxen	Placebo	Yes	N/A	Yes
Norris et al[98]	127	Diclofenac	Placebo	No	No	Yes
Pedersen et al[260]	87	Naproxen	Placebo	No	Yes	Yes
Morrow et al[261]	71	Diclofenac (D)	Ketorolac (K)	D = K	D = K	Yes
Berti et al[101]	45	Dexketoprofen	Ketoprofen	Yes	No	Yes
Dennis et al[100]	40	Ketorolac (K)	Diclofenac (D)	(K = D)	(K = D)	Yes
Van Lancker et al[106]	100	Tenoxicam	Placebo	No	No	Yes
Barber & Gladu[103]	125	Ketorolac (K)	Hydrocodone (H)	K > H	K > H	Yes
White et al[104]	252*	Ketorolac (K)	Hydrocodone (H) & placebo	K = H	K = H	Yes
Twersky et al[262]	69	Ketorolac (K)	Fentanyl (F)	Early F > K; late K > F	N/A	Yes
Laitenen et al[102]	75	Indomethacin (I)	Diclofenac & oxycodone (O)	D > I = O	D > I = O	Yes
McLoughlin et al[263]	60	Diclofenac	Fentanyl & placebo	D = F	D = F	Yes
Drez et al[264]	52	Naproxen (N)	Propoxyphene (P)	N > P	N = P	Yes
Morrow et al[265]	60	Piroxicam (P)	Bupivacaine (B)	P + B > P	P + B > P	Yes
Gurkan et al[266]	40	Diclofenac	Bupivacaine & placebo	Yes	Yes	Yes

*Included laparoscopy patients.
RCT, randomized controlled trial.

• In studies across analgesic classes, NSAIDs were equivalent to hydrocodone/acetaminophen combinations[103,104] and superior to oxycodone[102] and acetaminophen.[101,105,106] Barber and Gladu[103] found that ketorolac provided better pain relief than hydrocodone immediately after anterior cruciate ligament reconstruction. White et al[104] studied 68 patients with moderate to severe postarthroscopy pain who were randomly assigned to receive either ketorolac or hydrocodone/acetaminophen. No differences in analgesic efficacy of the two treatments were observed at any point.[104]

Intra-articular injection of NSAIDs has been compared with intra-articular placebo and local anesthetic with and without opiate as well as with intravenous administration of NSAIDs; findings are as follows:

• Intra-articular tenoxicam proved superior to the intravenous formulation in two studies involving nearly 150 patients.[107,108] The addition of intra-articular tenoxicam[108] or ketorolac[109] to intra-articular bupivacaine or morphine, respectively, reduced postoperative pain scores more than the non-NSAID individual treatments.

• Izdes et al[110] found a benefit from addition of intra-articular piroxicam to bupivacaine in patients with articular inflammation confirmed by synovial biopsy; no benefit was observed in patients with a biopsy result negative for inflammation.

Spine Surgery

NSAIDs are effective in various types of spine surgery, including diskectomy, laminectomy, and stabilization (Table 18–7); findings can be summarized as follows:

• Piroxicam,[111] tenoxicam,[112] and indomethacin[113,114] have been shown to provide superior pain relief and to reduce opioid requirements in comparison with placebo in spine surgery.

• Combination regimens consisting of an IV opioid (using PCA) plus ketorolac were superior to those using PCA alone in spine stabilization[115,116] and diskectomy.[117]

• The data on coxibs are inconsistent. Treatment with rofecoxib or celecoxib was no different from treatment with placebo in reducing postdiskectomy pain or opioid requirements[118,119]; however, a combination of either coxib plus opioid PCA provided better analgesia than opioid PCA alone after spine stabilization.[120]

Arthroplasty

NSAIDs and coxibs have been compared with placebo, with intrathecal and intravenous opiates, and with one another in joint replacement surgery (Table 18–8); data are as follows:

• Ibuprofen,[121] rofecoxib,[122] valdecoxib,[123] and parecoxib[124,125] provided better analgesia and reduced opiate use in comparison with placebo.

TABLE 18–7	Efficacy of NSAIDs in Spine Surgery					
Study	Number of Patients	NSAID	Comparator(s)	↓ Pain	↓ Opioid	RCT
Pookarnjanamorakot et al[111]	50	Piroxicam	Placebo	Yes	Yes	Yes
De Decker et al[112]	60	Piroxicam (P)	Tenoxicam (T) & placebo	Yes P, yes T	Yes P, yes T	Yes
Mack et al[267]	30	Ketorolac (K)	Bupivacaine (B)	K = B	K = B	Yes
Le Roux & Samudrala[117]	55	Ketorolac	Placebo	Yes	Yes	Yes
Reuben et al[115]	70	Ketorolac	Placebo	Yes	Yes	Yes
Rosenow et al[268]	96	Lomoxicam (L)	Morphine (M)	L = M	N/A	Yes
Reuben et al[116]	80	Ketorolac	Placebo	Yes	Yes	Yes
Fletcher et al[269]	60	Ketoprofen	Placebo	Yes	No	Yes
Nissen et al[114]	56	Indomethacin	Placebo	Yes	Yes	Yes
McGlew et al[113]	100	Indomethacin	Placebo	Yes	Yes	Yes
Thienthong et al[270]	56	Lomoxicam	Placebo	No	No	Yes

RCT, randomized controlled trial.

- Etches et al[126] treated 174 patients with a continuous ketorolac infusion; they reported better analgesia, less sedation, and reduced morphine and antiemetic requirements with ketorolac than with placebo.
- Intravenous ketorolac (30 mg) and parecoxib (20 or 40 mg) were compared with placebo and morphine (4 mg) in 208 patients undergoing total knee replacement.[125] The higher dose of parecoxib was equivalent to ketorolac and superior to both morphine and placebo.

NSAIDs have also been studied for joint surgery in conjunction with intrathecal and intravenous opiates; the findings can be summarized as follows:

- Addition of oral ibuprofen[127] to intrathecal morphine did not improve analgesia or diminish opiate requirements.

- Intravenous ketoprofen was as effective as epidural morphine (4 mg) for pain of total knee or total hip arthroplasty and produced fewer side effects.[128]
- Iohom et al[129] studied oral dexketoprofen before and after total hip arthroplasty under spinal anesthesia using bupivacaine plus morphine. Compared to placebo treatment, the NSAID group had less pain, lower opioid requirements, less nausea and sedation, and lower plasma interleukin-6 concentrations.
- Addition of NSAID to buprenorphine,[130] papaveretum,[131] and morphine PCA[132] resulted in better analgesia and lower opiate requirements than morphine PCA alone.

TABLE 18–8	Efficacy of NSAIDs in Joint Replacement					
Study	Number of Patients	NSAID	Comparator(s)	↓ Pain	↓ Opioid	RCT
Bugter et al[127]	50	Ibuprofen	Placebo	No	No	Yes
Iohom et al[129]	30	Dexketoprofen	Placebo	Yes	Yes	Yes
Silvanto et al[271]	64	Diclofenac (D)	Ketoprofen (Ke) & placebo	Yes D, yes Ke	Yes D, yes Ke	Yes
Zhou et al[272]	164	Ketorolac	Placebo	No	No	Yes
Kostamovaara et al[273]	85	Ketorolac (K)	Diclofenac & ketoprofen (Ke)	K = D = Ke	K = D = Ke	Yes
Eggers et al[274]	101	Tenoxicam	Placebo	No	Yes	Yes
Beattie et al[275]	130	Ketorolac	Placebo	Yes	Yes	Yes
Etches et al[126]	174	Ketorolac	Placebo	No	Yes	Yes
Fragen et al[276]	59	Ketorolac	Placebo	No	Yes	Yes
Dahl et al[121]	123	Ibuprofen	Placebo	Yes	Yes	Yes
Hommeril et al[128]	32	Ketoprofen (Ke)	Epidural morphine (M)	Ke = M	Ke = M	Yes
Boeckstyns et al[130]	81	Piroxicam	Placebo	Yes	Yes	Yes
Anderson et al[131]	60	Diclofenac	Placebo	Yes	Yes	Yes
Segstro et al[132]	50	Indomethacin	Placebo	Yes	Yes	Yes
Buvanendran et al[122]	70	Rofecoxib	Placebo	Yes	Yes	Yes
Malan et al[124]	201	Parecoxib	Placebo	Yes	Yes	Yes
Rasmussen et al[125]	208	Parecoxib (P)	Ketorolac (K) & placebo	Yes P, yes K	Yes P, yes K	Yes
Reuben et al[277]	100	Rofecoxib	Placebo	Yes	No	Yes

RCT, randomized controlled trial.

Toxicity

As discussed earlier, prostaglandin (PG) synthesis is both inducible and constitutive, the latter playing a key role in the homeostatic function of a variety of tissues. NSAIDs, by virtue of cyclooxygenase inhibition, can disrupt vital housekeeping functions of PGs and thereby have undesirable consequences. Given the important role of PGs in the kidney, vasculature, and gut, it is not surprising that NSAIDs have significant side effects in these tissues. The effects of NSAIDs on bone growth receive less attention, but they may have special relevance for orthopedic surgery. Adverse effects such as bronchospasm, CNS toxicity (headache, confusion, aseptic meningitis), hepatitis, cutaneous reactions, and allergy are not discussed here, because they have not been particularly related to perioperative use of NSAIDs.

RENAL TOXICITY

PGs are produced in the cortex and medulla of the kidney.[133] Cortical PGs are produced by the glomerulus as well as afferent and efferent arterioles, where they modulate the effects of norepinephrine, angiotensin II, and vasopressin on renal blood flow and glomerular filtration.[134] Medullary production of PGs occurs predominantly in the collecting tubules and serves to regulate fluid and electrolyte transport. Both cyclooxygenase isoforms are constitutively expressed in the kidney, although the exact contribution of Cox-2 to homeostatic function is unknown (Box 18–7).[135]

The glomerular arterioles represent the main point of resistance to glomerular plasma flow and are the major determinant of glomerular filtration rate (GFR). In conscious euvolemic patients with normal cardiovascular, hepatic, endocrine, and renal function, endogenous PG synthesis does not play a significant role in the regulation of GFR. Renal PG production is critical, however, in maintaining GFR in the presence of acute or chronic volume depletion.[136] In such a situation, preservation of renal blood flow and GFR becomes dependent on PG synthesis ("prostaglandin-dependent").[134] Most NSAIDs have been tested for their effects on urinary PG excretion. With the exception of sulindac, they reduce urinary PG excretion by more than 50% when administered at anti-inflammatory doses. Maximal suppression of renal PG synthesis occurs within 24 to 48 hours of treatment and is fully reversible within 72 hours of drug withdrawal[136]; no dose-response studies have been published.

Specific surgical populations are at increased risk for perioperative acute renal failure (ARF) and might therefore be more susceptible to NSAID-induced renal injury. In a systematic review of 10,865 patients undergoing cardiac, vascular, general, or biliary surgery, preexisting renal impairment, advanced age, and left ventricular dysfunction were most often associated with perioperative ARF.[137] A few small reports describe marked deterioration in renal function when NSAIDs are used in patients with cirrhosis/ascites or congestive heart failure (CHF).[138,139] This finding appears to confirm that PG-dependent patients are particularly susceptible to NSAID-associated renal toxicity. Thus far, similar toxicity has not been demonstrated in large perioperative populations; findings are summarized as follows:

- Parenteral ketorolac was evaluated retrospectively in a cohort study of 10,219 patients in comparison with opiate therapy in 10,145 controls.[140] Importantly, these groups were not matched for baseline renal status. The ketorolac and opioid groups had 109 versus 113 cases of postoperative ARF, respectively (1.07% versus 1.11%; not statistically significant). The overall risk for ARF in both groups was significantly raised by numerous factors (preexisting renal disease, cirrhosis, cancer, aminoglycoside therapy, medical or intensive care unit admission), but there were no interactions between ketorolac therapy and any predisposing factor. Prolonged ketorolac therapy (>5 days) was associated with an increased risk (odds ratio [OR] 2.08, 95% confidence interval [CI] 1.08–4.00; $P = .03$).
- A meta-analysis was conducted of data from 1204 patients with normal renal function who had been subjects in 19 NSAID studies.[141] There was an overall 18% reduction in creatinine clearance on the first postoperative day (16 mL · min^{-1} decrease; 95% CI 5–28 mL · min^{-1}) without an increase in serum creatinine concentration. The effect was significant after multiple doses but not after a single dose.

The renal effects of coxibs suggest that these compounds affect renal function similarly to the way their nonselective cousins do. Rofecoxib and indomethacin were studied in elderly patients (65–80 years). Compared with placebo, rofecoxib and indomethacin produced significant transient decreases in glomerular filtration and creatinine clearance, though there were no differences with regard to standard indices of kidney function.[142] Another study showed that treatment with celecoxib or naproxen had similar effects on renal electrolyte handling.[143]

GASTROINTESTINAL TOXICITY

Gastric PGs play a central role in maintaining the integrity of the gastrointestinal (GI) mucosal barrier through a variety of mechanisms. PGE_2 and PGI_2 stimulate bicarbonate ion secretion; increase mucus production and thickness, especially in response to injury; enhance mucosal blood flow; and decrease hydrogen ion production.[144] Prostaglandins reduce parietal cell hydrogen ion production by providing negative feedback inhibition of the hydrogen-potassium–adenosine triphosphatase ($H^+K^+ATPase$) pump.[145] They also increase mucosal blood flow, thereby rapidly removing hydrogen ions that penetrate the epithelial barrier. Gastric erosions

BOX 18–7	NSAIDS AND RENAL TOXICITY

Perioperative administration of NSAIDs to patients with normal renal function results in a transient decline in creatinine clearance but not usually a significant rise in serum creatinine concentration (level A evidence). Retrospective cohort data do not suggest that ketorolac raises the risk of acute renal failure (ARF) in comparison with opiates (level B evidence); however, several small reports suggest some association. Data on coxibs show that their effects on kidney function are similar to those of nonselective NSAIDs (level B evidence).

result when this compensatory vasodilatory response is absent.[146] Gastroduodenal PG synthesis is primarily a function of Cox-1.[147,148] However, Cox-2 mRNA is upregulated at the margins of healing ulcers and after exposure of gastric mucosa to noxious substances, suggesting a possible role for this isoform.[149]

NSAIDs damage the gastroduodenal mucosa by direct and indirect actions (the "dual-injury" hypothesis) (Box 18–8).[150] Direct damage occurs because NSAIDs are able to diffuse through the mucus layer and cause a "leaky" epithelial membrane. Injury occurs from protons that gain direct access to the gastroduodenal parenchyma. The indirect effects are due to PG inhibition and attenuation of the cytoprotective processes already described. In vitro PG inhibition correlates with the degree of gastric mucosal damage for several nonselective NSAIDs.[151] Gastroduodenal damage from long-term nonselective NSAID use can result in hemorrhage, ulceration, and perforation and is one of the most common adverse drug events reported in the United States.[152] Apart from a previous history of GI bleeding or peptic ulcer, the most important risk factors appear to be advanced age, cardiovascular disease, and concomitant use of corticosteroids.

There is reason to believe that some GI toxicity may also occur with acute perioperative NSAID therapy. Endoscopic evidence demonstrates that gastroduodenal damage rapidly accompanies oral administration of a single analgesic dose of aspirin (650 mg). In 12 healthy subjects, well-defined areas of gastric submucosal hemorrhage appeared within 2 hours and erosions within 24 hours in all subjects.[153] Administration of a second dose of aspirin caused only a slight enlargement of the area of hemorrhage. A separate study of 5 volunteers showed multiple petechiae in the gastric antrum and fundus within 1 hour, and 80% of the lesions were still present at 24 hours.[154]

Parenteral ketorolac was evaluated retrospectively in a cohort study covering 10,272 courses of therapy to assess the incidence of postoperative GI and operative site bleeding in comparison with parenteral opiate therapy given to matched controls.[155] The relative risk for GI bleeding in ketorolac-treated patients was 1.30 (95% CI 1.11–1.52). Increases in dose, duration of therapy, and patient age were also important factors. Cumulative data from 15 placebo-controlled trials of perioperative NSAID therapy (2 to 7 days

in duration) did not show an increased risk, although complications earlier than 48 hours were not measured.[156]

Protective strategies have been effective in limiting NSAID-induced GI damage during long-term administration, but their benefits during short-term administration are unknown. Misoprostol (PGE_1) serves as prostaglandin replacement therapy that can reduce the incidence of perforated ulcers and gastric obstructions by as much as 90%; however, patients frequently discontinue therapy because of diarrhea and flatulence.[157] Histamine type 2 antagonist therapy with ranitidine reduces the rate of duodenal, but not gastric, ulceration.[158,159] The proton-pump inhibitor, omeprazole, is superior to both ranitidine and misoprostol in preventing and healing peptic ulcers associated with long-term NSAID administration.[160,161] No evidence has been collected regarding this interaction in the perioperative setting.

The Vioxx Gastrointestinal Outcomes Research (VIGOR) study and the Celecoxib Long-term Arthritis Safety Study (CLASS) have demonstrated that coxibs preserve gastric PG synthesis and unquestionably produce less chronic GI toxicity than nonselective NSAIDs.[162,163] These data figure prominently in the ongoing debate about the risks and benefits of these agents. Because no significant GI risk has been demonstrated for acute perioperative NSAID administration, it is difficult to postulate an advantage for coxibs.

CARDIOVASCULAR TOXICITY

Thromboembolic Events

Both Cox-1 and Cox-2 are constitutively present in healthy endothelium, as well as in atherosclerotic plaques.[164,165] Systemic TXA_2 (including that derived from platelets) is exclusively produced by Cox-1,[166] whereas Cox-2 is the dominant source of PGI_2.[167] Cox-2 mRNA is upregulated by cytokines, shear and oxidative stress, and low-density lipoproteins (LDLs),[168] reflecting the chronic inflammatory nature of the atherosclerotic process.[169]

It is difficult to draw general conclusions about the cardiovascular toxicity of nonselective NSAIDs (Box 18–9). Naproxen has been found to be protective in animal models of myocardial ischemia, but other NSAIDs, such as

---

BOX 18–8   NSAIDS AND GASTROINTESTINAL TOXICITY

The potential for adverse gastrointestinal (GI) events accompanies even limited courses of NSAID therapy (level B evidence). Individuals at increased risk can be identified prospectively, and NSAIDs should be used with caution or avoided in these patients (level C evidence). Misoprostol, histamine type 2 blockers, and proton-pump inhibitors reduce the risk of adverse GI events in all patients (level A evidence). Coxibs decrease GI bleeding risk (level A evidence) associated with long-term administration; potential benefits in the perioperative period are unknown, and use of these agents must be balanced against possible problems with cardiovascular safety.

BOX 18–9   NSAIDS AND THROMBOEMBOLIC EVENTS

NSAIDs do not appear to raise cardiovascular risk, but only aspirin has been shown to have a cardioprotective effect (level A evidence). Some benefit may be possible with naproxen (level B evidence). Coxibs, including rofecoxib, celecoxib, and valdecoxib, have all been associated with increased risk of myocardial infarction, stroke, and cardiovascular death (level A evidence). The risk from parecoxib and valdecoxib is demonstrable after only 10 days of postoperative treatment in patients undergoing coronary revascularization. The evidence suggests that this is a class effect of coxibs, but the mechanism has not been well characterized. Because the coxibs are no more efficacious than other NSAIDs, evidence of their benefit must be compelling to justify their use in specific patient populations.

meclofenamate and indomethacin, have not.[170] Multiple case-controlled and retrospective observational studies have examined the relationship of naproxen and other NSAIDs to cardiovascular risk.[171-176] With the exception of one investigation by Solomon et al,[172] no studies identify a protective effect of naproxen in comparison with placebo, although two studies found naproxen to have a lower risk than other NSAIDs.[174,175] In the Solomon study, a cardioprotective effect for naproxen was identified in both sexes and for all ages, but no corresponding benefit was identified for other NSAIDs. Interestingly, the nonselective NSAIDs in the highest quintile for Cox-2 inhibition caused a rise in cardiovascular risk (OR 1.25, 95% CI 1.08–1.45).

The story of coxib-induced cardiovascular toxicity is still developing. As mentioned previously, both rofecoxib and valdecoxib have been withdrawn from the U.S. market, although there is a possibility that one or both might be reintroduced with significant restrictions. These drugs are clearly associated with excess cardiovascular morbidity and mortality (discussed later), but the magnitude of the problem and its mechanism are still undetermined. In the simplest of models, selective Cox-2 inhibition causes thrombosis and other cardiovascular morbidity because it spares TXA_2-mediated vasoconstriction and platelet aggregation, and it eliminates the beneficial effects of PGI_2. The findings are summarized as follows:

- Coxibs do decrease urinary excretion of prostacyclin metabolites in normal subjects,[177] but PGI_2 is not an important contributor to endothelial function in healthy individuals.[178] PGI_2 biosynthesis is increased in patients with severe atherosclerosis and evidence of platelet activation.[179] This finding suggests that Cox-2 may be part of a defense mechanism that limits the consequences of platelet activation by increasing PGI_2 production.
- Coxibs theoretically have some protective effects, because Cox-2 is responsible for producing inflammatory prostanoids like PGE_2 and PGH_2.[167,168] These PGs promote the release of matrix metalloproteinases that predispose to early plaque formation, plaque rupture, and platelet activation.[180,181]

The subsequent events in the coxib story have largely been driven by toxicity data from long-term administration, but a large 2005 study suggests that those findings are relevant for short-term perioperative use as well.[182] Questions concerning coxibs and cardiovascular safety were first raised by the VIGOR study, a large trial of long-term treatment with rofecoxib and naproxen.[162] Rofecoxib caused less GI toxicity but was associated with a significantly higher risk of all thrombotic events, including myocardial infarction. Because the trial did not have a placebo arm, many authorities believed that the data could also be explained by a protective effect of naproxen. The cardiovascular findings of the VIGOR study were subsequently not confirmed by CLASS,[163] another huge study that compared celecoxib with ibuprofen and diclofenac in 8059 patients with rheumatoid arthritis or osteoarthritis. It is important to stress that neither of these trials was designed with cardiovascular toxicity as a primary endpoint.

From 2000 to 2004, results of attempts to elucidate the cardiovascular safety of coxibs were inconclusive, as follows:

- Observational studies generally indicated an increased risk.[183,184]

- Studies of celecoxib and meloxicam in patients with severe coronary artery disease suggested beneficial effects.[185,186]
- Two large meta-analyses of rofecoxib reached dramatically different conclusions. Konstam et al[187] examined more than 28,000 patients (>14,000 patient-years at risk) and found no evidence for excess cardiovascular events for rofecoxib in comparison with placebo and non-naproxen NSAIDs.[187] Jüni et al[188] identified excess cardiovascular risk associated with rofecoxib in an analysis of 18 randomized controlled trials involving more than 20,000 patients.

In September 2004, the Adenomatous Polyp Prevention Trial on Vioxx (APPROVe) was stopped early. This placebo-controlled trial of 2586 patients unexpectedly showed that rofecoxib doubled the risk of cardiovascular events (hazard ratio 1.92, 95% CI 1.19–3.11), particularly myocardial infarction and ischemic stoke.[189] Importantly, the higher risk became apparent only after 18 months of treatment. When these results were announced, Merck, the manufacturer of Vioxx, withdrew the agent from the market, and a review was undertaken of a similar trial, the Adenoma Prevention with Celecoxib (APC) Study.[190] In the APC Study, a total of 2035 patients were given celecoxib, 200 or 400 mg twice daily, or placebo. Celecoxib caused a dose-related increase in deaths from all cardiovascular causes, myocardial infarction, stroke, and congestive heart failure (relative risk overall 2.8, 95% CI 1.3–6.3). This trial was also stopped prematurely.

Nussmeier et al[182] reported the results of a multicenter trial in which placebo or valdecoxib and its intravenous prodrug, parecoxib, were given to 1671 patients for 10 days after coronary artery bypass surgery.[182] Over the 30-day evaluation period, therapy with valdecoxib plus parecoxib was associated with a near quadrupling in cardiovascular events, including myocardial infarction, cardiac arrest, stroke, and pulmonary embolism (Table 18–9). This is the first clear evidence that even short-term perioperative administration of coxibs to a population at risk is associated with adverse outcomes.

Hypertension

The effects of NSAIDs on blood pressure (BP) have been well documented (Box 18–10). In volunteers, indomethacin infusions raise mean arterial blood pressure by approximately 10 mm Hg and cause a significant 30% rise in systemic vascular resistance.[191,192] This rise is almost completely explained by increases in renal and splanchnic tone, and it occurs within 2 to 3 minutes of the start of the infusion. Cardiac output drops significantly in these subjects, presumably from the combined effects of increased afterload and reduced heart rate.[193]

Many NSAIDs have been found to attenuate the effects of antihypertensive medications, including beta-blockers, angiotensin-converting enzyme (ACE) inhibitors, thiazide diuretics, prazosin, and hydralazine.[194,195] Coxibs appear to have a similar effect.[196] Rofecoxib-treated patients from the VIGOR study had a greater rise in BP than naproxen-treated controls.[162] In CLASS, the incidence of hypertension and aggravation of underlying hypertension were comparable in patients receiving celecoxib and those receiving ibuprofen

TABLE 18–9	Cardiovascular Events During 30 Days After Coronary Bypass			
Treatment*	Number of Patients	Number of Events (%)	Risk Ratio (95% CI)	P
Placebo	548	3 (0.5)	—	—
Placebo + valdecoxib	544	6 (1.1)	2.0 (0.5–8.1)	.31
Parecoxib + valdecoxib	544	11 (2.0)	3.7 (1.0–13.5)	.03
Coxib groups combined	1088	17 (1.6)	2.9 (0.8–9.9)	.08

*Patients received opioids and one of three study treatments starting the morning after surgery: (1) intravenous placebo through day 3, then oral placebo through day 10; (2) intravenous placebo through day 3, then oral valdecoxib through day 10; and (3) intravenous parecoxib through day 3, then oral valdecoxib through day 10.

CI, confidence interval.

Modified from Nussmeier NA, Whelton AA, Brown MT, et al: Complications of the COX-2 inhibitors parecoxib and valdecoxib after cardiac surgery. N Engl J Med 2005;352:1081–1091.

or diclofenac.[163,197] Six-week courses of rofecoxib and celecoxib were compared head-to-head in 1092 elderly patients receiving antihypertensive therapy. Significantly more patients in the rofecoxib group had a BP increase of >20 mm Hg (and absolute systolic BP ≥ 140 mm Hg) than in the celecoxib group; the effect was most pronounced in patients receiving angiotensin-converting enzyme inhibitors and beta-blockers.[198]

The contribution of elevated BP to perioperative cardiovascular (and cerebrovascular) risk has not been studied. A 5- to 6-mm Hg decline in diastolic BP has been estimated to reduce the incidences of stroke and coronary heart disease by 35% to 40% and 20% to 25%, respectively, over 5 years.[199] It is not clear, however, whether acute BP elevation of the magnitude produced by perioperative NSAIDs would result in incremental risk.

Congestive Heart Failure

NSAIDs have been associated with clinical decompensation in patients with left ventricular dysfunction. Impaired cardiac output reduces effective circulating blood volume,[200] in turn causing activation of renal sympathetic nerves and the renin-angiotensin system. In this situation, renal blood flow and GFR become dependent on PG synthesis.[134] Inhibition of Cox-1 and/or Cox-2 can increase preload by causing unopposed vasoconstriction or precipitating acute renal dysfunction.

No prospective data have correlated NSAID use with decompensated heart failure (Box 18–11). However, a number of observational studies suggest that NSAIDs elevate the risk of CHF in susceptible patients. In patients already diagnosed with CHF, the odds ratio for exacerbation requiring a hospital admission was 2.1 (95% CI 1.2–3.3) if they received an NSAID within the previous week.[201] Patients receiving an

NSAID prescription after the onset of CHF had an increased risk for clinical decompensation (3.8, 95% CI 1.1–12.7).[202] Similar data are not available for coxibs, although their effects may be comparable, given their equivalent effect on sodium and water handling at the kidney.

BLEEDING

Cyclooxygenase catalyzes the production of PGH_2, substrate for the generation of TXA_2. Cox-1 is constitutively present in platelets; NSAIDs inhibit Cox-1, decreasing platelet aggregation and prolonging bleeding time to varying degrees (Box 18–12). Because platelets have no nuclei, Cox-2 cannot be upregulated,[203] so selective Cox-2 inhibitors would not be expected to affect platelet activity. In general, NSAIDs produce a moderate, dose-dependent increase in bleeding time that may not exceed the upper limit of normal.[204] The majority of data relating cyclooxygenase inhibition to perioperative bleeding is derived from studies with aspirin. Although both NSAIDs and aspirin prevent PG formation, aspirin irreversibly acetylates a cyclooxygenase serine hydroxyl residue, so activation and TXA_2 production are inhibited for the life of the platelet. NSAIDs, in contrast, inhibit cyclooxygenase reversibly, so platelet function returns to baseline as the drugs are cleared.[203] Longer-acting NSAIDs such as piroxicam can inhibit aggregation for several days after treatment is discontinued.[205]

Patients at risk for increased bleeding associated with NSAID therapy in the perioperative period include those with an underlying coagulopathy, a history of alcohol abuse, or concomitant use of anticoagulants, as shown by the following findings[203]:

- Aspirin can provoke clinical bleeding in patients with borderline coagulopathy and has actually been used to improve the diagnosis of platelet–vessel wall

BOX 18–10	NSAIDS AND HYPERTENSION

Nonselective NSAIDs and coxibs can cause small rises in blood pressure in treated and untreated hypertensive individuals (level B evidence). No data are available linking this effect with long-term or short-term morbidity or mortality.

BOX 18–11	NSAIDS AND CONGESTIVE HEART FAILURE

Observational studies support an association between use of nonselective NSAIDs and exacerbation of the symptoms of congestive heart failure (level B evidence). No data are available on coxibs.

NSAIDs impair in vivo platelet aggregation and increase laboratory measures of bleeding time. Coxibs do not affect hemostasis. A large-scale prospective study found no difference in perioperative bleeding risk for patients treated with ketorolac, diclofenac, or ketoprofen (level A evidence), although urological and otolaryngological procedures appear to increase the bleeding risk with all three drugs (level B evidence). Patients undergoing tonsillectomy who are taking NSAIDs are not more likely to bleed, but they are more likely to need reoperation to control bleeding (level B evidence). A large surveillance study found no difference in bleeding between patients given ketorolac and those given opioids (level B evidence). Neuraxial analgesia and anesthesia are safe during short-term use of aspirin (level A evidence) and long-term use of NSAIDs (level B evidence).

abnormalities such as von Willebrand's disease[206] and myeloproliferative disorders.[207]

- Alcohol markedly potentiates the bleeding time prolongation due to aspirin and NSAIDs.[208] The mechanism by which this occurs is not clear but may be related to an increase in the inhibitory effect of prostacyclin on platelet aggregation.[209,210]
- Many NSAIDs are highly protein bound and displace warfarin from albumin-binding sites, thereby raising plasma concentrations of free warfarin. There are no studies definitely linking this effect to clinical bleeding.

Concerns about the adequacy of postoperative hemostasis in ketorolac-treated patients prompted a prospective 11,245-patient trial in 49 European centers.[211] Risk of surgical site bleeding was compared in patients given ketorolac, diclofenac, or ketoprofen for major procedures, including abdominal, orthopedic, gynecological, urological, and plastic/ear, nose, and throat (ENT) surgery. No differences were observed among the NSAIDs with regard to risk, and 117 of 11,245 patients (1.04% overall) had evidence of postoperative bleeding. Concomitant treatment with low-molecular-weight or unfractionated heparin was associated with greater risk, whereas plastic/ENT, gynecological, and urological procedures were independently associated with a higher risk of surgical site bleeding. The risk of perioperative bleeding has also been investigated for ketorolac in a postmarketing surveillance study of 10,272 courses of therapy.[155] The adjusted, multivariate odds ratio for operative site bleeding was no different from that in opiate-treated patients. Use of higher doses and administration to older patients may have slightly increased the risk (not statistically significant).

Additional studies have investigated whether the risk of NSAID-induced bleeding is influenced by the specific operative procedure. The oral cavity and genitourinary tract are areas of concentrated fibrinolytic activity, so the risk of antiplatelet agents may be greater for surgery at these sites.[203] In addition, for certain types of surgery (e.g., eye surgery), even minimal bleeding can cause major morbidity. The findings can be summarized as follows:

- A retrospective analysis in patients undergoing transurethral prostatectomy found a higher transfusion requirement among those taking aspirin and NSAIDs preoperatively.[212]
- Aspirin has been associated with increased bleeding after extracorporeal shock wave lithotripsy, prostate biopsy, and transurethral resection of bladder tumors.[213]
- A meta-analysis investigated NSAID use and bleeding risk in seven studies (505 patients) of tonsillectomy in a combined adult and pediatric population. There was no difference in the incidence of postoperative bleeding; however, more NSAID-treated patients needed reoperation to secure hemostasis (OR 3.8, 95% CI 1.3–11.5; $P = .02$). The number needed to harm was 29 (95% CI 17–144).[214]
- A second quantitative, systematic review of 25 tonsillectomy studies came to similar conclusions. NSAIDs did not increase rates of blood loss, postoperative bleeding, or hospital admission, but there was a significant rise in the need for reoperation (OR 2.3, 95% CI 1.12–4.83). The number need to harm was 60 (95% CI 34–227).[215]
- A review of NSAID use for all types of pediatric surgery identified four studies with significantly higher rates of postoperative bleeding.[216] Interestingly, three of these four studies involved ketorolac treatment for tonsillectomy pain.
- Continuation of aspirin therapy was not associated with greater intraoperative bleeding in cataract surgery.[217]

Orthopedic procedures commonly involve short- and long-term NSAID use, the latter typically in patients with chronic arthritis who present for surgical remedy. The data on bleeding risk are conflicting, as follows:

- A retrospective analysis in total hip arthroplasty compared 76 patients taking 11 different NSAIDs until 24 hours preoperatively with 89 patients who had discontinued NSAID treatment for at least 48 hours.[218] No difference between the groups was found with respect to intraoperative fluid administration, need for transfusion, postoperative wound drainage, maximal drop in hematocrit, or duration of hospital stay. However, the incidence of postoperative hypotension and GI bleeding was greater in individuals taking NSAIDs until 24 hours before operation, particularly the agents with half-lives longer than 6 hours.
- Another study of total hip surgery found that perioperative blood loss was an average of 45% higher (1161 ± 472 mL versus 796 ± 337 mL) in 25 patients randomly assigned to 2 weeks of preoperative treatment with ibuprofen than in those receiving placebo.[219]
- A final hip study in patients receiving aspirin did not demonstrate any increase in perioperative blood loss despite a significant elevation in bleeding time.[220]
- Preoperative treatment with nabumetone was found to have little impact on hemostasis in arthroscopic knee surgery.[221]

Finally, the American Society for Regional Anesthesia concluded that preoperative treatment with NSAIDs and aspirin is not associated with higher risk of spinal or epidural hematoma in patients undergoing regional anesthesia.[222] The Collaborative Low-dose Aspirin Study in Pregnancy (CLASP) involved 1422 high-risk obstetrical patients given 60 mg aspirin daily; all underwent epidural anesthesia without neurological sequelae.[223] In a study of epidural steroid injection, there were no reports of bleeding in 1214 patients, 32% of whom were taking NSAIDs.[224]

INHIBITION OF BONE GROWTH

Prostaglandins play a central role in bone repair after fracture. Bone healing comprises the following three main steps: (1) production of osteoid matrix, (2) mineralization of matrix to form woven bone, and (3) remodeling and resorption of the woven callus to produce cortical bone with the necessary shape and mechanical integrity.[225] In response to injury, local hypoxia and inflammation induce osteoblast proliferation and migration into the fracture site. Osteoblasts produce a collagenous matrix that serves as a scaffold for bone regrowth, and autocrine substances, such as PGs, determine the balance between bone formation and resorption.[226] In a rabbit model of traumatic fracture, PGE_2 was elevated; this elevation is thought to promote bone formation.[227] Rats treated with nonselective NSAIDs demonstrate delayed healing and a higher incidence of nonunion after experimental fracture,[228,229] an effect that can be observed after only 3 days of treatment.[230] Coxibs demonstrate a large effect in these models, suggesting that Cox-2 has a prominent role in the process.[231] Indeed, Cox-2 knockout mice (homozygous for the Cox-2 deletion) have a significant healing delay in stabilized tibia fractures compared with Cox-1 knockout and wild-type controls.[232]

The clinical data on bone healing and cyclooxygenase inhibition are mainly retrospective (Box 18–13). Giannoudis et al[233] found that NSAID users had more than a 10-fold higher risk of nonunion after intramedullary nailing for femoral diaphyseal fractures. Duration of NSAID use averaged 21 weeks, and longer exposure was associated with longer healing times among individuals with fractures that ultimately united.[234] Glassman et al[235] retrospectively assessed the effect of postoperative ketorolac administration on instrumented spinal fusion rates. The rate of nonunion among smokers and nonsmokers alike was significantly higher in the ketorolac group.

Flurbiprofen was studied in a prospective double-blind placebo-controlled fashion in 98 patients with displaced and nondisplaced Colles' fractures.[236] At 1-year follow-up, no differences were noted between the placebo and flurbiprofen groups regarding functional recovery and fracture union rates. However, individuals with nondisplaced fractures who had received placebo experienced a significantly higher rate of excellent outcomes than those who had received NSAIDs.

By far the largest clinical experience with NSAID treatment and bone growth has been in the prevention of heterotopic ossification, a condition that accompanies approximately one third of hip arthroplasties.[237] *Heterotopic ossification* is the abnormal formation of bone within extraskeletal tissue.

It occurs when surgical dissection activates dormant osteoprogenitor stem cells, with subsequent production of osteoid and heterotopic bone. A survey of 13 randomized trials found that perioperative NSAIDs may prevent 1 to 2 cases of severe heterotopic ossification and 10 to 20 cases of mild to moderate heterotopic bone formation for every 100 patients treated. Duration of treatment averaged nearly 5 weeks, a significantly longer time than that associated with poor bone healing in some animal models.[230]

The question remains whether NSAIDs' inhibitory effects on bone formation are a net benefit. Concerns have been raised that this effect might lead to aseptic loosening of prostheses, especially with cementless hip arthroplasties. A small amount of prospective data is reassuring in this regard. Wurnig et al[238] prospectively assessed heterotopic ossification in 80 patients receiving indomethacin prophylaxis and 82 controls. These investigators found no increase in radiolucency or other radiological change around a cementless stem after 6 years. Similar results were noted in another study, suggesting that NSAID treatment may not raise the risk of periprosthetic bone loss.[239]

Summary and Conclusions

NSAIDs have proved to be versatile and effective perioperative analgesics with a relatively low potential for serious side effects. Their therapeutic effects are due to their ability to suppress inflammation and to inhibit the development of a hyperalgesic state after painful stimuli. Inhibition of both cyclooxygenase isoforms in peripheral tissues and the CNS is probably necessary for the therapeutic effect. Of the many NSAIDs currently marketed, the ones with short half-lives and parenteral formulations tend to be most useful perioperatively. These drugs are sufficiently effective to be used as the sole analgesic therapy for many types of mild to moderate acute pain. For more severe pain, NSAIDs are generally used together with opioids or regional/local anesthesia.

There is good evidence for the analgesic efficacy of NSAIDs in treating pain after laparoscopy, vaginal and cesarean deliveries, and orthopedic procedures such as arthroscopy and total joint arthroplasty. They are much less consistently effective after thoracotomy or laparotomy and in other more severe pain states. NSAIDs do not appear to be useful for pain relief during surgical procedures.

Because prostaglandins play such an important role in the kidney, platelets, vasculature, and GI tract, it is not surprising that NSAIDs can have significant undesirable effects in these tissues. The clinical decision to use an NSAID often hinges on its anticipated toxicity, although the available literature suggests that serious toxicity is an infrequent occurrence during short-term perioperative treatment. The risk of acute renal failure is probably not increased with NSAID use, although care must be exercised in treating patients with hypovolemia or preexisting renal impairment. Similarly, the risk of GI toxicity is quite low in this setting if one avoids giving NSAIDS to patients who have previous ulcers or GI bleeding or are undergoing corticosteroid therapy. NSAIDs impair platelet aggregation and prolong bleeding time, but they do not produce significant bleeding in most surgical settings. The bleeding risk appears to be higher in urological

BOX 18–13	NSAIDS AND BONE HEALING

Evidence from animal models shows that NSAIDs and coxibs may have adverse effects on bone healing after fracture. Both cyclooxygenase-1 (Cox-1) and Cox-2 appear to be important. Clinical studies suggest a possible increase in bone nonunion rates, but the data are mostly retrospective (level B evidence). A single prospective study identified no effect of NSAID treatment on healing of Colles' fracture. Heterotopic bone formation after hip surgery and trauma is prevented by administration of NSAIDs (level A evidence).

and otolaryngological procedures, including tonsillectomy. Even though NSAIDs can raise blood pressure and exacerbate symptoms of congestive heart failure, perioperative use of the nonselective drugs is not associated with greater cardiovascular risk. Only aspirin has definitely been shown to have cardioprotective effects.

The coxibs unquestionably have fewer effects on platelets and the GI tract, but they increase the combined risk of myocardial infarction, stroke, and cardiovascular death, even after as little as 10 days of therapy in high-risk patients. These agents are now in a pharmaceutical limbo—the dose and indications for celecoxib are restricted, and it is unclear whether rofecoxib or valdecoxib will become available for use again. Now that toxicity has been demonstrated with several coxibs, it is reasonable to conclude that a class effect is being observed. Because coxibs have never been shown to produce better analgesia than other NSAIDs, the only logical reason to use them seems to be for long-term administration in patients at high risk of bleeding or GI toxicity. At present, there is no evidence that the benefits of coxib administration outweigh the risks in any surgical population.

Addendum

There are very few studies that directly compare the analgesic efficacy of an NSAID with that of an opioid. Drawing inferences from multiple placebo-controlled studies is prone to error, because different populations may not have comparable intensities of pain. Since the submission of this chapter, a randomized double-blind trial was published that directly compared intravenous morphine (0.1 mg/kg) and ketorolac (30 mg) in 1003 patients with moderate to severe postoperative pain.[278] Morphine was clearly more efficacious than ketorolac, although it produced more side effects. Addition of ketorolac to morphine significantly reduced the opioid dose and the side effects.

REFERENCES

1. Vane JR, Bakhle YS, Botting RM: Cyclooxygenases 1 and 2. Annu Rev Pharmacol Toxicol 1998;38:97–120.
2. Lim RK: Pain. Annu Rev Physiol 1970;32:269–288.
3. Chapman V, Dickenson AH: The spinal and peripheral roles of bradykinin and prostaglandins in nociceptive processing in the rat. Eur J Pharmacol 1992;219:427–433.
4. Biemond P, Swaak AG, Penders JA, et al: Superoxide production by polymorphonuclear leucocytes in rheumatoid arthritis and osteoarthritis: In vivo inhibition by the antirheumatic drug piroxicam due to interference with the activation of the NADPH-oxidase. Ann Rheum Dis 1986;45:249–255.
5. Bomalaski JS, Hirata F, Clark M: Aspirin inhibits phospholipase C. Biochem Biophys Res Commun 1986;139:115–121.
6. Abramson SB, Weissman G: The mechanisms of action of nonsteroidal anti-inflammatory drugs. Arthritis Rheum 1989;32:1–9.
7. McCormack K, Brune K: Dissociation between the antinociceptive and anti-inflammatory effects of the nonsteroidal anti-inflammatory drugs: A survey of their analgesic efficacy. Drugs 1991;41:533–547.
8. Gordon SM, Brahim JS, Rowan J, et al: Peripheral prostanoid levels and nonsteroidal anti-inflammatory drug analgesia: Replicate clinical trials in a tissue injury model. Clin Pharm Ther 2002;72:175–183.
9. Svensson CI, Yaksh TL: The spinal phospholipase-cyclooxygenase - prostanoid cascade in nociceptive processing. Annu Rev Pharmacol Toxicol 2002;42:553–583.
10. Dirig DM, Yaksh TL: In vitro prostanoid release from spinal cord following peripheral inflammation: Effects of substance P, NMDA and capsaicin. Br J Pharmacol 1999;126:1333–1340.
11. Malmberg AB, Yaksh TL: Cyclooxygenase inhibition and the spinal release of prostaglandin E2 and amino acids evoked by paw formalin injection: A microdialysis study in unanesthetized rats. J Neurosci 1995;15:2768–2776.
12. Minami T, Uda R, Horiguchi S, et al: Allodynia evoked by intrathecal administration of prostaglandin E2 to conscious mice. Pain 1994;57:217–223.
13. Ichitani Y, Shi T, Haeggstrom JZ, et al: Increased levels of cyclooxygenase-2 mRNA in the rat spinal cord after peripheral inflammation: An in situ hybridization study. Neuroreport 1997;8:2949–2952.
14. Samad TA, Moore KA, Sapirstein A, et al: Interleukin-1 beta-mediated induction of COX-2 in the CNS contributes to inflammatory pain hypersensitivity. Nature 2001;410:471–475.
15. Yaksh TL, Dirig DM, Conway CM, et al: The acute antihyperalgesic action of NSAIDs and release of spinal PGE2 is mediated by the inhibition of constitutive spinal COX-2 but not COX-1. J Neurosci 2001;21:5847–5853.
16. Malmberg AB, Yaksh TL: Hyperalgesia mediated by spinal glutamate or substance P receptor blocked by spinal cyclooxygenase inhibition. Science 1992;257:1276–1279.
17. Brooks PM, Day RO: Nonsteroidal anti-inflammatory drugs—differences and similarities. N Engl J Med 1991;324:1716–1725.
18. Moote C: Efficacy of nonsteroidal anti-inflammatory drugs in the management of postoperative pain. Drugs 1992;44(Suppl 5):14–30.
19. Cryer B, Feldman M: Cyclooxygenase-1 and cyclooxygenase-2 selectivity of widely used nonsteroidal anti-inflammatory drugs. Am J Med 1998;104:413–421.
20. Ebell MH, Siwek J, Weiss BD: Strength of recommendation taxonomy (SORT): A patient-centered approach to grading evidence in the medical literature. Am Fam Physician 2004;69:548-556.
21. Sandler AN: Post-thoracotomy analgesia and perioperative outcome. Minerva Anesthesiol 1999;65:267–274.
22. Scawn NDA, Pennefather SH, Soorae A, et al: Ipsilateral shoulder pain after thoracotomy with epidural analgesia: The influence of phrenic nerve infiltration. Anesth Analg 2001;93:260–264.
23. Loan WB, Morrison JD: The incidence and severity of postoperative pain. Br J Anesth 1967;39:695–698.
24. Perttunen K, Kalso E, Heinonen J, Salo J: IV diclofenac in post-thoracotomy pain. Br J Anesth 1992;68:474–480.
25. Rhodes M, Conacher I, Morritt G, Hilton C: Nonsteroidal antiinflammatory drugs for postthoracotomy pain: A prospective controlled trial after lateral thoracotomy. J Thorac Cardiovasc Surg 1992;103:17–20.
26. Murphy DF, Medley C: Preoperative indomethacin for pain relief after thoracotomy: Comparison with postoperative indomethacin. Br J Anaesth 1993;70:298–300.
27. Pavy T, Medley C, Murphy DF: Effect of indomethacin on pain relief after thoracotomy. Br J Anaesth 1990;65:624–627.
28. Power I, Bowler GMR, Pugh GC, Chambers WA: Ketorolac as a component of balanced analgesia after thoracotomy. Br J Anaesth 1994;72:224–226.
29. Singh H, Bossard RF, White PF, Yeatts RW: Effects of ketorolac versus bupivacaine coadministration during patient-controlled hydromorphone epidural analgesia after thoracotomy procedures. Anesth Analg 1997;84:564–569.
30. Puntillo K, Ley SJ: Appropriately timed analgesics control pain due to chest tube removal. Am J Crit Care 2004;13:292–301.
31. Merry AF, Wardall GJ, Cameron RJ, et al: Prospective, controlled, double-blind study of IV tenoxicam for analgesia after thoracotomy. Br J Anaesth 1992;69:92–94.
32. Merry AF, Sidebotham DA, Middleton NG, et al: Tenoxicam 20 mg or 40 mg after thoracotomy: A prospective, randomized, double-blind, placebo-controlled study. Anaesth Intensive Care 2002;30:160–166.
33. Bigler D, Moller J, Kamp-Jensen M, et al: Effect of piroxicam in addition to continuous thoracic epidural bupivacaine and morphine on postoperative pain and lung function after thoracotomy. Acta Anaesthesiol Scand 1992;36:647–650.
34. Landreneau RJ, Hazelrigg SR, Mack MJ, et al: Postoperative pain-related morbidity: Video-assisted thoracic surgery versus thoracotomy. Ann Thorac Surg 1993;56:1285–1289.
35. Perttunen K, Nilsson E, Kalso E: IV diclofenac and ketorolac for pain after thoracoscopic surgery. Br J Anaesth 1999;82:221–227.

36. McCrory C, Fitzgerald D: Spinal prostaglandin formation and pain perception following thoracotomy: A role for cyclooxygenase-2. Chest 2004;125:1321–1327.

37. Barkun JS, Barkun AN, Sampalis JS, et al: Randomized controlled trial of laparoscopic versus mini cholecystectomy: A national survey of 4292 hospitals and an analysis of 77604 cases. Lancet 1992;340: 1116–1119.

38. Tate JJ, Chung SCS, Dawson J, et al: Conventional versus laparoscopic surgery for acute appendicitis. Br J Surg 1993;80:761–764.

39. McMahon AJ, Russell IT, Baxter JN, et al: Laparoscopic versus minilaparotomy cholecystectomy: A randomized trial. Lancet 1994;343:135–138.

40. Stiff G, Rhodes M, Kelly A, et al: Long-term pain: Less common after laparoscopic than open cholecystectomy. Br J Surg 1994;81:1368–1370.

41. Laparoscopic cholecystectomy in PROSPECT: Procedure-specific pain management. Available at www.postoppain.org/frameset.htm

42. Willis VL, Hunt DR: Pain after laparoscopic cholecystectomy. Br J Surg 2000;87:273–284.

43. Joris J, Thiry E, Paris P, et al: Pain after laparoscopic cholecystectomy: Characteristics and effect of intraperitoneal bupivacaine. Anesth Analg 1995;81:379–384.

44. Chi IC, Cole LP: Incidence of pain among women undergoing laparoscopic sterilization by electrocoagulation, the spring-loaded clip, and the tubal ring. Obst Gynecol 1979;137:397–401.

45. Alexander JI. Pain after laparoscopy. Br J Anesth 1997;79:369–378.

46. Green CR, Pandit SK, Levy L, et al: Intraoperative ketorolac has an opioid-sparing effect in women after diagnostic laparoscopy but not after laparoscopic tubal ligation. Anesth Analg 1996;82:732–737.

47. Shapiro MH, Duffy BL: Intramuscular ketorolac for postoperative analgesia following laparoscopic sterilisation. Anaesth Intensive Care 1994; 22:22–24.

48. DeLucia JA, White PF: Effect of intraoperative ketorolac on recovery after outpatient laparoscopy. Anesthesiology 1991;75:A13.

49. Pandit SK, Kothary SP, Lebenbom-Mansour DO, et al: Failure of ketorolac to prevent severe post-operative pain following outpatient laparoscopy. Anesthesiology 1991;75:A33.

50. Campbell L, Plummer J, Owen H, et al: Effect of short-term ketorolac infusion on recovery following laparoscopic day surgery. Anaesth Intensive Care 2000;28:654–659.

51. Dunn TJ, Clark VA, Jones G: Preoperative oral naproxen for pain relief after day-case laparoscopic sterilization. Br J Anaesth. 1995;75:12–14.

52. Comfort VK, Code WE, Rooney ME, Yip RW: Naproxen premedication reduces postoperative tubal ligation pain. Can J Anaesth 1992;39: 349–352.

53. Van EE R, Hemrika DJ, van der Linden CT: Pain relief following day-case diagnostic hysteroscopy-laparoscopy for infertility: A double-blind randomized trial with preoperative naproxen versus placebo. Obstet Gynecol 1993;82:951–954.

54. Hovorka J, Kallela H, Kortilla K: Effect of intravenous diclofenac on pain and recovery profile after day-case laparoscopy. Eur J Anaesthesiol 1993;10:105–108.

55. Edwards ND, Barclay K, Catling SJ, et al: Day case laparoscopy: A survey of postoperative pain and an assessment of the value of diclofenac. Anaesthesia 1991;46:1077–1080.

56. Windsor A, McDonald P, Mumtaz T, Millar JM: The analgesic efficacy of tenoxicam versus placebo in day case laparoscopy: A randomised parallel double-blind trial. Anaesthesia 1996;51:1066–1069.

57. Colbert SA, McCrory C, O'Hanlon DM, et al: A prospective study comparing intravenous tenoxicam with rectal diclofenac for pain relief in day case surgery. Eur J Anaesthesiol 1998;15:544–548.

58. Phinchantra P, Bunyavehchevin S, Suwajanakorn S, Wisawasukmongchol W: The preemptive analgesic effect of celecoxib for day-case diagnostic laparoscopy. J Med Assoc Thai 2004;87:283–288.

59. Ng A, Temple A, Smith G, Emembolu J: Early analgesic effects of parecoxib versus ketorolac following laparoscopic sterilization: A randomized controlled trial. Br J Anaesth 2004;92:846–849.

60. Davie IT, Slawson KB, Burt RA: A double-blind comparison of parenteral morphine, placebo, and oral fenoprofen in management of postoperative pain. Anesth Analg 1982;61:1002–1005.

61. Aho MS, Erkola OA, Scheinin H, et al: Effect of intravenously administered dexmedetomidine on pain after laparoscopic tubal ligation. Anesth Analg 1991;73:112–118.

62. Putland AJ, McCluskey A: The analgesic efficacy of tramadol versus ketorolac in day-case laparoscopic sterilisation. Anaesthesia 1999;54: 382–385.

63. Cade L, Kakulas P: Ketorolac or pethidine for analgesia after elective laparoscopic sterilization. Anaesth Intensive Care 1995;23:158–161.

64. Rosenblum M, Weller RS, Conard PL, et al: Ibuprofen provides longer lasting analgesia than fentanyl after laparoscopic surgery. Anesth Analg 1991;73:255–259.

65. Salman MA, Yucebas ME, Coskun F, Aypar U: Day-case laparoscopy: A comparison of prophylactic opioid, NSAID or local anesthesia for postoperative analgesia. Acta Anaesthesiol Scand. 2000;44:536–542.

66. Crocker S, Paech M: Preoperative rectal indomethacin for analgesia after laparoscopic sterilization. Anesth Intensive Care 1992;20: 337–340.

67. Hong JY, Lee IH: Suprascapular nerve block or a piroxicam patch for shoulder tip pain after day case laparoscopic surgery. Eur J Anesthesiol 2003;20:426.

68. McMahon AJ, Russell IT, Ramsay G, et al: Laparoscopic and minilaparotomy cholecystectomy: A randomized trial comparing postoperative pain and pulmonary function. Surgery 1994;115:533–539.

69. Fredman B, Olsfanger D, Jedeikin R: A comparative study of ketorolac and diclofenac on post-laparoscopic cholecystectomy pain. Eur J Anaesthesiol 1995;12:501–504.

70. Lane GE, Lathrop JC, Boysen DA, Lane RC: Effect of intramuscular intraoperative pain medication on narcotic usage after laparoscopic cholecystectomy. Am Surg 1996;62:907–910.

71. Wilson YG, Rhodes M, Ahmed R, et al: Intramuscular diclofenac sodium for postoperative analgesia after laparoscopic cholecystectomy: A randomised, controlled trial. Surg Laparosc Endosc 1994;4:340–344.

72. Forse A, El-Beheiry H, Butler PO, Pace RF: Indomethacin and ketorolac given preoperatively are equally effective in reducing early postoperative pain after laparoscopic cholecystectomy. Can J Surg 1996;39: 26–30.

73. Horattas MC, Evans S, Sloan-Stakleff KD, et al: Does preoperative rofecoxib (Vioxx) decrease postoperative pain with laparoscopic cholecystectomy? Am J Surg 2004;188:271–276.

74. Gan TJ, Joshi GP, Zhao SZ, et al: Presurgical intravenous parecoxib sodium and follow-up oral valdecoxib for pain management after laparoscopic cholecystectomy surgery reduces opioid requirements and opioid-related adverse effects. Acta Anaesthesiol Scand 2004;48: 1194–1207.

75. Liu J, Ding Y, White PF, et al: Effects of ketorolac on postoperative analgesia and ventilatory function after laparoscopic cholecystectomy. Anesth Analg 1993;76:1061–1066.

76. Elhakim M, Amine H, Kamel S, Saad F: Effects of intraperitoneal lidocaine combined with intravenous or intraperitoneal tenoxicam on pain relief and bowel recovery after laparoscopic cholecystectomy. Acta Anaesthesiol Scand 2000;44:929–933.

77. Nagele F, Connor HO, Davies A, et al: 2500 outpatient diagnostic hysteroscopies. Obstet Gynecol 1996;88:87–92.

78. Nagele F, Lockwood G, Magos AL: Randomised placebo controlled trial of mefenamic acid for premedication at outpatient hysteroscopy: A pilot study. Br J Obstet Gynecol 1997;104:842–844.

79. Tam WH, Yuen PM: Use of diclofenac as an analgesic in outpatient hysteroscopy: A randomized, double-blind, placebo-controlled study. Fertil Steril 2001;76:1070–1072.

80. Mercorio F, De Simone R, Landi P, et al: Oral dexketoprofen for pain treatment during diagnostic hysteroscopy in postmenopausal women. Maturitas 2002;43:277–281.

81. Ding Y, Fredman B, White PF: Use of ketorolac and fentanyl during outpatient gynecologic surgery. Anesth Analg 1993;77:205–210.

82. De Lia JE, Rodman KC, Jolles CJ: Comparative efficacy of oral flurbiprofen, intramuscular morphine sulfate, and placebo in the treatment of gynecologic postoperative pain. Am J Med 1986 24;80:60–64.

83. Jones RDM, Miles W, Prankerd R, et al: Tenoxicam IV in major gynecologic surgery—pharmacokinetic, pain relief and hematologic effects. Anesth Intensive Care 2000;28:491–500.

84. Tang J, Li S, White PF, et al: Effect of parecoxib, a novel intravenous cyclooxygenase type-2 inhibitor, on the postoperative opioid requirement and quality of pain control. Anesthesiology 2002;96:1305–1309.

85. Bloomfield SS, Mitchell J, Cissell G, Barden TP: Analgesic sensitivity of two post-partum pain models. Pain 1986;27:171–179.

86. Bloomfield SS, Cissell GB, Mitchell J, Barden TP: Codeine and aspirin analgesia in postpartum uterine cramps: Qualitative aspects of quantitative assessments. Clin Pharmacol Ther 1983;34:488–495.

87. Bloomfield SS, Barden TP, Mitchell J: Naproxen, aspirin, and codeine in postpartum uterine pain. Clin Pharmacol Ther 1977;21:414–421.

88. Sunshine A, Zighelboim I, Olson NZ, et al: A comparative oral analgesic study of indoprofen, aspirin, and placebo in postpartum pain. J Clin Pharmacol 1985;25:374–380.

89. Sunshine A, Zighelboim I, Laska E, et al: A double-blind, parallel comparison of ketoprofen, aspirin, and placebo in patients with postpartum pain. J Clin Pharmacol 1986;26:706–711.

90. Sunshine A, Roure C, Olson N, et al: Analgesic efficacy of two ibuprofen-codeine combinations for the treatment of postepisiotomy and postoperative pain. Clin Pharmacol Ther 1987;42:374–379.

91. Kitterman JA: Patent ductus arteriosus: Current clinical status. Arch Dis Child 1980;55:106–109.

92. Zukerman H, Shaler E, Gilad G, Katzuni E: Further study of the inhibition of premature labor by indomethacin—part II double blind study. J Perinat Med 1984;12:25–29.

93. Spigset O: Anesthetic agents and excretion in breast milk. Acta Anesth Scand 1994;38:94–103.

94. Code WE, Yip RW, Rooney ME, et al: Preoperative naproxen sodium reduces postoperative pain following arthroscopic knee surgery. Can J Anaesth 1994;41:98–101.

95. Ogilvie-Harris DJ, Bauer M, Corey P: Prostaglandin inhibition and the rate of recovery after arthroscopic meniscectomy: A randomised double-blind prospective study. J Bone Joint Surg Br 1985;67:567–571.

96. Nelson WE, Henderson RC, Almekinders LC, et al: An evaluation of pre- and postoperative nonsteroidal antiinflammatory drugs in patients undergoing knee arthroscopy: A prospective, randomized, double-blinded study. Am J Sports Med 1993;21:510–516.

97. Sandin R, Sternlo JE, Stam H, et al: Diclofenac for pain relief after arthroscopy: A comparison of early and delayed treatment. Acta Anaesthesiol Scand 1993;37:747–750.

98. Norris A, Un V, Chung F, et al: When should diclofenac be given in ambulatory surgery: Preoperatively or postoperatively? J Clin Anesth 2001;13:11–15.

99. Reuben SS, Bhopatkar S, Maciolek H, et al: The preemptive analgesic effect of rofecoxib after ambulatory arthroscopic knee surgery. Anesth Analg 2002;94:55–59.

100. Dennis AR, Leeson-Payne CG, Hobbs GJ: A comparison of diclofenac with ketorolac for pain relief after knee arthroscopy. Anaesthesia 1995;50:904–906.

101. Berti M, Albertin A, Casati A, et al: A prospective, randomized comparison of dexketoprofen, ketoprofen or paracetamol for postoperative analgesia after outpatient knee arthroscopy. Minerva Anestesiol 2000;66:549–554.

102. Laitinen J, Nuutinen L, Kiiskila EL, et al: Comparison of intravenous diclofenac, indomethacin and oxycodone as post-operative analgesics in patients undergoing knee surgery. Eur J Anaesthesiol 1992;9:29–34.

103. Barber FA, Gladu DE: Comparison of oral ketorolac and hydrocodone for pain relief after anterior cruciate ligament reconstruction. Arthroscopy 1998;14:605–612.

104. White PF, Joshi GP, Carpenter RL, Fragen RJ: A comparison of oral ketorolac and hydrocodone-acetaminophen for analgesia after ambulatory surgery: Arthroscopy versus laparoscopic tubal ligation. Anesth Analg 1997;85:37–43.

105. Dahl V, Dybvik T, Steen T, et al: Ibuprofen vs. acetaminophen vs. ibuprofen and acetaminophen after arthroscopically assisted anterior cruciate ligament reconstruction. Eur J Anaesthesiol. 2004;21:471–475.

106. Van Lancker P, Vandekerckhove B, Cooman F: The analgesic effect of preoperative administration of propacetamol, tenoxicam or a mixture of both in arthroscopic, outpatient knee surgery. Acta Anaesthesiol Belg 1999;50:65–69.

107. Colbert ST, Curran E, O'Hanlon DM, et al: Intra-articular tenoxicam improves postoperative analgesia in knee arthroscopy. Can J Anaesth 1999;46:653–657.

108. Elhakim M, Fathy A, Elkott M, Said MM: Intra-articular tenoxicam relieves post-arthroscopy pain. Acta Anaesthesiol Scand 1996;40:1223–1236.

109. Gupta A, Axelsson K, Allvin R, et al: Postoperative pain following knee arthroscopy: The effects of intra-articular ketorolac and/or morphine. Reg Anesth Pain Med 1999;24:225–230.

110. Izdes S, Orhun S, Turanli S, et al: The effects of preoperative inflammation on the analgesic efficacy of intraarticular piroxicam for outpatient knee arthroscopy. Anesth Analg 2003;97:1016–1019.

111. Pookarnjanamorakot C, Laohacharoensombat W, Jaovisidha S: The clinical efficacy of piroxicam fast-dissolving dosage form for postoperative pain control after simple lumbar spine surgery: A double-blinded randomized study. Spine 2002;27:447–451.

112. De Decker K, Vercauteren M, Hoffmann V, et al: Piroxicam versus tenoxicam in spine surgery: A placebo controlled study. Acta Anaesthesiol Belg 2001;52:265–269.

113. McGlew IC, Angliss DB, Gee GJ, et al: A comparison of rectal indomethacin with placebo for pain relief following spinal surgery. Anaesth Intensive Care 1991;19:40–45.

114. Nissen I, Jensen KA, Ohrstrom JK: Indomethacin in the management of postoperative pain. Br J Anaesth 1992;69:304–306.

115. Reuben SS, Connelly NR, Lurie S, et al: Dose-response of ketorolac as an adjunct to patient-controlled analgesia morphine in patients after spinal fusion surgery. Anesth Analg 1998;87:98–102.

116. Reuben SS, Connelly NR, Steinberg R: Ketorolac as an adjunct to patient-controlled morphine in postoperative spine surgery patients. Reg Anesth 1997;22:343–346.

117. Le Roux PD, Samudrala S: Postoperative pain after lumbar disc surgery: A comparison between parenteral ketorolac and narcotics. Acta Neurochir (Wien) 1999;141:261–267.

118. Bekker A, Cooper PR, Frempong-Boadu A, et al: Evaluation of preoperative administration of the cyclooxygenase -2 inhibitor rofecoxib for the treatment of postoperative pain after lumbar disc surgery. Neurosurgery 2002;50:1053–1057.

119. Karst M, Kegel T, Lukas A, et al: Effect of celecoxib and dexamethasone on postoperative pain after lumbar disc surgery. Neurosurgery 2003;53:331–336.

120. Reuben SS, Connelly NR: Postoperative analgesic effects of celecoxib or rofecoxib after spinal fusion surgery. Anesth Analg 2000;91:1221–1225.

121. Dahl V, Raeder JC, Drosdal S, et al: Prophylactic oral ibuprofen or ibuprofen-codeine versus placebo for postoperative pain after primary hip arthroplasty. Acta Anaesthesiol Scand 1995;39:323–326.

122. Buvanendran A, Kroin JS, Tuman KJ, et al: Effects of perioperative administration of a selective cyclooxygenase 2 inhibitor on pain management and recovery of function after knee replacement: A randomized controlled trial. JAMA 2003;290:2411–2418.

123. Reynolds LW, Hoo RK, Brill RJ, et al: The COX-2 specific inhibitor, valdecoxib, is an effective, opioid-sparing analgesic in patients undergoing total knee arthroplasty. J Pain Symptom Manag 2003;25: 133–141.

124. Malan TP Jr, Marsh G, Hakki SI, et al: Parecoxib sodium, a parenteral cyclooxygenase-2 selective inhibitor, improves morphine analgesia and is opioid-sparing following total hip arthroplasty. Anesthesiology 2003;98:950–956.

125. Rasmussen GL, Steckner K, Hogue C, et al: Intravenous parecoxib sodium for acute pain after orthopedic knee surgery. Am J Orthop 2002;31:336–343.

126. Etches RC, Warriner CB, Badner N, et al: Continuous intravenous administration of ketorolac reduces pain and morphine consumption after total hip or knee arthroplasty. Anesth Analg 1995;81:1175–1180.

127. Bugter ML, Dirksen R, Jhamandas K, et al: Prior ibuprofen exposure does not augment opioid drug potency or modify opioid requirements for pain inhibition in total hip surgery. Can J Anaesth 2003;50:445–449.

128. Hommeril JL, Bernard JM, Gouin F, Pinaud M: Ketoprofen for pain after hip and knee arthroplasty. Br J Anaesth 1994;72:383–387.

129. Iohom G, Walsh M, Higgins G, Shorten G: Effect of perioperative administration of dexketoprofen on opioid requirements and inflammatory response following elective hip arthroplasty. Br J Anaesth 2002;88:520–526.

130. Boeckstyns ME, Backer M, Petersen EM, et al: Piroxicam spares buprenorphine after total joint replacement: Controlled study of pain treatment in 81 patients. Acta Orthop Scand 1992;63:658–660.

131. Anderson SK, al Shaikh BA: Diclofenac in combination with opiate infusion after joint replacement surgery. Anaesth Intensive Care 1991;19:535–538.

132. Segstro R, Morley-Forster PK, Lu G: Indomethacin as a postoperative analgesic for total hip arthroplasty. Can J Anaesth 1991;38:578–581.

133. Schlondorff D: Renal prostaglandin synthesis: Sites of production and specific actions of prostaglandins. Am J Med 1986;81:1–10.

134. Scharschmidt L, Simonson M, Dunn MJ: Glomerular prostaglandins, angiotensin II, and nonsteroidal anti-inflammatory drugs. Am J Med 1986;81:30–42.

135. Komhoff M, Grone HJ, Klein T, et al: Localization of cyclooxygenase -1 and -2 in adult and fetal human kidney: Implication for renal function. Am J Physiol 1997;272:F460–F468.

136. Dunn MJ, Zambraski EJ: Renal effects of drugs that inhibit prostaglandin synthesis. Kidney Int 1980;18:609–622.

137. Novis BK, Roizen MF, Aronson S, Thisted RA: Association of preoperative risk factors with postoperative acute renal failure. Anesth Analg 1994;78:143–149.
138. Zipser RD, Hoefs JC, Speckart PF, et al: Prostaglandins: Modulators of renal function and pressor resistance in chronic liver disease. J Clin Endocrinol Metab 1979;48:895–909.
139. Walshe JJ, Venuto RC: Acute oliguric renal failure induced by indomethacin: Possible mechanism. Ann Intern Med 1979;91:47–49.
140. Feldman HI, Kinman JL, Berlin JA, et al: Parenteral ketorolac: The risk for acute renal failure. Ann Intern Med 1997;126:193–199.
141. Lee A, Cooper MC, Craig JC, et al: The effects of nonsteroidal anti-inflammatory drugs (NSAIDs) on postoperative renal function. Cochrane Database Syst Rev 2004;(2):CD002765.
142. Swan SK, Rudy DW, Lasseter KC, et al: Effect of cyclooxygenase-2 inhibition on renal function in elderly persons receiving a low-salt diet. Ann Intern Med 2000;133:1–9.
143. Rossat J, Maillard M, Nussberger J, et al: Renal effects of selective cyclooxygenase -2 inhibition in normotensive salt-depleted subjects. Clin Pharmacol Ther 1999;66:76–84.
144. Lichtenstein DR, Syngal S, Wolfe MM: Nonsteroidal anti-inflammatory drugs and the gastrointestinal tract. Arthritis Rheum 1995;38:5–18.
145. Feldman M, Colturi TJ: Effect of indomethacin on gastric acid and bicarbonate secretion in humans. Gastroenterology 1984;87:1339–1343.
146. Soll AH, Weinstein WM, Kurata J, McCarthy D: Nonsteroidal antiinflammatory drugs and peptic ulcer disease. Ann Intern Med 1991;114:307–319.
147. Kargman S, Charleson S, Cartwright M, et al: Characterization of prostaglandin G/H synthase 1 and 2 in rat, dog, and human gastrointestinal tracts. Gastroenterology 1996;111:445–454.
148. Ristimaki A, Honkanen N, Jankala H, et al: Expression of cyclooxygenase -2 in human gastric carcinoma. Cancer Res 1997;57:1276–1280.
149. Halter F, Tarnaski AS, Schmassman A, Peskar BM: Cyclooxygenase 2—implications on maintenance of gastric mucosal integrity and ulcer healing: Controversial issues and perspectives. Gut 2001;49:443–453.
150. Schoen RT, Vender RJ: Mechanisms of nonsteroidal anti-inflammatory drug induced gastric damage. Am J Med 1989;86:449–458.
151. Whittle BJR, Higgs GA, Eakins KE, et al: Selective inhibition of prostaglandin production in inflammatory exudates and gastric mucosa. Nature 1980;284:271–273.
152. Raskin JB: Gastrointestinal effects of nonsteroidal anti-inflammatory therapy. Am J Med 1999;106:3S–12S.
153. Graham DY, Smith JL, Dobbs SM: Gastric adaptation occurs with aspirin administration in man. Dig Dis Sci 1983;28:1–6.
154. O'Laughlin JC, Hoftiezer JW, Ivey KJ: Effect of aspirin on the human stomach in normals: Endoscopic comparison of damage produced on hour, 24 hours, and 2 weeks after administration. Scand J Gastroenterol Suppl 1981;67:211–214.
155. Strom BL, Berlin JA, Kinman JL, et al: Parenteral ketorolac and risk of gastrointestinal and operative site bleeding: A postmarketing surveillance study. JAMA 1996;275:376–382.
156. Forrest JB, Camu F, Greer IA, et al: Ketorolac, diclofenac, and ketoprofen are equally safe for pain relief after major surgery. Br J Anaesth 2002;88:227–233.
157. Silverstein FE, Graham DY, Senior JR, et al: Misoprostol reduces serious gastrointestinal complications in patients with rheumatoid arthritis receiving nonsteroidal anti-inflammatory drugs. Ann Intern Med 1995;123:241–249.
158. Ehsanullah RSB, Page MC, Tildesley G, Wood JR: Prevention of gastroduodenal damage induced by nonsteroidal anti-inflammatory drugs: Controlled trial of ranitidine. BMJ 1988;297:1017–1021.
159. Robinson MG, Griffin JW, Bowers J, et al: Effect of ranitidine on gastroduodenal mucosal damage induced by nonsteroidal anti-inflammatory drugs. Dig Dis Sci 1989;34:424–428.
160. Yeomans ND, Tulassay Z, Juhasz L, et al: A comparison of omeprazole with ranitidine for ulcers associated with nonsteroidal anti-inflammatory drugs. N Engl J Med 1998;338:719–726.
161. Hawkey CJ, Karrasch JA, Szczepanski L, et al: Omeprazole compared with misoprostol for ulcers associated with nonsteroidal anti-inflammatory drugs. N Engl J Med 1998;338:727–734.
162. Bombardier C, Laine L, Reicin A, et al: Comparison of upper gastrointestinal toxicity of rofecoxib and naproxen in patients with rheumatoid arthritis. VIGOR Study Group. Engl J Med 2000;343:1520–1528.
163. Silverstein FE, Faich G, Goldstein JL, et al: Gastrointestinal toxicity with celecoxib vs. nonsteroidal anti-inflammatory drugs for osteoarthritis and rheumatoid arthritis: The CLASS study: A randomized controlled trial. Celecoxib Long-term Arthritis Safety Study. JAMA 2000;284:1247–1255.
164. Stemme V, Swedenborg J, Claesson H, Hansson GK: Expression of cyclooxygenase -2 in human atherosclerotic carotid arteries. Eur J Vasc Endovasc Surg 2000;20:146–152.
165. Schonbeck U, Sukhova GK, Graber P, et al: Augmented expression of cyclooxygenase -2 in human atherosclerotic lesions. Am J Pathol 1999;155:1281–1291.
166. Belton O, Byrne D, Kerney D, et al: Cyclooxygenase-1 and -2-dependent prostacyclin formation in patients with atherosclerosis. Circulation 2000;102:840–845.
167. Fitzgerald GA: Cardiovascular pharmacology of nonselective nonsteroidal antiinflammatory drugs and coxibs: Clinical considerations. Am J Cardiol 2002;89(Suppl):26D–32D.
168. Vila L: Cyclooxygenase and 5-lipoxygenase pathways in the vessel wall: Role in atherosclerosis. Med Res Rev 2004;24:399–424.
169. Ross R: Atherosclerosis: An inflammatory disease. N Engl J Med 1999;340:115–126.
170. Smith EF, Lefer AM: Stabilization of cardiac lysosomal and cellular membranes in protection of ischemic myocardium due to coronary occlusion: Efficacy of the nonsteroidal antiinflammatory agent, naproxen. Am Heart J 1981;101:394–402.
171. Garcia Rodriguez LA, Varas C, Patrono C: Differential effects of aspirin and nonaspirin nonsteroidal antiinflammatory drugs in the primary prevention of myocardial infarction in post-menopausal women. Epidemiology 2000;11:382–387.
172. Solomon DH, Glynn RJ, Levin R, Avorn J: Nonsteroidal antiinflammatory drug use and acute myocardial infarction. Arch Intern Med 2002;162:1099–1104.
173. Ray WA, Stein C, Hall K, et al: Nonsteroidal antiinflammatory drugs and risk of serious coronary heart disease. Lancet 2002;359:118–123.
174. Rahme E, Pilote L, Lelorier J: Association between naproxen use and protection against acute myocardial infarction. Arch Intern Med 2002;162:1111–1115.
175. Watson DJ, Rhodes T, Cai HB, Guess HA: Lower risk of thromboembolic events with naproxen among patients with rheumatoid arthritis. Arch Intern Med 2002;162:1105–1110.
176. Mamdani M, Rochon P, Juurlinl DN, et al: Effect of cyclooxygenase 2 inhibitors and naproxen on short-term risk of acute myocardial infarction in the elderly. Arch Intern Med 2003;163:481–486.
177. Fitzgerald GA, Patrono C: The coxibs, selective inhibitors of cyclooxygenase-2. N Engl J Med 2001;345:433–442.
178. Verma S, Raj SR, Shewchuk L, et al: Cyclooxygenase-2 blockade does not impair endothelial vasodilator function in healthy volunteers: Randomized evaluation of rofecoxib versus naproxen on endothelium-dependent vasodilation. Circulation 2001;104:2879–2882.
179. Fitzgerald GA, Smith B, Pedersen AK, Brash AR: Increased prostacyclin biosynthesis in patients with severe atherosclerosis and platelet activation. N Engl J Med 1984;310:1065–1068.
180. Cipollone F, Prontera C, Pini B, et al: Overexpression of functionally coupled cyclooxygenase-2 and prostaglandin E synthase in symptomatic atherosclerotic plaques as a basis of prostaglandin E2-dependent plaque instability. Circulation 2001;104:921–927.
181. Hankey GJ, Eikelboom JW: Cyclooxygenase-2 inhibitors: Are they really atherothrombotic, and if not, why not? Stroke 2003;34:2736–2740.
182. Nussmeier NA, Whelton AA, Brown MT, et al: Complications of the COX-2 inhibitors parecoxib and valdecoxib after cardiac surgery. N Engl J Med 2005;352:1081–1091.
183. Mukherjee D, Nissen SE, Topol EJ: Risk of cardiovascular events associated with selective COX-2 inhibitors. JAMA 2001;286:954–959.
184. Solomon DH, Schneeweiss S, Glynn RJ, et al: Relationship between selective cyclooxygenase inhibitors and acute myocardial infarction in older adults. Circulation 2004;109:2068–2073.
185. Chenevard R, Hürlimann D, Béchir M, et al: Selective COX-2 inhibition improves endothelial function in coronary artery disease. Circulation 2003;107:415–419.
186. Altman R, Luciardi HL, Muntaner J, et al: Efficacy assessment of meloxicam, a preferential cyclooxygenase -2 inhibitor, in acute coronary syndromes without ST-segment elevation: The Nonsteroidal Anti-Inflammatory Drugs in Unstable Angina Treatment-2 (NUT-2) Study. Circulation 2002;106:191–195.

187. Konstam MA, Weir MR, Reicin A, et al: Cardiovascular thrombotic events in controlled, clinical trials of rofecoxib. Circulation 2001;104:2280–2288.

188. Jüni P, Nartey L, Reichenbach S, et al: Risk of cardiovascular events and rofecoxib: Cumulative meta-analysis. Lancet 2004;364:2021–2029.

189. Bresalier RS, Sandler RS, Quan H, et al: Cardiovascular events associated with rofecoxib in a colorectal adenoma chemoprevention trial. N Engl J Med 2005;352:1092–1102.

190. Solomon SD, McMurray JJV, Pfeffer MA, et al, Adenoma Prevention with Celecoxib (APC) Study Investigators: Cardiovascular risk associated with celecoxib in a clinical trial for colorectal adenoma prevention. N Engl J Med 2005;352:1071–1080.

191. Wennmalm A: Influence of indomethacin on the systemic and pulmonary vascular resistance in man. Clin Sci 1978;54:141–145.

192. Nowak J, Wennmalm A: Influence of indomethacin and of prostaglandin E1 on total and regional blood flow in man. Acta Physiol Scand 1978;102:484–491.

193. Safar ME, Hornych AF, Levenson JA, et al: Central hemodynamics and plasma prostaglandin E2 in borderline and sustained essential hypertensive patients before and after indomethacin. Clin Sci 1981;61:323S–325S.

194. Brown J, Dollery C, Valdes G: Interaction of nonsteroidal anti-inflammatory drugs with antihypertensive and diuretic agents: Control of vascular reactivity by endogenous prostanoids. Am J Med 1986;81:43–57.

195. Pope JE, Anderson JJ, Felson DT: A meta-analysis of the effects of nonsteroidal anti-inflammatory drugs on blood pressure. Arch Intern Med 1993;153:477–484.

196. Muscara MN, Vergnolle N, Lovren F, et al: Selective cyclooxygenase-2 inhibition with celecoxib elevates blood pressure and promotes leukocyte adhesion. Br J Pharmacol 2000;129:1423–1430.

197. FDA CLASS Advisory Committee: CLASS Advisory Committee Briefing Document. Feb 7 2001. Available at www.fda.gov/ohrms/dockets/ac/01/briefing/3677_b1_searle.pdf

198. Whelton A, White WB, Bello AE, et al: Effects of celecoxib and rofecoxib on blood pressure and edema in patients ≥65 years of age with systemic hypertension and osteoarthritis. Am J Cardiol 2002;90:959–963.

199. Collins R, Peto R, MacMahon S, et al: Blood pressure, stroke, and coronary heart disease. Part 2: Short-term reductions in blood pressure: Overview of randomized drug trials in their epidemiological context. Lancet 1990;335:827–838.

200. Bleumink GS, Feenstra J, Sturkenboom MCJM, Stricker BH: Nonsteroidal anti-inflammatory drugs and heart failure. Drugs 2003;63:525–534.

201. Page J, Henry D: Consumption of NSAIDs and the development of congestive heart failure in elderly patients. Arch Intern Med 2000;160:777–784.

202. Feenstra J, Heerdink ER, Grobbee DE, Stricker BH: Association of nonsteroidal anti-inflammatory drugs with first occurrence of heart failure and with relapsing heart failure. Arch Intern Med 2002;162:265–270.

203. Schafer AI: Effects of nonsteroidal anti-inflammatory therapy on platelets. Am J Med 1999;106:25S–36S.

204. Schafer AI: Effects of nonsteroidal anti-inflammatory drugs on platelet function and systemic hemostasis. J Clin Pharmacol 1995;35:209–219.

205. Cronberg S, Wallmark E, Soderberg I: Effect on platelet aggregation of oral administration of 10 nonsteroidal analgesics to humans. Scand J Haematol 1984;33:155–159.

206. Stuart MJ, Miller ML, Davey FR, Wold JA: The post-aspirin bleeding time: A screening test for evaluating haemostatic disorders. Br J Haematol 1979;43:649–659.

207. Barbui T, Buelli M, Cortelazzo S, et al: Aspirin and risk of bleeding in patients with thrombocythemia. Am J Med 1987;83:265–268.

208. Deykin D, Janson P, McMahon L: Ethanol potentiation of aspirin-induced prolongation of bleeding time. N Engl J Med 1982;306: 852–854.

209. Jakubowski JA, Vaillancourt R, Deykin D: Interaction of ethanol, prostacyclin, and aspirin in determining human platelet reactivity in vitro. Arteriosclerosis 1988;8:436–441.

210. James MJ, Walsh JA: Effects of aspirin and alcohol on platelet thromboxane synthesis and vascular prostacyclin synthesis. Thromb Res 1985;39:587–593.

211. Forrest JB, Camu F, Greer IA, et al: Ketorolac, diclofenac, and ketoprofen are equally safe for pain relief after major surgery. Br J Anesth 2002;88:227–233.

212. Wierod FS, Frandsen NJ, Jacobsen JD, et al: Risk of haemorrhage from transurethral prostatectomy in acetylsalicylic acid and NSAID-treated patients. Scand J Urol Nephrol 1998;32:120–122.

213. Zhu JP, Davidsen MB, Meyhoff HH: Aspirin, a silent risk factor in urology. Scand J Urol Nephrol 1994;29:369–374.

214. Marret E, Flahault A, Samama CM, Bonnet F: Effects of postoperative, nonsteroidal, anti-inflammatory drugs on bleeding risk after tonsillectomy: Meta-analysis of randomized, controlled trials. Anesthesiology 2003;98:1497–1502.

215. Moiniche S, Romsing J, Dahl JB, Tramer MR: Nonsteroidal anti-inflammatory drugs and the risk of operative site bleeding after tonsillectomy: A quantitative systematic review. Anesth Analg 2003;96:68–77.

216. Romsing J, Walther-Larsen S: Peri-operative use of nonsteroidal anti-inflammatory drugs in children: Analgesic efficacy and bleeding. Anaesthesia 1997;52:673–683.

217. Assia EI, Raskin T, Kaiserman I, et al: Effect of aspirin intake on bleeding during cataract surgery. J Cataract Refract Surg 1998; 24:1243–1246.

218. Connelly CS, Panush RS: Should nonsteroidal anti-inflammatory drugs be stopped before elective surgery? Arch Intern Med 1991;151:1963–1966.

219. Slappendel R, Weber EW, Benraad B, et al: Does ibuprofen increase perioperative blood loss during hip arthroplasty? Eur J Anaesthesiol 2002;19:829–831.

220. Amrein PC, Ellman L, Harris WH: Aspirin-induced prolongation of bleeding time and perioperative blood loss. JAMA 1981;245: 1825–1828.

221. Schnitzer TJ, Donahue JR, Toomey EP, et al: Effect of nabumetone on hemostasis during arthroscopic knee surgery. Clin Ther 1998; 20:110–124.

222. Horlocker TT, Wedel DJ, Benzon H, et al: Regional anesthesia in the anticoagulated patient: Defining the risks (the second ASRA Consensus Conference on Neuraxial Anesthesia and Anticoagulation). Reg Anesth Pain Med 2003;28:172–197.

223. CLASP: A randomized trial of low-dose aspirin for the prevention and treatment of pre-eclampsia among 9364 pregnant women. CLASP (Collaborative Low-Dose Aspirin Study in Pregnancy) Collaborative Group. Lancet 1994;343:619–629.

224. Horlocker TT, Bajwa ZH, Ashraft Z, et al: Risk assessment of hemorrhagic complications associated with nonsteroidal anti-inflammatory medications in ambulatory pain clinic patients undergoing epidural steroid injection. Anesth Analg 2002;95:1691–1697.

225. Gajraj NM: The effect of cyclooxygenase -2 inhibitors on bone healing. Reg Anesth Pain Med 2003;28:456–465.

226. Kawaguchi H, Pilbeam CC, Harrison JR, Raisz LG: The role of prostaglandins in the regulation of bone metabolism. Clin Orthop 1995;313:36–46.

227. Dekel S, Lenthall G, Francis MJ: Release of prostaglandins from bone and muscle after tibial fracture: An experimental study in rabbits. J Bone Joint Surg Br 1981;63:185–189.

228. Allen HW, Wase A, Bear WT: Indomethacin and aspirin: Effect of nonsteroidal anti-inflammatory agents on the rate of fracture repair in the rat. Acta Orthop Scand 1980;51:595–600.

229. Altman RD, Latta LL, Keer R, et al: Effect of nonsteroidal anti-inflammatory drugs on fracture healing: A laboratory study in rats. J Orthop Trauma 1995;9:392–400.

230. Hogevold HE, Grogaard B, Reikeras O: Effects of short-term treatment with corticosteroids and indomethacin on bone healing. Acta Orthop Scand 1992;63:607–611.

231. Simon AM, Manigrasso MB, O' Connor JP: Cyclooxygenase 2 function is essential for bone fracture healing. J Bone Miner Res 2002; 17:963–976.

232. Zhang X, Schwarz EM, Young DA: Cyclooxygenase-2 regulates mesenchymal cell differentiation into the osteoblast lineage and is critically involved in bone repair. J. Clin Invest. 2002;109:1405–1415.

233. Giannoudis PV, MacDonald DA, Matthews SJ, et al: Nonunion of the femoral diaphysis: The influence of reaming and nonsteroidal anti-inflammatory drugs. J Bone Joint Surg Br 2000;82:655–658.

234. Smith RM: Personal communication, 2005.

235. Glassman SD, Rose SM, Dimar JR, et al: The effect of postoperative nonsteroidal anti-inflammatory drug administration on spinal fusion. Spine 1998;23:834–838.

236. Davis TRC, Ackroyd CE: Nonsteroidal anti-inflammatory agents in the management of Colles' fractures. Br J Clin Pract 1988;42:184–189.

237. Neal BC, Rodgers A, Clark T, et al: A systematic survey of 13 randomized trials of non-steroidal anti-inflammatory drugs for the prevention

of heterotopic bone formation after major hip surgery. Acta Orthop Scand 2000;71:122–128.

238. Wurnig C, Schwameis E, Bitzan P, Kainberger F: Six-year results of a cementless stem with prophylaxis against heterotopic bone. Clin Orthop 1998;361:150–158.

239. Persson E, Sodemann B, Nilsson OS: Preventive effects of ibuprofen on periarticular heterotopic ossification after total hip arthroplasty. Acta Orthop Scand 1998;69:111–115.

240. Carretta A, Zannini P, Chiesa G, et al: Efficacy of ketorolac tromethamine and extrapleural intercostals nerve block on post-thoracotomy pain: A prospective, randomized study. Int Surg 1996; 81:224–228.

241. Prados W, Blaylock S: The effect of ketorolac on the postoperative narcotic requirements of gynecological surgery outpatients. Anesthesiology 1991;75:A6.

242. Yeh CC, Wu CT, Lee MS, et al: Analgesic effects of preincisional administration of dextromethorphan and tenoxicam following laparoscopic cholecystectomy. Acta Anaesthesiol Scand 2004;48: 1049–1053.

243. Munro FJ, Young SJ, Broome IJ, et al: Intravenous tenoxicam for analgesia following laparoscopic cholecystectomy. Anaesth Intensive Care 1998;26:56–60.

244. Rorarius MG, Suominen P, Baer GA, et al: Diclofenac and ketoprofen for pain treatment after elective caesarean section. Br J Anaesth 1993;70:293–297.

245. Elhakim M, Nafie M: IV tenoxicam for analgesia during caesarean section. Br J Anaesth 1995;74:643–646.

246. Bush DJ, Lyons G, MacDonald R: Diclofenac for analgesia after caesarean section. Anaesthesia 1992;47:1075–1077.

247. Pavy TJ, Paech MJ, Evans SF: The effect of intravenous ketorolac on opioid requirement and pain after cesarean delivery. Anesth Analg 2001;92:1010–1014.

248. Lowder JL, Shackelford DP, Holbert D, Beste TM: A randomized, controlled trial to compare ketorolac tromethamine versus placebo after cesarean section to reduce pain and narcotic usage. Am J Obstet Gynecol. 2003;189:1559–1562.

249. Wilder-Smith CH, Hill L, Dyer RA, et al: Postoperative sensitization and pain after cesarean delivery and the effects of single IM doses of tramadol and diclofenac alone and in combination. Anesth Analg 2003;97:526–533.

250. Olofsson CI, Legeby MH, Nygards EB, Ostman KM: Diclofenac in the treatment of pain after caesarean delivery: An opioid-saving strategy. Eur J Obstet Gynecol Reprod Biol 2000;88:143–146.

251. Lim NL, Lo WK, Chong JL, Pan AX: Single dose diclofenac suppository reduces post-cesarean PCEA requirements. Can J Anaesth 2001;48:383–386.

252. Dennis AR, Leeson-Payne CG, Hobbs GJ: Analgesia after caesarean section: The use of rectal diclofenac as an adjunct to spinal morphine. Anaesthesia 1995;50:297–299.

253. Cardoso MM, Carvalho JC, Amaro AR, et al: Small doses of intrathecal morphine combined with systemic diclofenac for postoperative pain control after cesarean delivery. Anesth Analg 1998;86: 538–541.

254. Sun HL, Wu CC, Lin MS, et al: Combination of low-dose epidural morphine and intramuscular diclofenac sodium in postcesarean analgesia. Anesth Analg 1992;75:64–68.

255. Rautoma P, Santanen U, Avela R, et al: Diclofenac premedication but not intra-articular ropivacaine alleviates pain following day-case knee arthroscopy. Can J Anaesth 2000;47:220–224.

256. Hoe-Hansen C, Norlin R: The clinical effect of ketoprofen after arthroscopic subacromial decompression: A randomized double-blind prospective study. Arthroscopy 1999;15:249–252.

257. Rasmussen S, Thomsen S, Madsen SN, et al: The clinical effect of naproxen sodium after arthroscopy of the knee: A randomized, double-blind, prospective study. Arthroscopy 1993;9:375–380.

258. Smith I, Shively RA, White PF: Effects of ketorolac and bupivacaine on recovery after outpatient arthroscopy. Anesth Analg 1992;75: 208–212.

259. Arvidsson I, Eriksson E: A double blind trial of NSAID versus placebo during rehabilitation. Orthopedics 1987;10:1007–1014.

260. Pedersen P, Nielsen KD, Jensen PE: The efficacy of Na-naproxen after diagnostic and therapeutic arthroscopy of the knee joint. Arthroscopy 1993;9:170–173.

261. Morrow BC, Bunting H, Milligan KR: A comparison of diclofenac and ketorolac for postoperative analgesia following day-case arthroscopy of the knee joint. Anaesthesia 1993;48:585–587.

262. Twersky RS, Lebovits A, Williams C, Sexton TR: Ketorolac versus fentanyl for postoperative pain management in outpatients. Clin J Pain 1995;11:127–133.

263. McLoughlin C, McKinney MS, Fee JP, Boules Z: Diclofenac for day-care arthroscopy surgery: Comparison with a standard opioid therapy. Br J Anaesth 1990;65:620–623.

264. Drez D Jr, Ritter M, Rosenberg TD: Pain relief after arthroscopy: Naproxen sodium compared to propoxyphene napsylate with acetaminophen. South Med J 1987;80:440–443.

265. Morrow BC, Milligan KR, Murthy BV: Analgesia following day-case knee arthroscopy—the effect of piroxicam with or without bupivacaine infiltration. Anaesthesia 1995;50:461–463.

266. Gurkan Y, Kilickan L, Buluc L, et al: Effects of diclofenac and intra-articular morphine/bupivacaine on postarthroscopic pain control. Minerva Anestesiol 1999;65:741–745.

267. Mack PF, Hass D, Lavyne MH, et al: Postoperative narcotic requirement after microscopic lumbar discectomy is not affected by intraoperative ketorolac or bupivacaine. Spine 2001;26:658–661.

268. Rosenow DE, Albrechtsen M, Stolke D: A comparison of patient-controlled analgesia with lornoxicam versus morphine in patients undergoing lumbar disk surgery. Anesth Analg 1998;86:1045–1050.

269. Fletcher D, Negre I, Barbin C, et al: Postoperative analgesia with IV propacetamol and ketoprofen combination after disc surgery. Can J Anaesth 1997;44:479–485.

270. Thienthong S, Jirarattanaphochai K, Krisanaprakornkit W, et al: Treatment of pain after spinal surgery in the recovery room by single dose lornoxicam: A randomized, double blind, placebo-controlled trial. J Med Assoc Thai 2004;87:650–655.

271. Silvanto M, Lappi M, Rosenberg PH: Comparison of the opioid-sparing efficacy of diclofenac and ketoprofen for 3 days after knee arthroplasty. Acta Anaesthesiol Scand 2002;46:322–328.

272. Zhou TJ, Tang J, White PF: Propacetamol versus ketorolac for treatment of acute postoperative pain after total hip or knee replacement. Anesth Analg 2001;92:1569–1575.

273. Kostamovaara PA, Hendolin H, Kokki H, Nuutinen LS: Ketorolac, diclofenac and ketoprofen are equally efficacious for pain relief after total hip replacement surgery. Br J Anaesth 1998;81:369–372.

274. Eggers KA, Jenkins BJ, Power I: Effect of oral and IV tenoxicam in postoperative pain after total knee replacement. Br J Anaesth 1999;83:876–881.

275. Beattie WS, Warriner CB, Etches R, et al: The addition of continuous intravenous infusion of ketorolac to a patient-controlled analgetic morphine regime reduced postoperative myocardial ischemia in patients undergoing elective total hip or knee arthroplasty. Anesth Analg 1997;84:715–722.

276. Fragen RJ, Stulberg SD, Wixson R, et al: Effect of ketorolac tromethamine on bleeding and on requirements for analgesia after total knee arthroplasty. J Bone Joint Surg Am 1995;77:998–1002.

277. Reuben SS, Fingeroth R, Krushell R, Maciolek H: Evaluation of the safety and efficacy of the perioperative administration of rofecoxib for total knee arthroplasty. J Arthroplasty 2002;17:26–31.

278. Cepeda MS, Carr DB, Miranda N, et al: Comparison or morphine, ketorolac, and their combination for postoperative pain. Anesthesiology 2005;103:1225–1232.

19 Multimodal Analgesic Therapy

JOSEPH PERGOLIZZI • LEONARD M. WILLS

Toward Evidence-Based Multimodal Analgesia

Evidence-based medicine (EBM) can facilitate decision-making in the selection of the most appropriate treatment for the patient. The goal of this book is to apply principles of EBM to the treatment of acute pain. (The general concepts underlying EBM have been surveyed in Chapters 1 and 2.) This chapter focuses on *multimodal therapy*—the application of agents and techniques that act through different mechanisms. This method is now common clinical practice throughout the world, and not simply for the control of pain. In another context, multimodal therapy might mean, for example, the use of several chemotherapeutic agents, each of which acts via a different mechanism, along with radiation therapy or surgery to bring a cancer into remission. Multimodal pain therapy is therefore an adaptation of a broader concept already used to treat neoplasia, infections, hypertension, and many other conditions.[1]

The benefits of multimodal analgesia in terms of drug sparing have been reviewed in a perioperative setting by a multidisciplinary panel of experts who convened to evaluate the literature on postoperative nausea and vomiting (PONV) and to provide evidence-based guidelines for its management. The panel concluded that utilization of multimodal analgesic regimens in the perioperative setting may not only improve pain management but also reduce the incidence of PONV, particularly when opioid-sparing techniques are used.[2]

This chapter describes the rationale for multimodal analgesia, including its potential benefits and harms, and the use of fixed-dose combinations; applies the techniques of EBM relevant to synthesizing the literature on multimodal analgesia; notes the limitations of the current literature that preclude a quantitative synthesis; and presents results of a qualitative systematic review of this topic.

Rationale for Multimodal Analgesia

Pain may result from diverse etiologies and mechanisms—nociceptive, inflammatory, and neuropathic (Table 19–1; Fig. 19–1). Pain treatments target different receptors, enzymes, pathways, and processes. Because pain is commonly mediated by multiple concurrent mechanisms, it makes sense to combine drugs addressing several targets simultaneously for more complete inhibition of nociception. As well as improving efficacy, combining two or more analgesics with different mechanisms may also improve safety by inducing nonoverlapping

side effects or may even offer greater predictability of the time course of analgesia by providing complementary pharmacokinetic activity.[3,4] Agents commonly used for multimodal analgesia are listed in Box 19–1.

Potential Advantages of Multimodal Therapy

Although analgesic monotherapy can be successful, all analgesics induce adverse events. Nonsteroidal anti-inflammatory drugs (NSAIDs) cause gastrointestinal (GI) complaints and bleeding, whereas opioids cause nausea and vomiting, sedation, and constipation. Multimodal analgesia enables lower doses of individual agents to be used (drug sparing), thereby attenuating the severity of each drug's side effects while achieving pain relief that is either equianalgesic or synergistic with that of single components (Fig. 19–2). It also causes fewer adverse events (incidence, severity, type), provides better analgesia (onset, duration and quality), and improves convenience and compliance (Box 19–2). Each drug may contribute to an additive or synergistic action.[5] In order to achieve best results, a lower initial dosage of each component, prolonged dosage intervals, and slower dosage titrations are advisable when one is combining drugs.

The drug-sparing characteristics gained through the use of a combination have been shown in several models, including opioid-sparing, NSAID-sparing, and cyclooxygenase-2 (Cox-2) inhibitor–sparing combinations,[3,6–8] as discussed later. Positive attributes for multimodal analgesia have been demonstrated in, for example, opioid-sparing combinations that achieve a lower opioid dose, thereby avoiding sedation and respiratory depression, decreasing constipation and pruritus, and lowering risk of PONV. Patients also recover faster and are discharged earlier.[9–11]

Potential Disadvantages of Multimodal Therapy

Combining analgesics at lower doses has the following potential primary outcomes:

Best case—reduced incidence of adverse events and greater analgesia.

Very acceptable—reduced incidence of adverse events and equianalgesia.

Acceptable—no change in adverse-event profile and greater analgesia.

TABLE 19–1	Type of Stimulus and Processing		
Pain	**Stimulus**	**Mechanism(s)**	**Characteristics**
Nociceptive	Brief	"Activation," wide-dynamic-range neurons, "wind-up"	Pressure, heat, reversible
Inflammatory	Repeated	"Modulation," central and peripheral sensitization	Hyperalgesia, allodynia, slowly reversible
Neuropathic	Long-lasting	"Modification," trophic changes, central sensitization	Hyperalgesia, allodynia, spontaneous pain, persistent

From Woolf CJ, Salter MW: Neuronal plasticity: Increasing the gain in pain. Science 2000;288:1765–1769.

Not acceptable—higher incidence of adverse events and greater analgesia.

Not acceptable—higher incidence of adverse events and equianalgesia.

Safety is paramount: Combinations must at the very least not raise the incidence of adverse events. Even if they do reduce the incidence of adverse events, the reduction should be clinically meaningful to be considered useful. Several studies have demonstrated that multimodal therapy does not necessarily provide additive or synergistic analgesia. Some combinations tested show enhanced analgesia but also increased side effects.

In these cases, assessments must be made as to whether the combination is truly multimodal—that is, does the particular combination target multiple pain pathways, as opposed simply to being two drugs that target the same pain pathway? The simultaneous administration of two or more drugs does not guarantee that they interact clinically in a positive way. Furthermore, it is imperative that their use in special circumstances is considered as well as their pharmacokinetic and pharmacodynamic characteristics.

In certain circumstances, such as in the treatment of the elderly patient, multimodal therapy and polypharmacy can lead to

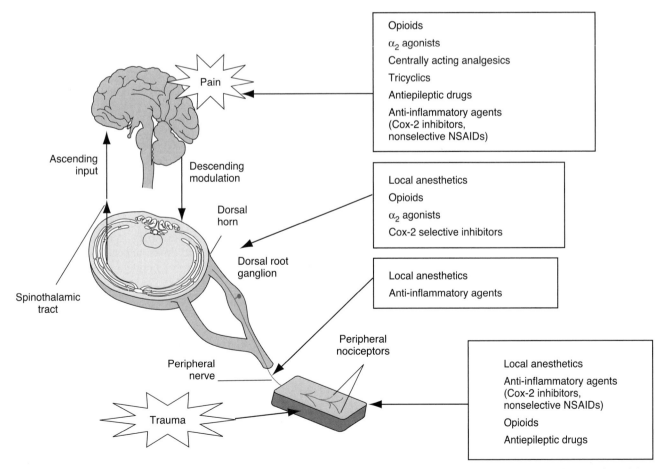

Figure 19–1   Analgesia and the pain pathway. Cox-2, cyclooxygenase-2; NSAIDs, nonsteroidal anti-inflammatory drugs. (Adapted from Gottschalk A. Smith DS: New concepts in acute pain therapy: Preemptive analgesia. Am Fam Physician 2001;63:1979–1984.)

- Local anesthetics
- Opioids
- Nonselective nonsteroidal anti-inflammatory drugs (NSAIDs)
- Cyclooxygenase 2 (Cox-2) selective inhibitors
- Acetaminophen
- Antihyperalgesics: Anti–N-methyl-D-aspartate (NMDA) (ketamine, dextromethorphan, amantadine, memantine), gabapentin, adenosine, α_2-adrenoreceptor agonists, etc.
- Other adjuvant therapies: complementary and alternative medicine (CAM), transcutaneous electrical nerve stimulation (TENS), etc.

| BOX 19–2 | POTENTIAL BENEFITS OF MULTIMODAL ANALGESIA |

- Synergistic analgesic effects: onset, duration of action, quality, etc.
- Pain prevention or attenuated nociception
- Diminished stress response
- Reduced sensitization
- Improved side-effect profile: incidence, severity, type, etc.
- Improved compliance: convenience, etc.
- Cost-effectiveness

increased risk of adverse events and multimorbidity because patients are already taking several drugs simultaneously, such as lipid-lowering drugs. Factors responsible for differential toxicity involve age-related pharmacokinetic, pharmacodynamic, and physiological factors as well as coincident disease states. Polypharmacy is a particular problem when physicians are unclear as to which drugs a patient is taking and may inadvertently prescribe drugs that compete or interfere with those drugs. Polypharmacy may even alter analgesic effects and pharmacokinetic or pharmacodynamic properties of combinations. An example of a successful multimodal analgesic is the triple combination of acetaminophen plus aspirin plus caffeine, which is commonly prescribed for migraine in the United States.

Fixed-Dose versus Flexible-Dose Combinations

Existing clinical data establish the equianalgesic dose of each component drug, enabling component doses to be lowered from this starting point to produce a fixed-dose combination (Table 19–2). The use of fixed-dose combinations can overcome problems associated with flexible-dose combinations, such as poor interaction indexes and an increase in adverse event rates, and can discourage self-titration of

drugs by patients. Fixed-drug combinations offer the potential to improve the analgesic effect, the spectrum of efficacy, the benefit-to-risk ratio, and compliance.

One means of showing how two drugs interact when combined is the *isobologram*, a commonly used graphical and statistical tool for analyzing the combined effects of simple chemical mixtures. To construct an isobologram, one first must decide on an endpoint that will be used to gauge the outcome of applying either a single dose of a particular drug or mixtures of two drugs in various proportions. Typically, in the evaluation of analgesics used for acute pain, the endpoint is 50% pain relief. Then one plots the dose of both agents given together that results in the same endpoint. As the dose ratios of both agents are varied, they may fall below the straight line connecting the dose of each single agent required to achieve the same endpoint. If that is the case, the interaction between the two agents is said to be *synergistic*. If the ratios of both agents' doses place them on the line, their interaction is termed *additive*, and if above the line, their action is termed *antagonistic*.

Tramadol is a centrally acting opioid analgesic with two complementary mechanisms: binding to μ opioid receptors and inhibition of reuptake of noradrenaline and serotonin. Acetaminophen is a nonopioid analgesic antipyretic and a weak inhibitor of prostaglandin biosynthesis. The isobologram for co-administration of tramadol plus acetaminophen is shown in Figure 19–3, which discloses a synergistic interaction for these agents at every dose combination studied. In this case, mice were pretreated with oral tramadol alone, acetaminophen alone, or fixed-ratio combinations of both. After 30 minutes, the mice were injected with a chemical

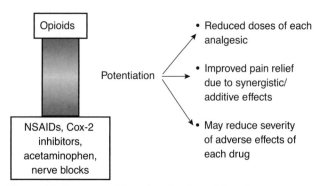

Figure 19–2 Potential benefits of multimodal analgesia. NSAIDs, nonsteroidal anti-inflammatory drugs. (From Kehlet H, Dahl JB: The value of "multimodal" or "balanced analgesia" in postoperative pain treatment. Anesth Analg 1993;77:1048–1056.)

TABLE 19–2	Combination Therapy
Why?	Establish optimal ratio of combination(s)
What?	Drugs with different mechanisms of action
How much?	Start combining ¹/₂ dose of each drug; then increase/decrease doses at fixed ratios
Other	Keep one drug at a fixed dose and increase the dose of the other
Which route(s)?	Least invasive
Variables	Analgesia and adverse events

Material taken from the first Meeting of the Working Group on Pain Management, Dec. 14, 2005, Taplow, UK. Courtesy of Professor M. Puig.

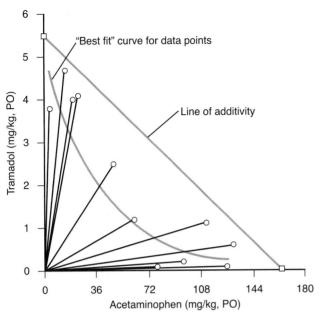

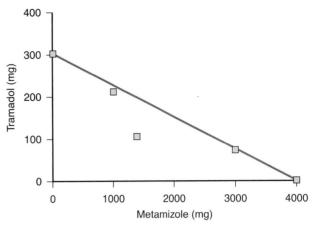

Figure 19–3 Isobologram of tramadol plus acetaminophen in various dose combinations. (From Tallarida RJ, Raffa RB. Testing for synergism over a range of fixed ratio drug combinations. Replacing the isobologram. Life Sci 1996;58:PL23—PL28.)

Figure 19–4 Isobologam showing tramadol–metamizole interaction. See text for explanation. (From Montes A, et al: Use of intravenous patient-controlled analgesia for the documentation of synergy between tramadol and metamizol. Brit J Anaesth 2000;85:217–223.)

irritant (acetylcholine). The absence of a specified behavioral response implies analgesia (actually, antinociception). In the isobologram, the straight line connects the individual drugs' mean effect dose (ED_{50}) values, which were determined using this method for tramadol and acetaminophen, individually, from a typical dose-response curve (only the ED_{50} values are plotted as the pair of points 0,y and x,0). The line represents all theoretical effects for the combination of tramadol and acetaminophen that are additive and is drawn by connecting the two ED_{50} values. The experiment is then conducted using actual fixed-ratio combinations of the two drugs, and the determined ED_{50} values from these dose-response curves are plotted as open circles, each of which represents the ED_{50} of a particular combination. ED_{50} values that "fall below" the line of additivity are in the region of synergy (above is the region of antagonism). The curve is a fit of the experimentally determined ED_{50} values.

Drug interactions can be assessed using isobolograms that help determine the optimal dose ratio for combining agents. Figure 19–4 shows an example of a study of tramadol plus metamizole at 8 hours. The axes indicate the mean cumulative doses (standard error of the mean [SEM]) of metamizole (abscissa) and tramadol (ordinate) that produce the same level of response (visual analogue scale pain intensity range 2.4–2.7). The diagonal line connects equally effective doses of each drug alone and designates additivity (zero interaction line). All other points in the graph were obtained by plotting each of the paired cumulative doses (SEM) in each treatment group.[12] These drugs are combined in a 1:1 efficacy ratio in post-hysterectomy pain for the specific dose used of each component. They show synergy for analgesia and adverse events, including nausea and vomiting, and sedation, with a therapeutic index of approximately 3.[12]

REGULATION OF COMBINATION THERAPIES

Currently, only a limited number of combinational analgesic compounds approved by regulatory authorities are available for the management of postoperative pain. The vast majority of analgesic combinations used are "loose" combinations that have not been tested by the rigors of regulatory agencies like the U.S. Food and Drug Administration (FDA) and the European Medicines Evaluation Agency (EMEA). As a result, their true pharmacological and clinical effects in all patient types are unknown.

Regulatory agencies such as FDA and EMEA have revised their procedures for the testing and approval of combination therapies. The FDA now requires single-dose studies to be conducted so that the "fixed" combination of analgesics is compared with individual components, with placebo, and with standards. Moreover, a novel analgesic combination must be proven to have more beneficial effects than either drug alone when being considered for all types of pain and patients.

In order to solve the problem of how analgesics should be combined, pharmaceutical companies have introduced several fixed-dose-combination preparations and are planning to introduce more. With industry-funded trials, however, there is a growing tendency to publish positive data, including those of fixed-dose combinations. To address this problem, De Angelis et al,[13] in a 2004 leading article in the *New England Journal of Medicine,* recommended that results from industry-sponsored clinical trials should not be published in a peer-reviewed journal unless the trial has first been registered. The registry must be electronically searchable and accessible to the public at no charge, open to all registrants, and incorporate a mechanism to ensure the validity of the registration data.[13] Moreover, they advocated that trial organizers should make a full endorsement of both the Consolidated Standards of Reporting Trials (CONSORT) Statement and the Cochrane Library. For balance, it is also equally important to study flexible-dose combinations, particularly in larger populations, and to further evaluate their pharmacokinetic and pharmacodynamic characteristics and clinical effects in special populations, such as pediatric and elderly patients.

Multimodal Analgesia/Antihyperalgesia

Adjuvant drugs (see later) and local anesthetic drugs used to decrease nociceptive sensitization (antihyperalgesics) that have been applied in the perioperative setting include anti–N-methyl-D-aspartate (NMDA) (ketamine, dextromethorphan, amantadine, memantine), gabapentin, adenosine, α_2-adrenoreceptor agonists, lidocaine, and mexiletine.[14] Treating postoperative patients with the antihyperalgesic ketamine, 0.5 mg/kg, led to an area of hyperalgesia for days 1 through 7 measuring less than 25 cm^2 (versus 175–200 cm^2 for placebo).[15] Gabapentin has demonstrated potential benefit in preemptive analgesia, preventing the greater neuronal sensitization associated with surgical stimuli, and has antihyperalgesic properties that can protect the patient's nociceptive system from pernicious sequelae of surgery, such as chronic pain.[16–18] In an arthroscopic anterior cruciate ligament repair study by Menigaux,[19] gabapentin 1200 mg on days 1 and 2 after operation achieved 76% and 84%, respectively, of maximal active flexion (versus 63% and 76% for placebo) (Fig. 19–5). Theoretically, the potentially protective effects of gabapentin could be heightened by combination with other drugs having different modes of action.

Fixed-dose combinations of traditional opioids and antihyperalgesics are currently being investigated in clinical trials. For example, ketamine has reduced the area of hyperalgesia around a surgical incision in patients also treated with morphine.[15] Further research has investigated intraoperative "subanesthetic doses" of ketamine for postoperative antihyperalgesia.[20]

Flexible-dose combinations are currently in use and are under investigation, yet no IA-type data exist (I indicating a large randomized controlled trial [RCT], $N \geq 100$ per group; A denoting good evidence to support the recommendation). An up-to-date, pertinent success in patients was reported by Panchal et al,[21] who implemented an analgesic/antihyperalgesic regimen for patients undergoing thoracotomy procedures (Table 19–3).

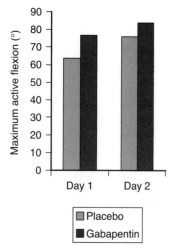

Figure 19–5 Antihyperalgesic properties of gabapentin in arthroscopic anterior cruciate ligament repair. (From Menigaux C, Adam F, Guignard B, et al: Preoperative gabapentin decreases anxiety and improves early functional recovery from knee surgery. Anesth Analg 2005;100:1394–1399.)

TABLE 19–3	Analgesic/Antihyperalgesic Regimen for Patients Undergoing Thoracotomy
Preoperatively and intraoperatively	(1) Valdecoxib 40 mg PO (oral) and gabapentin 1200 mg PO *PLUS* (2) 3-mL–5-mL bolus (depending on patient size) of 0.25% bupivacaine via thoracic epidural (T4–T5 or T3–T4) level prior to incision; repeat bolus every 2 hours intraoperatively
Postoperatively	Continue with: (1) Thoracic epidural using 0.0625% bupivacaine with sufentanil 1 μg/mL solution as patient-controlled epidural analgesia: bolus 3–5 mL; lockout interval 10 minutes; basal rate 3–4 mL/hour *AND* (2) Valdecoxib 40 mg PO daily for 14 days

Panchal SJ: Personal communication, January 2005.

Evidence-Based Review: Monotherapy and Multimodal Analgesia for Acute Pain

Most drugs have been studied as individual entities in isolation; however, as the term suggests, multimodal therapy incorporates combination of a variety of drugs of different drug classes. This situation leads to the question whether an evidence-based approach has been adopted to ascertain the risk-to-benefit ratios of multimodal analgesia, especially as there are problems associated with the way clinical trials are organized and their results reported.

MONOTHERAPY IS UNSATISFACTORY

Most patients receive monotherapy for postoperative pain,[18] and abundant data indicate the efficacy of single doses of many analgesic agents in this indication. This demonstration contrasts markedly with surveys indicating that patients are generally not happy with the management of their postoperative pain: Clinical audit data through decades of observation speak to the inadequacy of conventional therapy in this setting,[22] and results from later national audits and surveys suggest that postoperative pain continues to be undertreated.[23,24]

Undertreatment and patient dissatisfaction may be a result of the particular treatments chosen. For example, opioids are frequently used in this setting,[18] but it is known that patients with postoperative pain who are receiving monotherapy with a single analgesic prefer to be treated with nonopioid therapy (Fig. 19–6). [25] Nonopioid or opioid-sparing regimens may be preferable in this regard. Alternatively—or additionally—the fault may lie with the approach. Monotherapy will target only one of the many pathways that may be mediating the painful stimulus; multimodal analgesia, in addition to its presumptive dose-sparing effects, may be more effective by targeting multiple pain pathways.

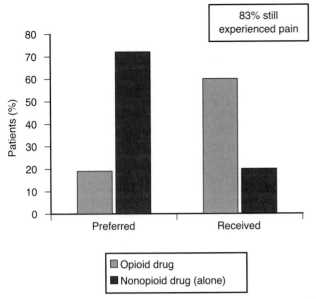

Figure 19–6 Postoperative pain: patient preferences versus actual treatments. (From Apfelbaum JL: Postoperative pain experience: Results from a national survey suggest postoperative pain continues to be undermanaged. Anesth Analg 2003;97:534–540.)

SYSTEMATIC REVIEW OF OUTCOMES OF MULTIMODAL THERAPY

In order to perform a systematic review of the outcomes of multimodal treatment of acute pain, I conducted a search of MedLine abstracts for the years 1995 through 2004 using the three most frequently applied terms from a selected list of ten terms (see Appendix) to describe multimodal treatment for pain. The search yielded 47 RCTs involving "multimodal pain treatment" or "multimodal pain therapy" and 35 RCTs for "multimodal analgesia." These postoperative analgesic trials assessed both fixed-dose and flexible-dose combinations, complementary and alternative medicine (CAM) interventions, and combinations of anesthetic techniques. A formal meta-analysis was not feasible because of the broad range of differences among the trials in terms of study populations, components of combinations, dosing schedules, and routes of administration as well as outcome measures and study durations.

Positive Results with Multimodal Therapy

Most studies from the MedLine search reported positive results. Several studies showed that opioid use increases the analgesic effects of a combination, whereas others demonstrated that in multimodal therapy the opioid dosage or the length of time an opioid is required can be reduced. Buvanendran et al[26] showed that opioid consumption could be reduced (opioid sparing) by using the Cox-2 inhibitor rofecoxib in multimodal analgesia, which also reduced pain, vomiting, and sleep disturbance and improved range of motion after total knee arthroplasty. Combining NSAIDs and opioids could result in synergistic analgesia because these agents act through different mechanisms. Hanna et al[27] showed a morphine-sparing effect and good analgesic efficacy with the use of dexketoprofen trometamol. A later comprehensive meta-analysis of the effect of adding NSAIDs to morphine given for patient-controlled analgesia (PCA) confirmed this opioid-sparing effect.[28]

Several studies have investigated the use of opioids in multimodal therapy regimens for treating postoperative pain after cesarean section. Cardoso et al,[29] evaluating the use of low-dose intrathecal morphine in combination with intramuscular diclofenac, demonstrated good analgesia with a low incidence of morphine-induced pruritus at morphine doses of 0.025 mg. Indeed, no added benefit was achieved when larger morphine doses were combined with systemic diclofenac. Another study showed that patients given intrathecal morphine, incisional bupivacaine, and ibuprofen plus acetaminophen experienced better early postoperative analgesia than those given conventional therapy with intravenous PCA (IV-PCA) morphine and weaned to an oral combination of acetaminophen plus codeine.[30]

For pain from ambulatory laparoscopic cholecystectomy, Michaloliakou et al[10] found that multimodal analgesia (local anesthetic plus NSAIDs plus opioids) significantly reduced the number of patients with pain, the pain severity (six-fold lower), and the incidence of nausea while satisfying discharge criteria significantly earlier in comparison with single-agent analgesia plus saline.

Several studies have demonstrated the Cox-2 inhibitor–sparing effects of multimodal analgesic regimens for the treatment of patients with osteoarthritis of more than 1 year's duration. Both Emkey et al[31] and Silverfield et al[32] reported that tramadol plus acetaminophen was effective and safe as an "add-on" to Cox-2 inhibitor therapy. A subanalysis of the Silverfield data in elderly patients showed the same positive results as those of the overall study.[33]

The nonbarbiturate, rapid-acting anesthetic (antihyperalgesic) ketamine has been used as an adjunct to multimodal therapy. Chia et al[34] proved that in patients undergoing major surgery, adding ketamine to a multimodal epidural PCA regimen (morphine, bupivacaine, and epinephrine) provided better postoperative pain relief, decreased analgesic consumption, and had an additive analgesic effect. Similarly, Menigaux et al[35] showed that addition of ketamine to a multimodal (morphine, naproxen sodium, di-antalvic) regimen improves both postoperative analgesia and functional outcome after knee arthroscopy.

Two Cochrane Library reviews have shown mixed conclusions regarding postoperative multimodal analgesia. The first was a quantitative assessment of oxycodone alone and oxycodone plus acetaminophen in RCTs of acute postoperative pain (77 reports). For efficacy, a significant benefit of active drug over placebo was seen for most oxycodone doses and for oxycodone plus acetaminophen. Oxycodone, with or without acetaminophen, appeared to be comparable in efficacy to intramuscular morphine and NSAIDs, although central nervous system (CNS) adverse events were common with its use.[36] The second Cochrane review compared dextropropoxyphene alone and combined with acetaminophen for moderate to severe postoperative pain in several trials and a meta-analysis. The efficacy of the combination of dextropropoxyphene 65 mg plus paracetamol 650 mg was similar to that of tramadol 100 mg in single-dose studies of postoperative pain but demonstrated a lower incidence of adverse events. However, acetaminophen 650 mg plus codeine 60 mg appeared to be more effective and had a similar incidence of adverse events.[37]

Tramadol Plus Acetaminophen Combination

As described earlier in this chapter, tramadol plus acetaminophen is an example of an FDA-approved fixed-dose combination. Both components are effective analgesics and have different pharmacokinetic characteristics that, when combined, affect three different and complementary pathways to achieve analgesia superior to that of the individual components while decreasing the risk for adverse events. The pharmacokinetic properties of tramadol plus acetaminophen result in a beneficial pharmacodynamic profile that combines the rapid onset of acetaminophen with the lasting effect of tramadol (Fig. 19–7) in both acute and chronic pain models.

Overall, multimodal therapy has shown positive analgesic effects in several acute pain situations. Combining NSAIDs, opioids, and/or Cox-2 inhibitors has led to additive or synergistic analgesia with a better balance and/or a lower incidence of adverse events, improved physical and psychological functioning, and a reduced period of immobilization and convalescence.[28,38–46] Accordingly, current evidence reviews and evidence-based guidelines endorse multimodal analgesic therapy as the default approach to postoperative pain control (e.g., see reference 47).

Positive Results with Preemptive Multimodal Analgesia

Surgical trauma induces nociceptive sensitization, leading to amplification and prolongation of postoperative pain. Preemptive multimodal therapy using opioids has proved successful. Rockemann et al[48] showed that a preemptive multimodal approach (diclofenac, metamizole, epidural morphine, and mepivacaine) before abdominal surgery significantly reduced the need for postoperative treatment when the drugs were administered prior to the surgical incision compared with their administration at the end of the operation, before wound closure. Rosaeg et al[49] demonstrated that preemptive multimodal analgesia for arthroscopic knee ligament repair, using ketorolac, intra-articular morphine/ropivacaine/epinephrine, and femoral nerve block with ropivacaine before surgery, achieved lower pain scores and less morphine consumption.

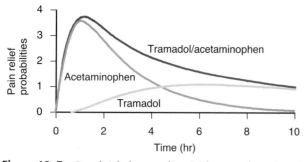

Figure 19–7 Beneficial pharmacokinetic/pharmacodynamic properties of the two-drug combination of tramadol plus acetaminophen. Relationship between the probability distribution of pain relief scores to tramadol and acetaminophen plasma concentration time profiles.

Negative or Equivocal Results with Multimodal Therapy

Clearly, not all agents that are effective as monotherapy are equally effective when used in a multimodal strategy. Combinational therapies do not always lead to an improved outcome for patients, as the isobologram data previously discussed have shown. Moreover, combining certain analgesic agents can result in an increase in side effects. Several double-blind RCTs of multimodal therapies have reported mixed or negative results. For example, in women undergoing cesarean section, Choi et al[50] showed that postoperative pain was not reduced by the addition of oral dextromethorphan to a multimodal approach based on intrathecal morphine. In a study of 240 women, Paech et al[51] demonstrated that combining subarachnoid bupivacaine, fentanyl, morphine, and clonidine provided better relief of cesarean section pain than morphine or clonidine alone, but it increased intraoperative sedation and possibly vomiting. Keita et al[52] compared saline, bupivacaine, and morphine individually with bupivacaine plus morphine for analgesia after gynecological laparoscopic surgery. The combination did not significantly improve postoperative analgesia.

Negative or Equivocal Results with Preemptive Multimodal Analgesia

Nagatsuka et al[53] reported that administration of diclofenac, butorphanol, and lidocaine did not obtain preemptive multimodal analgesia during sagittal split ramus osteotomy.[53] Doyle and Bowler[54] also showed that preemptive administration of analgesics (morphine, diclofenac and intercostal nerve block) before posterolateral thoracotomy had modest effects in terms of analgesia achieved, analgesic consumption, and long-term outcome. Reuben et al[55] showed that after ambulatory anterior cruciate ligament repair, patients receiving a multimodal analgesic regimen of perioperative NSAIDs, intra-articular bupivacaine, and external cooling did not receive any additional analgesia from the addition of intra-articular morphine.[55]

As of 2005, the Cochrane Library did not have an assessment available on the use of multimodal analgesia/antihyperalgesic combinations in a postoperative setting. However, a report by Bell[56] from the Cochrane Library quantitatively assessed four RCTs and 32 case studies of multimodal analgesia/antihyperalgesic combinations examining the use of ketamine as an adjuvant to opioids in treating cancer pain. Ketamine was found to improve the effectiveness of morphine. However, pooling of data was inappropriate, and some patients experienced hallucinations with both ketamine plus morphine and morphine alone. Bell concluded that current evidence was insufficient for the use of ketamine as an adjuvant to opioid therapy.

Multimodal Therapy: Current Options and Dilemmas

Various agents within several major analgesic classes can currently be combined to provide enhanced adverse-event profiles and achieve equianalgesic or synergistic analgesia,

TABLE 19–4	Analgesic Agents Used in Multimodal Analgesic Regimens*
Nonsteroidal anti-inflammatory drugs	Acetaminophen Cyclooxygenase-2 inhibitors Diclofenac Ibuprofen Ketoprofen Ketorolac Naproxen
Opioids	Butorphanol Codeine Fentanyl Morphine Oxycodone Tramadol
Local anesthetics	Bupivacaine Lidocaine Mepivacaine Ropivacaine
Adjuvants	α_2 agonists Antiepileptics Antidepressants Ketamine

*See text.

including local anesthetics, opioids, nonselective NSAIDs, Cox-2 inhibitors, α_2 agonists, and acetaminophen (Table 19–4). The most common combinations are opioid + NSAID ± local anesthetic ± adjuvant drugs. *Adjuvant drugs* typically have weak or no analgesic effects in humans for nociceptive pain but do enhance the effects of standard analgesics for nociceptive pain. Some adjuvant drugs are first-line agents for the treatment of neuropathic pain.

Examples of combinations used for acute postoperative pain (systemic pain) are as follows:
- Opioids + NSAIDs or α_2 agonists
- Morphine + ketamine
- Acetaminophen + NSAIDs

An example of combinations used for acute postoperative pain (spinal pain) is local anesthetic + opioid ± α_2 agonist.

SELECTING PRACTICAL DRUG COMBINATIONS FOR POSTOPERATIVE PAIN

Individually, analgesic drugs have positive and negative effects. Selecting the appropriate drug components for multimodal therapy is key to practical success in treating postoperative pain. Some positive and negative attributes of NSAIDs, Cox-2 inhibitors, and opioids are listed in Table 19–5.

NSAIDs in particular provide a foundation for multimodal pharmacotherapy. These agents enhance the analgesic actions of opioids in several regions of the CNS in combination therapy while reducing adverse events, most commonly urinary, respiratory, and CNS effects. Opioids are commonly used for managing postoperative pain because they have no ceiling for analgesia. However, raising doses of opioids induces intolerable adverse events, thereby limiting their usefulness as sole or even principal agents for treating acute pain.[57] The role of NSAIDs in multimodal analgesia and their advantages are listed in Box 19–3.

TABLE 19–5	Comparison of Different Analgesic Classes	
Analgesic Class	**Pros**	**Cons**
Nonselective NSAIDs	Effective in relieving inflammation associated with musculoskeletal pain Short-term (<1 wk) use for acute postoperative pain carries minimal GI or cardiac risk	Nonselective NSAIDS are associated with increased upper and lower GI adverse events with long-term use OTC availability of nonselective NSAIDs provides risk of patient misuse or overdose, alone or in combination with prescription nonselective NSAIDs All nonselective NSAIDs should be used with caution in patients with renal insufficiency
Cox-2 inhibitors	Effective in relieving inflammation associated with musculoskeletal pain	Cost may present managed care access issues Cardiovascular risks (myocardial infarction, edema, hypertension) with rofecoxib >25 mg/day over long term Postoperative cardiovascular risk led to FDA caution against use of any Cox-2 inhibitor for postoperative pain (April 2005) Celecoxib and valdecoxib are contraindicated in patients with known sulfonamide allergy All NSAIDs and Cox-2 inhibitors should be used with caution in patients with renal insufficiency
Opioids	Effective for most patients	Up to 38% rate of no response, even with liberal use, in some studies Efficacy may differ according to whether pain is neuropathic or nociceptive Adverse events: constipation, sedation, nausea, neurotoxic effects, respiratory depression Potential for abuse, addiction, or tolerance

Cox-2, cyclooxygenase-2; FDA, U.S. Food and Drug Administration; GI, gastrointestinal; NSAID, nonsteroidal anti-inflammatory drug; OTC, over-the-counter.

<table>
<tr><td>**BOX 19–3**</td><td>**NONSTEROIDAL ANTI-INFLAMMATORY DRUGS (NSAIDS) IN MULTIMODAL ANALGESIA**</td></tr>
</table>

Role of NSAIDs in multimodal analgesia:
- Reduce the activation and sensitization of peripheral nociceptors
- Attenuate the inflammatory response
- Possible central effect
- Possible action on N-methyl-D-aspartate (NMDA) receptor
- No dependence/addiction potential
- Synergistic effects with opioids
- Opioid-sparing effect (20-50%)
- No effect on sleep
- Used as part of a "balanced technique" multimodal analgesia

Advantages of NSAIDs over opioids:
- Preemptive analgesia (decreased neuronal sensitization)
- Pain prophylaxis (decreased postoperative pain)
- No respiratory depression
- Less nausea and vomiting than with opioids
- Decreased postoperative ileus and time to oral feeding
- Less dose variability than with opioids
- Cover some pain types better than with opioids (bone pain, incident pain, breathing, movement)
- No pupillary changes (neurological assessment)
- No cognitive impairment (consent, confusion in elderly)

THE COX-2 DILEMMA

Cox-2 is induced both peripherally and centrally in response to pain, and Cox-2 inhibition represents an excellent target for analgesia. Using Cox-2 inhibitors after painful injury may prevent latent development of central sensitization, hyperalgesia, and persistent, pathological pain.

Three studies have shown that administering Cox-2 inhibitors as part of a multimodal regimen results in lower pain scores, better respiratory function, and a reduced need for morphine (opioid sparing) compared with placebo and also prolongs the time to first use of opioids.[8,58,59]

In a study by Reuben et al,[8] 60 patients undergoing arthroscopic meniscectomy were randomly assigned to receive rofecoxib 50 mg, either 1 hour prior to incision (preoperative group) or at completion of surgery (postoperative group). A third group received placebo tablets. At 24 hours, use of acetaminophen/oxycodone was lower in the preoperative rofecoxib group (1.5 ± 0.6 tablets) than in both the postoperative rofecoxib group (3.3 ± 1.3 tablets) and the placebo group (5.5 ± 1.6 tablets). Patients who received preoperative rofecoxib needed significantly fewer tablets of acetaminophen/oxycodone at 24 hours after knee surgery and had a significantly longer mean time to first opioid use (preoperative group, 803 minutes; postoperative group, 461 minutes; placebo group, 318 minutes). In addition, pain scores with movement were lower in the preoperative group at all postoperative intervals. More patients in the preoperative group reported not using opioids than patients in the other two groups.[8]

The dilemma with the use of Cox-2 inhibitors is that although they promise fewer GI and hemorrhagic side effects,

they do raise concerns in respect to long-term treatment—namely deleterious renal and cardiovascular effects, particularly in the elderly. Accordingly, the long-term use of Cox-2 inhibitors has been called into question by both EMEA and FDA. In general the adverse effect profile of NSAIDs and, by extension, Cox-2 inhibitors that is evident during long-term use has been viewed as distinct from that associated with short-term use. The safety of the injectable Cox-2 inhibitor valdecoxib for immediate postoperative use has now been questioned, however, owing to the finding of higher rates of cardiovascular complications in a large RCT of its use after coronary artery bypass graft surgery.[60] Therefore, as of June 2005, the position of FDA's Center for Drug Evaluation and Research, based on a "thorough review of the available data," is that the "short-term use of NSAIDs to relieve acute pain, particularly at low doses, does not appear to confer an increased risk of serious adverse cardiovascular events (with the exception of valdecoxib in hospitalized patients immediately post-operative from coronary artery bypass surgery)."[61] Valdecoxib was withdrawn by its manufacturer in early 2005 but may well be reinstated; if this drug class continues to be used for chronic pain, its co-administration with other drugs (e.g., opioids such as tramadol and dextropropoxyphene) to lessen the risk of adverse events may become the subject of study.

Thus, the use of multimodal analgesia may diffuse outward from the short-term to the long-term setting, such as during rehabilitation after surgery. For the time being, especially in light of ample multinational data referring to the GI, renal, and cardiac safety of nonselective NSAIDs given for brief courses (<1 week) to control postoperative pain after major surgery,[62] it would seem most prudent to employ these more well-established agents rather than Cox-2 inhibitors for routine postoperative multimodal analgesia.

Complementary and Alternative Medicine in Pain Management

Modalities for acute pain control need not be limited to drug therapy. Optimal pain management can also encompass non-pharmacological and holistic/complementary approaches to pain management, such as neuromodulation, ablative and decompressive techniques, and physical rehabilitation techniques (exercise, transcutaneous electrical nerve stimulation, acupuncture). Psychological methods such as relaxation and imagery may help postoperative patients with pain management. Trials of behavioral approaches to postoperative pain control have produced mixed results.

Evidence from RCTs and systematic literature reviews led Astin[63] to make the following recommendations for alternative therapies:
- Postsurgical pain—mind-body therapies (e.g., imagery, hypnosis, relaxation) employed presurgically can improve recovery time and pain.
- Pain amelioration during invasive procedures—mind-body approaches can be used as adjunctive therapies.

Astin[63] also summarized evidence for the use of these therapies in chronic conditions, such as chronic low back pain, rheumatoid arthritis, osteoarthritis, and recurrent headache.

Potential Cost-Effectiveness and Reduction in Side Effects with Drug-Sparing Techniques

Negative clinical outcomes of inadequately managed acute postoperative pain include extended hospitalization, compromised prognosis, higher morbidity and mortality, and the development of a chronic pain state. The economic burden of postoperative pain is considerable and results from direct costs due to excess healthcare resources as well as indirect costs from reduced patient functionality and productivity. For example, the economic burden of treating a 30-year-old person with chronic postsurgical pain over a lifetime could be up to $1 million.[25] Undertreated acute pain appears, from the extensive epidemiological work of Macrae et al and Perkins and Kehlet,[18] to be a risk factor for the development for chronic postsurgical pain. Chronic postsurgical pain, in addition to its significant adverse impact on patients' quality of life, may be associated with the development of depression and anxiety.[2,6] On the other hand, patients are willing to trade pain relief for a reduction in severity of the side effects of analgesic drugs, such as nausea and vomiting.[2]

In answer to these problems, a multimodal approach incorporating different drugs and techniques can be effective in reducing postoperative pain but is limited by currently available therapies. As monotherapy, opioids have well-established efficacy, but there are concerns about dependency and side effects. NSAIDs, too, are effective as adjunctive medications in a multimodal regimen but are associated with side effects. Cox-2 inhibitors such as celecoxib, rofecoxib, and valdecoxib were developed to provide the efficacy of nonspecific NSAIDs while limiting associated toxicity and have shown an opioid-sparing effect in surgical procedures,[6] yet studies have now shown their potential for higher risks of cardiovascular adverse events, casting doubt on their future role. Combining drugs from these classes at lower doses enables drug sparing and a resultant reduction in adverse events for each drug or drug class.

Future Directions

Many data from clinical trials are unpublished even though their conclusions may be important. Inadequate reporting of RCTs that reach negative conclusions about tested agents introduces a publication bias that tends to overestimate the efficacy of interventions. Furthermore, positive reports of research sponsored by pharmaceutical companies may be widely disseminated—for example, through reprints—and may further skew appraisal of the benefits of such interventions in a positive direction. This skewing of clinical trial results, including those of analgesics, particularly in relation to publication bias, may influence conclusions drawn from meta-analyses.

To address these reporting and publication biases, an international group of clinical trialists, media journal editors, and statisticians developed the CONSORT statement to improve reporting through use of a standardized checklist and flow diagram.[64] These experts suggested that to achieve a more balanced approach, all RCTs should be registered in a fully accessible database. Noting that the heterogeneity of analgesic trial design, enrollment, and outcomes assessment has led to an unfortunate situation in which the majority of the published RCTs for both acute and other types of pain cannot be combined through meta-analysis, many in the field of pain studies have called for a more conscientious application of the CONSORT statement to the publication of analgesic trials. Further positive developments include establishment of the Cochrane Library to solve the problem of inherent publishing bias by providing the best available information about healthcare interventions, both for and against the effectiveness and appropriateness of treatments. Cochrane Collaborative Review Groups have now been established for anesthesia as well as pain, palliative care, and supportive care.

In the future, testing drugs with low number-needed-to-treat (NNT) values may provide a basis for identifying combinations of drugs on the basis of their efficacy as monotherapy. Optimizing a combination by sourcing analgesics—including

Figure 19–8 Comparison of NNT (number-needed-to-treat) values for analgesics as monotherapy for acute postoperative pain. All listed doses are given orally in mg except morphine (intramuscular [IM] administration). *Recommended dose of celecoxib for acute pain is 400 mg. NOTE: Rofecoxib was withdrawn from the market by its manufacturer in 2005. (Data from Barden J, Edwards J, Moore RA, McQuay HJ: Single dose oral diclofenac for postoperative pain. Cochrane Database Syst Rev 2004, Issue 2, article no. CD004768. DOI: 10.1002/14651858.CD004768; Edwards et al: Cochrane Database Syst Rev 2000, article no. CD00276; Edwards et al: The Cochrane Library 2004, Issue 2; Moore et al: Cochrane Database Syst Rev 2004, article no. CD004234; Barden et al: Cochrane Database Syst Rev 2004, Issue 1, article no. CD004604.)

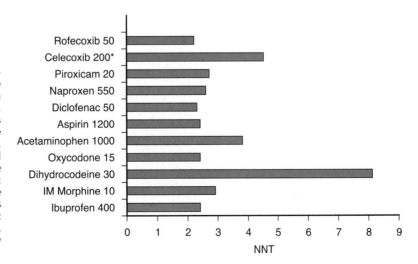

those of different class or mode of action—with the lowest NNT values might enable not only additive but also synergistic analgesia to be achieved (Fig. 19–8). Maximum analgesia can be gained while reducing the dose of each component and their associated side effects.

Although some analgesic combinations may show negative results, these conclusions are not necessarily a reflection of the approach, but instead show that some drugs do not work well together pharmacologically; for instance, they may interact with the same receptor or enzyme. The challenge remains to find an a priori basis to identify those analgesics that are likely to work well when combined. As ongoing preclinical research leads to a better understanding of the pathophysiology of pain transmission, drugs introduced into future analgesic trials will likely include NMDA receptor antagonists, bradykinin receptor antagonists, neuronal nicotinic acetylcholine receptor agonists, inhibitors of glutamate release, substance P inhibitors, superoxide dismutase agonists, and nitric oxide synthase inhibitors. Assessment of these drugs, perhaps in fixed-dose combinations, will likely reinforce multimodal analgesia as the gold standard for managing many types of pain, particularly acute pain.

REFERENCES

1. Walker SM, Goudas LC, Cousins MJ, Carr DB: Combination spinal analgesic chemotherapy: A systematic review. Anesth Analg 2002; 95:674–715.
2. Gan TJ: Consensus guidelines for managing postoperative nausea and vomiting. Anesth Analg 2003;97:62–71.
3. Kehlet H, Dahl JB: The value of "multimodal" or "balanced analgesia" in postoperative pain treatment. Anesth Analg 1993;77:1048–1056.
4. Gottschalk A, Smith DS: New concepts in acute pain therapy: Preemptive analgesia. Am Fam Physician 2001;63:1979–1984.
5. Raffa RB: Pharmacology of oral combination analgesics: Rational therapy for pain. J Clin Pharm Ther 2001;26:257–264.
6. Stephens J, et al: The burden of acute postoperative pain and the potential role of the COX-2-specific inhibitors. Rheumatology 2003; (Suppl 3):iii40–iii52.
7. Siddik SM, et al: Diclofenac and/or propacetamol for postoperative pain management after cesarean delivery in patients receiving patient controlled analgesia morphine. Reg Anesth Pain Med 2001;26:310–315.
8. Reuben SS, et al: The preemptive analgesic effect of rofecoxib after ambulatory arthroscopic knee surgery. Anesth Analg 2002;94:55–59.
9. Olofsson CI, et al: Diclofenac in the treatment of pain after caesarean delivery: An opioid-saving strategy. Eur J Obstet Gynecol Reprod Biol 2000;88:143–146.
10. Michaloliakou C, et al: Preoperative multimodal analgesia facilitates recovery after ambulatory laparoscopic cholecystectomy. Anesth Analg 1996;82:44–51.
11. Scuderi P, et al: Multimodal antiemetic management prevents early postoperative vomiting after outpatient laparoscopy. Anesth Analg 2000;91:1408–1414.
12. Montes A, et al: Use of intravenous patient-controlled analgesia for the documentation of synergy between tramadol and metamizol. Brit J Anaesth 2000;85:217–223.
13. De Angelis C, et al: Clinical trial registration: A statement from the International Committee of Medical Journal Editors. N Engl J Med 2004;351:1250–1251.
14. Fassoulaki A, Patris K, Sarantopoulos C, Hogan Q: The analgesic effect of gabapentin and mexiletine after breast surgery for cancer. Anesth Analg 2002;95:985–991.
15. Stubhaug A, et al: Mapping of punctate hyperalgesia around a surgical incision demonstrates that ketamine is a powerful suppressor of central sensitization to pain following surgery. Acta Anaesthesiol Scand 1997; 41:1124–1132.
16. Pertunnen K, Tasmuth T, Kalso E: Chronic pain after thoracic surgery: A follow-up study [comment in Acta Anaesthesiol Scand 2000;44: 220]. Acta Anaesthesiol Scand 1999;43:563–567.
17. Poobalan AS, Bruce J, King PM, et al:. Chronic pain and quality of life following open inguinal hernia repair. Br J Surg 2001;88:1122–1126.
18. Perkins FM, Kehlet H: Chronic pain as an outcome of surgery: A review of predictive factors. Anesthesiology 2000;93:1123–1133.
19. Menigaux C, Adam F, Guignard B, et al: Preoperative gabapentin decreases anxiety and improves early functional recovery from knee surgery. Anesth Analg 2005;100:1394–1399.
20. De Kock M, Lavand'homme P, Waterloos H: 'Balanced analgesia' in the perioperative period: Is there a place for ketamine? Pain 2001;92: 373–380.
21. Panchel SJ: Personal communication, January 2005.
22. Carr DB, Jacox AK, Chapman CR, et al: 1992 Acute pain management in infants, children, and adolescents: Operative and medical procedures: Quick reference guide for clinicians (AHCPR Publication No. 92-0020). Rockville, MD: Agency for Health Care Policy and Research. September 2002. Available at http://www.ahcpr.gov/gils/00000052.htm/
23. Dolin SJ, Cashman JN, Bland JM: Effectiveness of acute postoperative pain management. I: Evidence from published data. Br J Anaesth 2002;89:409–423.
24. Powell AE, Davies HT, Bannister J, Macrae WA: Rhetoric and reality on acute pain services in the UK: A national postal questionnaire survey. Br J Anaesth 2004;92:689–693.
25. Apfelbaum JL: Postoperative pain experience: Results from a national survey suggest postoperative pain continues to be undermanaged. Anesth Analg 2003;97:534–540.
26. Buvanendran A, et al: Effects of perioperative administration of a selective cyclooxygenase 2 inhibitor on pain management and recovery of function after knee replacement: A randomized controlled trial. JAMA 2003;290:2411–2418.
27. Hanna MH, et al: Comparative study of analgesic efficacy and morphine-sparing effect of intramuscular dexketoprofen trometamol with ketoprofen or placebo after major orthopaedic surgery. Br J Clin Pharmacol 2003;55:126–133.
28. Marret E, Kurdi O, Zufferey P, Bonnet F: Effects of nonsteroidal antiinflammatory drugs on patient-controlled analgesia morphine side effects: Meta-analysis of randomized controlled trials. Anesthesiology 2005;102:1249–1260.
29. Cardoso MM, et al: Small doses of intrathecal morphine combined with systemic diclofenac for postoperative pain control after cesarean delivery. Anesth Analg 1998;86:538–541.
30. Rosaeg OP, et al: Peri-operative multimodal pain therapy for caesarean section: Analgesia and fitness for discharge. Can J Anaesth 1997;44: 803–809.
31. Emkey R, et al: Efficacy and safety of tramadol/acetaminophen tablets (Ultracet) as add-on therapy for osteoarthritis pain in subjects receiving a COX-2 nonsteroidal antiinflammatory drug: A multicenter, randomized, double-blind, placebo-controlled trial. J Rheumatol 2004;31: 150–156.
32. Silverfield JC, et al: Tramadol/acetaminophen combination tablets for the treatment of osteoarthritis flare pain: A multicenter, outpatient, double-blind, placebo-controlled, parallel-group, add-on study. Clin Ther 2002;24:282–297.
33. Rosenthal NR, et al: Tramadol/acetaminophen combination tablets for the treatment of pain associated with osteoarthritis flare in an elderly patient population. J Am Geriatr Soc 2004;52:374–380.
34. Chia YY, et al: Adding ketamine in a multimodal patient-controlled epidural regimen reduces postoperative pain and analgesic consumption. Anesth Analg 1998;86:1245–1249.
35. Menigaux C, et al: Intraoperative small-dose ketamine enhances analgesia after outpatient knee arthroscopy. Anesth Analg 2001;93:606–612.
36. Edwards JE, Moore RA, McQuay HJ: Single dose oxycodone and oxycodone plus paracetamol (acetaminophen) for acute postoperative pain (Cochrane Review). In The Cochrane Library, Issue 4. Chichester, UK, John Wiley & Sons, Ltd., 2004.
37. Collins SL, Edwards JE, Moore RA, McQuay HJ: Single dose dextropropoxyphene, alone and with paracetamol (acetaminophen), for postoperative pain (Cochrane Review). In The Cochrane Library, Issue 4. Chichester, UK:, John Wiley & Sons, Ltd., 2004.
38. Lauretti GR, et al: Tramadol and beta-cyclodextrin piroxicam: Effective multimodal balanced analgesia for the intra- and postoperative period. Reg Anesth 1997;22:243–248.
39. Anderson AD, et al: Randomized clinical trial of multimodal optimization and standard perioperative surgical care. Br J Surg 2003;90: 1497–1504.

40. Barratt SM, et al: Multimodal analgesia and intravenous nutrition preserves total body protein following major upper gastrointestinal surgery. Reg Anesth Pain Med 2002;27:15–22.

41. Bisgaard T, et al: Multi-regional local anesthetic infiltration during laparoscopic cholecystectomy in patients receiving prophylactic multimodal analgesia: A randomized, double-blinded, placebo-controlled study. Anesth Analg 1999;89:1017–1024.

42. Liu SS, et al: Effects of perioperative analgesic technique on rate of recovery after colon surgery. Anesthesiology 1995;83:757–765.

43. Mulroy MF, et al: Femoral nerve block with 0.25% or 0.5% bupivacaine improves postoperative analgesia following outpatient arthroscopic anterior cruciate ligament repair. Reg Anesth Pain Med 2001;26:24–29.

44. Rasmussen S, et al: Intra-articular glucocorticoid, bupivacaine and morphine reduces pain, inflammatory response and convalescence after arthroscopic meniscectomy. Pain 1998;78:131–134.

45. Van Ee R, et al: Effects of ketoprofen and mesosalpinx infiltration on postoperative pain after laparoscopic sterilization. Obstet Gynecol 1996;88:568–572.

46. Schumann R, et al: A comparison of multimodal perioperative analgesia to epidural pain management after gastric bypass surgery. Anesth Analg 2003;96:469–474.

47. Australian and New Zealand College of Anaesthetists and Faculty of Pain Medicine: Acute Pain Management: Scientific Evidence, 2nd ed (Publication No. CP104). Canberra, National Health and Medical Research Council, 2005. Available at http://www.nhmrc.gov.au/publications/_files/cp104.pdf/

48. Rockemann MG, et al: Prophylactic use of epidural mepivacaine/morphine, systemic diclofenac, and metamizole reduces postoperative morphine consumption after major abdominal surgery. Anesthesiology 1996;84:1027–1034.

49. Rosaeg OP, et al: Effect of preemptive multimodal analgesia for arthroscopic knee ligament repair. Reg Anesth Pain Med 2001;26:125–130.

50. Choi DM, et al: Dextromethorphan and intrathecal morphine for analgesia after Caesarean section under spinal anaesthesia. Br J Anaesth 2003;90:653–658.

51. Paech MJ, et al: Postcesarean analgesia with spinal morphine, clonidine, or their combination. Anesth Analg 2004;98:1460–1466.

52. Keita H, et al: Prophylactic IP injection of bupivacaine and/or morphine does not improve postoperative analgesia after laparoscopic gynecologic surgery. Can J Anaesth 2003;50:362–367.

53. Nagatsuka C, et al: Preemptive effects of a combination of preoperative diclofenac, butorphanol, and lidocaine on postoperative pain management following orthognathic surgery. Anesth Prog 2000;47:119–124.

54. Doyle E, Bowler GM: Pre-emptive effect of multimodal analgesia in thoracic surgery. Br J Anaesth 1998;80:147–151.

55. Reuben SS, et al: Intraarticular morphine in the multimodal analgesic management of postoperative pain after ambulatory anterior cruciate ligament repair. Anesth Analg 1998;86:374–378.

56. Bell R: Ketamine as an adjuvant to opioids for cancer pain (Cochrane Review). The Cochrane Library, Issue 4. Chichester, UK, Wiley & Sons, 2004.

57. Cashman JN, Dolin SJ: Respiratory and haemodynamic effects of acute postoperative pain management: Evidence from published data. Br J Anaesth 2004;93:212–223.

58. Sinatra RS, et al: Preoperative rofecoxib oral suspension as an analgesic adjunct after lower abdominal surgery: The effects on effort-dependent pain and pulmonary function. Anesth Analg 2004;98:135–140.

59. Camu F, et al: Valdecoxib, a COX-2-specific inhibitor, is an efficacious, opioid-sparing analgesic in patients undergoing hip arthroplasty. Am J Ther 2002;9:43–51.

60. Nussmeier NA, Whelton AA, Brown MT, et al: Complications of the COX-2 inhibitors parecoxib and valdecoxib after cardiac surgery. N Engl J Med 2005;352:1081–1091.

61. U.S. Food and Drug Administration, Office of New Drugs and Office of Pharmacoepidemiology and Statistical Science: Analysis and recommendation for Agency action regarding non-steroidal anti-inflammatory drugs and cardiovascular risk. Memorandum, April 6, 2005. Available at http://www.fda.gov/cder/drug/infopage/COX2/NSAIDdecisionMemo.pdf/

62. Forrest JB, Camu F, Greer IA, et al: Ketorolac, diclofenac, and ketoprofen are equally safe for pain relief after major surgery. Br J Anaesth 2002;88:2227–2233.

63. Astin JA: Mind-body therapies for the management of pain. Clin J Pain 2004;20:27–32.

64. Moher D, et al: The CONSORT statement: Revised recommendations for improving the quality of reports of parallel-group randomised trials. Lancet 2001;357:1191–1194.

Appendix: Medline Search of Multimodal Analgesic Treatment Between 1995 and 2005

The following reports the results of the Medline search described in the text of this chapter, followed by the reference "hits" for the top three search terms used.

Medline Search of Multimodal Analgesic Treatment Between 1995 and 2005			
Search Terms (1995–2005)	No. of Hits	No. of Clinical Trials	No. of Randomized Clinical Trials
Multimodal treatment pain*	217	55	47
Multimodal therapy pain*	210	55	47
Multimodal analgesia*	123	38	35
Multidisciplinary intervention pain	109		
Multimodal pain management	98		
Multidisciplinary approach pain	77		
Multimodal perioperative analgesia	29		
Multimodal pain relief	8		
Multimodal preemptive approach pain	3		
Multimodal optimization pain	2		

*Appendix references list the hits for this search term.

REFERENCES FOR TOP THREE SEARCH TERMS

"MULTIMODAL TREATMENT PAIN"

1. Atlantis E, Chow CM, Kirby A, Singh MF: An effective exercise-based intervention for improving mental health and quality of life measures: a randomized controlled trial. Prev Med 2004;39:424–434.
2. Paech MJ, Pavy TJ, Orlikowski CE, et al: Postcesarean analgesia with spinal morphine, clonidine, or their combination. Anesth Analg 2004; 98:1460–1466.
3. Brown DR, Hofer RE, Patterson DE, et al: Intrathecal anesthesia and recovery from radical prostatectomy: A prospective, randomized, controlled trial. Anesthesiology 2004;100:926–934.
4. Ma H, Tang J, White PF, et al: Perioperative rofecoxib improves early recovery after outpatient herniorrhaphy. Anesth Analg 2004;98:970–975.
5. Anderson AD, McNaught CE, MacFie J, et al: Randomized clinical trial of multimodal optimization and standard perioperative surgical care. Br J Surg 2003;90:1497–1504.
6. Buvanendran A, Kroin JS, Tuman KJ, et al: Effects of perioperative administration of a selective cyclooxygenase 2 inhibitor on pain management and recovery of function after knee replacement: A randomized controlled trial. JAMA 2003;290:2411–2418.
7. Bisgaard T, Klarskov B, Kehlet H, Rosenberg J: Preoperative dexamethasone improves surgical outcome after laparoscopic cholecystectomy: A randomized double-blind placebo-controlled trial. Ann Surg 2003;238:651–660.
8. Choi DM, Kliffer AP, Douglas MJ: Dextromethorphan and intrathecal morphine for analgesia after Caesarean section under spinal anaesthesia. Br J Anaesth 2003;90:653–658.
9. Keita H, Benifla JL, Le Bouar V, et al: Prophylactic IP injection of bupivacaine and/or morphine does not improve postoperative analgesia after laparoscopic gynecologic surgery. Can J Anaesth 2003;50: 362–367.
10. Hanna MH, Elliott KM, Stuart-Taylor ME, et al: Comparative study of analgesic efficacy and morphine-sparing effect of intramuscular dexketoprofen trometamol with ketoprofen or placebo after major orthopaedic surgery. Br J Clin Pharmacol 2003;55:126–133.
11. Schumann R, Shikora S, Weiss JM, et al: A comparison of multimodal perioperative analgesia to epidural pain management after gastric bypass surgery. Anesth Analg 2003;96:469–474.
12. Issioui T, Klein KW, White PF, et al: Cost-efficacy of rofecoxib versus acetaminophen for preventing pain after ambulatory surgery. Anesthesiology 2002;97:931–937.
13. Carli F, Mayo N, Klubien K, et al: Epidural analgesia enhances functional exercise capacity and health-related quality of life after colonic surgery: Results of a randomized trial. Anesthesiology 2002;97:540–549.
14. Ekman EF, Fiechtner JJ, Levy S, Fort JG: Efficacy of celecoxib versus ibuprofen in the treatment of acute pain: A multicenter, double-blind, randomized controlled trial in acute ankle sprain. Am J Orthop 2002; 31:445–451.
15. Hammas B, Thorn SE, Wattwil M: Superior prolonged antiemetic prophylaxis with a four-drug multimodal regimen—comparison with propofol or placebo. Acta Anaesthesiol Scand 2002;46:232–237.
16. Boisseau N, Rabary O, Padovani B, et al: Improvement of 'dynamic analgesia' does not decrease atelectasis after thoracotomy. Br J Anaesth 2001;87:564–569.
17. Henriksen MG, Jensen MB, Hansen HV, et al: Enforced mobilization, early oral feeding, and balanced analgesia improve convalescence after colorectal surgery. Nutrition 2002;18:147–152.
18. Barratt SM, Smith RC, Kee AJ, et al: Multimodal analgesia and intravenous nutrition preserves total body protein following major upper gastrointestinal surgery. Reg Anesth Pain Med 2002;27:15–22.
19. Camu F, Beecher T, Recker DP, Verburg KM: Valdecoxib, a COX-2-specific inhibitor, is an efficacious, opioid-sparing analgesic in patients undergoing hip arthroplasty. Am J Ther 2002;9:43–51.
20. Menigaux C, Guignard B, Fletcher D, et al: Intraoperative small-dose ketamine enhances analgesia after outpatient knee arthroscopy. Anesth Analg 2001;93:606–612.
21. Siddik SM, Aouad MT, Jalbout MI, et al: Diclofenac and/or propacetamol for postoperative pain management after cesarean delivery in patients receiving patient controlled analgesia morphine. Reg Anesth Pain Med 2001;26:310–315.
22. Nagatsuka C, Ichinohe T, Kaneko Y: Preemptive effects of a combination of preoperative diclofenac, butorphanol, and lidocaine on postoperative pain management following orthognathic surgery. Anesth Prog 2000; 47:119–124.
23. Brodner G, Van Aken H, Hertle L, et al: Multimodal perioperative management—combining thoracic epidural analgesia, forced mobilization, and oral nutrition—reduces hormonal and metabolic stress and improves convalescence after major urologic surgery. Anesth Analg 2001;92:1594–1600.
24. Rosaeg OP, Krepski B, Cicutti N, et al: Effect of preemptive multimodal analgesia for arthroscopic knee ligament repair. Reg Anesth Pain Med 2001;26:125–130.
25. Taylor D: More than personal change: Effective elements of symptom management. Nurse Pract Forum 2000;11:79–86.
26. Mulroy MF, Larkin KL, Batra MS, et al: Femoral nerve block with 0.25% or 0.5% bupivacaine improves postoperative analgesia following outpatient arthroscopic anterior cruciate ligament repair. Reg Anesth Pain Med 2001;26:24–29.
27. Scuderi PE, James RL, Harris L, Mims GR 3rd: Multimodal antiemetic management prevents early postoperative vomiting after outpatient laparoscopy. Anesth Analg 2000;91:1408–1414.
28. Reuben SS, Connelly NR: Postoperative analgesic effects of celecoxib or rofecoxib after spinal fusion surgery. Anesth Analg 2000;91: 1221–1225.
29. Bisgaard T, Klarskov B, Trap R, et al: Pain after microlaparoscopic cholecystectomy: A randomized double-blind controlled study. Surg Endosc 2000;14:340–344.
30. Taimela S, Takala EP, Asklof T, et al: Active treatment of chronic neck pain: A prospective randomized intervention. Spine 2000;25:1021–1027.
31. Olofsson CI, Legeby MH, Nygards EB, Ostman KM: Diclofenac in the treatment of pain after caesarean delivery: An opioid-saving strategy. Eur J Obstet Gynecol Reprod Biol 2000;88:143–146.
32. Bisgaard T, Klarskov B, Kristiansen VB, et al: Multi-regional local anesthetic infiltration during laparoscopic cholecystectomy in patients receiving prophylactic multi-modal analgesia: A randomized, double-blinded, placebo-controlled study. Anesth Analg 1999;89:1017–1024.
33. Petersen-Felix S, Luginbuhl M, Schnider TW, et al: Comparison of the analgesic potency of xenon and nitrous oxide in humans evaluated by experimental pain. Br J Anaesth 1998;81:742–747.
34. Rasmussen S, Larsen AS, Thomsen ST, Kehlet H: Intra-articular glucocorticoid, bupivacaine and morphine reduces pain, inflammatory response and convalescence after arthroscopic meniscectomy. Pain 1998;78: 131–134.
35. Lauretti GR, Mattos AL, Reis MP, Pereira NL: Combined intrathecal fentanyl and neostigmine: Therapy for postoperative abdominal hysterectomy pain relief. J Clin Anesth 1998;10:291–296.
36. Chia YY, Liu K, Liu YC, et al: Adding ketamine in a multimodal patient-controlled epidural regimen reduces postoperative pain and analgesic consumption. Anesth Analg 1998;86:1245–1249.
37. Doyle E, Bowler GM: Pre-emptive effect of multimodal analgesia in thoracic surgery. Br J Anaesth 1998;80:147–151.
38. Haldorsen EM, Kronholm K, Skouen JS, Ursin H: Multimodal cognitive behavioral treatment of patients sicklisted for musculoskeletal pain: A randomized controlled study. Scand J Rheumatol 1998;27:16–25.
39. Reuben SS, Steinberg RB, Cohen MA, et al: Intraarticular morphine in the multimodal analgesic management of postoperative pain after ambulatory anterior cruciate ligament repair. Anesth Analg 1998;86:374–378.
40. Rosaeg OP, Lui A, Cicutti NJ, et al: Peri-operative multimodal pain therapy for caesarean section: Analgesia and fitness for discharge. Can J Anaesth 1997;44:803–809.
41. Lauretti GR, Mattos AL, Lima IC: Tramadol and beta-cyclodextrin piroxicam: Effective multimodal balanced analgesia for the intra- and postoperative period. Reg Anesth 1997;22:243–248.
42. Van Ee R, Hemrika DJ, De Blok S, et al: Effects of ketoprofen and mesosalpinx infiltration on postoperative pain after laparoscopic sterilization. Obstet Gynecol 1996;88:568–572.
43. Provinciali L, Baroni M, Illuminati L, Ceravolo MG: Multimodal treatment to prevent the late whiplash syndrome. Scand J Rehabil Med 1996;28:105–111.
44. Rockemann MG, Seeling W, Bischof C, et al: Prophylactic use of epidural mepivacaine/morphine, systemic diclofenac, and metamizole reduces postoperative morphine consumption after major abdominal surgery. Anesthesiology 1996;84:1027–1034.
45. Katz J, Jackson M, Kavanagh BP, Sandler AN: Acute pain after thoracic surgery predicts long-term post-thoracotomy pain. Clin J Pain 1996;12:50–55.

46. Michaloliakou C, Chung F, Sharma S: Preoperative multimodal analgesia facilitates recovery after ambulatory laparoscopic cholecystectomy. Anesth Analg 1996;82:44–51.
47. Jensen I, Nygren A, Gamberale F, et al: The role of the psychologist in multidisciplinary treatments for chronic neck and shoulder pain: A controlled cost-effectiveness study. Scand J Rehabil Med 1995;27:19–26.

"MULTIMODAL THERAPY PAIN"

1. Atlantis E, Chow CM, Kirby A, Singh MF: An effective exercise-based intervention for improving mental health and quality of life measures: A randomized controlled trial. Prev Med 2004;39:424–434.
2. Paech MJ, Pavy TJ, Orlikowski CE, et al: Postcesarean analgesia with spinal morphine, clonidine, or their combination. Anesth Analg 2004;98:1460–1466.
3. Brown DR, Hofer RE, Patterson DE, et al: Intrathecal anesthesia and recovery from radical prostatectomy: A prospective, randomized, controlled trial. Anesthesiology 2004;100:926–934.
4. Ma H, Tang J, White PF, et al: Perioperative rofecoxib improves early recovery after outpatient herniorrhaphy. Anesth Analg 2004;98:970–975.
5. Anderson AD, McNaught CE, MacFie J, et al: Randomized clinical trial of multimodal optimization and standard perioperative surgical care. Br J Surg 2003;90:1497–1504.
6. Buvanendran A, Kroin JS, Tuman KJ, et al: Effects of perioperative administration of a selective cyclooxygenase 2 inhibitor on pain management and recovery of function after knee replacement: A randomized controlled trial. JAMA 2003;290:2411–2418.
7. Bisgaard T, Klarskov B, Kehlet H, Rosenberg J: Preoperative dexamethasone improves surgical outcome after laparoscopic cholecystectomy: A randomized double-blind placebo-controlled trial. Ann Surg 2003;238:651–660.
8. Choi DM, Kliffer AP, Douglas MJ: Dextromethorphan and intrathecal morphine for analgesia after Caesarean section under spinal anaesthesia. Br J Anaesth 2003;90:653–658.
9. Keita H, Benifla JL, Le Bouar V, et al: Prophylactic IP injection of bupivacaine and/or morphine does not improve postoperative analgesia after laparoscopic gynecologic surgery. Can J Anaesth 2003;50:362–367.
10. Hanna MH, Elliott KM, Stuart-Taylor ME, et al: Comparative study of analgesic efficacy and morphine-sparing effect of intramuscular dexketoprofen trometamol with ketoprofen or placebo after major orthopaedic surgery. Br J Clin Pharmacol 2003;55:126–133.
11. Schumann R, Shikora S, Weiss JM, et al: A comparison of multimodal perioperative analgesia to epidural pain management after gastric bypass surgery. Anesth Analg 2003;96:469–474.
12. Issioui T, Klein KW, White PF, et al: Cost-efficacy of rofecoxib versus acetaminophen for preventing pain after ambulatory surgery. Anesthesiology 2002;97:931–937.
13. Carli F, Mayo N, Klubien K, et al: Epidural analgesia enhances functional exercise capacity and health-related quality of life after colonic surgery: Results of a randomized trial. Anesthesiology 2002;97:540–549.
14. Ekman EF, Fiechtner JJ, Levy S, Fort JG: Efficacy of celecoxib versus ibuprofen in the treatment of acute pain: A multicenter, double-blind, randomized controlled trial in acute ankle sprain. Am J Orthop 2002;31:445–451.
15. Hammas B, Thorn SE, Wattwil M: Superior prolonged antiemetic prophylaxis with a four-drug multimodal regimen—comparison with propofol or placebo. Acta Anaesthesiol Scand 2002;46:232–237.
16. Boisseau N, Rabary O, Padovani B, et al: Improvement of 'dynamic analgesia' does not decrease atelectasis after thoracotomy. Br J Anaesth 2001;87:564–569.
17. Henriksen MG, Jensen MB, Hansen HV, et al: Enforced mobilization, early oral feeding, and balanced analgesia improve convalescence after colorectal surgery. Nutrition 2002;18:147–152.
18. Barratt SM, Smith RC, Kee AJ, et al: Multimodal analgesia and intravenous nutrition preserves total body protein following major upper gastrointestinal surgery. Reg Anesth Pain Med 2002;27:15–22.
19. Camu F, Beecher T, Recker DP, Verburg KM: Valdecoxib, a COX-2-specific inhibitor, is an efficacious, opioid-sparing analgesic in patients undergoing hip arthroplasty. Am J Ther 2002;9:43–51.
20. Menigaux C, Guignard B, Fletcher D, et al: Intraoperative small-dose ketamine enhances analgesia after outpatient knee arthroscopy. Anesth Analg 2001;93:606–612.
21. Siddik SM, Aouad MT, Jalbout MI, et al: Diclofenac and/or propacetamol for postoperative pain management after cesarean delivery in patients receiving patient controlled analgesia morphine. Reg Anesth Pain Med 2001;26:310–315.
22. Nagatsuka C, Ichinohe T, Kaneko Y: Preemptive effects of a combination of preoperative diclofenac, butorphanol, and lidocaine on postoperative pain management following orthognathic surgery. Anesth Prog 2000;47:119–124.
23. Brodner G, Van Aken H, Hertle L, et al: Multimodal perioperative management—combining thoracic epidural analgesia, forced mobilization, and oral nutrition—reduces hormonal and metabolic stress and improves convalescence after major urologic surgery. Anesth Analg 2001;92:1594–1600.
24. Rosaeg OP, Krepski B, Cicutti N, et al: Effect of preemptive multimodal analgesia for arthroscopic knee ligament repair. Reg Anesth Pain Med 2001;26:125–130.
25. Taylor D: More than personal change: Effective elements of symptom management. Nurse Pract Forum 2000;11:79–86.
26. Mulroy MF, Larkin KL, Batra MS, et al: Femoral nerve block with 0.25% or 0.5% bupivacaine improves postoperative analgesia following outpatient arthroscopic anterior cruciate ligament repair. Reg Anesth Pain Med 2001;26:24–29.
27. Scuderi PE, James RL, Harris L, Mims GR 3rd: Multimodal antiemetic management prevents early postoperative vomiting after outpatient laparoscopy. Anesth Analg 2000;91:1408–1414.
28. Reuben SS, Connelly NR: Postoperative analgesic effects of celecoxib or rofecoxib after spinal fusion surgery. Anesth Analg 2000;91:1221–1225.
29. Bisgaard T, Klarskov B, Trap R, et al: Pain after microlaparoscopic cholecystectomy: A randomized double-blind controlled study. Surg Endosc 2000;14:340–344.
30. Taimela S, Takala EP, Asklof T, et al: Active treatment of chronic neck pain: A prospective randomized intervention. Spine 2000;25:1021–1027.
31. Olofsson CI, Legeby MH, Nygards EB, Ostman KM: Diclofenac in the treatment of pain after caesarean delivery: An opioid-saving strategy. Eur J Obstet Gynecol Reprod Biol 2000;88:143–146.
32. Bisgaard T, Klarskov B, Kristiansen VB, et al: Multi-regional local anesthetic infiltration during laparoscopic cholecystectomy in patients receiving prophylactic multi-modal analgesia: A randomized, double-blinded, placebo-controlled study. Anesth Analg 1999;89:1017–1024.
33. Petersen-Felix S, Luginbuhl M, Schnider TW, et al: Comparison of the analgesic potency of xenon and nitrous oxide in humans evaluated by experimental pain. Br J Anaesth 1998;81:742–747.
34. Rasmussen S, Larsen AS, Thomsen ST, Kehlet H: Intra-articular glucocorticoid, bupivacaine and morphine reduces pain, inflammatory response and convalescence after arthroscopic meniscectomy. Pain 1998;78:131–134.
35. Lauretti GR, Mattos AL, Reis MP, Pereira NL: Combined intrathecal fentanyl and neostigmine: Therapy for postoperative abdominal hysterectomy pain relief. J Clin Anesth 1998;10:291–296.
36. Chia YY, Liu K, Liu YC, et al: Adding ketamine in a multimodal patient-controlled epidural regimen reduces postoperative pain and analgesic consumption. Anesth Analg 1998;86:1245–1249.
37. Doyle E, Bowler GM: Pre-emptive effect of multimodal analgesia in thoracic surgery. Br J Anaesth 1998;80:147–151.
38. Haldorsen EM, Kronholm K, Skouen JS, Ursin H: Multimodal cognitive behavioral treatment of patients sicklisted for musculoskeletal pain: A randomized controlled study. Scand J Rheumatol 1998;27:16–25.
39. Reuben SS, Steinberg RB, Cohen MA, et al: Intraarticular morphine in the multimodal analgesic management of postoperative pain after ambulatory anterior cruciate ligament repair. Anesth Analg 1998;86:374–378.
40. Rosaeg OP, Lui AC, Cicutti NJ, et al: Peri-operative multimodal pain therapy for caesarean section: Analgesia and fitness for discharge. Can J Anaesth 1997;44:803–809.
41. Lauretti GR, Mattos AL, Lima IC: Tramadol and beta-cyclodextrin piroxicam: Effective multimodal balanced analgesia for the intra- and postoperative period. Reg Anesth 1997;22:243–248.
42. Van Ee R, Hemrika DJ, De Blok S, et al: Effects of ketoprofen and mesosalpinx infiltration on postoperative pain after laparoscopic sterilization. Obstet Gynecol 1996;88:568–572.
43. Provinciali L, Baroni M, Illuminati L, Ceravolo MG: Multimodal treatment to prevent the late whiplash syndrome. Scand J Rehabil Med 1996;28:105–111.
44. Rockemann MG, Seeling W, Bischof C, et al: Prophylactic use of epidural mepivacaine/morphine, systemic diclofenac, and metamizole reduces postoperative morphine consumption after major abdominal surgery. Anesthesiology 1996;84:1027–1034.

45. Katz J, Jackson M, Kavanagh BP, Sandler AN: Acute pain after thoracic surgery predicts long-term post-thoracotomy pain. Clin J Pain 1996;12:50–55.

46. Michaloliakou C, Chung F, Sharma S: Preoperative multimodal analgesia facilitates recovery after ambulatory laparoscopic cholecystectomy. Anesth Analg 1996;82:44–51.

47. Jensen I, Nygren A, Gamberale F, et al: The role of the psychologist in multidisciplinary treatments for chronic neck and shoulder pain: A controlled cost-effectiveness study. Scand J Rehabil Med 1995;27:19–26.

"MULTIMODAL ANALGESIA"

1. Paech MJ, Pavy TJ, Orlikowski CE, et al: Postcesarean analgesia with spinal morphine, clonidine, or their combination. Anesth Analg 2004;98:1460–1466.

2. Brown DR, Hofer RE, Patterson DE, et al: Intrathecal anesthesia and recovery from radical prostatectomy: A prospective, randomized, controlled trial. Anesthesiology 2004;100:926–934.

3. Buvanendran A, Kroin JS, Tuman KJ, et al: Effects of perioperative administration of a selective cyclooxygenase 2 inhibitor on pain management and recovery of function after knee replacement: A randomized controlled trial. JAMA 2003;290:2411–2418.

4. Basse L, Madsen JL, Billesbolle P, et al: Gastrointestinal transit after laparoscopic versus open colonic resection. Surg Endosc 2003;17:1919–1922.

5. Choi DM, Kliffer AP, Douglas MJ: Dextromethorphan and intrathecal morphine for analgesia after Caesarean section under spinal anaesthesia. Br J Anaesth 2003;90:653–658.

6. Keita H, Benifla JL, Le Bouar V, et al: Prophylactic IP injection of bupivacaine and/or morphine does not improve postoperative analgesia after laparoscopic gynecologic surgery. Can J Anaesth 2003;50:362–367.

7. Hanna MH, Elliott KM, Stuart-Taylor ME, et al: Comparative study of analgesic efficacy and morphine-sparing effect of intramuscular dexketoprofen trometamol with ketoprofen or placebo after major orthopaedic surgery. Br J Clin Pharmacol 2003;55:126–133.

8. Schumann R, Shikora S, Weiss JM, et al: A comparison of multimodal perioperative analgesia to epidural pain management after gastric bypass surgery. Anesth Analg 2003;96:469–474.

9. Issioui T, Klein KW, White PF, et al: Cost-efficacy of rofecoxib versus acetaminophen for preventing pain after ambulatory surgery. Anesthesiology 2002;97:931–937.

10. Carli F, Mayo N, Klubien K, et al: Epidural analgesia enhances functional exercise capacity and health-related quality of life after colonic surgery: Results of a randomized trial. Anesthesiology 2002;97:540–549.

11. Boisseau N, Rabary O, Padovani B, et al: Improvement of 'dynamic analgesia' does not decrease atelectasis after thoracotomy. Br J Anaesth 2001;87:564–569.

12. Henriksen MG, Jensen MB, Hansen HV, et al: Enforced mobilization, early oral feeding, and balanced analgesia improve convalescence after colorectal surgery. Nutrition 2002;18:147–152.

13. Barratt SM, Smith RC, Kee AJ, et al: Multimodal analgesia and intravenous nutrition preserves total body protein following major upper gastrointestinal surgery. Reg Anesth Pain Med 2002;27:15–22.

14. Camu F, Beecher T, Recker DP, Verburg KM: Valdecoxib, a COX-2-specific inhibitor, is an efficacious, opioid-sparing analgesic in patients undergoing hip arthroplasty. Am J Ther 2002;9:43–51.

15. Menigaux C, Guignard B, Fletcher D, et al: Intraoperative small-dose ketamine enhances analgesia after outpatient knee arthroscopy. Anesth Analg 2001;93:606–612.

16. Siddik SM, Aouad MT, Jalbout MI, et al: Diclofenac and/or propacetamol for postoperative pain management after cesarean delivery in patients receiving patient controlled analgesia morphine. Reg Anesth Pain Med 2001;26:310–315.

17. Nagatsuka C, Ichinohe T, Kaneko Y: Preemptive effects of a combination of preoperative diclofenac, butorphanol, and lidocaine on postoperative pain management following orthognathic surgery. Anesth Prog 2000;47:119–124.

18. Brodner G, Van Aken H, Hertle L, et al: Multimodal perioperative management—combining thoracic epidural analgesia, forced mobilization, and oral nutrition—reduces hormonal and metabolic stress and improves convalescence after major urologic surgery. Anesth Analg 2001;92:1594–1600.

19. Rosaeg OP, Krepski B, Cicutti N, et al: Effect of preemptive multimodal analgesia for arthroscopic knee ligament repair. Reg Anesth Pain Med 2001;26:125–130.

20. Mulroy MF, Larkin KL, Batra MS, et al: Femoral nerve block with 0.25% or 0.5% bupivacaine improves postoperative analgesia following outpatient arthroscopic anterior cruciate ligament repair. Reg Anesth Pain Med 2001;26:24–29.

21. Reuben SS, Connelly NR: Postoperative analgesic effects of celecoxib or rofecoxib after spinal fusion surgery. Anesth Analg 2000;91:1221–1225.

22. Olofsson CI, Legeby MH, Nygards EB, Ostman KM: Diclofenac in the treatment of pain after caesarean delivery: An opioid-saving strategy. Eur J Obstet Gynecol Reprod Biol 2000;88:143–146.

23. Bisgaard T, Klarskov B, Kristiansen VB, et al: Multi-regional local anesthetic infiltration during laparoscopic cholecystectomy in patients receiving prophylactic multi-modal analgesia: A randomized, double-blinded, placebo-controlled study. Anesth Analg 1999;89:1017–1024.

24. Petersen-Felix S, Luginbuhl M, Schnider TW, et al: Comparison of the analgesic potency of xenon and nitrous oxide in humans evaluated by experimental pain. Br J Anaesth 1998;81:742–747.

25. Lauretti GR, Mattos AL, Reis MP, Pereira NL: Combined intrathecal fentanyl and neostigmine: Therapy for postoperative abdominal hysterectomy pain relief. J Clin Anesth 1998;10:291–296.

26. Chia YY, Liu K, Liu YC, et al: Adding ketamine in a multimodal patient-controlled epidural regimen reduces postoperative pain and analgesic consumption. Anesth Analg 1998;86:1245–1249.

27. Doyle E, Bowler GM: Pre-emptive effect of multimodal analgesia in thoracic surgery. Br J Anaesth 1998;80:147–151.

28. Cardoso MM, Carvalho JC, Amaro AR, et al: Small doses of intrathecal morphine combined with systemic diclofenac for postoperative pain control after cesarean delivery. Anesth Analg 1998;86:538–541.

29. Reuben SS, Steinberg RB, Cohen MA, et al: Intraarticular morphine in the multimodal analgesic management of postoperative pain after ambulatory anterior cruciate ligament repair. Anesth Analg 1998;86:374–378.

30. Rosaeg OP, Lui AC, Cicutti NJ, et al: Peri-operative multimodal pain therapy for caesarean section: Analgesia and fitness for discharge. Can J Anaesth 1997;44:803–809.

31. Lauretti GR, Mattos AL, Lima IC: Tramadol and beta-cyclodextrin piroxicam: Effective multimodal balanced analgesia for the intra- and postoperative period. Reg Anesth 1997;22:243–248.

32. Rockemann MG, Seeling W, Bischof C, et al: Prophylactic use of epidural mepivacaine/morphine, systemic diclofenac, and metamizole reduces postoperative morphine consumption after major abdominal surgery. Anesthesiology 1996;84:1027–1034.

33. Katz J, Jackson M, Kavanagh BP, Sandler AN: Acute pain after thoracic surgery predicts long-term post-thoracotomy pain. Clin J Pain 1996;12:50–55.

34. Michaloliakou C, Chung F, Sharma S: Preoperative multimodal analgesia facilitates recovery after ambulatory laparoscopic cholecystectomy. Anesth Analg 1996;82:44–51.

35. Liu SS, Carpenter RL, Mackey DC, et al: Effects of perioperative analgesic technique on rate of recovery after colon surgery. Anesthesiology 1995;83:757–765.

20 Nonconventional and Adjunctive Analgesia

KATE FITZGERALD • DONAL BUGGY

Postoperative analgesia requires a balance between pain relief and unwanted side effects. This balance is especially important in ambulatory (outpatient) surgery, for which growing numbers of patients and procedures are now deemed suitable. The ideal postoperative analgesic agent would provide complete pain relief without side effects. Because such an analgesic does not yet exist, attempts to find an agent or combination of agents that could optimize analgesia and minimize deleterious side effects have continued. Conventional paradigms, such as the World Health Organization's analgesic ladder, are long established and widely accepted. Conventional analgesia has limitations, however—principally, the adverse effects of systemic opioids (nausea, vomiting, oversedation, respiratory depression) and of nonsteroidal anti-inflammatory drugs (NSAIDs) (gastrointestinal mucosal bleeding, renal impairment, increased risk of thromboembolism).

Postoperative pain is feared by patients yet frequently undertreated. This situation has increased patients' demand for and acceptance of unconventional therapies. *Complementary medicine*, often termed *alternative medicine*, encompasses a heterogeneous mix of agents and techniques not widely accepted by the medical community. A study published in 1998 found that 42% of American adults use some form of unconventional therapy.[1] A wide variety of unconventional alternatives to traditional analgesic drugs and techniques have been described, including physical, pharmacological, and psychological modalities of analgesia (Table 20–1). In this chapter, we consider the evidence supporting the use of some of these alternatives in the postoperative setting.

Nonpharmacological Modalities

TRANSCUTANEOUS ELECTRICAL NERVE STIMULATION

The mode of action of transcutaneous electrical nerve stimulation (TENS) is based on the gate control theory of pain as described by Melzack and Wall.[2] TENS is a vibratory sensation produced by a small electrical current. The current is produced between plastic pads that are applied to the skin at the affected area, through which a low-voltage electrical stimulus is passed (Fig. 20–1). The frequency and amplitude of the current used may be varied. The mode of action of TENS is activation of A-beta peripheral nerve fibers, leading to a reduction in central nociceptive cell activity.[3] A systematic review of the use of TENS in postoperative pain judged it to be ineffective in this area.[4] The Bandolier evidence-based website[4a] states, "TENS is not effective in the relief of postoperative pain." It is possible, however, that suboptimal frequencies were studied.

A later meta-analysis of randomized controlled trials (RCTs) of TENS and acupuncture-like transcutaneous electrical nerve stimulation (ALTENS) has been conducted.[5] Subgroup analysis for adequate treatment was performed, which involved electrode placement in the area of the incision. For all trials, the mean reduction in analgesic consumption after TENS/ALTENS was 26.5% (range, −6% to +51%), better than that for placebo. Twenty-one trials were studied, involving a total of 1350 surgical patients having predominantly abdominal and orthopedic procedures. Eleven of the trials, involving 964 patients, reported that a strong, subnoxious electrical stimulation with adequate frequency was administered. The investigators reported a mean reduction in analgesic consumption of 36% (range, 14% to 51%), again better than that for placebo. In nine trials without explicit confirmation of sufficient current intensity and adequate frequency, the mean weighted analgesic consumption was 4% (range, −10% to +29%) in favor of active treatment. The median frequency used in trials with optimal treatment was 85 Hz for TENS and 2 Hz in the only trial investigating ALTENS.[6] The researchers in this meta-analysis concluded that TENS can significantly reduce analgesic consumption for postoperative pain. The use of this technique is associated with only minor side effects, such as discomfort at the electrode site.

Therefore, there exists credible evidence that TENS may be useful for postoperative pain in some patients. However, much more, properly controlled clinical research in different surgical settings must be conducted before more widespread use of TENS as an adjunctive analgesic technique can be advocated in the perioperative period.

ACUPUNCTURE

Acupuncture is a traditional Chinese medical practice in use for three millennia. Very thin needles are inserted at specific acupuncture points on the body (Fig. 20–2). Manual, thermal, or electrical stimulation can then be applied to the needles.

TABLE 20–1	Unconventional Analgesic Agents and Techniques for Postoperative Pain
Pharmacological agents	Adenosine
	Anticonvulsants
	Antihistamines
	Baclofen
	Caffeine
	Cannabinoids
	Capsaicin
	Clonidine
	Dantrolene
	Dextroamphetamine
	Ketamine
	Lignocaine (intravenous)
	Midazolam
	Neostigmine
	Ondansetron
	Orphenadrine
Nonpharmacological modalities	Acupuncture
	Behavioral therapy
	Cold and heat
	Hypnosis
	Iontophoresis
	Music
	Transcutaneous electrical nerve stimulation (TENS)

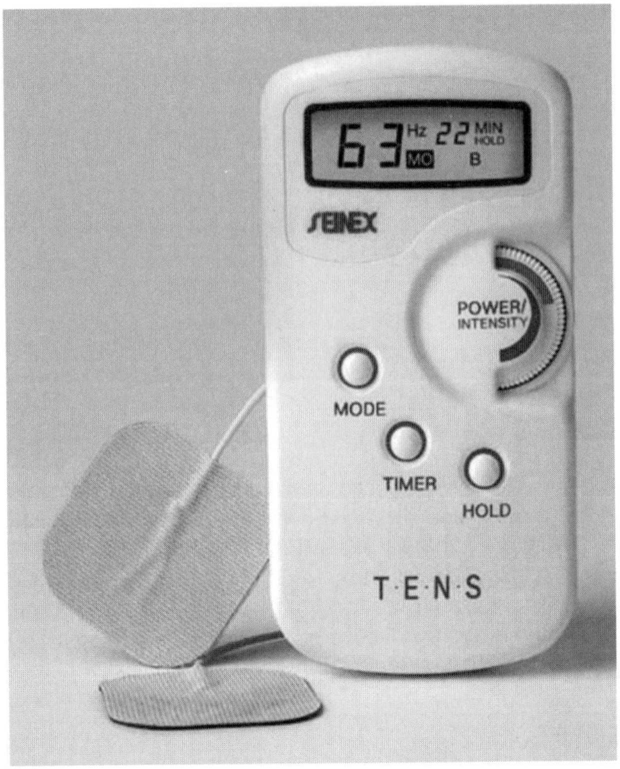

Figure 20–1 A transcutaneous electrical nerve stimulation (TENS) machine, the Seinex SE33 TENS, with electrodes. (Source: http://www.medisave.co.uk/popup_image.php/pID/761/)

In the most widely accepted acupuncture model, needling of nerve fibers in muscle sends impulses to the spinal cord. Three centers are activated—the spinal cord, the midbrain, and the hypothalamic-pituitary system. Pain inhibition is mediated by endorphins and monoamine neurotransmitters. When performed by an experienced practitioner, acupuncture is rarely associated with complications.

The U.S. National Institutes of Health Consensus Statement on Acupuncture, published in 1997, concluded that sufficient evidence exists to support the efficacy of acupuncture for acute postoperative dental pain.[7] Much of the published literature on acupuncture is case reports. A few RCTs have been carried out despite obvious research challenges, such as blinding of subjects.

In a 2002 review, Akca et al[8] examined four RCTs evaluating the perioperative use of acupuncture and whether it would reduce the dose of anesthetic agent needed to maintain an adequate depth of anesthesia. Three studies did not demonstrate a clinically important reduction in anesthetic requirement. In contrast, Kotani et al[9] showed that at least some acupuncture techniques provide substantial postoperative analgesia and significantly reduce opioid requirements after abdominal surgery. Patients undergoing upper and lower abdominal surgery using both general and epidural anesthesia techniques were studied. Preoperative intradermal acupuncture was found to decrease incisional and visceral pain.

Although acupuncture may offer some benefit in the perioperative setting, the evidence for improved postoperative analgesia with the use of preoperative intradermal acupuncture is limited to a single RCT showing reduced opioid requirements. Further studies are warranted to evaluate the mechanism of this observation and determine whether this effect is applicable to a range of surgical procedures. Acupuncture cannot be recommended for perioperative use at present.

HYPNOSIS

Hypnosis is induction of a heightened state of concentration characterized by a markedly greater receptivity to suggestion and the capacity for an alteration of perception. Hypnosis has been found to activate and attenuate a triple hierarchical pain control system: the nociceptive reflex (spinal and descending control mechanisms), the perceived intensity of evoked pain sensations (spinal and supraspinal inhibitory mechanisms), and the unpleasantness of the pain sensation (sensory and affective inhibitory systems).[10]

The usefulness of hypnosis as an adjunctive technique for postoperative pain is clear from the literature. Initial evidence came from case reports and case series, suggesting a role in both adult and pediatric patients undergoing surgery ranging from orthopedic hand procedures to laminectomy,[11] dental surgery, and cervical endocrine surgery.[12] A retrospective study evaluating hypnosis as an adjunct to intravenous conscious sedation with local anesthesia for 337 patients undergoing plastic surgery concluded that lower doses of intraoperative alfentanil and midazolam, better pain relief, and improved patient satisfaction were obtained in the hypnosis group.[13]

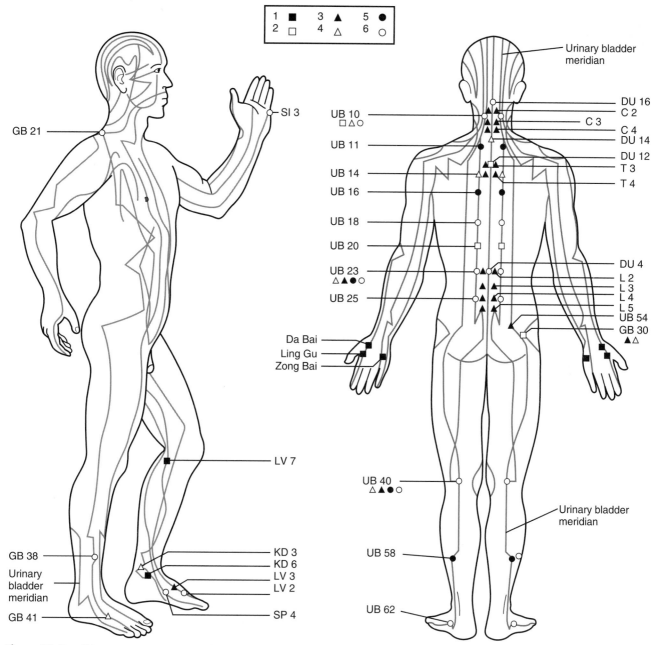

Figure 20–2 Chinese acupuncture points diagram, corresponding to specific visceral stimulation points. (Source: http://www.medscape.com/content/2001/00/41/07/410779/art-smj9405.08.fig.jpg/)

There would seem to be a potential role for hypnosis in carefully selected patients, in conjunction with analgesia, for certain procedures. Clinical RCTs are needed before the potential of hypnosis, combined with conventional balanced analgesia, can be more fully evaluated.

IONTOPHORESIS

Iontophoresis is the transdermal administration of ionized drugs in which electrically charged molecules are propelled through the skin by an external electrical field. Transfer can be facilitated by a small current across two electrodes, the rate of drug delivery being proportional to the current applied.

Greater drug delivery to specific sites is thus achieved. Local anesthetic agents and steroids are among the agents that can be delivered to tissues by iontophoresis.

The transdermal administration of morphine has been used to reduce postoperative intravenous opioid requirement, attaining serum morphine concentrations of 20 to 50 ng • mL^{-1}. The results of a single-blind prospective RCT published in 1992 suggest a potential role for iontophoretic delivery of morphine.[14] Thirty-eight patients who had undergone joint replacement surgery were randomly assigned to receive either placebo or iontophoretic transdermal morphine in addition to morphine delivered using a patient-controlled analgesia (PCA) device for a period of 6 hours.

Significantly lower consumption of PCA morphine was observed in the study group during this time. Further evaluation of iontophoretic methods of analgesic drug delivery is needed before any progress can be made in developing its role in the perioperative setting.

COLD AND HEAT

Physical therapies such as cold and heat may have a potential role in managing postoperative pain. Cold therapy is commonly used in acute injuries to reduce swelling and pain. The reduction in edema and pain with cold therapy occurs because of vasoconstriction and diminution of nerve conduction velocity. A reduction in opioid requirements was found in a group of patients undergoing anterior cruciate ligament reconstruction when a cooling unit was put on the operated knee and used for the first 4 days after surgery.[15]

Heat therapy may be delivered as conductive, convective, or converted heat—as infrared treatment, shortwave diathermy, and ultrasound. There is a role for these treatments in soft tissue injury and chronic pain states. As yet, no evidence exists for their role in acute postoperative pain.

MUSIC

Music is a nursing intervention that has the potential to decrease patients' pain perception in the post-anesthesia care unit.[16] Greater patient satisfaction and alleviation of anxiety have been observed.[17,18] More substantial evidence from an RCT concludes that the use of intraoperative music combined with general anesthesia may have beneficial effects on postoperative recovery.[19] In a separate paper the researchers of the RCT found that perioperative music therapy had a short-term pain-reducing effect.[20]

MIND-BODY THERAPIES

A rather heterogeneous group of nonpharmacological techniques may be classified as *mind-body therapies*. Most are aimed at promoting calm and general well-being rather than reducing postoperative pain specifically. In a 2004 review of the literature, Astin[21] reports some evidence that these approaches could influence postoperative pain. Studies addressing postoperative pain may be classified into two groups, relaxation techniques taught preoperatively and positive suggestions played to the patient on audiotapes during general anesthesia.

Relaxation Training

In 1984, Scott and Clum[22] investigated the merits of training patients preoperatively in relaxation techniques and suggested that the results depended on the individual's pain coping style, with "sensitizers" benefiting but "avoiders" showing no reduction in postoperative pain. Mogan et al[23] found no difference in postoperative pain or analgesia requirement with relaxation training in 72 patients having abdominal surgery,[23] and Daltroy et al[24] demonstrated no difference in pain with or without a preoperative psychoeducational program for 222 patients undergoing hip or knee replacement.[24]

One specific relaxation technique, guided imagery, has shown benefits. In the Cleveland Clinic, patients randomly assigned to receive guided imagery training had a substantially lower pain score (59% of control) and smaller morphine requirements after surgery (58%) than their control group counterparts ($P < .001$ for both outcomes).[25] Similarly, Halpin et al[26] demonstrated reduced postoperative analgesic consumption after cardiac surgery,[26] and Laurion and Fetzer[27] demonstrated that patients experienced less pain after laparoscopy, with guided imagery. Overall, though, relaxation training can at best be a measure to reduce anxiety in the preoperative period, thus reducing postoperative analgesic requirements in anxious patients.

Intraoperative Suggestion

Playing tapes of positive suggestions to patients under general anesthesia in order to influence their postoperative pain has little biological plausibility or face validity. In a 1990 trial with 60 participants, McLintock et al[28] showed modestly reduced morphine consumption after abdominal hysterectomy in the group receiving positive suggestion ($P = .028$), but the patients' postoperative pain scores were the same in the treatment and control groups. Subsequent studies in patients undergoing general and gynecological procedures did not confirm any beneficial effect of intraoperative positive suggestion on postoperative pain relief.[29–31]

Pharmacological Agents

Table 20–2 summarizes dosage ranges and adverse effects of the pharmacological agents discussed here.

ADENOSINE

A ubiquitous endogenous purine nucleoside, adenosine is primarily useful in cardiology. It also has neuromodulatory effects at the presynaptic receptor[32] and in the spinal cord[33] via the A1 and A3 receptors, which downregulate cyclic adenosine monophosphate (cAMP) through inhibitory G protein.[34] Intrathecal adenosine showed a postoperative analgesic effect in a rat model.[35] In a randomized placebo-controlled trial of 48 women undergoing abdominal hysterectomy, however, Rane et al[36] demonstrated no advantage for intrathecal adenosine (500 µg).[36] Apan et al[37] randomly assigned 60 patients undergoing surgery with brachial plexus block anesthesia to receive either placebo or adenosine infusion; they found a prolonged duration of blockade in the adenosine-treated group, although clinical outcome measures (time to first requirement of supplemental analgesia, analgesic consumption, visual analogue scale scores) were similar in the two groups, and two of the treated patients had adverse effects—chest pain and palpitations.[37]

By contrast, in two RCTs, Segerdahl et al[38,39] reported reductions in both anesthetic and postoperative morphine requirements after peripheral adenosine infusion (80 µg • kg^{-1} • min^{-1}) during breast surgery and abdominal hysterectomy. Fukunaga et al[40] randomly assigned 62 patients undergoing major surgery to receive infusion of either remifentanil (0.05–0.5 µg • kg^{-1} • min^{-1}; total dose 2.5 mg) or adenosine

TABLE 20–2	Dose Ranges and Adverse Effects of Pharmacological Agents for Postoperative Pain		
Pharmacological Agents	**Dose or Range**	**Adverse Effect(s)**	**Chapter Reference(s)**
Adenosine	Intrathecal: 500 µg Infusion: 50–500 µg	Chest pain, palpitations, flushing, bronchospasm	36–40
Anticonvulsants		Liver dysfunction	
Pregabalin	50–300 mg	Sedation	132
Antihistamines		Sedation	
Phenyltoloxamine	60 mg		149
Cannabinoids		Dependence potential, increased awareness	
delta-9-Tetrahydrocannabinol	5 mg		152
Capsaicin	0.025–0.075% (topical)	Initial burning sensation	146, 147
Clonidine	Systemic: 0.3–5 µg/kg Intra-articular: 150 µg Regional: 1 µg/kg Epidural: 3 µg/kg Intrathecal: 15–150 µg	Hypotension, bradycardia, sedation	43–63, 159–166
Dantrolene	1.5 mg/kg, 50–150 mg	Muscle weakness, allergy	124–126
Dextroamphetamine	5–10 mg	Dependence potential	153
Ketamine	Bolus: 300 µg/kg Infusion: 1–14 µg/kg Caudal: 250–500 µg/kg Intramuscular: 0.5–1 mg/kg	Cardiovascular stimulation, spinal toxicity	89, 90, 105, 167
Lignocaine (intravenous)	1.5 mg/kg/hour	Cardiac failure, arrhythmias	123
Midazolam	Intramuscular: 5-mg bolus Caudal: 50 µg/kg Epidural: 150 µg/kg	Sedation, hypotension	116, 119, 121
Neostigmine	Intrathecal: 1–50 µg/kg Intra-articular: 500 µg	Nausea, vomiting	68–73, 79
Nefopam	0.4 mg/kg, 15–30 mg	Sweating, tachycardia	110–113, 168
Ondansetron	—	Antalgesia in combination with tramadol	157, 158
Orphenadrine	25–30 mg	Nausea, vomiting	128, 129

(50–500 $\mu g \cdot kg^{-1} \cdot min^{-1}$; total dose 2500 mg) during surgery and general anesthesia, with the doses titrated against cardiovascular responses. These researchers found a major difference in postoperative pain and morphine requirements in favor of adenosine.[40] Cumulative morphine consumption in the first 48 hours was significantly lower in the adenosine group than in the remifentanil group (53 ± 26 mg versus 92 ± 35 mg, P = .001).[40]

Synthetic adenosine receptor agonists have been investigated, but the only RCT involving such an agent for postoperative pain showed no benefit.[41]

On balance, there is RCT evidence supporting a role for systemic adenosine during general anesthesia to improve postoperative analgesia and reduce opioid requirements,[38-40] although its widespread application may be limited by cardiovascular side effects such as those reported by Apan et al.[37]

CLONIDINE

Clonidine is an α_2-adrenergic agonist. These agents, originally used for their centrally acting antihypertensive action, are now widely used in anesthesia for their analgesic, sedative, anxiolytic, sympatholytic, anesthesia-sparing, and hemodynamics-stabilizing properties. Agents such as clonidine, dexmedetomidine, and tizanidine act both centrally and peripherally. The four receptor subtypes that have been

identified by molecular genetic technology are 2A, 2B, 2C, and 2D. The 2A subtype mediates the antinociceptive action of α_2 agonists.

It has been widely demonstrated that clonidine, whether given by the intravenous,[42,43] epidural, caudal,[44,45] intramuscular, oral, transdermal, peripheral, or intra-articular[46] route, enhances analgesia for acute postoperative pain.

Happily, although there is a synergistic and additive analgesic effect between the α agonists and opioids, no such synergism exists with regard to respiratory depression. This makes α agonists desirable adjuvant analgesics, enhancing analgesia and reducing adverse side effects. Hypotension, bradycardia, and sedation, the important side effects of the α agonists, are dose related. Premedication with oral clonidine and intraoperative use of a clonidine transdermal patch reduce postoperative morphine requirements.[47-49]

Intravenous clonidine is given as a bolus, followed by infusion on the order of 45 $\mu g \cdot kg^{-1} \cdot hr^{-1}$, because of its pharmacokinetic profile and short half-life. High doses result in sedation and hypotension.[43]

The addition of clonidine to both local anesthetic[50] and opioids in epidural infusions has been examined. The combination of epidural clonidine and morphine provides longer-lasting and more potent analgesia.[51-53] One meta-analysis was unsuccessful, however, in identifying the optimal dose for epidural administration.[54]

Intrathecal clonidine, 15 to 30 μg added to bupivacaine for inguinal repair, decreases postoperative pain.[55] The intrathecal combination of morphine and clonidine has implications for patients undergoing cardiac surgery.[56] For parturients having cesarean section, multimodal analgesia with intrathecal bupivacaine, opioid, and clonidine provides the best postoperative pain relief.[57]

Intra-articular clonidine achieves analgesia comparable to that of intra-articular morphine.[58] When co-delivered with local anesthetic into the knee joint, clonidine also improves postoperative pain for ambulatory patients who have had knee arthroscopy.[59]

Added to local anesthetic agents in peripheral nerve blockade, clonidine has short-term analgesic-sparing properties. In peripheral nerve blockade, it is useful only in combination with local anesthetic.[60,61] Clonidine has been used for intercostal nerve blockade after thoracotomy[62] and for foot surgery.[63]

As an adjunct to intravenous regional anesthesia, clonidine enhances postoperative analgesia in a dose of $1 \ \mu g \cdot kg^{-1}$,[64] but it has been shown to be of limited benefit.[65]

In summary, clonidine is of proven benefit as an adjunctive analgesic agent both in regional anesthetic techniques and for systemic analgesia. It deserves more widespread use as part of a balanced analgesic regimen.

NEOSTIGMINE

Widely used in anesthetic practice for its muscarinic anticholinesterase properties, reversing the effects of nondepolarizing muscle relaxants, neostigmine has also been used for its analgesic effects. Intrathecal, epidural, caudal, and intra-articular administration routes for neostigmine have all been investigated.

The analgesic benefit of neuraxial neostigmine is well described, but side effects such as nausea, vomiting, sedation, and hypotension limit its use.[66,67]

There is a clear case for the use of epidural or caudal neostigmine as a local anesthetic–sparing agent in pediatric practice. For children undergoing genitourinary surgery, a single caudal injection of $2 \ \mu g \cdot kg^{-1}$ added to local anesthetic resulted in lower pain scores ($P < .005$) and a longer time to first analgesia ($P < .05$).[68] In a separate study, addition of neostigmine $2 \ \mu g \cdot kg^{-1}$ to caudal bupivacaine provided comparable analgesia, extended postoperative analgesia, and reduced the need for supplementary analgesia, yet was associated with an increased rate of vomiting.[69] A third study found that dose-dependent analgesia was provided by caudal neostigmine 20 to $50 \ \mu g \cdot kg^{-1}$, with doses greater than $30 \ \mu g \cdot kg^{-1}$ having a higher incidence of nausea and vomiting.[70]

In adult gynecological surgery, neostigmine as an analgesic has limitations. Intrathecal neostigmine 25 to 75 μg does have a sparing effect on morphine consumption after major gynecological surgery.[71] Intrathecal neostigmine, 1 to 5 μg added to bupivacaine and morphine, doubled the time to rescue analgesia and reduced consumption in the first 24 hours after gynecological procedures without raising the incidence of postoperative nausea and vomiting.[72] A significant reduction in postoperative PCA requirement was found after cesarean section with intraoperative use of intrathecal neostigmine and morphine; the combination provided better

analgesia than either agent alone, and neostigmine alone had a higher incidence of nausea.[73]

In patients undergoing knee replacement surgery, intrathecal neostigmine prolonged motor blockade compared with morphine, which was associated with more pruritus, a later onset of postoperative pain, and longer time to rescue analgesia.[74]

Therefore, epidural neostigmine produces prolonged postoperative analgesia either alone or in combination with local anesthetic, when it has a local anesthetic–sparing effect.[74–76] Intrathecal neostigmine is effective when combined with local anesthetic but produces unacceptable postoperative nausea and vomiting when used alone.[77]

The intra-articular administration of neostigmine 500 μg in the knee joint after meniscus repair produces a better analgesic effect than 2 mg of morphine, with no difference in side effects.[78]

In summary, neostigmine has the potential to enhance postoperative analgesia. Epidural neostigmine is perhaps best used in combination with local anesthetic. Intrathecal neostigmine also has a local anesthetic–sparing effect. Its main drawback is postoperative nausea and vomiting, which can be minimized through the use of this agent in combination with local anesthetic. There is no role for systemic neostigmine, but intra-articular neostigmine is promising.

KETAMINE

Ketamine is an induction agent for general anesthesia that acts as a noncompetitive antagonist at the N-methyl-D-aspartate (NMDA) receptor. NMDA receptor activation is considered to be one of the mechanisms involved in postoperative pain and hypersensitivity. Ketamine has potent analgesic properties; however, its usefulness has been limited by psychic emergence phenomena and cardiovascular stimulating properties. Elucidation of the role of the NMDA receptor in the processing of nociceptive input has led to renewed interest in ketamine as an analgesic agent.[79] One hypothesis is that the analgesic effect of ketamine is mediated by a nonopioid mechanism possibly involving phencyclidine receptor–mediated blockade of the NMDA receptor–operated ion channel.[80] Ketamine blocks sodium channels, both in the periphery and in the central nervous system.[81] It also interacts with μ, δ, and κ opioid receptors[82] and with monoaminergic-sensitive and voltage-sensitive calcium channels[83] as well as nicotinic and muscarinic receptors.[81]

Ketamine is available as a racemic mixture, containing equal amounts of the two isomers, S^+ ketamine and R^- ketamine, and also as pure S^+ ketamine, which is three to four times more potent than R^- ketamine for pain relief. Current evidence suggests that low-dose ketamine may play an important role in postoperative pain management as an adjunct to local anesthetic, opioid, and other agents and reduces opioid-related adverse effects.

Clinical trials to date have evaluated oral, parenteral,[84] subcutaneous, neuraxial, intra-articular, and transdermal[85] administration of ketamine. A systematic review of ketamine given preemptively before surgery found a significant preventive analgesic benefit in postoperative pain.[86]

Intraoperative low-dose ketamine has been investigated using the hypothesis that subanesthetic doses lead to postoperative antihyperalgesia and analgesia.[87] Studies can be categorized according to route of ketamine administration as follows: bolus injection, bolus plus continuous infusion, continuous infusion, and PCA. The analgesic efficacy of ketamine depends on infusion rate, initial loading dose, and whether concomitant opioids are administered. Effective short-acting analgesia is produced when ketamine is given as a single bolus of more than 300 $\mu g \cdot kg^{-1}$ At infusions less than 4 $\mu g \cdot kg^{-1}$ without a loading dose, ketamine has no effect on postoperative pain. With a loading dose, ketamine infusion rates of 1 to 6 $\mu g \cdot kg^{-1} \cdot min^{-1}$ provide evidence of analgesic effects. A value for the analgesic potency of ketamine has not yet been determined. When ketamine (1–14 $\mu g \cdot kg^{-1} \cdot min^{-1}$ following a loading dose) is combined with an opioid, an opioid-sparing effect as large as 50% is seen. It may also be given as a bolus followed by infusion, in combination with regional techniques,[88,89] to reduce opioid requirement postoperatively[90,91] and hasten mobilization.[92]

In combination with morphine for PCA, ketamine provides effective postoperative analgesia, reducing morphine consumption.[93] This effect can be evident up to 48 hours postoperatively; cumulative morphine consumption for post-laparotomy pain in one group was significantly lower at 48 hours (28 mg versus 54 mg, $P = .0003$)[94] with a ketamine dose of 2.5 $\mu g \cdot kg^{-1} \cdot min^{-1}$. Some researchers have found no benefit, however, in adding ketamine to morphine PCA,[95] probably because inadequate doses were used.

Epidural preservative-free ketamine with morphine improves pain relief[96,97] and lowers morphine consumption[98,99] with a prolongation of analgesia.[100] Patients undergoing upper abdominal surgery who were given preincisional epidural bupivacaine, ketamine, and morphine had better postoperative pain relief and significantly less morphine requirement—6.0 mg (range, 1 to 200 mg) versus 12.5 mg (range, 3 to 42 mg) ($P = .005$).[101] Patient-controlled epidural analgesia (PCEA) with ketamine has been investigated, with promising results.[102,103] In pediatric practice, adding ketamine to caudal local anesthetic prolongs block for subumbilical surgery[104,105] in doses on the order of 0.25 mg $\cdot kg^{-1}$.[106]

Intrathecal administration of ketamine is to be avoided owing to potential spinal toxicity. This is true of both preservative-free ketamine and the preservative itself.[107] Intra-articular ketamine has been shown to be less effective than intramuscular ketamine for patients undergoing arthroscopic surgery.[108]

In conclusion, intravenous ketamine has proven benefit as an adjunctive analgesic in the intraoperative setting, especially when used preemptively. Ketamine is also effective as a local anesthetic–sparing agent when used in an epidural or caudal technique. It appears that the analgesic potential of ketamine in the perioperative setting is underutilized.

NEFOPAM

Nefopam, a nonopiate, centrally acting analgesic, is unrelated to other drugs and has an unclear mechanism of action. It does not influence prostaglandin synthesis but does inhibit neuronal reuptake of the neurotransmitters serotonin, dopamine, and noradrenaline. A number of RCTs of nefopam have been published. Tigerstedt et al[109] compared nefopam with pethidine after abdominal surgery in 100 patients and showed that the analgesic effect of 15-mg or 30-mg doses of

nefopam was intermediate between the effects of 50 mg and 100 mg of pethidine.[109] In 49 patients who had undergone upper abdominal surgery, McLintock et al[110] demonstrated a significant morphine-sparing effect for nefopam 20 mg.[110] Similarly, Moffat et al[111] showed that nefopam had morphine-sparing analgesic effects, particularly when combined with diclofenac, in 42 patients receiving PCA after abdominal surgery.[111] A placebo-controlled RCT of 201 patients who had undergone hip replacement surgery again demonstrated a morphine-sparing effect of nefopam (20 mg oral). Studies to determine equipotent postoperative analgesic doses of nefopam and morphine have estimated equivalencies between nefopam 0.4 mg $\cdot kg^{-1}$ and morphine 0.1 mg $\cdot kg^{-1}$ and between nefopam 18 mg and morphine 5 mg.[112] Nefopam appears to be effective in reducing opiate requirements when used as part of a balanced postoperative analgesic regimen, yet it is rarely used in clinical practice. Perhaps nefopam deserves more careful consideration as an adjunctive analgesic in a balanced analgesia regimen.

MIDAZOLAM

An intermediate-acting benzodiazepine, midazolam is used primarily for sedation but also has antinociceptive properties. It is useful in ameliorating the affective component of acute pain.

Used systemically as a bolus intramuscular injection 30 minutes preoperatively, midazolam reduced postoperative pain in patients undergoing outpatient surgery ($P = .035$).[113] Sedation with midazolam in addition to local anesthesia for third molar extraction was associated with a significant reduction in postoperative pain intensity ($P < .005$) and in analgesia consumption ($P < .001$).[114] A preoperative bolus dose and intraoperative infusion of midazolam reduced pain scores and morphine requirements in women undergoing abdominal hysterectomy ($P < .002$).[115] Spinal administration of midazolam has also been investigated. Bupivacaine and midazolam combined produced better postoperative analgesia than spinal bupivacaine alone after knee arthroscopy ($P < .05$)[116] and cesarean section.[117] Similarly, in caudal blocks in children, midazolam added to bupivacaine produced a doubling of postoperative analgesia duration ($P < .001$).[118] Midazolam alone is also effective when given caudally, reducing analgesia requirements after herniotomy ($P < .05$).[119] Nishiyama[120] has produced a series of papers showing the effectiveness of midazolam as part of epidural analgesia after abdominal surgery, both as a one-shot rescue analgesia method[120] and as a continuous postoperative infusion.[121]

Spinal or epidural administration of midazolam appears to have a definite postoperative analgesic effect. There are, however, concerns regarding the potential for neurotoxicity.[122] Further studies are needed to define more clearly the dose and timing of midazolam in postoperative analgesia, but it seems to have the potential for more widespread use in a balanced analgesic regimen.

LIGNOCAINE

The ubiquitous local anesthetic agent lignocaine has many clinical uses. Interest has focused on the potential analgesic role of intravenous lignocaine. Blockade of sodium channels in peripheral mechanosensitive nociceptors has been linked to central sensitization of pain. For patients undergoing major abdominal surgery, a preincisional lignocaine bolus of 1.5 mg • kg^{-1}, followed by infusion of 1.5 mg • kg^{-1} • hr, caused a significant reduction in morphine requirement (103 ± 72 mg versus 159 ± 73.3 mg, P = .05) that persisted up to 72 hours postoperatively.[123] Clearly, further work in this area is warranted, but initial results are encouraging.

DANTROLENE

Dantrolene sodium has a known myorelaxant action owing to partial inhibition of calcium ion release from the lateral sacs of the sarcoplasmic reticulum in muscle cells. Its use is contraindicated in acute liver disease. A number of studies have examined the use of dantrolene in alleviating muscle pains postoperatively.

In one RCT, single-dose oral dantrolene (100–150 mg) given 2 hours preoperatively was found to significantly reduce the incidence of muscle pains after suxamethonium administration from 56% to 4% in 48 patients without affecting the duration of action of suxamethonium.[124] This effect is less relevant now that the use of suxamethonium is declining. For tonsillectomy pain, oral dantrolene in a dose of 1.5 mg/kg/day in 4 doses was compared with placebo in a group of 113 patients for 5 days after tonsillectomy. The investigators concluded that dantrolene was effective in reducing the analgesic requirements after tonsillectomy.[125] However, a double-blind, placebo-controlled trial of 40 patients who had undergone surgery for hemorrhoidal prolapse found no significant difference in analgesia between patients receiving oral dantrolene and controls.[126]

In summary, dantrolene seems to be effective in reducing muscle pain after suxamethonium administration[124] but otherwise not to have clinically useful analgesic properties in the postoperative setting.

ORPHENADRINE

Orphenadrine is a centrally acting anticholinergic muscle relaxant for which there is sparse literature regarding use in the postoperative setting. In 1979, Fry[127] reported preliminary experience with a papaveretum-orphenadrine combination. He claimed that orphenadrine administered toward the end of surgery delayed the requirement for postoperative analgesia by extending the analgesic effect of papaveretum. No follow-up paper ensued. The same year, Winter and Post[128] studied the effects of orphenadrine alone (25 mg), paracetamol alone (325 mg), the two drugs together, and placebo in a double-blind trial involving 200 patients undergoing oral surgery. The group given both drugs fared best, and those given orphenadrine alone also had better analgesia than those given placebo.[128] Later in the Czech Republic, Malek et al[129] randomly assigned patients to receive intravenous piroxicam, placebo, or a combination of diclofenac 75 mg and orphenadrine 30 mg after outpatient knee arthroscopy. The diclofenac-orphenadrine group had the best pain relief and fewest adverse effects.[129] Overall, the two good-quality trials in the literature, reported 25 years apart, suggest a potential modest benefit for orphenadrine. This suggestion must be validated by further larger trials before orphenadrine can be recommended as an adjunctive analgesic agent.

ANTICONVULSANTS

Anticonvulsants are membrane-stabilizing agents that have an established role in managing neuropathic pain by preventing spontaneous neuronal firing[130] but have been little investigated in the postoperative setting. Most have a significant side effect profile and, in the chronic pain setting, are introduced at low doses that are gradually increased to the point of effectiveness. This is an obvious limitation of their use for postoperative pain. Nevertheless, Field et al[131] demonstrated a postoperative analgesic effect of gabapentin and S-+3-isobutylgaba in a rat hindlimb model. In a clinical study, the gamma-aminobutyric acid (GABA) precursor pregabalin was superior to ibuprofen and placebo after dental extraction.[132] Although further investigation of perioperative pregabalin is perhaps justified, anticonvulsants do not appear to be useful for postoperative pain control at present.

TRICYCLIC AND TETRACYCLIC ANTIDEPRESSANTS

Tricyclic and tetracyclic antidepressants, which are primarily psychoactive drugs, are thought to exert a secondary analgesic effect by modulating the levels of serotonin and noradrenaline in the brain and spinal cord.[133] Animal studies lend support to the idea that the antidepressants have a distinct biochemical analgesic effect rather than simply reducing the distress associated with pain by elevating mood.[134,135] There are few clinical studies in the postoperative setting. Iacono et al[136] claim that tricyclic antidepressants are effective in preventing and treating phantom limb pain after lower extremity amputation.

Most investigators have concentrated on the setting of chronic pain, in which antidepressants are now well-established, mainstream therapeutic agents. It is generally accepted in this context that the onset of analgesic effect of antidepressants takes weeks. This is obviously a major limitation to their use for postoperative analgesia. The major analgesic role of the tricyclic and tetracyclic antidepressants remains the treatment of chronic neuropathic pain.

CAFFEINE

Caffeine has long been used as an adjunct in various analgesic medications. The best evidence for its effectiveness comes from a 1984 meta-analysis of 30 trials involving 10,000 patients that concluded that the pooled relative potency of analgesics with caffeine was 1.4 times greater than their potency without caffeine.[137] RCTs of ibuprofen[138] and aspirin[139] with and without caffeine for postoperative dental pain showed a beneficial effect of caffeine. Later systematic reviews question the benefit of using low-dose caffeine with paracetamol[140] or aspirin[141] and raise concerns about an association between analgesic nephropathy and caffeine-enhanced analgesics.[142] Despite being supported by level IA evidence (I indicating a large RCT, N ≥ 100 per group; A denoting good evidence to support the recommendation),[137] caffeine has failed to gain popularity as a credible component of balanced analgesic regimens. Further studies of the optimum dose and surgical settings for its use are warranted to evaluate whether its potential as an analgesic may be more fully exploited.

CAPSAICIN

The red pepper extract capsaicin has been used topically for relief of pain in a variety of conditions.[143] It is thought to desensitize unmyelinated C-fiber nociceptors and thinly myelinated A-delta sensory neurons by depleting stores of the neurotransmitters substance P and calcitonin gene–related peptide (CGRP).[144,145] Although the initial topical application of capsaicin causes burning pain, repeated application leads to desensitization, which is a reversible calcium-dependent process. Neurotoxicity may result from high-dose capsaicin. An RCT of 23 women with postmastectomy pain syndrome demonstrated a 62% response to topical capsaicin (0.075%), compared with a 30% response to placebo.[146] The investigators in this study mention the difficulty of blinding patients to their treatment owing to the characteristic burning sensation produced by capsaicin; this problem may partly explain the large proportion of capsaicin studies that involve no control group. For example, in a cohort of 21 women with postmastectomy pain syndrome who were treated for 2 months with topical capsaicin cream (0.025%), Dini et al[147] found that 13 (62%) responded to treatment and 11 (52%) were pain free 3 months after finishing treatment. Although this result appears good in isolation, it is less impressive if a placebo response rate of 18% to 30% is extrapolated from other studies.[143,146,148] Therefore, a clinical role for capsaicin in postoperative pain management appears unlikely.

ANTIHISTAMINES

Used mostly for their sedative, antiemetic, and antimuscarinic properties, antihistamines have also been shown to possess analgesic actions, potentiating the effect of more traditional analgesic drugs. This effect may be partly explained by the sedative properties of most antihistamines. One RCT of 200 gynecological inpatients found significantly better pain relief with the use of paracetamol 650 mg and phenyltoloxamine 60 mg than with paracetamol alone after episiotomy.[149] This single study is hardly sufficient, however, to suggest a role for antihistamines in postoperative pain control.

BACLOFEN

The muscle relaxant baclofen is an agonist at the $GABA_\beta$ receptor. It acts presynaptically by preventing the influx of calcium ions and inhibiting neurotransmitter release. Baclofen is commonly used to treat neuropathic pain, but its use is limited by side effects such as sedation and confusion. It has an antispasmodic effect after spinal surgery that is not associated with pain relief. In a single experimental study, preoperative baclofen appeared to have a synergistic analgesic effect when combined with morphine that was not observed when baclofen was combined with pentazocine. Baclofen alone is no better than placebo and is inferior to paracetamol in relieving postoperative dental pain.[150] Baclofen has no role in relieving acute postoperative pain.

CANNABINOIDS

Active constituents of cannabis, cannabinoids are postulated to have anxiolytic and analgesic effects. They act at the cannabinoid receptors CB1 and CB2 to inhibit adenylyl cyclase and inhibit N-type calcium currents.[151] Cannabinoids are likely to produce antinociception at both spinal and supraspinal sites. CB1 receptors predominate in the brain and spinal cord and are the likely site of analgesic effect. CB1-selective agonists have shown some promise as analgesics. They may have a role in the management of chronic pain, especially in terminal illness.[151] In the latest RCT of these agents for postoperative pain, the cannabinoid δ-9-tetrahydrocannabinol showed no benefit over placebo when given 2 days after abdominal hysterectomy.[152]

DEXTROAMPHETAMINE

Dextroamphetamine, a psychostimulant, was evaluated for postoperative pain in an RCT in 1977. A dose of 10 mg was shown to double the analgesic effect of morphine when the two drugs were co-administered. Common adverse opiate effects of oversedation and drowsiness were reduced.[153] The addictive potential of the amphetamines is better understood now, and they are no longer likely to be prescribed for postoperative pain.

ONDANSETRON

A competitive 5-hydroxytryptamine type 3 ($5HT_3$) receptor antagonist, ondansetron is an effective antiemetic.[154] Its involvement with serotonin pathways led some investigators to speculate about analgesic properties. There are two double-blind RCTs in the literature. Doenicke et al[155] gave intravenous ondansetron or placebo to 100 patients after minor surgery and found no analgesic effect.[155] Broome et al,[156] co-administering either ondansetron or metoclopramide orally with either diclofenac or tramadol after dental extractions, showed no difference in pain relief.[156] Furthermore, ondansetron competes with tramadol at the $5HT_3$ receptor, demonstrably reducing tramadol's analgesic effect.[157,158] The published evidence not only fails to show a beneficial effect of ondansetron as an analgesic but actually shows that it interferes with the effects of the established analgesic tramadol.

Conclusion

Of the various nonconventional drugs and other therapies advocated for postoperative pain management over the years, some have moved toward conventional use because of supportive evidence, others have been discarded on the basis of evidence of no or a negative effect, and still others have continued in use but remain nonconventional because of insufficient or conflicting evidence. The first group includes agents such as ketamine, clonidine, and neostigmine. Discarded agents include dextroamphetamine. The third group, the largest, comprises most of the remaining agents discussed in this chapter. Definitive evidence is difficult to obtain in many cases, with a dearth of evidence from properly conducted

RCTs in the literature. There are obvious research limitations in obtaining evidence from rigorously conducted trials for some of the techniques of complementary medicine, but until this challenge is met, the usefulness or futility of some of these methods cannot be assumed by medical practitioners.

This review has discussed many of the agents and strategies that have been used to enhance the quality of postoperative analgesia. Evidence-based medicine seems to support a role for a greater use of many of them. In certain patient subgroups, particularly those who have previously had a positive experience with them, hypnosis, acupuncture, and TENS may be helpful.

A number of pharmacological agents not known for their conventional analgesia seem to have significant evidence supporting their greater use. Neostigmine and clonidine in low doses have definite local anesthetic–sparing effects when used in epidural analgesia, with tolerable side effects if doses are kept to the levels outlined. Ketamine has a demonstrable preemptive effect when given intravenously at doses of $0.2 \text{ mg} \bullet \text{kg}^{-1}$, which seems to minimize side effects, while adjunctive roles for midazolam, orphenadrine, and adenosine are also suggested by clinical analgesia studies. We emphasize that opioids, NSAIDs and paracetamol are, and are likely to remain, the mainstays of acute postoperative pain management, but a number of the agents discussed here have the potential to enhance postoperative analgesia with acceptable adverse effects.

Enhancing awareness of these agents among anesthetists, perioperative nurses, pharmacists, and surgeons—in addition to further clinical research to more clearly define dosage and route of administration—remains the outstanding challenge to be overcome before the potential of these adjunctive agents to improve acute postoperative analgesia can be realized.

REFERENCES

1. Eisenberg DM, Davis RB, Ettner SL: Trends in alternative medicine use in the United States, 1990–1997: Results of a follow-up national survey. JAMA 1998;280:246–252.
2. Melzack R, Wall PD: Pain mechanisms: A new theory. Science 1965;150:971–979.
3. Garrison DW, Foreman RD: Decreased activity of spontaneous and noxiously evoked dorsal horn cells during transcutaneous electrical nerve stimulation (TENS). Pain 1994;58:309–315.
4. Carroll D, Tramer M, McQuay H, et al: Randomization is important in studies with pain outcomes: Systematic review of transcutaneous electrical nerve stimulation in acute postoperative pain. Br J Anaesth 1996;77:798–803.
4a. www.jr2ox.ac.uk/bandolier/booth/booths/ebmstor.html
5. Bjordal JM, Johnson MI, Ljunggreen AE: Transcutaneous electrical nerve stimulation (TENS) can reduce postoperative analgesic consumption: A meta-analysis with assessment of optimal treatment parameters for postoperative pain. Eur J Pain 2003;7:181–188.
6. Hamza MA, White PF, Ahmed HE, Ghoname EA: Effect of the frequency of transcutaneous electrical nerve stimulation on the postoperative analgesic requirement and recovery profile. Anesthesiology 1999; 91:1232–1328.
7. Acupuncture. MH Consensus Statement. 1997, Nov. 3–5;15(5):1–34.
8. Akca O, Sessler DI: Acupuncture: A useful complement of anesthesia? Minerva Anestesiol 2002;68:147–151.
9. Kotani N, Hashimoto H, Sato Y, et al: Preoperative intradermal acupuncture reduces postoperative pain, nausea and vomiting, analgesic requirement, and sympathoadrenal responses. Anesthesiology 2001; 95:349–356.
10. Gracely RH: Hypnosis and hierarchical pain control systems. Pain 1995;60:1–2.
11. Snow BR: The use of hypnosis in the management of preoperative anxiety and postoperative pain in a patient undergoing laminectomy. Bull Hosp Jt Dis Orthop Inst 1985;45:143–149.
12. Meurisse M: [Thyroid and parathyroid surgery under hypnosis: from fiction to clinical application.] Bull Mem Acad R Med Belg 1999; 154:142–150.
13. Faymonville ME, Fissette J, Mambourg PH, et al: Hypnosis as adjunct therapy in conscious sedation for plastic surgery. Reg Anesth 1995; 20:145–151.
14. Ashburn MA, Stephen RL, Ackerman E, et al: Iontophoretic delivery of morphine for postoperative analgesia. J Pain Symptom Manag 1992;7:27–33.
15. Cohn BT, Draeger RI, Jackson DW: The effects of cold therapy in the postoperative management of pain in patients undergoing anterior cruciate ligament reconstruction. Am J Sports Med 1989;17:344–349.
16. Heitz L, Symreng T, Scamman FL: Effect of music therapy in the postanesthesia care unit: A nursing intervention. J Post Anesth Nurs 1992;7:22–31.
17. Good M, Anderson GC, Stanton-Hicks M, et al: Relaxation and music reduce pain after gynecologic surgery. Pain Manage Nursing 2002; 3:61–70.
18. Koch ME, Kain ZN, Ayoub C, Rosenbaum SH: The sedative and analgesic sparing effect of music. Anesthesiology 1998;89:300–306.
19. Nilsson U, Rawal N, Unestahl LE, et al: Improved recovery after music and therapeutic suggestions during general anaesthesia: A double-blind randomised controlled trial. Acta Anaesth Scand 2001;45:812–817.
20. Nilsson U, Rawal N, Unosson M: A comparison of intra-operative or postoperative exposure to music—a controlled trial of the effects on postoperative pain. Anaesthesia 2003;58:699–703.
21. Astin JA: Mind-body therapies for the management of pain. Clin J Pain 2004;20:27–32.
22. Scott LE, Clum GA: Examining the interaction effects of coping style and brief interventions in the treatment of postsurgical pain. Pain 1984;20:279–291.
23. Mogan J, Wells N, Robertson E: Effects of preoperative teaching on postoperative pain: A replication and expansion. Int J Nurs Stud 1985;22:267–280.
24. Daltroy LH, Morlino CI, Eaton HM, et al: Preoperative education for total hip and knee replacement patients. Arthritis Care Res 1998;11:469–478.
25. Tusek DL, Church JM, Strong SA, et al: Guided imagery: A significant advance in the care of patients undergoing elective colorectal surgery. Dis Colon Rectum 1997;40:172–178.
26. Halpin LS, Speir AM, CapoBianco P, Barnett SD: Guided imagery in cardiac surgery. Outcomes Manag 2002;6:132–137.
27. Laurion S, Fetzer SJ: The effect of two nursing interventions on the postoperative outcomes of gynecologic laparoscopic patients. J Perianesth Nurs 2003;18:254–261.
28. McLintock TT, Aitken H, Downie CF, Kenny GN: Postoperative analgesic requirements in patients exposed to positive intraoperative suggestions. BMJ 1990;301:788–790.
29. Block RI, Ghoneim MM, Sum Ping ST, Ali MA: Efficacy of therapeutic suggestions for improved postoperative recovery presented during general anesthesia. Anesthesiology 1991;75:746–755.
30. Lebovits AH, Twersky R, McEwan B: Intraoperative therapeutic suggestions in day-case surgery: Are there benefits for postoperative outcome? Br J Anaesth 1999;82:861–866.
31. Dawson P, Van Hamel C, Wilkinson D, et al: Patient-controlled analgesia and intra-operative suggestion. Anaesthesia 2001;56:65–69.
32. Sawynok J: Adenosine receptor activation and nociception. Eur J Pharmacol 1998;347:1–11.
33. Sollevi A: Adenosine for pain control. Acta Anaesthesiol Scand Suppl 1997;110:135–136.
34. Gordh T, Karlsten R, Kristensen J: Intervention with spinal NMDA, adenosine, and NO systems for pain modulation. Ann Med 1995;27: 229–234.
35. Chiari AI, Eisenach JC: Intrathecal adenosine: Interactions with spinal clonidine and neostigmine in rat models of acute nociception and postoperative hypersensitivity. Anesthesiology 1999;90:1413–1421.
36. Rane K, Sollevi A, Segerdahl M: Intrathecal adenosine administration in abdominal hysterectomy lacks analgesic effect. Acta Anaesthesiol Scand 2000;44:868–872.
37. Apan A, Ozcan S, Buyukkocak U, et al: Perioperative intravenous adenosine infusion to extend postoperative analgesia in brachial plexus block. Eur J Anaesthesiol 2003;20:916–919.

38. Segerdahl M, Ekblom A, Sandelin K, et al: Perioperative adenosine infusion reduces the requirements for isoflurane and postoperative analgesics. Anesth Analg 1995;80:1145–1149.

39. Segerdahl M, Irestedt L, Sollevi A: Antinociceptive effect of perioperative adenosine infusion in abdominal hysterectomy. Acta Anaesthesiol Scand 1997;41:473–479.

40. Fukunaga AF, Alexander GE, Stark CW: Characterization of the analgesic actions of adenosine: Comparison of adenosine and remifentanil infusions in patients undergoing major surgical procedures. Pain 2003; 101:129–138.

41. Seymour RA, Hawkesford JE, Hill CM, et al: The efficacy of a novel adenosine agonist (WAG 994) in postoperative dental pain. Br J Clin Pharmacol 1999;47:675–680.

42. Bernard JM, Hommeril JL, Passuti N, Pinaud M: Postoperative analgesia by intravenous clonidine. Anesthesiology 1991;75:577–582.

43. Marinangeli F, Ciccozzi A, Donatelli F, et al: Clonidine for treatment of postoperative pain: A dose-finding study. Eur J Pain 2002;6:35–42.

44. Van Elstraete AC, Pastureau F, Lebrun T, Mehdaoui H: Caudal clonidine for postoperative analgesia in adults. Br J Anaesth 2000;84:401–402.

45. Constant I, Gall O, Gouyet L, et al: Addition of clonidine or fentanyl to local anaesthetics prolongs the duration of surgical analgesia after single shot caudal block in children. Br J Anaesth 1998;80:294–298.

46. De Kock M, Wiederkher P, Laghmiche A, Scholtes JL: Epidural clonidine used as the sole analgesic agent during and after abdominal surgery: A dose-response study. Anesthesiology 1997;86:285–292.

47. Park J, Forrest J, Kolesar R, et al: Oral clonidine reduces postoperative PCA morphine requirements. Can J Anaesth 1996;43:900–906.

48. Goyagi T, Tanaka M, Nishikawa T: Oral clonidine premedication enhances postoperative analgesia by epidural morphine. Anesth Analg 1999;89:1487–1491.

49. Yu HP, Hseu SS, Yien HW, et al: Oral clonidine premedication preserves heart rate variability for patients undergoing laparoscopic cholecystectomy. Acta Anaesthesiol Scand 2003;47:185–190.

50. Milligan KR, Convery PN, Weir P, et al: The efficacy and safety of epidural infusions of levobupivacaine with and without clonidine for postoperative pain relief in patients undergoing total hip replacement. Anesth Analg 2000;91:393–397.

51. Anzai Y, Nishikawa T: Thoracic epidural clonidine and morphine for postoperative pain relief. Can J Anaesth 1995;42:292–297.

52. Capogna G, Celleno D, Zangrillo A, et al: Addition of clonidine to epidural morphine enhances postoperative analgesia after cesarean delivery. Reg Anesth 1995;20:57–61.

53. Carabine UA, Milligan KR, Mulholland D, Moore J: Extradural clonidine infusions for analgesia after total hip replacement. Br J Anaesth 1992; 68:338–343.

54. Armand S, Langlade A, Boutros A, et al: Meta-analysis of the efficacy of extradural clonidine to relieve postoperative pain: An impossible task. Br J Anaesth 1998;81:126–134.

55. Dobrydnjov I, Axelsson K, Thorn SE, et al: Clonidine combined with small-dose bupivacaine during spinal anesthesia for inguinal herniorrhaphy: A randomized double-blinded study. Anesth Analg 2003;96:1496–1503.

56. Lena P, Balarac N, Arnulf JJ, et al: Intrathecal morphine and clonidine for coronary artery bypass grafting. Br J Anaesth 2003;90:300–303.

57. Paech MJ, Pavy TJ, Orlikowski CE, et al: Postcesarean analgesia with spinal morphine, clonidine, or their combination. Anesth Analg 2004;98:1460–1466.

58. Joshi W, Reuben SS, Kilaru PR, et al: Postoperative analgesia for outpatient arthroscopic knee surgery with intraarticular clonidine and/or morphine. Anesth Analg 2000;90:1102–1106.

59. Reuben SS, Connelly NR: Postoperative analgesia for outpatient arthroscopic knee surgery with intraarticular clonidine. Anesth Analg 1999;88:729–733.

60. Sia S, Lepri A: Clonidine administered as an axillary block does not affect postoperative pain when given as the sole analgesic. Anesth Analg 1999;88:1109–1112.

61. Singelyn FJ, Gouverneur JM, Robert A: A minimum dose of clonidine added to mepivacaine prolongs the duration of anesthesia and analgesia after axillary brachial plexus block. Anesth Analg 1996;83:1046–1050.

62. Tschernko EM, Klepetko H, Gruber E, et al: Clonidine added to the anesthetic solution enhances analgesia and improves oxygenation after intercostal nerve block for thoracotomy. Anesth Analg 1998;87:107–111.

63. Reinhart DJ, Wang W, Stagg KS, et al: Postoperative analgesia after peripheral nerve block for podiatric surgery: Clinical efficacy and chemical stability of lidocaine alone versus lidocaine plus clonidine. Anesth Analg 1996;83:760–765.

64. Reuben SS, Steinberg RB, Klatt JL, Klatt ML: Intravenous regional anesthesia using lidocaine and clonidine. Anesthesiology 1999; 91:654–658.

65. Kleinschmidt S, Stockl W, Wilhelm W, Larsen R: The addition of clonidine to prilocaine for intravenous regional anaesthesia. Eur J Anaesthesiol 1997;14:40–46.

66. Klamt JG, Slullitel A, Garcia IV, Prado WA: Postoperative analgesic effect of intrathecal neostigmine and its influence on spinal anaesthesia. Anaesthesia 1997;52:547–551.

67. Lauretti GR, Mattos AL, Gomes JM, Pereira NL: Postoperative analgesia and antiemetic efficacy after intrathecal neostigmine in patients undergoing abdominal hysterectomy during spinal anesthesia. Reg Anesth 1997;22:527–533.

68. Turan A, Memis D, Basaran UN, et al: Caudal ropivacaine and neostigmine in pediatric surgery. Anesthesiology 2003;98:719–722.

69. Abdulatif M, El Sanabary M: Caudal neostigmine, bupivacaine, and their combination for postoperative pain management after hypospadias surgery in children. Anesth Analg 2002;95:1215–1218.

70. Batra YK, Arya VK, Mahajan R, Chari P: Dose response study of caudal neostigmine for postoperative analgesia in paediatric patients undergoing genitourinary surgery. Paediatr Anaesth 2003;13:515–521.

71. Lauretti GR, Hood DD, Eisenach JC, Pfeifer BL: A multi-center study of intrathecal neostigmine for analgesia following vaginal hysterectomy. Anesthesiology 1998;89:913–918.

72. Almeida RA, Lauretti GR, Mattos AL: Antinociceptive effect of low-dose intrathecal neostigmine combined with intrathecal morphine following gynecologic surgery. Anesthesiology 2003;98:495–498.

73. Chung CJ, Kim JS, Park HS, Chin YJ: The efficacy of intrathecal neostigmine, intrathecal morphine, and their combination for postcesarean section analgesia. Anesth Analg 1998;87:341–346.

74. Kaya FN, Sahin S, Owen MD, Eisenach JC: Epidural neostigmine produces analgesia but also sedation in women after cesarean delivery. Anesthesiology 2004;100:381–385.

75. Omais M, Lauretti GR, Paccola CA: Epidural morphine and neostigmine for postoperative analgesia after orthopedic surgery. Anesth Analg 2002;95:1698–1701.

76. Nakayama M, Ichinose H, Nakabayashi K, et al: Analgesic effect of epidural neostigmine after abdominal hysterectomy. J Clin Anesth 2001;13:86–89.

77. Lauretti GR, de Oliveira R, Reis MP, et al: Study of three different doses of epidural neostigmine coadministered with lidocaine for postoperative analgesia. Anesthesiology 1999;90:1534–1538.

78. Yang LC, Chen LM, Wang CJ, Buerkle H: Postoperative analgesia by intra-articular neostigmine in patients undergoing knee arthroscopy. Anesthesiology 1998;88:334–339.

79. Ilkjaer S, Petersen KL, Brennum J, et al: Effect of systemic NMDA receptor antagonist (ketamine) on primary and secondary hyperalgesia in humans. Br J Anaesth 1996;76:829–834.

80. Willets J, Balster RL, Leander P: The behavioural pharmacology of NMDA receptor antagonists. Trends Pharmacol Sci 1990;11:423–428.

81. Scheller M, Bufler J, Hertle I, et al: Ketamine blocks currents through mammalian nicotinic acetylcholine receptor channels by interaction with both the open and the closed state. Anesth Analg 1996; 83:830–836.

82. Hustveit O, Maurset A, Oye I: Interaction of the chiral forms of ketamine with opioid, phencyclidine, sigma and muscarinic receptors. Pharmacol Toxicol 1995;77:355–359.

83. Smith DJ, Pekoe GM, Martin LL, Coalgate B: The interaction of ketamine with the opiate receptor. Life Sci 1980;26:789–795.

84. Dich-Nielsen JO, Svendsen LB, Berthelsen P: Intramuscular low-dose ketamine versus pethidine for postoperative pain treatment after thoracic surgery. Acta Anaesthesiol Scand 1992;36:583–587.

85. Azevedo VM, Lauretti GR, Pereira NL, Reis MP: Transdermal ketamine as an adjuvant for postoperative analgesia after abdominal gynecological surgery using lidocaine epidural blockade. Anesth Analg 2000; 91:1479–1482.

86. Schmid RL, Sandler AN, Katz J: Use and efficacy of low-dose ketamine in the management of acute postoperative pain: A review of current techniques and outcomes. Pain 1999;82:111–125.

87. De Kock M, Lavand'homme P, Waterloos H: 'Balanced analgesia' in the perioperative period: Is there a place for ketamine? Pain 2001;92:373–380.

88. Argiriadou H, Himmelseher S, Papagiannopoulou P, et al: Improvement of pain treatment after major abdominal surgery by intravenous S+-ketamine. Anesth Analg 2004;98:1413–14˙8.

89. Aida S, Yamakura T, Baba H, et al: Preemptive analgesia by intravenous low-dose ketamine and epidural morphine in gastrectomy: A randomized double-blind study. Anesthesiology 2000;92:1624–1630.

90. Guignard B, Coste C, Costes H, et al: Supplementing desflurane-remifentanil anesthesia with small-dose ketamine reduces perioperative opioid analgesic requirements. Anesth Analg 2002;95:103–108.

91. Kararmaz A, Kaya S, Karaman H, et al: Intraoperative intravenous ketamine in combination with epidural analgesia: Postoperative analgesia after renal surgery. Anesth Analg 2003;97:1092–1096.

92. Menigaux C, Fletcher D, Dupont X, et al: The benefits of intraoperative small-dose ketamine on postoperative pain after anterior cruciate ligament repair. Anesth Analg 2000;90:129–135.

93. Sveticic G, Gentilini A, Eichenberger U, et al: Combinations of morphine with ketamine for patient-controlled analgesia: a new optimization method. Anesthesiology 2003;98:1195–1205.

94. Adriaenssens G, Vermeyen KM, Hoffmann VL, et al: Postoperative analgesia with i.v. patient-controlled morphine: Effect of adding ketamine. Br J Anaesth 1999;83:393–396.

95. Reeves M, Lindholm DE, Myles PS, et al: Adding ketamine to morphine for patient-controlled analgesia after major abdominal surgery: A double-blinded, randomized controlled trial. Anesth Analg 2001;93:116–120.

96. Subramaniam K, Subramaniam B, Pawar DK, Kumar L: Evaluation of the safety and efficacy of epidural ketamine combined with morphine for postoperative analgesia after major upper abdominal surgery. J Clin Anesth 2001;13:339–344.

97. Himmelseher S, Ziegler-Pithamitsis D, Argiriadou H, et al: Small-dose S(+)-ketamine reduces postoperative pain when applied with ropivacaine in epidural anesthesia for total knee arthroplasty. Anesth Analg 2001;92:1290–1295.

98. Wong CS, Lu CC, Cherng CH, Ho ST: Pre-emptive analgesia with ketamine, morphine and epidural lidocaine prior to total knee replacement. Can J Anaesth 1997;44:31–37.

99. Xie H, Wang X, Liu G, Wang G: Analgesic effects and pharmacokinetics of a low dose of ketamine preoperatively administered epidurally or intravenously. Clin J Pain 2003;19:317–322.

100. Taura P, Fuster J, Blasi A, et al: Postoperative pain relief after hepatic resection in cirrhotic patients: The efficacy of a single small dose of ketamine plus morphine epidurally. Anesth Analg 2003;96:475–480.

101. Wu CT, Yeh CC, Yu JC, et al: Pre-incisional epidural ketamine, morphine and bupivacaine combined with epidural and general anaesthesia provides pre-emptive analgesia for upper abdominal surgery. Acta Anaesthesiol Scand 2000;44:63–68.

102. Tan PH, Kuo MC, Kao PF, et al: Patient-controlled epidural analgesia with morphine or morphine plus ketamine for post-operative pain relief. Eur J Anaesthesiol 1999;16:820–825.

103. Chia YY, Liu K, Liu YC, et al: Adding ketamine in a multimodal patient-controlled epidural regimen reduces postoperative pain and analgesic consumption. Anesth Analg 1998;86:1245–1249.

104. Marhofer P, Krenn CG, Plochl W, et al: S(+)-ketamine for caudal block in paediatric anaesthesia. Br J Anaesth 2000;84:341–345.

105. De Negri P, Ivani G, Visconti C, De Vivo P: How to prolong postoperative analgesia after caudal anaesthesia with ropivacaine in children: S-ketamine versus clonidine. Paediatr Anaesth 2001;11:679–683.

106. Lee HM, Sanders GM: Caudal ropivacaine and ketamine for postoperative analgesia in children. Anaesthesia 2000;55:806–810.

107. Malinovsky JM, Lepage JY, Cozian A, et al: Is ketamine or its preservative responsible for neurotoxicity in the rabbit. Anesthesiology 1993;78:109–115.

108. Rosseland LA, Stubhaug A, Sandberg L, Breivik H: Intra-articular (IA) catheter administration of postoperative analgesics: A new trial design allows evaluation of baseline pain, demonstrates large variation in need of analgesics, and finds no analgesic effect of IA ketamine compared with IA saline. Pain 2003;104:25–34.

109. Tigerstedt I, Sipponen J, Tammisto T, Turunen M: Comparison of nefopam and pethidine in postoperative pain. Br J Anaesth 1977;49:1133–1138.

110. McLintock TT, Kenny GN, Howie JC, et al: Assessment of the analgesic efficacy of nefopam hydrochloride after upper abdominal surgery: A study using patient controlled analgesia. Br J Surg 1988;75:779–781.

111. Moffat AC, Kenny GN, Prentice JW: Postoperative nefopam and diclofenac: Evaluation of their morphine-sparing effect after upper abdominal surgery. Anaesthesia 1990;45:302–305.

112. Beloeil H, Delage N, Negre I, et al: The median effective dose of nefopam and morphine administered intravenously for postoperative pain after minor surgery: A prospective randomized double-blinded isobolographic study of their analgesic action. Anesth Analg 2004;98:395–400.

113. Kain ZN, Sevarino F, Pincus S, et al: Attenuation of the preoperative stress response with midazolam: Effects on postoperative outcomes. Anesthesiology 2000;93:141–147.

114. Ong CK, Seymour RA, Tan JM: Sedation with midazolam leads to reduced pain after dental surgery. Anesth Analg 2004;98:1289–1293.

115. Gilliland HE, Prasad BK, Mirakhur RK, Fee JP: An investigation of the potential morphine sparing effect of midazolam. Anaesthesia 1996;51:808–811.

116. Batra YK, Jain K, Chari P, et al: Addition of intrathecal midazolam to bupivacaine produces better post-operative analgesia without prolonging recovery. Int J Clin Pharmacol Ther 1999;37:519–523.

117. Shah FR, Halbe AR, Panchal ID, Goodchild CS: Improvement in post-operative pain relief by the addition of midazolam to an intrathecal injection of buprenorphine and bupivacaine. Eur J Anaesthesiol 2003;20:904–910.

118. Bano F, Haider S, Sultan ST: Comparison of caudal bupivacaine and bupivacaine-midazolam for peri and postoperative analgesia in children. J Coll Physicians Surg Pak 2004;14:65–68.

119. Naguib M, el Gammal M, Elhattab YS, Seraj M: Midazolam for caudal analgesia in children: Comparison with caudal bupivacaine. Can J Anaesth 1995;42:758–764.

120. Nishiyama T: The post-operative analgesic action of midazolam following epidural administration. Eur J Anaesthesiol 1995;12:369–374.

121. Nishiyama T, Matsukawa T, Hanaoka K: Effects of adding midazolam on the postoperative epidural analgesia with two different doses of bupivacaine. J Clin Anesth 2002;14:92–97.

122. Murphy TM: Psychoactive drugs for pain control. Pain Reviews 1994;1:9–14.

123. Koppert W, Weigand M, Neumann F, et al: Perioperative intravenous lidocaine has preventive effects on postoperative pain and morphine consumption after major abdominal surgery. Anesth Analg 2004;98:1050–1055.

124. Collier CB: Dantrolene and suxamethonium: The effect of pre-operative dantrolene on the action of suxamethonium. Anaesthesia 1979;34:152–158.

125. Salassa JR, Seaman SL, Ruff T, et al: Oral dantrolene sodium for tonsillectomy pain: A double-blind study. Otolaryngol Head Neck Surg 1988;98:26–33.

126. Morganti I: [Evaluation of the mechanism determining the painful symptomatology after proctological interventions.] Minerva Med 1988;79:463–466.

127. Fry EN: Postoperative analgesia using papaveretum and orphenadrine: A preliminary trial. Anaesthesia 1979;34:281–283.

128. Winter LJ., Post A: Analgesic combinations with orphenadrine in oral post-surgical pain. J Int Med Res 1979;7:240–246.

129. Malek J, Nedelova I, Lopourova M, et al: [Diclofenac 75mg. and 30 mg. orfenadine (Neodolpasse) versus placebo and piroxicam in postoperative analgesia after arthroscopy.] Acta Chir Orthop Traumatol Cech 2004;71:80–83.

130. Hays H, Woodroffe MA: Using gabapentin to treat neuropathic pain. Can Fam Physician 1999;45:2109–2112.

131. Field MJ, Holloman EF, McCleary S, et al: Evaluation of gabapentin and S-(+)-3-isobutylGABA in a rat model of postoperative pain. J Pharmacol Exp Ther 1997;282:1242–1246.

132. Hill CM, Balkenohl M, Thomas DW, et al: Pregabalin in patients with postoperative dental pain. Eur J Pain 2001;5:119–124.

133. Onghena P, Van Houdenhove B: Antidepressant-induced analgesia in chronic non-malignant pain: A meta-analysis of 39 placebo-controlled studies. Pain 1992;49:205–219.

134. Archid D, Eschalier A, Lavarenne J: Evidence for a central but not peripheral analgesic effect of clomipramine in rats. Pain 1991;45:100.

135. Archid D, Guilbaud G: Antinociceptive effects of acute and chronic injections of tricyclic antidepressant drugs in a new model of mononeuropathy in rats. Pain 1992;49:279–287.

136. Iacono RP, Linford J, Sandyk R: Pain management after lower extremity amputation. Neurosurgery 1987;20:496–500.

137. Laska EM, Sunshine A, Mueller F, et al: Caffeine as an analgesic adjuvant. JAMA 1984;251:1711–1718.
138. Forbes JA, Beaver WT, Jones KF, et al: Effect of caffeine on ibuprofen analgesia in postoperative oral surgery pain. Clin Pharmacol Ther 1991;49:674–684.
139. Forbes JA, Jones KF, Kehm CJ, et al: Evaluation of aspirin, caffeine, and their combination in postoperative oral surgery pain. Pharmacotherapy 1990;10:387–393.
140. Zhang WY, Li Wan PA: Analgesic efficacy of paracetamol and its combination with codeine and caffeine in surgical pain—a meta-analysis. J Clin Pharm Ther 1996;21:261–282.
141. Zhang WY, Po AL: Do codeine and caffeine enhance the analgesic effect of aspirin? A systematic overview. J Clin Pharm Ther 1997;22:79–97.
142. Zhang WY: A benefit-risk assessment of caffeine as an analgesic adjuvant. Drug Saf 2001;24:1127–1142.
143. Watson CP: Topical capsaicin as an adjuvant analgesic [review; 69 refs]. J Pain Symptom Manag 1994;9:425–433.
144. Dubner R: Pain and hyperalgesia following tissue injury: New mechanisms and new treatments. Pain 1991;44:213–214.
145. Jagger SI, Rice ASC: Novel vistas in analgesic pharmacology for the treatment of chronic pain. Anaesth Pharmacol Physiol Rev 1996;4:66–73.
146. Watson CP, Evans RJ: The postmastectomy pain syndrome and topical capsaicin: A randomized trial. Pain 1992;51:375–379.
147. Dini D, Bertelli G, Gozza A, Forno GG: Treatment of the postmastectomy pain syndrome with topical capsaicin. Pain 1993;54:223–226.
148. Ellison N, Loprinzi CL, Kugler J, et al: Phase III placebo-controlled trial of capsaicin cream in the management of surgical neuropathic pain in cancer patients. J Clin Oncol 1997;15:2974–2980.
149. Sunshine A, Zighelboim I, De Castro A, et al: Augmentation of acetaminophen analgesia by the antihistamine phenyltoloxamine. J Clin Pharmacol 1989;29:660–664.
150. Terrence CF, Potter DM, Fromm GH: Is baclofen an analgesic? Clin Neuropharmacol 1983;6:241–245.
151. Hirst RA, Lambert DG, Notcutt WG: Pharmacology and the potential therapeutic uses of cannabis. Br J Anaesth 1998;81:77–84.
152. Buggy DJ, Toogood L, Maric S, et al: Lack of analgesic efficacy of oral delta-9-tetrahydrocannabinol in postoperative pain. Pain 2003;106:169–172.
153. Forrest WH Jr, Brown BW Jr, Brown CR, et al: Dextroamphetamine with morphine for the treatment of postoperative pain. N Engl J Med 1977;296:712–715.
154. Sung YF, Wetchler BV, Duncalf D, Joslyn AF: A double-blind, placebo-controlled pilot study examining the effectiveness of intravenous ondansetron in the prevention of postoperative nausea and emesis. J Clin Anesth 1993;5:22–29.
155. Doenicke A, Mayer M, Vogginger T: [Postoperative pain therapy: The efficacy of a serotonin antagonist (GR 38032F;ondansetron) and the prostaglandin synthesis inhibitor lysin acetylsalicylate (Aspisol).] Anaesthesist 1993;42:800–806.
156. Broome IJ, Robb HM, Raj N, et al: The use of tramadol following day—case oral surgery. Anaesthesia 1999;54:289–292.
157. De Witte JL, Schoenmaekers B, Sessler DI, Deloof T: The analgesic efficacy of tramadol is impaired by concurrent administration of ondansetron. Anesth Analg 2001;92:1319–1321.
158. Arcioni R, della RM, Romano S, et al: Ondansetron inhibits the analgesic effects of tramadol: A possible 5-HT(3) spinal receptor involvement in acute pain in humans. Anesth Analg 2002;94:1553–1557.
159. Alayurt S, Memis D, Pamukcu Z: The addition of sufentanil, tramadol or clonidine to lignocaine for intravenous regional anaesthesia. Anaesth Intensive Care 2004;32:22–27.
160. Buerkle H, Huge V, Wolfgart M, et al: Intra-articular clonidine analgesia after knee arthroscopy. Eur J Anaesthesiol 2000;17:295–299.
161. Casati A, Magistris L, Beccaria P, et al: Improving postoperative analgesia after axillary brachial plexus anesthesia with 0.75% ropivacaine: A double-blind evaluation of adding clonidine. Minerva Anestesiol 2001;67:407–412.
162. Casati A, Magistris L, Fanelli G, et al: Small-dose clonidine prolongs postoperative analgesia after sciatic-femoral nerve block with 0.75% ropivacaine for foot surgery. Anesth Analg 2000;91:388–392.
163. Gentili M, Houssel P, Osman M, et al: Intra-articular morphine and clonidine produce comparable analgesia but the combination is not more effective. Br J Anaesth 1997;79:660–661.
164. Gentili M, Juhel A, Bonnet F: Peripheral analgesic effect of intra-articular clonidine. Pain 1996;64:593–596.
165. Gentili M, Enel D, Szymskiewicz O, et al: Postoperative analgesia by intraarticular clonidine and neostigmine in patients undergoing knee arthroscopy. Reg Anesth Pain Med 2001;26:342–347.
166. Sung CS, Lin SH, Chan KH, et al: Effect of oral clonidine premedication on perioperative hemodynamic response and postoperative analgesic requirement for patients undergoing laparoscopic cholecystectomy. Acta Anaesthesiol Sin 2000;38:23–29.
167. Hagelin A, Lundberg D: Ketamine for postoperative analgesia after upper abdominal surgery. Clin Ther 1981;4:229–233.
168. Phillips G, Vickers MD: Nefopam in postoperative pain. Br J Anaesth 1979;51:961–965.

21

Postoperative Pain Management in Infants and Children

YUAN-CHI LIN

Pain sensation is a universal protective mechanism that is essential for survival. Pain causes suffering and physiological abnormalities in infants and children that are similar to those that occur in adults. Pain and stress can induce significant physiological and behavioral reactions even in infants. Numerous myths, inadequate knowledge among caregivers, and insufficient application of knowledge contribute to ineffective pain management.

Postoperative pain is one of the most common adverse stimuli, occurring as a result of surgery, underlying diseases, and medical diagnostic procedures. It is associated with anxiety and distress among pediatric patients, family, and care providers. Infants and children frequently receive inadequate treatment for pain.[1,2] A thorough understanding of the physiological, developmental, and situational factors relevant to pain is necessary to provide optimal care of children in the perioperative period—including adequate psychological preparation of both the children and their relatives. Children and their families should also receive detailed descriptions of their options for postoperative analgesia. The striving for more humane patient treatment and economic concerns have been the driving forces behind improvements in pediatric pain management. Over the past few years, the quality of pain management for children undergoing surgery has changed remarkably.[3]

A 2002 Swedish nationwide survey evaluated the prevalence of acute postoperative pain in children. The majority of the surgical procedures were performed as outpatient operations. Despite treatment, moderate to severe pain occurred in 23% of patients with postoperative pain and 31% of patients with pain of other origin. Postoperative pain seemed to be a greater problem in the surgical units where children were treated along with adults and in departments where fewer children were treated. Unsatisfactory pain treatment frequently seemed to be related to inadequate dosing. Anxiety in children or parents also contributed to ineffective pain treatment.[4]

Pain is the most common complication after outpatient surgery. When a child returns home after outpatient surgery, the parent becomes responsible for the assessment and treatment of that pain. In a study of 189 parents of children 2 to 12 years old who had undergone outpatient surgery, each parent completed a 3-day diary of the child's pain and the methods used to alleviate it. There were clear differences in pain reported according to the type of surgery performed. About half of children undergoing tonsillectomy, circumcision, or strabismus repair experienced clinically significant pain. Sixty-eight percent of the parents of these children reported that they had been instructed to use acetaminophen for pain "if necessary," 13% had been told to use acetaminophen regularly, and 8% recalled no instructions. Some types of "minor" surgery cause significant postoperative pain. Even when parents recognize that their children are in pain, most give inadequate doses of medication to control the pain.[5]

In a study of 100 parents of children who underwent outpatient surgery, the parents were contacted by telephone in their own homes 24 hours postoperatively. The parents were able to manage their child's pain in the home if they had been provided with information and suitable analgesia upon discharge.[6]

New discoveries help us to understand the mechanisms of pain and develop better tools for the treatment of postoperative pain in infants and children. Effective and safe postoperative pain management requires the selection of proper analgesic techniques and medications, administered in appropriate doses to selected patients, and in a suitable environment.[7] Substantial creativity and initiative is required when practicing pediatric pain management. Randomized controlled trials (RCTs) in the treatment of pediatric pain are lacking. Recommendations for pediatric pain therapy are commonly not based on the best evidence. Using a critical analysis of the peer-reviewed literature, this chapter presents an evidence-based approach to pediatric pain management.

Developmental Pain

Afferent nociceptive sensory input is present at birth. The sensory responses to painful procedures in the immature nervous system in neonates can cause distress. The immaturity of sensory processing within the newborn spinal cord leads to lower thresholds for excitation and sensitization, potentially maximizing the central effects of these tissue-damaging inputs. The plasticity of both peripheral and central sensory connections in the neonatal period means that early damage in infancy can lead to prolonged structural and functional alterations in pain pathways that can last into adult life.[8] The cutaneous flexor reflexes in newborns are exaggerated compared with those in adults.[9] The thresholds for the reflexes are lower, and reflex muscle contractions are more synchronized and long-lasting in newborns. Repeated skin stimulation results in considerable hyperexcitability or central sensitization. The flexor reflex thresholds are particularly low in preterm infants but increase with postconceptional age.[10] At birth, the skin is innervated by both large myelinated A fibers and small unmyelinated C fibers.[11] During development, 70% to 80% of small C fiber nociceptors express nerve growth factor.[12]

The pain system undergoes major reorganization during the perinatal period. The organization and function of the immature pain system may be influenced by exposure to light or rigorous painful stimulation in the neonatal period. The basic excitatory processes develop early, whereas the development of the inhibitory processes is delayed. The behavioral responses of newborns exposed to painful stimuli are not always predictable. Absence of adequate inhibitory mechanisms may lead to exaggerated and generalized responses to all sensory inputs. Neonates undergo considerable maturation of peripheral, spinal, and supraspinal afferent pain transmission over the early postnatal period but are able to respond to tissue injury with specific behavior and with autonomic, hormonal, and metabolic signs of stress and distress. The changing morphine sensitivity in the postnatal period may be part of a general reorganization in the structure and function of primary afferent synapses, neurotransmitter/receptor expression and function, and excitatory and inhibitory modulation from higher brain centers.[13] An understanding of the developmental aspects of the neurotransmission highlights the importance of a specialized approach to the pharmacological treatment of neonatal pain.[14]

Pain Measurement

Pain assessment is difficult in infants and children, but regular assessment of the existence and severity of pain and the child's response to treatment[15] are essential for pediatric pain management. Pain can be assessed by psychological methods, physiological measures, or behavioral observation, depending on the age of the child and his or her ability to communicate. Acceptable postoperative pain assessment requires consideration of the complexity of children's pain perception and psychological as well as developmental factors. Age-appropriate pain assessment is essential for managing pediatric patients with pain. Both subjective and objective assessment tools may be used, depending on the patient's age and clinical status.

Because pain is a subjective experience, individual self-report is often preferred. Children between the ages of 3 and 7 years are competent to provide information regarding the location, quality, intensity, and tolerability of pain.

Observation of behavior should be used to complement self-report and can be an acceptable alternative when valid self-report is not available. The pain assessment tools should be introduced before the operation or before the pain occurs. Each institution must adapt a uniform tool for pain assessment in pediatric patients.

The six-face Faces Pain Scale–Revised is useful in the assessment of acute pain intensity in children 4 years and older. It has the advantage of being suitable for use with the most widely applied metric scoring system (0–10) and conforms closely to a linear interval scale.[16] In a study of 276 children, Baxt et al[17] demonstrated the feasibility of assessing pain after pediatric injury with the use of two validated scales, the Bieri Faces Pain Scale and the Color Analogue Scale. They also established the worth of parental reports of pain when the child is not able to provide a self-report.[17]

Pain assessment at home is an especially difficult task for parents postoperatively. The findings of Chambers et al[18] supported the reliability and validity of the 15-item Parents' Postoperative Pain Measure (PPPM) as a measurement of postoperative pain among children ages 2 to 12 years. Koh et al[19] compared 152 children with cognitive impairment and 138 nonimpaired children. They showed that children with cognitive impairment who underwent surgery received less opioid in the perioperative period than children without cognitive impairment. The Face, Legs, Activity, Cry, Consolability (FLACC) pain assessment tool may facilitate reliable and valid observational pain assessment in children with cognitive impairment.[20]

Pain Therapies

ACETAMINOPHEN AND NONSTEROIDAL ANTI-INFLAMMATORY DRUGS

Acetaminophen and the nonsteroidal anti-inflammatory drug (NSAID) ibuprofen are the most widely available over-the-counter drugs on the market for relief of pain. They are commonly used for mild to moderate postoperative pain. Single doses of ibuprofen (4–10 mg/kg) and acetaminophen (7–15 mg/kg) have similar efficacy for relieving moderate to severe pain and similar safety as analgesics or antipyretics. Ibuprofen (5–10 mg/kg) has been shown to be a more effective antipyretic than acetaminophen (10–15 mg/kg) at 2, 4, and 6 hours after treatment.[21] The adverse effects of ibuprofen include gastritis, potential gastrointestinal bleeding, and platelet and renal function impairment. The mechanism of action of NSAIDs is inhibition of prostaglandin synthesis by inhibition of cyclooxygenase (Cox). Aspirin is not recommended for pediatric patients because of its association with Reye's syndrome. Cox-2 selective inhibitors, such as celecoxib, can also be administered to children.

Ketorolac, a parenteral NSAID, is frequently administered as an adjuvant for acute pediatric pain management.[22] Intravenous ketorolac (0.3–0.5 mg/kg) is recommended for children. Parenteral ketorolac (0.5 mg/kg every 4 to 6 hours for 5 days or less) is generally well tolerated and has opioid-sparing effects in children.[23] The maintenance dose requirements of ketorolac are similar in children, adolescents, and adults.[24]

SYSTEMIC OPIOID ANALGESIA

Opioids are commonly administered for pediatric postoperative pain treatment. Except for the neonatal period, the pharmacokinetics and pharmacodynamics of opioid analgesics in infants and children are not markedly different from those in adults, and the associated risks are not higher. Morphine is the standard opioid analgesic, and its pharmacology is well studied in pediatric patients. The volume of distribution appears to be smaller in neonates than in adults, but adult values are reached in slightly older children. For all the opioids studied, elimination is slower in neonates than in adults. The rate of elimination generally reaches and even exceeds adult values within the first year of life. The high rate of drug metabolism leads to greater dose requirements. Infants and children do not appear to be more sensitive to the effects of opioids than adults.[25]

Patient-controlled analgesia (PCA) can be safely used in children older than 6 years. Morphine, hydromorphone, and fentanyl are equally effective (Table 21–1). Nurse-controlled analgesia can allow greater flexibility and is commonly employed for children too young to use PCA. The PCA bolus plus basal rate continuous-infusion mode can improve night-time sleep for children. Loading doses may be needed in some patients to establish analgesia. The lockout interval (time during which no drug is administered when PCA device is activated) can be as short as 5 minutes.

For patients in whom PCA is not appropriate, bolus and continuous infusion can be used. Morphine infusion (10–30 μg/kg/hr) results in serum concentration of 10 to 22 ng/mL and adequate analgesia.[26]

If patients can tolerate oral medication, it is the preferred route of administration. Adjustments to account for oral bioavailability of drugs are required. Medication should be titrated to appropriate analgesic effect. Oral opioid preparations (codeine, oxycodone, morphine) and combinations of opioid plus NSAID are widely and effectively administered for acute postoperative pain management in children. Tramadol hydrochloride is an analgesic with μ receptor activity; in children ages 4 to 7 years, oral tramadol 1.5 mg/kg is an effective analgesic for 7 hours.[27]

REGIONAL ANESTHESIA

Regional techniques compare favorably with systemic analgesic techniques in infants and children.[28] Regional infusion techniques are most successful in the context of perioperative pain management. The overall morbidity of regional anesthesia in children is low. Sound selection of local anesthetics, insertion routes, and block procedures together with appropriate and careful monitoring should prevent any major undesirable effects and enable regional anesthesia to be a well-tolerated and effective tool for overcoming pain in children.[29]

Caudal Epidural Block

Caudal epidural block is one of the most common regional anesthetic techniques for pediatric ambulatory surgical procedures performed below the umbilicus. It is used for procedures involving the lower thorax, hip, pelvis, urogenital/perianal regions, and lower extremity. It also provides effective analgesia after bone marrow harvest.

Caudal blocks are easy to perform. A single injection achieves long-lasting postoperative analgesia in pediatric ambulatory patients. Alternatively, an epidural catheter can be placed through a standard intravenous (IV) cannula (e.g., Angiocath) to deliver prolonged postoperative analgesia. Conroy et al[30] compared the effectiveness of caudal epidural block with surgical wound infiltration in providing postoperative analgesia after inguinal herniorrhaphy in 35 children. Patients who had received caudal epidural block had shorter emergence times from anesthesia, less pain-related behavior, and lower opiate requirements postoperatively. General contraindications to caudal epidural block include uncorrected coagulopathy and localized infection at the injection site. Specific contraindications are spinal deformities such as myelomeningocele and abnormalities in sacral anatomy.

In general, caudal epidural block is safe. Rare complications include subcutaneous injection, dural puncture, subarachnoid injection, intravascular injection, intraosseous injection, hematoma, infection, and urinary retention. Broadman[31] reported that in 1154 consecutive uses of the block for pediatric operations, no serious complication occurred. One dural puncture occurred and was detected by aspiration prior to injection of local anesthetics. Fisher et al[32] demonstrated that the time to postoperative micturition in 82 children undergoing herniorrhaphy and orchiopexy was independent of whether caudal epidural block or ilioinguinal nerve block was used. Caudal anesthesia seems to be an inexpensive, simple, and effective technique not only as a supplement to postoperative analgesia but also as the sole method of anesthesia.[33]

Lumbar Epidural Block

Lumbar epidural block is used for surgical procedures in the hip, pelvis, and lower extremity. For patients with previous surgery involving the rectal and sacral areas or with anatomical abnormalities in the sacral area, lumbar epidural block is a practical alterative to caudal epidural block. Epidural anesthesia reduces the requirement for general anesthesia

TABLE 21–1	Agents Useful for Patient-Controlled Analgesia (PCA) in Children		
Agent	**Loading Dose**	**Basal Rate**	**PCA Demand**
Morphine (1 or 5 mg/mL)	0.03 mg/kg	0.01 mg/kg/hr	0.02–0.03 mg/kg
Hydromorphone (100 μg/mL)	5 μg/kg	1 μg/kg/hr	2 μg/kg
Fentanyl (50 μg/mL)	0.3 μg/kg	0.1 μg/kg/hr	0.2–0.3 μg/kg/hr

and alleviates postoperative pain.[34] Most pediatric patients require sedation or general anesthesia before the block. The depth of the epidural space can be predicted from a modification of the Dohi formula, as follows:

$$\text{Depth (mm)} = 18 + (1.5 \times \text{Age [yr]})$$

Before the injection of local anesthetics, results of aspiration for blood and cerebrospinal fluid (CSF) must be negative. Epidural anesthesia is accomplished through single injection or continuous infusion of local anesthetics via an epidural catheter. Complications include accidental dural puncture, direct trauma to the spinal cord, embolism from air introduced during epidural needle placement, and seizures in patients receiving continuous bupivacaine infusion.

Epidural analgesics are effective in alleviating intense localized pain, somatic pain, and visceral pain. They provide greater pain relief at lower doses and with less sedation than parenteral narcotics. Epidural techniques in children are associated with cardiovascular safety and analgesic efficacy,[35] reduction of the stress response to abdominal surgery in infants,[36] and improved outcome after patent ductus arteriosus ligation.[37] Continuous epidural infusions are currently recommended and used with epidural analgesia for infants,[38] children, and adolescents.[39,40] Patient-controlled epidural analgesia (PCEA) can also be used in some patients.[41] This technique avoids periodic pain and is more manageable for the anesthesia and nursing staffs.

The most common insertion sites for epidural analgesia are (1) caudal route for patients younger than 12 months, (2) lumbar approach for patients older than 12 months, and (3) thoracic route for patients with specific indications, such as thoracic or upper abdominal procedures. In addition, single-shot caudal blockade is very useful for minor procedures.

It is best to avoid using an air-filled syringe for detection of loss of resistance to locate the epidural space. This technique causes air embolism in some pediatric patients. Epidural catheter placement using electrical stimulation guidance is an alternative approach for positioning the catheter into the thoracic region via the caudal space. This easily performed clinical assessment provides optimization of catheter tip positioning to achieve effective pain control.[42]

For small infants, an epidural solution of 0.1% bupivacaine with 3 μg/mL hydromorphone can be administered at 0.2 to 0.4 mL/kg/hr. In neonates, the recommended rate for continuous epidural infusion of bupivacaine is 0.2 to 0.3 mg/kg/hr.[43–45] Continuous thoracic epidural infusion for postoperative analgesia is effective after pectus deformity repair, decreases the requirement for intravenous opioid, and, in one study, was associated with no catheter-related complications.[46] Continuous regional techniques, including epidural infusions, are effective in pediatric patients. Because of their potential complications, these blocks should be performed, monitored, and cared for by staff experienced with and trained in them.[47]

PERIPHERAL NERVE BLOCK

Axillary Brachial Plexus Block

The axillary brachial plexus block, indicated for procedures on the forearm and the hand, can be performed safely in children. The technique is similar to that for adults, except that children are usually sedated or anesthetized, making the use of a nerve stimulator advantageous. The axillary artery serves as the landmark for the axillary sheath, which contains the axillary artery and vein, the median nerve, the radial nerve, and the ulnar nerve. A 23- or 25-gauge needle is inserted and directed toward the axillary arterial pulsation. The needle is advanced slowly until nerve stimulation elicits distal muscle twitching at a current less than 0.5 mA. A needle that is directed proximally parallel to the axillary sheath achieves a higher level of analgesia than one that is directed perpendicular to the axillary sheath. After result of aspiration for blood and CSF are negative, the entire volume of local anesthetic is injected. Alternatively, a double-injection technique may be used, with half the dose injected cephalic to the artery at the median nerve, and half injected caudal to the artery at the ulnar nerve.

Commonly used local anesthetics are lidocaine, mepivacaine, and bupivacaine, all of which are given as 0.5 to 0.75 mL/kg of local anesthetic solution. Alternatively, a mixture of 1% lidocaine (for rapid onset) plus 0.1% tetracaine (for long duration) in a volume of 0.5 mL/kg may be used. This mixture is made by dissolving 20 mg of tetracaine crystals in 20 mL of 1% lidocaine. Ivani and Tonnetti[48] reported administering a bolus dose of 0.5 to 1 mL/kg of ropivacaine 0.2% or levobupivacaine 0.25% with clonidine 2 μg/kg followed by a continuous infusion of 0.1 to 0.3 mL/kg/hr of 0.2% ropivacaine or 0.25% levobupivacaine with clonidine 3 μg/kg/24hr for 48 to 72 hours. Complications of axillary brachial plexus block include intravascular injection, direct injury to the nerve or artery, hematoma, and infection.[49]

Interscalene Block

The interscalene block is indicated for procedures on the clavicle, shoulder, and upper arm. The patient is placed in the supine position. Having the patient voluntarily lift the head off the operating table accentuates the interscalene groove, which is marked prior to induction of general anesthesia. Because patient cooperation is necessary, this block may not be feasible in younger patients. At the level of the cricoid cartilage, a 22- to 25-gauge needle is inserted into the interscalene groove and directed medially, caudally, and posteriorly toward the C6 transverse process. Nerve stimulation can assist in confirming correct needle placement. A mixture of 1% lidocaine 0.5 mL/kg and 0.1% tetracaine or 0.5 mL/kg of 0.25% to 0.5% bupivacaine can be used for the interscalene block. A continuous catheter technique can also be used.[50]

Complications of interscalene block include intravascular injection, hematoma, and infection. Phrenic nerve block with unilateral diaphragmatic paralysis, subarachnoid injection with total spinal anesthesia, and basilar artery injection has also been reported.

Femoral Nerve Block and 3-in-1 Block (Inguinal Paravascular Technique)

The femoral nerve block and the 3-in-1 block (inguinal paravascular technique) are indicated for femoral osteotomy, quadriceps and vastus lateralis muscle biopsy, and harvesting of donor skin from the anterior thigh. Both blocks relieve muscle spasm in femoral shaft fractures.

The femoral artery lies medial to the femoral nerve and serves as the anatomical landmark. For the femoral nerve block, a short-beveled needle is inserted perpendicular to the skin at the level of the inguinal ligament and lateral to the femoral artery pulsation. Paresthesia is not necessary. A nerve stimulator aids in localizing the nerve.[51] After results of aspiration for blood and CSF are negative, local anesthetics are injected in a fanlike manner lateral and deep to the femoral artery to anesthetize the lateral femoral cutaneous nerve. The 3-in-1 block is performed much like the femoral nerve block. The needle is inserted while pointed rostrally at a 30-degree angle from the anterior thigh. Local anesthetics are injected with compression of the femoral canal distal to the needle.

For femoral nerve block, 0.2 to 0.3 mL/kg of 0.25 to 0.5% bupivacaine is recommended. For the 3-in-1 block, 0.5 to 0.7 mL/kg of 0.25% to 0.5% bupivacaine is recommended (maximum dose: 2.5 mg/kg). The duration of analgesia for both blocks is 3 to 6 hours. Complications include sympathetic nerve block, injury to adjacent blood vessels, and hematoma. Sympathetic nerve block is transient and improves peripheral circulation to the lower extremity.[52–54]

Lateral Femoral Cutaneous Nerve Block

The lateral femoral cutaneous nerve block is indicated for muscle biopsy at the thigh, skin graft harvesting, and lateral thigh incision.[55,56] The lateral femoral cutaneous nerve has no motor component, and the block does not interfere with lower extremity motor function. The lateral femoral cutaneous nerve (L2–L3) passes under the fascia iliaca and enters the thigh deep to the inguinal ligament and medial to the anterior superior iliac spine. At the level of the inguinal ligament, a 22-gauge, short-beveled needle is inserted—at a distance equal to one or two of the patient's fingerbreadths—medial to the anterior superior iliac spine. Resistance is felt as the needle penetrates, in turn, the external oblique aponeurosis, the internal oblique muscle, and the fascia iliaca.

Fascia Iliaca Compartment Block

Fascia iliaca compartment block is used for femoral osteotomies, femur fracture repair, hip surgery, knee arthroscopy, and muscle biopsy. The patient is placed in the supine position. Landmarks consist of the anterior superior iliac spine, the pubic tubercle, and the inguinal ligament. At 0.5 cm caudal to the junction of the lateral third and the medial two thirds of the inguinal ligament, the needle is inserted perpendicular to the skin. Distinctive losses of resistance occur when the needle punctures the fascia lata and the fascia iliaca. Then, local anesthetics are injected with firm pressure applied caudal to the needle. This technique favors cephalad spread of local anesthetics in the fascia iliaca compartment. Dalens et al[57] compared 60 children who received fascia iliaca compartment block with 60 children who received 3-in-1 block. Ninety percent of patients who received fascia iliaca compartment block had adequate analgesia, compared with 20% of patients who received 3-in-1 block.[57] One effective local anesthetic combination is

a 50:50 mixture of 1% lidocaine and 0.5% bupivacaine with 1:200,000 epinephrine. The volume is based on patient weight: 0.7 mL/kg for weight less than 20 kg, 15 mL for 20 to 30 kg, 20 mL for 30 to 40 kg, 25 mL for 40 to 50 kg, and 27.5 mL for weight more than 50 kg. The fascia iliaca compartment block lasts 12 to 15 hours.

Popliteal Fossa Nerve Block

The popliteal fossa nerve block anesthetizes the sciatic nerve and its two branches, the tibial and peroneal nerves. The block is indicated for procedures below the knee, such as hallux valgus surgery, tendon surgery, synovectomy of the metatarsal joint, toe amputation, foreign body removal, and tumor excision. The popliteal fossa is a diamond-shaped area bound superiorly by the biceps femoris muscle, the semitendinosus muscle, and the semimembranosus muscle and inferiorly by the medial and lateral heads of the gastrocnemius muscle. The sciatic nerve bifurcates at the apex of the popliteal fossa into the tibial nerve, which runs medially, and the common peroneal nerve, which runs laterally. A nerve stimulator assists in accurate localization.[58] The patient is placed in the prone or lateral position with the knee slightly flexed, allowing the upper borders of the popliteal fossa to become more palpable. When the patient is in the prone position, the needle is introduced at the apex of the popliteal fossa, and the sciatic nerve is blocked, resulting in complete anesthesia of the foreleg and the foot, except for the skin around the medial malleolus. Individual blocks of the tibial nerve and the common peroneal nerve are easily performed. When the fascia covering the popliteal fossa is penetrated, loss of resistance is felt. Subsequently, the needle is advanced an additional 5 mm. This technique is a safe and reliable alternative to the more common forms of anesthesia for surgery below the knee.[58,59]

Penile Nerve Block

The penis receives innervation from the dorsal penile nerves, the genitofemoral nerve, and the iliohypogastric nerve. The distal two thirds of the penis is innervated by the paired dorsal penile nerves, which emerge caudal to the symphysis pubis and run down the penile shaft beneath Buck's fascia at 1 o'clock and 11 o'clock. Penile nerve block is indicated for patients undergoing circumcision or distal hypospadias repair. A comparison of penile block with caudal block for circumcision showed that penile block is equally effective without the associated motor blockade produced by caudal block.[60,61]

Three approaches to penile nerve block have been described. In the first, a 22-gauge, short-beveled needle is inserted perpendicular to the midline at the inferior edge of the symphysis pubis and advanced until loss of resistance indicates penetration of Buck's fascia. After results of aspiration for blood and CSF are negative, local anesthetics are injected. In the second approach, sites at 1 o'clock and 11 o'clock deep to Buck's fascia are injected with local anesthetics. The third approach consists of subcutaneous infiltration ring block at the penile base. The most successful technique combines injection of the dorsal penile nerves at 1 o'clock and 11 o'clock with subcutaneous infiltration at the penile base dorsally from 3 o'clock to 9 o'clock.[62] Epinephrine-containing solution is never used. Complications of penile nerve block include intravascular injection, hematoma, infection, and ischemia.

Ilioinguinal and Iliohypogastric Nerve Blocks

Ilioinguinal and iliohypogastric nerve blocks are commonly performed for inguinal hernia repair and orchiopexy. The blocks provide effective operative and postoperative analgesia. Cross and Barrett[63] compared the use of iliohypogastric and ilioinguinal nerve blocks using 0.25% bupivacaine and 1:200,000 epinephrine with caudal anesthesia using 0.25% bupivacaine in children undergoing herniorrhaphy and orchiopexy. The two techniques did not differ in duration and quality of analgesia, incidence of vomiting, or time to first micturition. The principal anatomic landmark is the anterior superior iliac spine. At a distance equal to one patient's fingerbreadth medial to the anterior superior iliac spine, a 22- to 25-gauge, short-beveled needle is inserted perpendicular to the skin. A subtle loss of resistance occurs as the needle penetrates the external oblique aponeurosis and the internal oblique muscle fascia. After results of aspiration for blood and CSF are negative, local anesthetics are injected. With a single-injection technique, ilioinguinal and iliohypogastric nerve block provides adequate analgesia for children undergoing hernia repair.[64]

Treatment of Side Effects and Postoperative Monitoring

Preprinted orders for PCA, continuous infusion narcotics, epidural analgesia, and PCEA that include the treatment of side effects as well as standard monitoring are helpful for managing acute postoperative pain in children.[65] The use of pulse oximetry is recommended for the first 24 hours after an infusion is begun or the rate is increased. Nausea and vomiting can be treated with metoclopramide, 0.1 to 0.2 mg/kg/dose (maximum 10 mg) IV given every 6 hours as needed (PRN), or ondansetron, 0.1 mg/kg/dose (maximum 2 mg) IV given every 4 to 8 hours PRN. Pruritus can be treated with nalbuphine, 0.01 to 0.02 mg/kg/dose (maximum 1.5 mg) IV given every 6 hours PRN, or diphenhydramine, 0.25 to 0.5 mg/kg/dose (maximum 25 mg) IV given every 6 hours PRN. Respiratory depression should be treated immediately; the dosage for naloxone is 1 µg/kg (maximum 80 µg) IV PRN.

Epidural infection is rare in pediatric patients who undergo short-term postoperative catheterization.[66] Kost-Byery et al[67] studied bacterial colonization and infection rates of continuous epidural catheters in children. They reported that in patients treated with caudal epidural catheters, children ages 3 years and older were less likely to have colonized epidural catheters than younger children. Age did not affect the probability of development of cellulitis at the insertion site. Despite bacterial colonization of caudal and lumbar epidural catheters, these investigators observed that serious systemic and local infection after short-term epidural analgesia did not occur.[67] Seth et al[68] studied postoperative epidural analgesia in 100 consecutive children ages 1 day to 15 years. They showed that minor local signs of inflammation and infection are common in pediatric patients during continuous epidural infusion. Epidural catheter tips are also frequently culture positive in patients both with and without local signs who may not go on to have further signs or symptoms of infection.[68]

Other Pain Treatment Approaches

Intraoperative regional blockade or local infiltration for postoperative analgesia in children should be considered whenever possible.[69] Nonpharmacological treatments are also helpful adjuvants; for example, hypnosis, relaxation, biofeedback, transcutaneous electrical nerve stimulation (TENS), art therapy, and acupuncture may offer pain relief for children and adolescents.[70,71] Both children and adolescents benefit from coordinated efforts to manage their acute pain. Anesthesiologists who manage perioperative pain in pediatric patients should be familiar with the special characteristics of this population and should use the appropriate pharmacological and nonpharmacological strategies.

Postoperative Pediatric Pain Management Service

The majority of patients managed by an acute pain service are inpatients who have undergone surgery. Ideally, an institution's pediatric pain management service integrates physicians from the department of pediatric anesthesia with dedicated staff from the departments of nursing, pediatric psychiatry, and pediatric physical therapy. Collaboration will be established with the departments of pediatrics, pediatric general surgery, pediatric urology, pediatric orthopedic surgery, pediatric plastic surgery, pediatric cardiac surgery, pediatric neurosurgery, pediatric otolaryngology, and complementary medical services[72] for optimization of care. The American Society of Anesthesiologists has published practice guidelines for acute pain management in the perioperative setting.[73] Standard protocols for acute pediatric pain management have been established for the purposes of patient care, as well as ongoing education and training to ensure that hospital personnel are knowledgeable and skilled with regard to the effective and safe use of the available treatment options in the hospital. Optimal pain management for pediatric patients requires reliable assessment tools and aggressive management of the pain and side effects with consideration of the emotional as well as social factors contributing to the pain.[74]

Although methods for the safe and effective management of pain in children are now known, this knowledge has not been widely used in routine clinical practice. Pain in early life may have long-term behavioral consequences. The timing, the extent of injury, and the administration and nature of analgesics may be important determinants of the long-term outcome in children and infants who experience pain perioperatively. The assessment and management of this pain and understanding its functional consequences present considerable and important challenges to those who care for children who need surgery.[75]

REFERENCES

1. Anand K, Hickey P: Pain and its effects on the human neonates and fetus. N Engl J Med 1987;317:1321–1329.
2. Anand KJ, Hickey P: Halothane-morphine compared with high dose sufentanil for anesthesia and postoperative analgesia in neonatal cardiac surgery. N Engl J Med 1992;326:1–9.
3. Lloyd-Thomas AR: Modern concepts of paediatric analgesia. Pharmacol Ther 1999;83:1–20.
4. Karling M, Renstrom M, Ljungman G: Acute and postoperative pain in children: A Swedish nationwide survey. Acta Paediatr 2002;91:660–666.
5. Finley GA, McGrath PJ, Forward SP, et al: Parents' management of children's pain following 'minor' surgery. Pain 1996;64:83–87.
6. Jonas DA: Parent's management of their child's pain in the home following day surgery. J Child Health Care 2003;7:150–162.
7. Berde CB, Sethna NF: Analgesics for the treatment of pain in children. N Engl J Med 2002;347:1094–1103.
8. Fitzgerald M, Beggs S: The neurobiology of pain: developmental aspects. Neuroscientist 2001;7:246–257.
9. Andrews K, Fitzgerald M: Cutaneous flexion reflex in human neonates: A quantitative study of threshold and stimulus-response characteristics after single and repeated stimuli. Dev Med Child Neurol 1999;41:696–703.
10. Fitzgerald M: A physiological study of the prenatal development of cutaneous sensory inputs to dorsal horn cells in the rat. J Physiol 1991;432:473–482.
11. Jackman A, Fitzgerald M: Development of peripheral hindlimb and central spinal cord innervation by subpopulations of dorsal root ganglion cells in the embryonic rat. J Comp Neurol 2000;418:281–298.
12. Ruit KG, Elliott JL, Osborne PA, et al: Selective dependence of mammalian dorsal root ganglion neurons on nerve growth factor during embryonic development. Neuron 1992;8:573–587.
13. Nandi R, Fitzgerald M: Opioid analgesia in the newborn. Eur J Pain 2005;9:105–108.
14. Pattinson D, Fitzgerald M: The neurobiology of infant pain: Development of excitatory and inhibitory neurotransmission in the spinal dorsal horn. Reg Anesth Pain Med 2004;29:36–44.
15. Bulloch B, Tenenbein M: Assessment of clinically significant changes in acute pain in children. Acad Emerg Med 2002;9:199–202.
16. Hicks CL, von Baeyer CL, Spafford PA, et al: The Faces Pain Scale–Revised: Toward a common metric in pediatric pain measurement. Pain 2001;93:173–183.
17. Baxt C, Kassam-Adams N, Nance ML, et al: Assessment of pain after injury in the pediatric patient: Child and parent perceptions. J Pediatr Surg 2004;39:979–983.
18. Chambers CT, Finley GA, McGrath PJ, Walsh TM: The parents' postoperative pain measure: Replication and extension to 2-6-year-old children. Pain 2003;105:437–443.
19. Koh JL, Fanurik D, Harrison RD, et al: Analgesia following surgery in children with and without cognitive impairment. Pain 2004;111:239–244.
20. Voepel-Lewis T, Merkel S, Tait AR, et al: The reliability and validity of the Face, Legs, Activity, Cry, Consolability observational tool as a measure of pain in children with cognitive impairment. Anesth Analg 2002;95:1224–1229.
21. Perrott DA, Piira T, Goodenough B, Champion GD: Efficacy and safety of acetaminophen vs ibuprofen for treating children's pain or fever: A meta-analysis. Arch Pediatr Adolesc Med 2004;158:521–526.
22. Vetter T, Heiner E: Intravenous ketorolac as an adjuvant to pediatric patient-controlled analgesia with morphine. J Clin Anesth 1994;6:110–113.
23. Rusy L, Houck C, Sullivan L, et al: A double-blind evaluation of ketorolac tromethamine versus acetaminophen in pediatric tonsillectomy: Analgesia and bleeding. Anesth Analg 1995;80:226–229.
24. Hamunen K, Maunuksela EL, Sarvela J, et al: Stereoselective pharmacokinetics of ketorolac in children, adolescents and adults. Acta Anaesthesiol Scand 1999;43:1041–1046.
25. Olkkola KT, Hamunen K, Maunuksela EL: Clinical pharmacokinetics and pharmacodynamics of opioid analgesics in infants and children. Clin Pharmacokinet 1995;28:385–404.
26. Lynn A, Opheim, Tyler D: Morphine infusion after pediatric cardiac surgery. Crit Care Medi 1984;12:863–866.
27. Payne KA, Roelofse JA, Shipton EA: Pharmacokinetics of oral tramadol drops for postoperative pain relief in children aged 4 to 7 years—a pilot study. Anesth Prog 2002;49:109–112.
28. Bösenberg AT, Handley GP, Murray W: Epidural analgesia reduces postoperative ventilation requirements following esophageal atresia repair. J Pain Symptom Manag 1991;6:209A.
29. Dalens BJ, Mazoit JX: Adverse effects of regional anaesthesia in children. Drug Saf 1998;19:251–268.
30. Conroy JM, Othersen HB Jr, Dorman BH, et al: A comparison of wound instillation and caudal block for analgesia following pediatric inguinal herniorrhaphy. J Pediatr Surg 1993;28:565–567.
31. Broadman LM: Blocks and other techniques pediatric surgeons can employ to reduce postoperative pain in pediatric patients. Semin Pediatr Surg 1999;8:30–33.
32. Fisher QA, McComiskey CM, Hill JL, et al: Postoperative voiding interval and duration of analgesia following peripheral or caudal nerve blocks in children. Anesth Analg 1993;76:173–177.
33. Uguralp S, Mutus M, Koroglu A, et al: Regional anesthesia is a good alternative to general anesthesia in pediatric surgery: Experience in 1,554 children. J Pediatr Surg 2002;37:610–613.
34. Dalens B, Tanguy A, Haberer JP: Lumbar epidural anesthesia for operative and postoperative pain relief in infants and young children. Anesth Analg 1986;65:1069–1073.
35. Murat I, Delleur MM, Esteve C, et al: Continuous extradural anaesthesia in children: Clinical and haemodynamic implications. Br J Anaesth 1987;59:1441–1450.
36. Wolf AR, Eyres RL, Laussen PC, et al: Effect of extradural analgesia on stress responses to abdominal surgery in infants. Br J Anaesth 1993;70:654–660.
37. Lin YC, Sentivany-Collins SK, Peterson KL, et al: Outcomes after single injection caudal epidural versus continuous infusion epidural via caudal approach for postoperative analgesia in infants and children undergoing patent ductus arteriosus ligation. Paediatr Anaesth 1999;9:139–143.
38. Murrell D, Gibson P, Cohen R: Continuous epidural analgesia in newborn infants undergoing major surgery. J Pediatr Surg 2 1993;28:548–552.
39. Desparmet J, Meistelman C, Bare J: Continuous epidural infusion of bupivacaine for postoperative pain relief in children. Anesthesiology 1987;67:108–110.
40. Ecoffey D, Dubousset A, Samii K: Lumbar and thoracic epidural anesthesia for urologic and upper abdominal surgery in infants and children. Anesthesiology 1986;65:87–90.
41. Caudle C, Freid E, Baley A, et al: Epidural fentanyl infusion with patient-controlled epidural analgesia for postoperative analgesia in children. J Pediatr Surg 1993;28:554–558.
42. Tsui BC, Seal R, Koller J, et al: Thoracic epidural analgesia via the caudal approach in pediatric patients undergoing fundoplication using nerve stimulation guidance. Anesth Analg 2001;93:1152–1155.
43. Berde CB: Convulsions associated with pediatric regional anesthesia. Anesth Analg 1992;75:164–166.
44. Lin Y, Krane E: Comparison of continuous epidural infusion using low dose bupivacaine with or without morphine for postoperative analgesia in neonates. Anesth Analg 1997;84:S441.
45. McCloskey J, Haun S, Deshpande J: Bupivacaine toxicity secondary to continuous caudal infusion in children. Anesth Analg 1992;75:287–290.
46. McBride WJ, Dicker R, Abajian JC, Vane DW: Continuous thoracic epidural infusions for postoperative analgesia after pectus deformity repair. J Pediatr Surg 1996;31:105–108.
47. Williams DG, Howard RF: Epidural analgesia in children: A survey of current opinions and practices amongst UK paediatric anaesthetists. Paediatr Anaesth 2003;13:769–776.
48. Ivani G, Tonetti F: Postoperative analgesia in infants and children: New developments. Minerva Anestesiol 2004;70:399–403.
49. Fisher WJ, Bingham RM, Hall R: Axillary brachial plexus block for perioperative analgesia in 250 children. Paediatr Anaesth 1999;9:435–438.
50. Ilfeld BM, Morey TE, Wright TW, et al: Interscalene perineural ropivacaine infusion: A comparison of two dosing regimens for postoperative analgesia. Reg Anesth Pain Med 2004;29:9–16.
51. Bosenberg AT: Lower limb nerve blocks in children using unsheathed needles and a nerve stimulator. Anaesthesia 1995;50:206–210.
52. Grossbard GD, Love BR: Femoral nerve block: A simple and safe method of instant analgesia for femoral shaft fractures in children. Aust N Z J Surg 1979;49:592–594.

53. Denton JS, Manning MP: Femoral nerve block for femoral shaft fractures in children: Brief report. J Bone Joint Surg Br 1988;70:84.

54. Ronchi L, Rosenbaum D, Athouel A, et al: Femoral nerve blockade in children using bupivacaine. Anesthesiology 1989;70:622–624.

55. Maccani RM, Wedel DJ, Melton A, Gronert GA: Femoral and lateral femoral cutaneous nerve block for muscle biopsies in children. Paediatr Anaesth 1995;5:223–227.

56. Khan ML, Hossain MM, Chowdhury AY, et al: Lateral femoral cutaneous nerve block for split skin grafting. Bangladesh Med Res Counc Bull 1998;24:32–34.

57. Dalens B, Vanneuville G, Tanguy A: Comparison of the fascia iliaca compartment block with the 3-in-1 block in children. Anesth Analg 1989;69:705–713.

58. Singelyn FJ, Gouverneur JM, Gribomont BF: Popliteal sciatic nerve block aided by a nerve stimulator: A reliable technique for foot and ankle surgery. Reg Anesth 1991;16:278–281.

59. Tobias JD, Mencio GA: Popliteal fossa block for postoperative analgesia after foot surgery in infants and children. J Pediatr Orthop 1999;19:511–514.

60. Vater M, Wandless J: Caudal or dorsal nerve block? A comparison of two local anaesthetic techniques for postoperative analgesia following day case circumcision. Acta Anaesthesiol Scand 1985;29:175–179.

61. Yeoman P, Cooke R, Hain W: Penile block for circumcision? A comparison with caudal blockade. Anaesthesia 1983;38:862–866.

62. Dalens B, Vanneuville G, Dechelotte P: Penile block via the subpubic space in 100 children. Anesth Analg 1989;69:41–45.

63. Cross GD, Barrett RF: Comparison of two regional techniques for postoperative analgesia in children following herniotomy and orchidopexy. Anaesthesia 1987;42:845–849.

64. Lim SL, Ng Sb A, Tan GM: Ilioinguinal and iliohypogastric nerve block revisited: Single shot versus double shot technique for hernia repair in children. Paediatr Anaesth 2002;12:255–260.

65. Brenn B, Rose J: Pediatric pain services: Monitoring for epidural analgesia in the non-intensive care unit setting. Anesthesiology 1995;83:432.

66. Strafford MA, Wilder RT, Berde CB: The risk of infection from epidural analgesia in children: A review of 1620 cases. Anesth Analg 1995;80:234–238.

67. Kost-Byerly S, Tobin J, Greenberg R, et al: Bacterial colonization and infection rate of continuous epidural catheters in children. Anesth Analg 1998;86:712–716.

68. Seth N, Macqueen S, Howard RF: Clinical signs of infection during continuous postoperative epidural analgesia in children: The value of catheter tip culture. Paediatr Anaesth 2004;14:996–1000.

69. Lin Y, Krane EJ: Regional anesthesia for the pediatric outpatient. Refesher Courses in Anesthesiology 1996;24:163–175.

70. Chambliss CR, Heggen J, Copelan DN, Pettignano R: The assessment and management of chronic pain in children. Paediatr Drugs 2002;4:737–746.

71. Hobbie C: Relaxation techniques for children and young people. J Pediatr Health Care 1989;3:83–87.

72. Cohen MH, Kemper KJ: Complementary therapies in pediatrics: A legal perspective. Pediatrics 2005;115:774–780.

73. Ready L, Ashburn M, Caplan R, et al: Practice guidelines for acute pain management in the peri-operative setting. Anesthesiology 1995;82:1071–1081.

74. Lin Y: Analgesics and sedatives for critical ill infants and children. J Intensive Care Med 1992;7:221–222.

75. Howard RF: Current status of pain management in children [erratum appears in JAMA 2004;291:695]. JAMA 2003;290:2464–2469.

22 Postoperative Pain Management in the Elderly

DIARMUID McCOY • DOMINIC HARMON

Poor postoperative pain control can lead to slower recovery and an increase in postoperative complications. This statement is especially true for the elderly patient.[1] The severity of perioperative pain can influence the development of chronic postsurgical pain.[2] This possibility has significant implications for older patients, for whom the impact of chronic pain can be considerable. The management of postoperative pain in this population is complicated not only by the nature of the operation but also by intercurrent illness, concurrent medications, and difficulty in assessment of pain.

The number of elderly patients as a proportion of the population presenting for surgery is growing; a third of all inpatient procedures has been reported as being performed in elderly patients.[3] Similarly, the surgery performed on these patients is becoming more complex. A 2000 publication has estimated that the proportion of the Australian population 65 years and older is projected to rise from 12% (2000) to 18% in 2020 and 25% in 2050.[4] This trend is similar to that seen in Europe and North America.

Advances in surgical techniques and anesthetic management mean that increasingly elderly patients are presenting for more major surgery,[5] creating an acute pain management problem. This issue is an addition to pain from conditions that are common in the elderly, such as acute exacerbation of arthritis, fractures secondary to osteoporosis, and intermittent acute pain such as angina. In addition to these confounding factors, changes in physiology, pharmacodynamics, and kinetics; alterations in pain perceptions and processing; and the problem of accurate assessment of pain make acute postoperative pain management in the elderly challenging.

The barriers to good pain control in the older postoperative patient are little different from those in any other population. They include (1) the idea that pain is merely a symptom and not harmful in itself, (2) a lack of understanding of the pharmacology of analgesic agents, (3) fear of addiction to opioids, and (4) patients' difficulties in communicating their need for analgesia. Specific barriers in the elderly may be due to patient factors such as fear of being bothersome or discomfort with unfamiliar equipment such as patient-controlled analgesia (PCA) devices. Healthcare provider factors, such as belief that the elderly are unable to tolerate opioids and that pain perception decreases with age, are also barriers. Other barriers are factors common to the patient's family and healthcare provider, such as fear of drug side effects and the belief that pain is an inevitable consequence of aging. A common lament in the pain literature is that the treatment of acute pain is poor and that patients are suffering unnecessarily; this may still be true, but the improvements that have been made must be appreciated, and further strides taken toward ideal pain management, particularly in the elderly population.

Physiology of Pain Perception in the Elderly

Evidence has now recognized important changes in the central nervous system as humans age. These include changes in neurochemistry, anatomy, and function, with some deterioration in opioid systems. The pain inhibitory system becomes impaired, leading to important changes in pain processing.[6] $A\delta$ fibers appear to be more impaired than C fibers, leading to alteration in early pain perception. Decreased conduction velocities and concentrations of neurotransmitters, including substance P, along with decreases in peripheral nerve fibers, alter the quality and experience of pain. Experimentally induced pain demonstrates increased pain thresholds for thermal stimuli; however, the changes found in thresholds for mechanical stimuli are equivocal, and thresholds for electrical stimuli are unchanged.[7] Studies using a variety of experimental pain stimuli suggest that the reduced ability of elderly patients to endure pain means that severe pain in this population may have a greater impact.

Pharmacological Changes in the Elderly

Changes in physiology alter the handling of drugs in the elderly (Table 22–1). Cardiac output and cerebral, renal, and hepatic blood flow decrease with age. Hepatic function, particularly phase 1 oxidative enzyme function, may be reduced by 25% and, along with a possible decrease in glomerular filtration rate and creatinine clearance of between 30% and 50%, leads to diminished clearance of drugs or active metabolites.[8] Alterations in fat content result in a greater volume of distribution, and a drop in albumin concentration alters the free fraction of drug, leading to variability in bolus dosing.

In one study, measuring changes in electroencephalographic (EEG) values in response to the effects of fentanyl demonstrated little alteration in the pharmacokinetics with increasing age, but the brain was 50% more sensitive to this drug.[9]

TABLE 22–1	Changes in Physiological Variables in the Elderly and Their Effects on Pharmacokinetic Variables		
Physiological Process	**Direction and Magnitude of Change (%)**	**Dose Strategy**	
Whole body:			
Cardiac output	↓ 0–20	Smaller initial dose	
		Slower injection rate	
Fat	↑ 10–50	↓ Maintenance dose	
Muscle mass/blood flow	↓ 20		
Plasma volume	Little change	↓ Maintenance dose	
Total body water	↓ 10		
Plasma albumin	↓ 20	Variable effect on bolus dose	
α_1-Glycoprotein	↑ 30–50	Little effect on maintenance dose	
Drug binding	↑ (variable)		
Liver:			
Hepatic blood flow	↓ 25–40	↓ Maintenance dose	
Hepatic enzymes:			
Phase I	↓ 25		
Phase II	Little change		
Kidney:			
Renal blood flow	↓ 10 per decade	↓ Maintenance dose, renally excreted drugs	
Glomerular filtration rate	↓ 50	Monitor for accumulation of active metabolites	
Creatinine clearance	↓ 50–70		
Central nervous system:			
Cerebral blood flow	↓ 20	Little net effect on dose	
Cerebral volume	↓ 20		

Adapted from Macintyre PE, Upton RN, Ludbrook GL: Acute pain management in the elderly: In Rowbotham D, Macintyre PE, Breivik H, et al (eds): Clinical Pain Management: Acute Pain. London, Arnold, 2002.

This greater sensitivity may be due to altered sensitivity of opioid receptors, a higher free fraction of the drug, or a combination of factors. Animal studies show fewer numbers of some opioid receptors with age.[10]

Assessment of Pain in the Elderly

Except those individuals who lack sensory perception, every human being experiences acute pain. Normally, pain is a well-defined, quite intense sensation (nociceptive) or is poorly localized and dull (visceral). The problem of pain description and measurement has attended both the diagnosis and treatment of pain and research into pain for generations. Most researchers use the 100-mm visual analogue pain score (VAPS) as the standard measurement tool. However, pain is a multidimensional experience, with the nociceptive experience being modulated by environment circumstance, disease, both medical and psychiatric comorbidities, and cognition. It is estimated that cognitive impairment may be present in 15% of older adults and is characterized by deterioration in memory, attention, spatial skill, language, and behavior.[11] Acute pain is more likely to be untreated or undertreated in patients with cognitive impairment.[12] Delirium in the elderly population is a common form of cognitive impairment; risk factors for its development include advancing age, pyrexia and infection, preexisting dementia, depression, anemia, medication or drug withdrawal (including alcohol), fluid and electrolyte abnormalities, hypoxia, and unrelieved pain.[13] Assessment of pain in the elderly should be conducted like it is in younger patients (Box 22–1). Alterations in approaches

may be necessary, depending on the patient's cognitive status. A baseline preoperative pain assessment should be performed, involving a physical examination, pain history, past pain experience and knowledge, medication history, and a self-report of pain.

Many elderly patients have chronic conditions and other causes for pain that must be distinguished from the pain associated with surgery. Past pain experience and knowledge, including previous use of analgesics, their effectiveness and adverse effects, and nonpharmacological methods previously used to relieve pain, can guide postoperative pain management. The patient's attitudes and beliefs about pain, as well as fears of addiction and analgesic side effects, should be addressed. A medication history is important to identify medications that may interfere with analgesics in the analgesic treatment plan.

BOX 22–1	POSTOPERATIVE PAIN ASSESSMENT IN THE ELDERLY

1. Consider various etiologies of pain, not just the surgical incision.
2. Obtain patient self-reports of pain with adapted instruments if necessary.
3. If patient is unable to give a self-report, use behavioral observations.
4. Obtain opinions from caregivers regarding changes in behavior.
5. Document and assess at regular and frequent intervals.
6. Use the same pain scale throughout a patient's care.

Self-reports of pain are the most reliable indicators of the existence and intensity of pain.[14] Alterations in assessment approaches may be necessary to obtain a self-report in the elderly. It is important not to assume that the cognitively impaired patient cannot provide a report of his or her pain. Most elderly patients, including those with mild to moderate cognitive impairment, can use some form of pain-rating scale to report pain intensity.[15] There is no universal pain assessment tool suitable for all elderly patients. Once an assessment tool that matches an elderly patient's preferences and cognitive/functional abilities has been chosen, it should be used consistently throughout the patient's hospital stay.

The pain team should consider ways to adapt approaches to assessment to enhance success with their use in the elderly. Auditory or visual impairments can be compensated by ensuring that a patient's eyeglasses or hearing aid is readily available. Caregivers can speak slowly, decrease extraneous noises, and provide written as well as verbal instructions. Assessment tools can also be altered to make them more easily read and understood.

A study comparing the five pain scales commonly used in elderly patients in the acute care setting found that the verbal descriptor scale (VDS) was the most reliable and sensitive, although it was ranked second to the numerical rating scale for patient preference.[16] The VDS is considered the most suitable for elderly adults, including those with mild cognitive impairment.[16] Observations of facial grimacing and sounds are an accurate measure of the presence of pain but not the intensity in patients with advanced dementia.[16] Behavioral indicators must be observed during activity and not only at rest.[17] Cognitively impaired patients may demonstrate fewer obvious behavioral pain indicators, such as agitation and aggression.

Patient Education

Patient education is an important component of postoperative pain management. Patients and their families need information about the harmful effects of unrelieved pain. They should be informed about how the pain will be managed, the importance of reporting pain, and the benefits of pain control to recovery. Adverse effects of analgesics and nonpharmacological strategies should be explained. It is important to avoid words such as *narcotic*, which contributes to fears about drug addiction.[18]

Analgesic Drugs in the Postoperative Elderly Patient

Physical and psychological strategies should always be employed in association with medication for the treatment of pain in all postoperative patients, including the elderly. Individualization of the analgesic dose is an important concept in effective postoperative pain management in the elderly. Around-the-clock analgesic administration is recommended in the initial postoperative period. This approach increases efficacy, reduces side effects, and avoids the reluctance of elderly patients to ask for pain medication. Preexisting polypharmacy in the elderly must also be considered. Beneficial effects of multimodal analgesia have been established in the postoperative pain management of the elderly patient.[19] Recommended treatment for acute pain involves the use of simple analgesics for mild to moderate pain and addition of an opioid for moderate to severe pain.[20]

OPIOIDS

The older postoperative patient requires less opioid than younger patients, but there is wide inter-individual variability. Doses must be tailored to effect for the individual patient. The decrease in opioid requirement is much greater than age-related changes in physiology would predict.[8] The overall reduction in morphine and fentanyl requirements of approximately two- to fourfold is not associated with increased reported pain.[21] Tramadol, though not strictly a pure opioid, demonstrates slightly prolonged elimination half-life, so lower doses are required. Impaired renal function can lead to accumulation of active opioid metabolites (norpethidine, morphine-3-glucuronide, morphine-6-glucuronide, desmethyltramadol).

The fear of respiratory depression in elderly patients, especially those with preexisting respiratory disease, is the most common reason for inadequate opioid analgesia. As with other patient groups, this problem can largely be avoided with appropriate monitoring of sedation. The rate of postoperative nausea, vomiting, and pruritus decreases with rising age.[22] Less depression of cognitive function and less confusion may be associated with fentanyl than with morphine. One must remember that some antiemetics are more likely to cause side effects in the elderly.

LOCAL ANESTHETICS

The elderly are more sensitive to the effects of local anesthetics. Pharmacokinetic and pharmacodynamic changes in intrinsic neuronal sensitivity explain these differences in the elderly.[23] The terminal half-life of lidocaine and bupivacaine lengthens, whereas the total plasma clearance of these local anesthetics decreases with age after a single epidural administration.[24] Reduced clearance is important during continuous infusions, with higher plasma concentrations of local anesthetics occurring in elderly patients.[23]

PARACETAMOL

There is no evidence that doses of paracetamol must be altered in the elderly, and this drug has a useful role in multimodal analgesia. Daily doses should be decreased (50%) in the frail elderly and patients with hepatic or renal impairment.

NONSTEROIDAL ANTI-INFLAMMATORY DRUGS

Elderly patients are more prone to gastritis, gastric erosions, and renal dysfunction after administration of nonsteroidal anti-inflammatory drugs (NSAIDs). Some may also demonstrate cognitive impairment with these drugs.[25] Preexisting renal impairment makes renal failure a particular concern. This situation may be compounded by coexisting cirrhosis, cardiac failure, and the use of diuretics and antihypertensive medications. Adverse drug interactions between NSAIDs and warfarin, oral hypoglycemic agents, phenytoin, and aminoglycosides create further risks for the elderly patient's renal function.

Selective cyclooxygenase-2 (Cox-2) inhibitors show promise of significantly fewer adverse effects in the elderly population. There is good evidence, however, that adverse effects of Cox-2 inhibitors are no different from those of conventional NSAIDs. Evidence has demonstrated that Cox-2 inhibitors are better avoided in the elderly, even for short periods such as the postoperative setting.

KETAMINE

There is no evidence to suggest changes in dosing for ketamine in the elderly. However, the NMDA receptor on which ketamine is an antagonist undergoes structural changes and a decrease in binding, thus requiring lower dosing in the elderly.

PATIENT-CONTROLLED ANALGESIA

PCA is an effective mode of delivering postoperative analgesia in the elderly (Table 22–2).[26] Cognitive dysfunction is a relative contraindication to this technique. In elderly patients, PCA results in significantly lower pain scores than those seen with intermittent subcutaneous morphine. Vision, hearing, and motor impairment may be barriers to the successful use of PCA in the elderly postoperative patient; however, clear repeated instruction in the preoperative stage will overcome these barriers. Some devices can be modified to be activated by foot if manual dexterity is impaired by surgery or arthritis. PCA has been shown to result in less pulmonary morbidity, less confusion, and better pain control in elderly men than intramuscular morphine.[27] Some patients may be taking oral opioids for chronic painful conditions, and this medication must be factored into the postoperative pain management plan. Background infusions of the equivalent daily dose of oral opioid should be included for such patients. Background infusions in conjunction with PCA opioids should be avoided in opioid-naive patients.

REGIONAL ANESTHETIC TECHNIQUES

Outcome studies suggest that there is no difference in mortality or major morbidity between general and regional anesthesia techniques in most patient populations.[28] Regional anesthesia is frequently recommended in elderly patients on the basis of clinical observation that patients with minimal sedation remain more oriented and return to normal functioning more rapidly.[29] The incidence of thrombolytic events,[30] blood loss,[31] and deep venous thrombosis[32] is reduced after hip surgery performed with regional anesthesia rather than general anesthesia in elderly patients. Regional anesthesia provides superior postoperative analgesia and reduces the incidence of adverse cardiac events in the postoperative period.[33] Other advantages of regional anesthesia are a quicker return of bowel function[34] and integrity of the immune system in the postoperative period.[35] In order to obtain these benefits in the elderly, careful consideration must be given to age-related physiological changes.

Spinal anesthesia, despite its technical simplicity and overall effectiveness, is not without risks, particularly in the elderly. Patient positioning and needle insertion can be more difficult in the elderly. Bony landmarks are more recognizable in elderly patients, but calcification of spinal ligaments prevents easy entry of needles into the epidural and intrathecal spaces. Paramedian approaches are thus recommended.[36] Changes in the spinal column and neural tissues and their effects on the absorption, distribution, and duration of local anesthetics must be considered. The total volume of cerebrospinal fluid is decreased, and its specific gravity increased.[24] There are inconsistencies among studies that correlate age and spread of analgesia after spinal block.[24] The elderly patient is also at greater risk of associated adverse perioperative events and thus must be monitored carefully. High spinal blocks can have more significant effects in the elderly.

The area of the epidural space is smaller in the elderly because the intervertebral foramina become more dense with age. This situation results in a higher cephalad spread of injected local anesthetics.[38] The effect is exacerbated by arteriosclerosis and diabetes.[38] The elderly can also experience rapid onset of epidural anesthesia owing to increased permeability of the dura and larger size of arachnoid villi.[39] It is also important to reduce the dose of local anesthetic because of the greater risk of cardiovascular events. Spinal stenosis is more common in the elderly. Large doses of local anesthetics with prolonged epidural anesthesia can thus be associated with cauda equina syndrome in the elderly.[40] Elderly patients

TABLE 22–2	Daily Satisfaction and PCA Survey Scores by Age Group		
	Young Patients (39 ± 9) (n = 45)	Older Patients (67 ± 8) (n = 44)	P Value*
Satisfaction day 1 (cm)†	8.2 ± 1.9	8.4 ± 1.8	NS
Satisfaction day 2 (cm)†	8.0 ± 2.0	8.2 ± 2.1	NS
PCA survey subscale (%):			
Satisfaction with PCA	81 ± 9	82 ± 11	NS
Satisfaction with pain relief	49 ± 16	43 ± 11	NS
Satisfaction with level of control	32 ± 12	32 ± 9	NS
Concerns about addiction and adverse effects	47 ± 12	46 ± 11	NS
Concerns about equipment use or malfunction	40 ± 11	38 ± 10	NS

NS, not significant; PCA, patient-controlled analgesia.
*Values are mean ± standard deviation (SD).
†0- to 10-cm analogue scale: 0 = totally dissatisfied; 10 = totally satisfied.
Adapted from Gagliese L Jackson M, Ritvo P, et al: Age is not an impediment to effective use of patient controlled analgesia by surgical patients. Anaesthesiology 2000;93:601–610.

given epidural bupivacaine and sufentanil report lower pain scores both at rest and on movement than those using PCA intravenous opioids. In addition, epidural analgesia is associated with higher patient satisfaction and quicker return of gastrointestinal function.[41] Epidural opioid requirements diminish with increasing age (Table 22–3).

A wide variety of peripheral nerve blocks are suitable in elderly patients.[42] As already mentioned, bony landmarks are more readily identifiable but arthritic changes may hinder optimal patient positioning. Age-related changes in the neural and perineural tissues can alter features of peripheral nerve blocks. The diameter and number of myelinated fibers decrease with age.[37] More sodium channels are available to local anesthetic drugs because the distances between Schwann cells in myelinated fibers diminish with age.[37] Deterioration of the mucopolysaccharides in connective tissue sheaths allows more local anesthetic solution to infiltrate nerve sheaths.[37] Nerves also become more sensitive to local anesthetics with age; this change is related to a decline in the neuronal population and slower peripheral nerve conduction velocity.[43] Cumulative toxicity can occur in older patients owing to a decline in drug clearance. Large doses of local anesthetics should be avoided, and further doses administered with caution.

Despite the advantages of regional anesthesia, controversy still remains about whether patient outcome is better with general or regional anesthesia. Several issues confound this clinical question, such as the type and duration of operation, coexisting medical conditions, and the skill or experience of the anesthetist and surgeon. Poorly conducted regional anesthesia can be more hazardous in an elderly patient than well-conducted general anesthesia.[36] The quality of the anesthesia administered rather than the type of anesthetic is most important.

Nonpharmacological Techniques in the Elderly

Multiple nonpharmacological techniques have been studied in the management of postoperative pain.[44] These techniques can be divided into cutaneous stimulation interventions and cognitive-behavioral interventions. Cutaneous stimulation interventions involve stimulating the skin and underlying tissues to moderate pain transmission.[45] Cognitive-behavioral

interventions modify thoughts and behaviors that exacerbate pain or interfere with coping.[45] Patients must have the mental and physical capacity to participate in these interventions. Pain must be well controlled with analgesics so that patients can concentrate and participate in cognitive-behavioral interventions.

Conclusion

Elderly patients will continue to present in ever-increasing numbers for surgery. Physiological changes, multiple comorbidities, and cognitive impairment make acute postoperative pain management more challenging in such patients. Visual, hearing, language, and cognitive impairment may make the task of pain assessment, measurement, and treatment more difficult. Postoperative pain management should be planned well in advance of surgery. Regional anesthetic techniques are appropriate techniques to use. Safe regional anesthesia in elderly patients requires modified regional techniques and reduced local anesthetic doses for the same effect. Good analgesia in the postoperative period, in conjunction with multidisciplinary rehabilitation, will aid the successful recovery of the elderly patient.

REFERENCES

1. Feldt KS, Oh HL: Pain and hip fracture outcomes for older adults. Orthop Nurs 2000;19:35–44.
2. Katz J, Jackson M, Kavanagh BP, et al: Acute pain after thoracic surgery predicts long-term post-thoracotomy pain. Clin J Pain 1996;12:50–55.
3. Hall MJ, Owings MF: 2000 National Hospital Discharge Survey, vol 329. Hyattsville, MD, National Cancer Center for Health Statistics, 2002.
4. Australian Bureau of Statistics: Population Deaths 2000. Published ABS. Canberra, Australia.
5. Richardson J, Bresland K: The management of post surgical pain in the elderly population. Drugs Aging 1998;13:17–31.
6. Gibson SJ, Farrell M: A review of age differences in neurophysiology of nociception and the perceptual experience of pain. Clin J Pain 2004; 20:227–239.
7. Gibson SJ: Pain and ageing the pain experience over the adult life span. In Proceedings of the 10th World Congress in Pain. Seattle, IASP Press, 2003, pp 767–790.
8. Macintyre PE, Upton R, Ludbrook GL: Pain in the elderly. In Rowbotham DJ, Macintyre PE, Breivik H, et al (eds): Clinical Pain Management: Acute Pain. London, Arnold, 2002.
9. Scott JC, Stanski DR: Decreased fentanyl and alfentanyl requirements with age: A simultaneous pharmacokinetic and pharmacodynamic evaluation. J Pharmacol Exp Ther 1987;240:159–166.
10. Vuyk J: Pharmacodynamics in the elderly. Best Pract Res Clin Anaesthesiol 2003;17:207–218.
11. Ferrell B, Ferrell B (eds): Pain in the Elderly: Task Force on Pain in the Elderly. Seattle, IASP Press, 1996.
12. Morrison RS, Siu AL: A comparison of pain and its treatment in advanced dementia and cognitively intact patients with hip fracture. J Pain Symptom Manag 2000;19:240–248.
13. Bekker AY, Weeks EJ: Cognitive function after anaesthesia in the elderly. Best Pract Res Clin Anaesthesiol 2003;17:259–272.
14. American Geriatrics Society Panel on Persistent Pain in Older Persons: Clinical Practice Guidelines: The management of chronic pain in older persons. J Am Geriatr Soc 2002;50:S205–S224.
15. Chibnall J, Tait R: Pain assessment in cognitively and non cognitively impaired older adults: A comparison of four scales. Pain 2001; 92:173–186.
16. Herr KA, Spratt K, Mobily PR, Richardson G: Pain intensity in older adults: Use of experimental pain to compare psychometric properties and usability of selected pain scales with younger adults. Clin J Pain 2004;20:207–219.

TABLE 22–3	Age-Based Infusion Rates for Lumbar Epidural Analgesia Using Mixtures of 0.1% Bupivacaine and 5 mg • mL⁻¹ Fentanyl*	
	Younger Patients (≤40 years)	**Elderly Patients (>70 years)**
Infusion rate (mL/hr)	7–14	4–8
Bolus doses (mL) as needed	4–7	2 or 3

*Doses are individually titrated in all cases.
Adapted from Macintyre PE, Ready LB: Acute Pain Management: A Practical Guide, 2nd ed. London, WB Saunders, 2001.

17. Feldt K: The Checklist of Nonverbal Pain Indicators (CNPI). Pain Manage Nurs 2000;1:13–21.

18. Herr KA, Titler MG, Soroform BA, et al: Acute Pain Management in the Elderly. Iowa City, IA, University of Iowa Gerontological Nursing Interventions Resource Center, 2000.

19. Adrienssens G, Vermeyen KM, Hoffman VL, et al: Postoperative analgesia with I.V. patient-controlled morphine: Effect of adding ketamine. Br J Anaesth 1999;83:393–396.

20. American Pain Society: Principles of Analgesic Use in the Treatment of Acute Pain And Cancer Pain. Glenview, IL, American Pain Society, 2003.

21. Macintyre PE, Jarvis DA: Age is the best predictor of postoperative morphine requirement. Pain 1996;64:357–364.

22. Quinn AC, Brown JH, Wallace PG, et al: Studies in postoperative sequelae: Nausea and vomiting still a problem. Anaesthesia 1994;49:62–65.

23. Sadean MR, Glass PSA: Pharmacokinetics in the elderly. Best Pract Res Clin Anaesthesiol 2003;17:191–205.

24. Veering BT: The role of aging in regional anaesthesia. Pain Rev 1999;6:167–173.

25. Phillips AC, Polisson RP, Simon LS: NSAIDS and the elderly: Toxicity and economic implications. Drugs Aging 1997;10:119–130.

26. Gagliese L Jackson M, Ritvo P, et al: Age is not an impediment to effective use of patient controlled analgesia by surgical patients. Anaesthesiology 2000;93:601-610.

27. Egbert AM, Parks LH, Short LM, et al: Randomized trial of postoperative patient controlled analgesia vs intramuscular narcotics in elderly frail men. Arch Intern Med 1990;150:1897–1903.

28. Roy RC: Choosing general versus regional anesthesia for the elderly. Anesthesiol Clin North Am 2000;18:91:104.

29. Chung F, Meier R, Lautenshlager E, et al: General or spinal anesthesia: Which is better in the elderly? Anesthesiology 1987;67:422–427.

30. Modig J, Borg T, Karlstrom G, et al: Thromboembolism after total hip replacement: Role of epidural and general anesthesia. Anesth Analg 1983;62:174–180.

31. Keith J: Anesthesia and blood loss in total hip replacement. Anesthesia 1977;32:444–450.

32. Sorensen RM, Pace NL: Anesthetic techniques during surgical repair of femoral neck fractures. Anesthesiology 1992;77:1095–1104.

33. Matot I, Oppenheim-Eden A, Ratrot R, et al: Preoperative cardiac events in elderly patients with hip fracture randomized to epidural or conventional analgesia. Anesthesiology 2003;98:156–163.

34. Breen P, Park KW: General anesthesia versus regional anesthesia. Int Anesthesiol Clin 2002;40:61–71.

35. Nielson KC, Steele SM: Outcome after regional anaesthesia in the ambulatory setting: Is it really worth it? Best Prac Res Clin Anaesthesiol 2002;16:145–157.

36. Mulroy MF: Modification of regional anesthetic techniques. In McLesky CH (ed): Geriatric Anesthesiology. Baltimore, Williams & Wilkins, 1997, pp 381–388.

37. Bromage PR: Epidural Analgesia. Philadelphia, WB Saunders, 1978, pp 40–42.

38. Bromage PR: Exaggerated spread of epidural analgesia in arteriosclerotic patients: Dosage in relation to biological and chronological ageing. BMJ 1962;5320:1634–1638.

39. Veering BT, Braun AG, van Kleef JW, et al: Epidural anesthesia with bupivacaine: Effects of age on neural blockade and pharmacokinetics. Anesth Analg 1987;66:589–593.

40. Faccenda KA, Finucane BT: Complications of regional anaesthesia: Incidence and prevention. Drug Saf 2001;24:13–42.

41. Mann C, Pouzeratte Y, Boccara G: Comparison of intravenous or epidural patient-controlled analgesia in the elderly after major abdominal surgery. Anaesthesiology 2000;92:433–441.

42. Raj PP: Conduction blocks. In Textbook of Regional Anesthesia. Philadelphia, Churchill Livingstone, 2002, pp 285–306.

43. Dorfman LJ, Bosley TM: Age-related changes in peripheral and central nerve conduction in man. Neurology 1979;29:38–44.

44. Agency for Healthcare Research and Quality: System to Rate the Strength of Scientific Evidence. Rockville, MD, U.S. Department of Health and Human Services, 2003.

45. Herr KA, Kwekkeboom KL: Assisting older clients with pain management in the home. Home Health Care Manage Pract 2003;15:237–250.

23 Postoperative Pain Management after Cesarean Section

RACHEL A. FARRAGHER • JOHN G. LAFFEY

Cesarean section is the most commonly performed surgical procedure in the United States,[1] with more than 1 million patients undergoing this procedure annually. It is a major surgical procedure, for which substantial postoperative discomfort and pain can be anticipated. The provision of effective postoperative analgesia is of key importance in facilitating early ambulation, infant care including breast-feeding, and maternal-infant bonding as well as preventing postoperative morbidity (pneumonias, thromboses, etc.). In addition, the potential for drug transfer to breast milk must be considered. The analgesic regimen needs to meet the goals of providing safe, effective analgesia with minimal side effects for the mother and her child. It should at best facilitate, and at worst not interfere with, early maternal-infant bonding. A multimodal analgesic regimen is the approach most likely to achieve these goals.

The choice of postoperative analgesic technique is influenced by the anesthetic technique chosen for cesarean section. Regional anesthesia is the predominant technique used, accounting for anesthesia in 78% of cesarean sections in the United Kingdom.[2] This technique facilitates the administration of neuraxial agents as a principal component of the postoperative analgesic regimen. Intravenous patient-controlled analgesia (IV-PCA) is widely used, either as a sole technique or in combination with neuraxial agents, and constitutes the mainstay of analgesia after cesarean section performed with general anesthesia. A variety of adjuvant agents—nonsteroidal anti-inflammatory drugs (NSAIDs) and simple analgesics— are commonly combined with the modalities just described and have clearly been demonstrated to decrease opioid requirements and opioid-induced side effects.

The very rapid rate at which advances in the management of pain after cesarean section have occurred has led to uncertainty among clinicians as to which advances truly justify a change in practice. This chapter aims to address these issues by providing a comprehensive, current source of information on what practices are (or are not) justified by existing evidence.

Epidural Analgesic Techniques

The use of the epidural route for the provision of analgesia for both labor and cesarean section[1] renders the epidural administration of agents, particularly opioids, an attractive option for the provision of postoperative pain relief (Box 23–1).

EPIDURAL OPIOID ADMINISTRATION

Epidural narcotic administration provides high-quality analgesia, with single doses of morphine providing effective and prolonged analgesia after cesarean section. In randomized controlled trials, single-dose epidural morphine provides more effective analgesia than intramuscular morphine and has a similar side effect profile.[3] Meperidine (pethidine) produces better analgesia when administered via patient-controlled epidural analgesia (PCEA) devices than by the intramuscular route.[4] Negre et al[5] demonstrated that 5 mg epidural morphine improved postoperative analgesia and markedly decreased IV-PCA opioid for up to 3 days after cesarean section (Fig. 23–1). Duale et al[6] showed that 2 mg epidural morphine provides better analgesia and leads to lower supplemental opioid requirement, with a comparable side effect profile, than 75 μg intrathecal (IT) morphine during the first 24 postoperative hours.

The presence of an epidural catheter facilitates epidural opioid administration after delivery of the infant, removing any risk of fetoplacental drug transmission. The importance of this advantage is underlined by the finding that administration

BOX 23–1	ADVANTAGES OF NEURAXIAL OPIOID ANALGESIA

"Potency gain"—greater-intensity analgesia than similar doses administered parenterally, more pronounced with hydrophilic opioids. Allows use of very small doses and a decrease in total opioid administration.
Lower dose means virtually no placental transfer, minimum accumulation in breast milk, and less sedation than with parenteral opioids.
Selective analgesia—no motor or sympathetic blockade in comparison with local anesthetics.
Facilitates patient ambulation while minimizing the risk of hypotension.
Improved intraoperative comfort with lipid-soluble agents.
Excellent, prolonged postoperative analgesia.

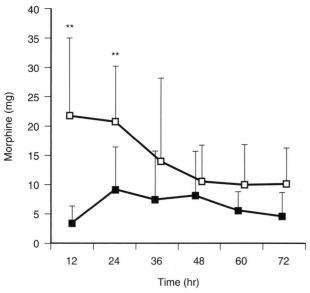

Figure 23–1 Intravenous patient-controlled analgesia (IV-PCA) morphine consumption for 3 days after operation. *Open boxes* indicate controls; *solid boxes* indicate epidural morphine group. *P* < .01. (From Negre I, Gueneron JP, Jamali SJ, et al: Preoperative analgesia with epidural morphine. Anesth Analg 1994;79:298–302.)

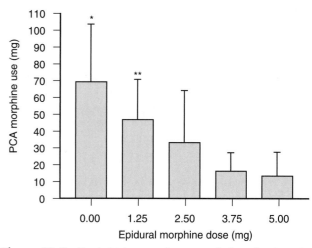

Figure 23–2 Total 24-hour patient-controlled analgesia (PCA) morphine use with varying doses of epidural morphine. Groups were significantly different; *P* < .001. *Group 0.0 mg was significantly different from Groups 2.5, 3.75, and 5.0 mg. **Group 1.25 mg was significantly different from groups 3.75 and 5.0 mg. (From Palmer CM, Nogami WM, Van Maren G, Alves DM: Postcesarean epidural morphine: A dose-response study. Anesth Analg 2000;90:887–891.)

of epidural sufentanil before surgical incision did produce mild transient neurobehavioral depression in neonates.[7]

Morphine

Morphine, the first opioid to receive approval from the U.S. Food and Drug Administration (FDA) for neuraxial administration, has been widely investigated and extensively used clinically. The optimal dose range for epidural morphine is 2.5 to 3.75 mg (Fig. 23–2).[8,9] The peak effect of morphine occurs 60 to 90 minutes after epidural injection and produces analgesia for up to 24 hours (Table 23–1). Continuous epidural morphine infusion offers no advantage over a single bolus dose of morphine after cesarean section.[10]

The choice of local anesthetic used for epidural anesthesia may affect the subsequent efficacy of epidural morphine. 2-Chloroprocaine decreases the quality and duration of analgesia produced by epidural morphine.[11,12] The mechanism is unknown, although an anti-μ opioid receptor–specific antagonist effect of chloroprocaine and its metabolites has been suggested.[13]

A novel single-dose, sustained-release formulation of morphine has been approved by the FDA. A phase 3 trial demonstrated a significant improvement in postoperative analgesia and functional ability with 10-mg and 15-mg single epidural doses of DepoDur in comparison with a single dose of unencapsulated morphine sulfate for the 48-hour period following elective cesarean section.[14]

Short-Acting Lipophilic Opiates

Fentanyl is not FDA-approved for neuraxial administration, but it has been demonstrated in several studies to provide effective analgesia, with limited duration of action.[15–22] The analgesic effects of epidural fentanyl and sufentanil are mediated by a direct spinal action rather than an indirect action from systemic absorption.[15–17] The relative analgesic potency of epidural sufentanil to fentanyl is 5:1. Grass et al[19] reported that the optimal doses of epidural fentanyl and sufentanil are 100 µg and 20 µg, respectively, for provision of analgesia after cesarean section. At equianalgesic doses, there are no differences between the opioids in terms of onset and duration of analgesia. However, PCEA sufentanil is associated with a higher incidence of vomiting than PCEA fentanyl[20] and hence offers no advantages over epidural fentanyl. The volume of diluent solution influences the quality

TABLE 23–1	Characteristics of Epidural Opioids for Cesarean Delivery			
Drug	**Dose**	**Onset (min)**	**Peak Effect (min)**	**Duration (hr)**
Morphine	2–4 mg	45–60	60–120	12–24
Fentanyl	50–100 µg	5	20	2–3
Sufentanil	25–50 µg	5	15–20	2–4
Meperidine	50 mg	15	30	4–6
Morphine/fentanyl	3 mg/50 µg	10	15	12–24

of analgesia produced by lipophilic opioids, faster onset and greater duration of action being seen with diluent volumes of 10 mL or more.[18] In summary, although epidural fentanyl and sufentanil produce effective analgesia of rapid onset, their short duration of action (mean, 117–138 min) renders them of little use as sole agents for postoperative pain management (Fig. 23–3; see Table 23–1).[19,21,22]

Other Opioids

Epidural meperidine provides effective postoperative analgesia of relatively short duration (median, 165 min with 25 mg). A single 25-mg dose of meperidine provides better analgesia than 12.5 mg, but doses of 50 mg or more offer no further improvement in the quality or duration of analgesia.[23]

Hydromorphone, a hydroxylated derivative of morphine, is more lipid soluble, with a faster onset of action and shorter duration of analgesia. The analgesic ratio of epidural morphine to hydromorphone is 5:1. However, at equianalgesic doses, hydromorphone provides no clinical advantage, with regard to analgesia or severity of side effects, over epidural morphine for postoperative analgesia after cesarean section.[24]

Epidural tramadol prolongs the time to first request for analgesia and decreases postoperative opioid and NSAID consumption compared with placebo.[25] There is no difference in efficacy between 100-mg and 200-mg doses of tramadol.

Diamorphine is a lipid-soluble derivative of morphine. It produces rapid and effective epidural analgesia, but its systemic absorption is high, and its duration of activity is limited to 6 to 8 hours. The addition of epinephrine to epidural diamorphine improves the quality of analgesia at 8 hours but does not reduce supplemental morphine consumption.[26] Diamorphine has a better analgesic profile than hydromorphone.[27]

The mixed agonist-antagonist opioids offer two theoretical advantages when administered into the epidural space. First, they may selectively activate κ opioid receptors that modulate visceral nociception. Second, a ceiling effect for respiratory depression may exist, which should limit the reduction in respiratory drive even if molecules spread rostrally to the brainstem. However, Camann et al[28] were unable to demonstrate any clinical advantage of given epidural over intravenous administration of butorphanol.[28] Abboud et al[29] reported that epidural butorphanol provided comparable analgesia with less pruritus and respiratory depression than epidural morphine; they used a high dose of morphine, which may have influenced the incidence of side effects.

Opioid Combinations

The administration of morphine in combination with a lipophilic opioid may offer some advantages. The rapid onset of analgesia with the lipophilic opioids may compensate for the latency of morphine, providing better intraoperative analgesia and a smooth transition during regression of regional anesthesia. The combination of epidural morphine (2–4 mg) with either fentanyl (100 μg) or sufentanil (20–30 μg) provides effective analgesia of rapid onset and extended duration without any increase in unwanted effects.[30–32] Nalbuphine used in combination with hydromorphone produces effective analgesia with less nausea than hydromorphone alone.[33] The addition of butorphanol to epidural morphine significantly reduces pruritus and nausea and tends to decrease the incidence of respiratory depression without altering the analgesic profile.[34]

NONOPIOID AGENTS

Epidural neostigmine produces modest dose-independent analgesia in women after cesarean delivery.[35] Neostigmine also produces mild sedation for several hours, limiting its role for single-bolus administration after cesarean delivery.

PCEA clonidine in combination with sufentanil reduces opiate requirements and tends to improve postoperative analgesia.[36]

The addition of 1/200,000 epinephrine to a single dose of epidural opioid hastens the onset and prolongs the duration of analgesia after cesarean section.[37,38] However, addition of epinephrine to PCEA meperidine does not improve analgesia but does increase side effects.[39]

PATIENT-CONTROLLED EPIDURAL ANALGESIA

The prolonged latency and risk of delayed respiratory depression with morphine render it less suitable for PCEA. For this reason, the more lipophilic opioids have been evaluated for use in this setting. PCEA with meperidine produces effective analgesia and is superior to IV-PCA using meperidine, epidural morphine, and PCEA with fentanyl.[40–42] In one study, PCEA fentanyl produced better analgesia with less postoperative nausea and drowsiness, but had an earlier onset of pruritus, in comparison with IV-PCA morphine.[43] In contrast, PCEA with fentanyl alone offered no analgesic advantage over a single dose of 3 mg epidural morphine.[44] The addition of a background infusion to PCEA has no clinical benefit; drug consumption is increased without improving analgesia (Table 23–2).[45–47]

The use of local anesthetic agents as sole agents for PCEA results in significant motor effects.[48,49] In contrast, PCEA

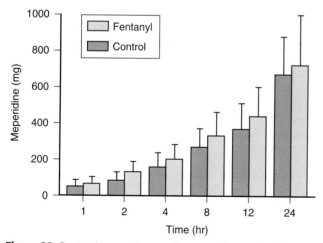

Figure 23–3 Total meperidine requirements after epidural fentanyl or normal saline injection. Epidural fentanyl produces analgesia of limited duration and does not influence IV-PCA requirements after cesarean section. (From Sevarino FB, McFarlane C, Sinatra RS: Epidural fentanyl does not influence intravenous PCA requirements in the post-caesarean patient. Can J Anaesth 1991;39:450–453.)

TABLE 23–2	Advantages of Patient-Controlled Epidural Analgesia
Over epidural opioid bolus/infusion	Patient control and autonomy Greater patient satisfaction Less anxiety Reduced opioid requirement
Over intravenous patient-controlled analgesia	Increased efficacy of analgesia Greater patient satisfaction Less sedation Reduced opioid requirement

with a combination of fentanyl, bupivacaine, and epinephrine produces greater analgesia with fewer side effects than PCEA with fentanyl alone.[50] PCEA with bupivacaine and sufentanil was found to produce better-quality analgesia with less nausea and vomiting than IT morphine.[51] These findings demonstrate the superior analgesic and side effect profile of a multidrug approach to neuraxial analgesia, compared with the use of opioids alone. However, these techniques are more expensive, mainly because of the more expensive equipment required for PCEA.[51]

Intrathecal Analgesic Agents

The emergence of spinal anesthesia as the first-choice anesthetic technique for cesarean section[2] renders IT opioid administration an attractive option for the provision of postoperative pain relief (see Box 23–1). The knowledge that 50% of patients who are given local anesthetic alone for both spinal and epidural analgesia experience visceral pain further promotes the use of IT opioids.[52]

INTRATHECAL OPIOID ADMINISTRATION

Morphine produces high-quality analgesia, with an onset time of 30 minutes, peak analgesic effect at 45-60 minutes, and duration of action of 18 to 24 hours (Table 23–3; Fig. 23–4).[53–55] The side effect profile is similar to that seen with epidural morphine, but the dose requirements are lower, reflecting the potency gain associated with subarachnoid injection of drug. This feature is of particular benefit for women in whom accumulation of opioids in breast milk may be of concern.

Multiple studies and a meta-analysis report that the IT administration of morphine 100 μg produces excellent analgesia with a minimal side effect profile (Fig. 23–5).[54–59] Raising the dose above 100 μg does not enhance analgesia (see Fig. 23–4)[55–58] and may increase the incidence of side effects, particularly pruritus (Fig. 23–6).[55,56,58] Minimal evidence of respiratory depression has been reported with 100 μg IT morphine.[54] In contrast, the incidence of nausea and vomiting after intrathecal morphine does not appear to be dose related,[55,56] although findings of some studies disagree.[57,58] There appears to be little advantage to decreasing the dose of intrathecal morphine below 100 μg. Although 75 μg IT morphine does produce significant analgesia, 50 μg does not appear to produce a clinically relevant analgesic effect (see Fig. 23–4).[55,56] The provision of optimal analgesia in this patient group appears to require opioid agonism at both spinal and supraspinal sites. In this regard, the provision of IV-PCA morphine facilitates the supraspinal opioid agonism necessary for maximal opioid-induced analgesia.[56]

Diamorphine

A lipid-soluble derivative of morphine, diamorphine is commonly used in the United Kingdom. It provides a rapid onset and long duration of analgesia owing to the action of its active metabolites, 6 mono-acetylmorphine and morphine. Diamorphine is similar in duration of action to morphine within the spinal cord, and similar in potency.[60] The lipid solubility of diamorphine decreases its onset of action and the likelihood of rostral spread's causing respiratory depression. The intrathecal administration of 200 μg of diamorphine produced comparable analgesia but less pruritus and drowsiness than 200 μg morphine.[60] A dose-finding study reported that both 250 μg and 375 μg IT diamorphine produced greater analgesia than did 125 μg.[61] The incidence and severity of pruritus and vomiting were dose related, but no evidence of respiratory depression was detected.[61] The use of 0.5-mg and 1-mg doses of IT diamorphine as sole postoperative opiate analgesic in combination with rectal diclofenac has been reported.[62]

Short-Acting Lipophilic Opioids

The primary advantage of spinally administered lipid-soluble opioids such as fentanyl and sufentanil is that they improve analgesia during cesarean section, because the duration of postoperative analgesia is limited (see Fig. 23–4).[55] In a meta-analysis, Dahl et al[55] found that although intrathecal doses of fentanyl greater than 6.25 μg did increase the time to requirement for supplemental analgesia, neither fentanyl nor sufentanil provided clinically useful postoperative analgesia.[55]

TABLE 23–3	Characteristics of Intrathecal Opioids for Cesarean Delivery			
Opioid	**Dose**	**Onset (min)**	**Peak Effect (min)**	**Duration (hr)**
Morphine	0.1–0.3 mg	30	60	18–24
Fentanyl	10–20 μg	5	10	2–4
Sufentanil	5–10 μg	5	10	2–4
Meperidine	10 mg	10	15	4–5

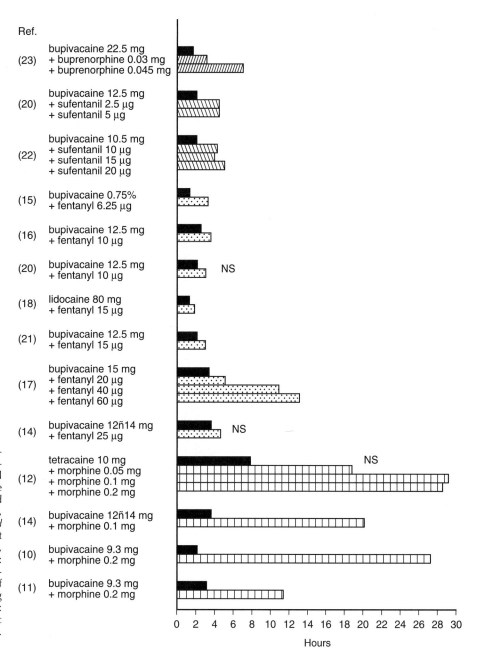

Figure 23–4 Time to first administration (hours) of postoperative supplemental analgesia in patients receiving spinal anesthesia with local anesthetic alone (*solid bars*) or local anesthetic combined with buprenorphine, sufentanil, fentanyl, or morphine in varying doses (*patterned bars*). NS, no statistically significant difference from control. (From Dahl JB, Jeppesen IS, Jorgensen H, et al: Intraoperative and postoperative analgesic efficacy and adverse effects of intrathecal opioids in patients undergoing cesarean section with spinal anesthesia: A qualitative and quantitative systematic review of randomized controlled trials. Anesthesiology 1999;91:1919–1927.)

The quality of postoperative analgesia provided by the IT administration of 25 μg fentanyl is inferior to that with 100 μg morphine and not different from that of placebo.[63] Fentanyl may produce meaningful analgesia at doses of 40 μg and 60 μg, but greater sedation and pruritus are seen in this higher dose range.[64] IT sufentanil, at doses of 2.5 μg and 5 μg, has been demonstrated to diminish the consumption of postoperative supplemental analgesics in the first 6 hours postoperatively but has no effect thereafter.[65]

Meperidine

IT meperidine 10 mg provides effective postoperative analgesia of intermediate duration (4-5 hours) after cesarean section.[66]

Although data are limited, there appears to be no advantage to the use of 20 mg versus 10 mg of IT meperidine.[67]

Other Opioids

The demonstration that IT butorphanol is neurotoxic in sheep has limited its clinical use.[68] To our knowledge, there are no reports of IT methadone use in this patient population after cesarean section.

Opioid Combinations

The administration of a highly lipid soluble drug together with IT morphine allows the advantageous combination of a short onset time of lipophilic drug and the longer duration

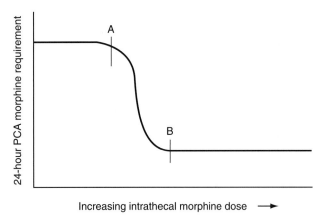

Figure 23–5 Hypothetical shape of the dose-response curve for intrathecal morphine dose plotted against patient-controlled analgesia (PCA) morphine use. A, 0.075 mg morphine; B, 0.1 mg morphine. (From Palmer CM, Emerson S, Volgoropolous D, Alves D: Dose-response relationship of intrathecal morphine for postcesarean analgesia. Anesthesiology 1999;90:437–444.)

of a hydrophilic drug.[69] This is disputed, and use of these opioid combinations by the IT route may increase the incidence of side effects with little analgesic benefit.[63] Furthermore, the combination of morphine and fentanyl does not appear to provide better postoperative analgesia than morphine alone.[69] In contrast, the IT administration of morphine 150 μg in combination with the more rapidly acting meperidine 10 mg may provide more uniform analgesia without any period of inadequate pain relief between the

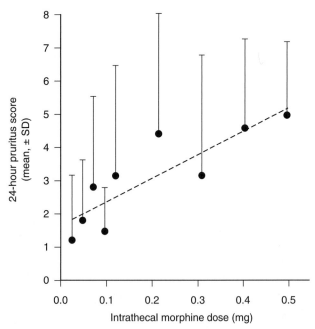

Figure 23–6 Mean 24-hour pruritus score for the different intrathecal morphine doses (mean, ± SD). Groups were significantly different; P = .003. The *dashed line* represents the trend toward a higher pruritus score with rising intrathecal morphine dose (linear regression analysis; P = .001). (From Palmer CM, Emerson S, Volgoropolous D, Alves D: Dose-response relationship of intrathecal morphine for postcesarean analgesia. Anesthesiology 1999;90:437–444.)

regression of local anesthetic block and the onset of morphine's analgesic effect.[66]

NONOPIOID AGENTS

IT administration of neostigmine inhibits the metabolism of spinally released acetylcholine and produces analgesia without pruritus or respiratory depression. Doses of 10, 30, and 100 μg produced dose-independent decreases in morphine use for 10 hours postoperatively in an open-label dose-finding study.[70] No adverse fetal effects were detected.[70] In another study, the IT administration of neostigmine 25 μg provided analgesia similar to that of morphine 100 μg.[71] Of interest, the combination of neostigmine 12.5 μg and morphine 50 μg appeared to provide superior pain relief with the most favorable side effect profile.[71] Unfortunately, the incidence and severity of postoperative nausea and vomiting may well limit the clinical utility of IT neostigmine in this population.[70-72]

The addition of 0.2 mg epinephrine to a combination of hyperbaric bupivacaine with 200 μg morphine has been demonstrated to enhance intraoperative and postoperative analgesia.[73] The mechanism of action of epinephrine is unclear but appears to be independent of a vasoconstriction-mediated reduction in the absorption of bupivacaine from the subarachnoid space.[73]

IT administration of clonidine produces analgesia by inhibiting release of substance P, which attenuates nociceptive neuron activation in response to noxious stimuli. Clonidine provides effective postoperative analgesia when used either as a sole agent[74] or in combination with IT opioids[75] or neostigmine.[76] When used as a sole agent, clonidine 75 μg does not produce postoperative analgesia,[77] although 150 μg produces effective analgesia for several hours.[74] However, the side effects of IT clonidine, which include hypotension, postoperative nausea and vomiting, and sedation, are more likely with the higher dose.[74] The combination of morphine 100 μg and clonidine 60 μg produces superior postoperative analgesia than morphine 100 μg or clonidine 150 μg alone[75] but may increase intraoperative sedation and vomiting.[75] The combination of clonidine 150 μg and neostigmine 50 μg produces better postoperative analgesia that either agent alone.[76]

ADVERSE EFFECTS OF NEURAXIAL OPIOIDS

Pruritus, nausea, and vomiting are increased in patients receiving epidural and IT opioids. Pruritus is more common in the obstetrical patient than in any other patient group and constitutes the most common cause of patient dissatisfaction after the administration of neuraxial opioids. The incidence and severity of pruritus after IT morphine use is dose related, being more likely at doses greater than 100 μg.[55,56] Nausea may result from either rostral spread of the drug in the cerebrospinal fluid (CSF) to the brainstem or vascular uptake to the vomiting center and chemoreceptor trigger zone. Evidence for a dose-response relationship is unclear. For every 100 women receiving 0.1 mg IT morphine added to a spinal anesthetic, 43 patients experience pruritus, 10 experience nausea, and 12 experience nausea postoperatively.[55]

Respiratory depression is the most feared complication of neuraxial opioid administration. Delayed respiratory depression results from rostral spread of hydrophilic morphine to the brainstem through the CSF and may occur 6 to 10 hours after IT drug administration. Early-onset respiratory depression, occurring within 30 minutes, results from vascular uptake of lipophilic opioids; it is usually of lesser significance because it is more likely to occur in a high-visibility setting (operating room, post-anesthesia care unit).

Fortunately, respiratory depression is a rare event in this setting. Parturients have higher levels of the respiratory stimulant progesterone and are usually healthy. In their meta-analysis, Dahl et al[55] reported respiratory depression in one of 485 patients receiving IT opioids. Consequently, the pooled figure for numbers-needed-to-harm (NNH) due to IT opioid–induced respiratory depression was 476, which was not significantly different from that for the control group.[55] Another study reported respiratory depression only in markedly obese patients while asleep.[78] Abboud et al[54] reported no respiratory depression after IT administration of 100 µg morphine.[54] In contrast, significant respiratory depression was seen after parenteral administration of morphine in this study.[54] Notwithstanding these reassuring data, all patients receiving neuraxial opioids must be appropriately monitored in the postoperative period (Box 23–2).

Intravenous Patient-Controlled Analgesia

IV-PCA may be used either as a sole technique or in combination with administration of neuraxial agents. IV-PCA is the method of choice for the delivery of parenteral opiates, constituting the predominant analgesic technique after cesarean section performed with the use of general anesthesia.

EFFICACY

IV-PCA with morphine has been clearly demonstrated to provide superior postoperative analgesia in comparison with traditional intramuscular (IM) morphine regimens, as well as greater patient satisfaction, improved ambulation, and reduced sedation levels.[79–82] Although the quality of postoperative analgesia with IV-PCA may be inferior to that with

---

BOX 23–2 | **MONITORING OF RESPIRATORY FUNCTION AFTER NEURAXIAL OPIOIDS**

No universally accepted method.
Several noninvasive monitors have been advocated, e.g., pulse oximetry, end-tidal partial pressure carbon dioxide (P_{CO_2}), and apnea monitors.
Hourly assessment of respiratory rate is the most common form of monitoring.[48]
Onset of respiratory depression is more often slowly progressive, typically preceded by somnolence.
Greater surveillance needed in patients who are morbidly obese and in parturients receiving magnesium sulfate.
Vigilant nursing observation and documentation of an inadequate respiratory effort, a slow RR, or unusual somnolence is probably the best form of monitoring.

---

neuraxial techniques,[81–83] patient satisfaction tends to be higher with IV-PCA. In a comparison of IV-PCA diamorphine with PCEA diamorphine, pain scores fell more rapidly with PCEA and patients were less sedated during the first postoperative day, but overall satisfaction scores were higher with IV-PCA.[84] In fact, of all analgesic regimens, patient satisfaction levels tend to be the highest with IV-PCA. Most parturients who have undergone cesarean delivery appear to use IV-PCA to achieve adequate, but not complete, analgesia. Parturients seem willing to accept a lesser degree of analgesia in order to be more alert, have less nausea, and thus feel better able to interact with their infants. Other important benefits of IV-PCA appear to be a lower incidence of opioid-mediated side effects, such as pruritus,[81–83] and a greater degree of patient control over these side effects.[84]

Significant pain may rapidly supervene after regression of the neuraxial blockade in patients receiving IV-PCA after they have undergone cesarean section with regional anesthesia.[85] An opioid "loading dose" should be administered to provide a baseline effective opioid plasma concentration in these patients. Serum levels can subsequently be maintained within a narrow therapeutic range by self-administered IV-PCA boluses. Otherwise, patients may not be able to generate sufficient plasma opioid levels to control their pain with IV-PCA alone, which may therefore fail to provide analgesia for them (Table 23–4).

OPIOID DRUG ALTERNATIVES

Morphine, the opioid of choice for IV-PCA, has been clearly demonstrated to be more effective than either meperidine[86,87] or fentanyl (Table 23–5).[88] In a nonrandomized study of IV-PCA and IM morphine and meperidine analgesic regimens after cesarean delivery, morphine was more effective than meperidine regardless of route of administration. Pain relief was superior with the morphine regimens used and was positively associated with breast-feeding and infant rooming-in.[86] IV-PCA fentanyl provides inferior postoperative analgesia in comparison with IV-PCA morphine and consequently is not recommended for routine PCA use after cesarean section.[88]

In a randomized trial of IV-PCA with morphine, meperidine, or oxymorphone after cesarean delivery, patients receiving IV-PCA morphine had the lowest pain scores beyond 8 hours postoperatively but also had greater maternal sedation.[87] Oxymorphone produced rapid analgesia but had a high incidence of nausea and vomiting. Meperidine was associated with the worst pain on movement. In a small study of IV-PCA buprenorphine and morphine, buprenorphine was demonstrated to produce comparable analgesia with less sedation.[89] Therefore, oxymorphone and buprenorphine constitute useful alternatives for IV-PCA in situations in which one might wish to avoid morphine.

BASAL BACKGROUND INFUSION

The use of basal background infusions in combination with standard IV-PCA bolus regimens appears to be safe but does not confer any particular advantage after cesarean section.[90] In a comparison of IV-PCA bolus alone with bolus plus infusion in patients receiving either morphine or hydromorphone, the use of infusions decreased pain scores but did not

TABLE 23–4 **Troubleshooting Problems with IV-PCA Therapy**

Problem	Potential Causes	Solution to Cause	Comments
Failure to produce satisfactory analgesia	Failure to attain therapeutic plasma opioid concentrations	Administer a loading dose of opioid prior to or at the commencement of IV-PCA therapy Use adjunctive agents to reduce overall opioid consumption	IV-PCA alone generally insufficient to produce therapeutic levels of narcotic within a reasonable time frame, especially if no intraoperative narcotics administered[85]
	Failure to maintain therapeutic plasma opioid concentrations	Administer a background infusion of opioid Use adjunctive agents such as NSAIDs to cover periods of anticipated reduced use, e.g., sleep	Demonstrated to reduce pain scores but does not improve overall satisfaction score[90] Efficacy clearly demonstrated in the setting of post–cesarean section, e.g., for rectal diclofenac[96]
Discontinuation due to intolerable side effects	Severe PONV	Administer antiemetic therapy intraoperatively and on regular rather than on PRN basis during postoperative period Add antiemetics to PCA narcotic Use adjunctive agents to reduce overall opioid consumption	Produces superior PONV prophylaxis
	Severe pruritus	Administer antipruritic therapy on regular rather than PRN basis during postoperative period Use adjunctive agents to reduce overall opioid consumption	

IV, intravenous; NSAIDs, nonsteroidal anti-inflammatory drugs; PCA, patient-controlled analgesia; PONV, postoperative nausea and vomiting; PRN, as needed.

TABLE 23–5 **Advantages and Disadvantages of Different Opioids for Intravenous Patient-Controlled Analgesia**

Drug	Advantages	Disadvantages	Comments*
Morphine	High-quality analgesia[86,117] Little accumulation of morphine or its active metabolite, morphine-6-glucuronide, in colostrum[94] Little or no impairment of neonatal neurobehavior[91]	Associated with more maternal sedation than meperidine or oxymorphone[87]	Agent most commonly used Effective analgesic profile Maternal sedation is a disadvantage Safety in neonates of breast-feeding mothers well established
Buprenorphine	Analgesic profile comparable to morphine's[7]	Produces less sedation than morphine[7]	Potential alternative to morphine Advantage of causing less sedation
Meperidine	Maternal analgesia and overall satisfaction equivalent to morphine's in certain studies[93]	Less effective analgesic than morphine or oxymorphone in other studies[87] Concerns about normeperidine accumulation resulting in transient impairment of neonatal neurobehavior[93]	Should be avoided in breast-feeding mothers

influence patient satisfaction or diminish the requirement for self-administered boluses of opioids.[90]

USE IN COMBINATION WITH NEURAXIAL OPIOIDS

The use of neuraxial opioids at cesarean section followed by IV-PCA constitutes a common analgesic regimen that appears safe and well tolerated, with minimal effects on the neonates of breast-feeding mothers.[91]

SAFETY ISSUES

Maternal

The potential for IV-PCA techniques to cause respiratory depression is clear. Brose et al[92] studied oxyhemoglobin saturation in the first 24 hours after cesarean section in patients receiving epidural morphine, IV-PCA meperidine, or IM meperidine analgesia. Patients receiving IV-PCA meperidine spent the longest cumulative time with pulse oximetry oxygen saturation (SpO_2) values between 91% and 95% and between 86% and 90%. However, the incidence of severe desaturation episodes, defined as SpO_2 less than or equal to 85% for more than 30 seconds, was lowest in the IV-PCA group and highest in the epidural morphine group.[92]

Neonatal

The use of systemic opioids carries the potential for adverse fetal effects, most importantly respiratory depression, if the mother is breast-feeding. However, these risks appear to be low with IV-PCA. In this regard, IV-PCA morphine appears to possess advantages over meperidine.[93] The concentration of morphine and its active metabolite, morphine-6-glucuronide, in the colostrum of mothers receiving IV-PCA morphine is

very small.[94] In a randomized controlled clinical trial comparing IV-PCA morphine and IV-PCA meperidine after cesarean section, nursing infants exposed to meperidine were significantly less alert and less responsive to human orientation cues on their third day of life.[93] These findings were postulated to be due to accumulation of normeperidine, which may be of importance in low-birth-weight babies already prone to seizures.[91] In a follow-up study, the use of IV-PCA morphine, in combination with epidural morphine, resulted in no impairment of neonatal neurobehavior compared with neurobehavior in normal infants experiencing no drug exposure after vaginal delivery (Fig. 23–7).[91] The neonatal neurobehavioral effects of meperidine were transient, but IV-PCA morphine may be a better choice for the breast-feeding mother.

Nonsteroidal Anti-inflammatory Drugs

NSAIDs constitute an effective component of analgesic regimens for patients who have undergone cesarean section. These drugs exert an anti-inflammatory effect at the incision site and reduce uterine cramping pain via a depressant effect on uterine contractility. Multiple NSAIDs given by various routes of administration have been studied in this context, and considerable evidence supports their efficacy in terms of reduced postoperative pain (Fig. 23–8), decreased consumption of other analgesic agents, particularly opioid agents (Fig. 23–9), and diminished opioid-induced side effects.

Diclofenac is the best-studied NSAID in this context, and considerable evidence supports its analgesic efficacy. Diclofenac decreases both postoperative wound pain and uterine cramping pain in a dose-dependent manner after cesarean section.[95] The regular rectal administration of diclofenac (e.g., 150 mg daily in divided doses) is the most effective regimen; it has been demonstrated to improve

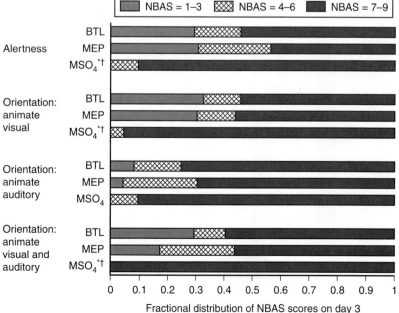

Figure 23–7 Four neurobehavioral outcomes (alertness; orientation: animate visual; orientation: animate auditory; and orientation: animate visual and auditory) among three neonatal groups. BTL, bottle-fed; MEP, exposed to meperidine in breast milk; MSO_4, exposed to morphine in breast milk. *Gray* represents the proportion of neonates within each group that achieved a Brazelton Neonatal Behavioral Assessment Scale (NBAS) score of 1–3; *cross-hatched bars* represent the proportion of neonates within each group that achieved a NBAS score of 4–6; *black bars* represent the proportion of neonates within each group that achieved a NBAS score of 7–9. *$P < .05$ versus meperidine group; †$P < .05$ versus bottle-fed group. (From Wittels B, Glosten B, Faure EA, et al: Postcesarean analgesia with both epidural morphine and intravenous patient-controlled analgesia: Neurobehavioral outcomes among nursing neonates. Anesth Analg 1997;85:600–606.)

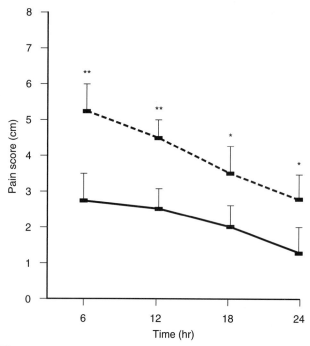

Figure 23–8 Mean (±SD) pain scores in patients in the tenoxicam (*solid line*) and control (*dashed line*) groups. *$P < .05$; **$P < .001$. (From Elhakim M, Nafie M: I.V. tenoxicam for analgesia during caesarean section. Br J Anaesth 1995;74:643–646.)

postoperative pain relief and to decrease morphine usage (by 39% to 46%, depending on dose) and opioid-induced side effects in the first 24 hours after cesarean section.[96–98] Single-dose rectal diclofenac, administered immediately postoperatively, is beneficial but less effective; it reduces supplemental analgesic requirements by 33% but does not improve postoperative pain relief or patient satisfaction, in the first 24 postoperative hours.[99,100] In contrast, the preoperative administration of single-dose rectal diclofenac 100 mg was found in one study to decrease postoperative wound pain and uterine cramping pain and to reduce supplemental opioid use in the first 24 hours after cesarean section.[95] In another study, the postoperative IM administration of 75 mg diclofenac improved pain relief and decreased sedation and opioid use by 33% in the first 18 hours postoperatively.[101] When combined, IM tramadol 100 mg and diclofenac 75 mg appear to act synergistically by preventing both primary and secondary hyperalgesia after cesarean section.[102]

Ketorolac may be administered either IV or IM, in doses up to 120 mg over 24 hours. It decreases postoperative pain and reduces narcotic usage by 30% to 50%, depending on dose and specific study, in the first 24 hours after cesarean section (Fig. 23–10).[103,104] Gin et al[105] found that administration of 30 mg IM ketorolac in the post-anesthesia care unit provided duration and quality of analgesia comparable to that provided by 75 mg IM meperidine with fewer side effects (nausea, dizziness) after elective cesarean section with general anesthesia.[105] Ketorolac (60 mg IV 1 hour after

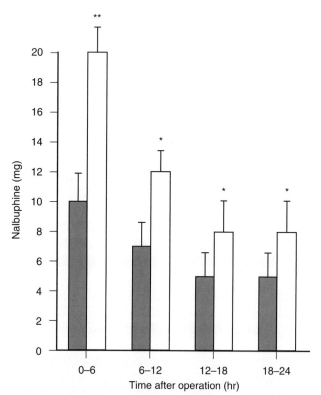

Figure 23–9 Mean (±SD) hourly consumption of nalbuphine in the tenoxicam (*shaded bar*) and control (*open bar*) groups. *$P < .05$; **$P < .01$. (From Elhakim M, Nafie M: I.V. tenoxicam for analgesia during caesarean section. Br J Anaesth 1995;74:643–646.)

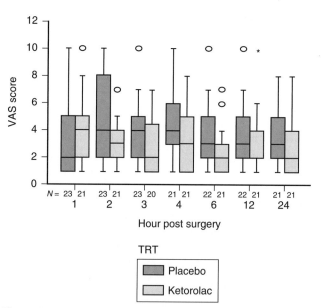

Figure 23–10 Box plot of visual analogue scales (VAS) postoperatively showing the median scores at each of the individual data collection points. The top and bottom of each box are the upper and lower quartiles. The *black line* between the top and bottom of the box is at the median. The area represents the range of scores for the middle 50% of subjects from the top to the bottom of the box. *Vertical lines* extend to the extremes, with outliers plotted separately. (From Lowder JL, Shackelford DP, Holbert D, Beste TM: A randomized, controlled trial to compare ketorolac tromethamine versus placebo after cesarean section to reduce pain and narcotic usage. Am J Obstet Gynecol 2003;189:1559–1562.)

spinal injection, and 30 mg IV every 6 hours for three doses) achieved a postoperative analgesic profile comparable to that seen with spinal morphine 0.1 mg, but with fewer opioid-induced side effects.[106]

Rectal indomethacin (200 mg immediately postoperatively followed by 100 mg 12 hourly for six doses) improved postoperative pain relief, increased the time to first request for supplemental analgesia, and decreased supplemental analgesic requirements on the first postoperative day after cesarean delivery performed with spinal anesthesia.[107] A retrospective study found that rectal indomethacin resulted in a 28% reduction in narcotic use after cesarean delivery with regional anesthesia.[108]

Intravenous tenoxicam (20 mg immediately after clamping of the umbilical cord) decreased 24-hour morphine consumption by approximately 30% and reduced the intensity of uterine cramping pain, but did not diminish wound pain at rest or with movement.[109] Preoperative administration of tenoxicam, however, improved postoperative analgesic profile, increased the time to first request for supplemental analgesia, reduced opioid consumption by 50%, and decreased sedation in the first 24 hours after cesarean delivery (see Figs. 23–8 and 23–9).[110]

Oral ketoprofen (100 mg postoperatively and for up to 7 days) has been demonstrated to provide superior analgesia with fewer side effects than the combination of 650 mg acetaminophen plus 10 mg oxycodone hydrochloride.[111] Ketoprofen 50 mg has also been demonstrated to provide effective analgesia in this population.[112] Ketoprofen (200 mg over 24 hours) has been demonstrated to be as effective as diclofenac (150 mg over 24 hours) after elective cesarean section.[113] Indoprofen[114] and naproxen[115] have also been shown to provide effective analgesia in this population.

In summary, the effectiveness of NSAIDs as part of a multimodal analgesia strategy is clear. Diclofenac and ketorolac are best-studied in this regard. Unfortunately, the relative efficacies of different NSAIDs in this context are unclear, given the relative lack of comparative trials of different agents. The available evidence clearly supports the regular use of NSAIDs for all patients after cesarean section, in the absence of contraindications to their use. However, the potential for NSAIDs to contribute to uterine atony and hemorrhage, particularly when important risk factors are already present (e.g., twin gestation and performance of myomectomy)[110,113,116] must be borne in mind. Therefore, it may be preferable to wait until sustained uterine tone has been confirmed and intraoperative hemostasis secured before NSAIDs are administered.

Other Oral Adjunctive Agents

Acetaminophen is widely used as an adjunct for postoperative pain relief and may have benefits after cesarean section, although there are few studies of its use in this context. One small study did not demonstrate morphine-sparing effects with acetaminophen after cesarean section.[96] A systematic review of randomized controlled trials, however, demonstrated acetaminophen to decrease opioid analgesic use by 30% in postoperative patients.[117] In patients undergoing elective abdominal gynecological surgery, administration of acetaminophen in combination with an NSAID has a higher analgesic effect than administration of either drug alone.[118]

Conclusions

A large number of studies have focused on optimizing postoperative pain therapy for cesarean section. The use of single-shot neuraxial morphine, hydromorphone, or diamorphine, and PCEA opioid administration produces effective analgesia. However, the high incidence of side effects with these techniques, particularly nausea, vomiting, and pruritus, reduces overall patient satisfaction. IV-PCA morphine produces incomplete analgesia, but the lower incidence of opioid-mediated side effects and the greater degree of patient control with IV-PCA results in high patient satisfaction levels. The optimal approach to the provision of postoperative analgesia is to use a balanced multimodal approach. The use of low dose and/or combinations of short-acting and long-acting neuraxial opioids, with or without IV-PCA, further supplemented by NSAIDs and simple analgesics, may best provide high-quality analgesia with a low incidence of side effects.

REFERENCES

1. Gaiser RR: Changes in the provision of anesthesia for the parturient undergoing cesarean section. Clin Obstet Gynecol 2003;46:646–656.
2. Shibli KU, Russell IF: A survey of anaesthetic techniques used for caesarean section in the UK in 1997. Int J Obstet Anesth 2000;9:160–167.
3. Daley MD, Sandler AN, Turner KE, et al: A comparison of epidural and intramuscular morphine in patients following cesarean section. Anesthesiology 1990;72:289–294.
4. Yarnell RW, Polis T, Reid GN, et al: Patient-controlled analgesia with epidural meperidine after elective cesarean section. Reg Anesth 1992;17:329–333.
5. Negre I, Gueneron JP, Jamali SJ, et al: Preoperative analgesia with epidural morphine. Anesth Analg 1994;79:298–302.
6. Duale C, Frey C, Bolandard F, et al: Epidural versus intrathecal morphine for postoperative analgesia after Caesarean section. Br J Anaesth 2003;91:690–694.
7. Capogna G, Celleno D, Tomassetti M: Maternal analgesia and neonatal effects of epidural sufentanil for cesarean section. Reg Anesth 1989;14:282–287.
8. Palmer CM, Nogami WM, Van Maren G, Alves DM: Postcesarean epidural morphine: A dose-response study. Anesth Analg 2000;90:887–891.
9. Chumpathong S, Santawat U, Saunya P, et al: Comparison of different doses of epidural morphine for pain relief following cesarean section. J Med Assoc Thai 2002;(Suppl 3):S956–S962.
10. Sharar SR, Ready LB, Ross BK, et al: A comparison of postcesarean epidural morphine analgesia by single injection and by continuous infusion. Reg Anesth 1991;16:232–235.
11. Eisenach JC, Schlairet TJ, Dobson CE 2nd, Hood DH: Effect of prior anesthetic solution on epidural morphine analgesia. Anesth Analg 1991;73:119–123.
12. Karambelkar DJ, Ramanathan S: 2-Chloroprocaine antagonism of epidural morphine analgesia. Acta Anaesthesiol Scand 1997;41:774–778.
13. Camann WR, Hartigan PM, Gilbertson LI, et al: Chloroprocaine antagonism of epidural opioid analgesia: A receptor-specific phenomenon? Anesthesiology 1990;73:860–863.
14. Carvalho B, Riley E, Manvelian G, Gambling D: Management of postoperative pain following cesarean section with epidural sustained-release morphine (SKY0401). Anesthesiology 2003;99:A1165.
15. Cooper DW, Ryall DM, Desira WR: Extradural fentanyl for postoperative analgesia: Predominant spinal or systemic action? Br J Anaesth 1995;74:184–187.
16. Cohen S, Pantuck CB, Amar D, et al: The primary action of epidural fentanyl after cesarean delivery is via a spinal mechanism. Anesth Analg 2002;94:674–679.

17. Joris JL, Jacob EA, Sessler DI, et al: Spinal mechanisms contribute to analgesia produced by epidural sufentanil combined with bupivacaine for postoperative analgesia. Anesth Analg 2003;97:1446–1451.

18. Birnbach DJ, Johnson MD, Arcario T, et al: Effect of diluent volume on analgesia produced by epidural fentanyl. Anesth Analg 1989;68:808–810.

19. Grass JA, Sakima NT, Schmidt R, et al: A randomized, double-blind, dose-response comparison of epidural fentanyl versus sufentanil analgesia after cesarean section. Anesth Analg 1997;85:365–371.

20. Cohen S, Amar D, Pantuck CB, et al: Postcesarean delivery epidural patient-controlled analgesia: Fentanyl or sufentanil? Anesthesiology 1993;78:486–491.

21. Sevarino FB, McFarlane C, Sinatra RS: Epidural fentanyl does not influence intravenous PCA requirements in the post-caesarean patient. Can J Anaesth 1991;39:450–453.

22. Paech MJ: Epidural pethidine or fentanyl during caesarean section: A double-blind comparison. Anaesth Intensive Care 1989;17:157–165.

23. Ngan Kee WD, Lam KK, Chen PP, Gin T: Epidural meperidine after cesarean section: A dose-response study. Anesthesiology 1996;85:289–294.

24. Halpern SH, Arellano R, Preston R, et al: Epidural morphine vs hydromorphone in post-caesarean section patients. Can J Anaesth 1996;43:595–598.

25. Siddik-Sayyid S, Aouad-Maroun M, Sleiman D, et al: Epidural tramadol for postoperative pain after Cesarean section. Can J Anaesth 1999;46:731–735.

26. Roulson CJ, Bennett J, Shaw M, Carli F: Effect of extradural diamorphine on analgesia after caesarean section under subarachnoid block. Br J Anaesth 1993;71:810–813.

27. Haynes SR, Davidson I, Allsop JR, Dutton DA: Comparison of epidural methadone with epidural diamorphine for analgesia following caesarean section. Acta Anaesthesiol Scand 1993;37:375–380.

28. Camann WR, Loferski BL, Fanciullo GJ, et al: Does epidural administration of butorphanol offer any clinical advantage over the intravenous route? A double-blind, placebo-controlled trial. Anesthesiology 1992;76:216–220.

29. Abboud TK, Moore M, Zhu J, et al: Epidural butorphanol or morphine for the relief of post-cesarean section pain: Ventilatory responses to carbon dioxide. Anesth Analg 1987;66:887–893.

30. Tanaka M, Watanabe S, Endo T, et al: Combination of epidural morphine and fentanyl for postoperative analgesia. Reg Anesth 1991;16:214–217.

31. Dottrens M, Rifat K, Morel DR: Comparison of extradural administration of sufentanil, morphine and sufentanil-morphine combination after caesarean section. Br J Anaesth 1992;69:9–12.

32. Sinatra RS, Goldstein R, Sevarino FB: The clinical effectiveness of epidural bupivacaine, bupivacaine with lidocaine, and bupivacaine with fentanyl for labor analgesia. J Clin Anesth 1991;3:219–225.

33. Parker RK, Holtmann B, White PF: Patient-controlled epidural analgesia: Interactions between nalbuphine and hydromorphone. Anesth Analg 1997;84:757–763.

34. Lawhorn CD, McNitt JD, Fibuch EE, et al: Epidural morphine with butorphanol for postoperative analgesia after cesarean delivery. Anesth Analg 1991;72:53–57.

35. Kaya FN, Sahin S, Owen MD, Eisenach JC: Epidural neostigmine produces analgesia but also sedation in women after cesarean delivery. Anesthesiology 2004;100:381–385.

36. Vercauteren MP, Saldien V, Bosschaerts P, Adriaensen HA: Potentiation of sufentanil by clonidine in PCEA with or without basal infusion. Eur J Anaesthesiol 1996;13:571–576.

37. Dougherty TB, Baysinger CL, Henenberger JC, Gooding DJ: Epidural hydromorphone with and without epinephrine for post-operative analgesia after cesarean delivery. Anesth Analg 1989;68:318–322.

38. Ngan Kee WD, Ma ML, Khaw KS: Addition of adrenaline to pethidine for epidural analgesia after caesarean section. Anaesthesia 1997;52:853–857.

39. Ngan Kee WD, Khaw KS, Ma ML: The effect of the addition of adrenaline to pethidine for patient-controlled epidural analgesia after caesarean section. Anaesthesia 1998;53:1012–1016.

40. Goh JL, Evans SF, Pavy TJ: Patient-controlled epidural analgesia following caesarean delivery: A comparison of pethidine and fentanyl. Anaesth Intensive Care 1996;24:45–50.

41. Fanshawe MP: A comparison of patient controlled epidural pethidine versus single dose epidural morphine for analgesia after caesarean section. Anaesth Intensive Care 1999;27:610–614.

42. Paech MJ, Moore JS, Evans SF: Meperidine for patient-controlled analgesia after cesarean section: Intravenous versus epidural administration. Anesthesiology 1994;80:1268–1276.

43. Cooper DW, Saleh U, Taylor M, et al: Patient-controlled analgesia: Epidural fentanyl and i.v. morphine compared after caesarean section. Br J Anaesth 1999;82:366–370.

44. Yu PY, Gambling DR: A comparative study of patient-controlled epidural fentanyl and single dose epidural morphine for post-caesarean analgesia. Can J Anaesth 1993;40:416–420.

45. Ngan Kee WD, Khaw KS, Ma ML: Patient-controlled epidural analgesia after caesarean section using meperidine. Can J Anaesth 1997;44:702–706.

46. Vercauteren MP, Coppejans HC, ten Broecke PW, et al: Epidural sufentanil for postoperative patient-controlled analgesia (PCA) with or without background infusion: A double-blind comparison. Anesth Analg 1995;80:76–80.

47. Parker RK, Sawaki Y, White PF: Epidural patient-controlled analgesia: Influence of bupivacaine and hydromorphone basal infusion on pain control after cesarean delivery. Anesth Analg 1992;75:740–746.

48. Buggy DJ, Hall NA, Shah J, et al: Motor block during patient-controlled epidural analgesia with ropivacaine or ropivacaine/fentanyl after intrathecal bupivacaine for caesarean section. Br J Anaesth 2000;85:468–470.

49. Cooper DW, Ryall DM, McHardy FE, et al: Patient-controlled extradural analgesia with bupivacaine, fentanyl, or a mixture of both, after Caesarean section. Br J Anaesth 1996;76:611–615.

50. Cohen S, Lowenwirt I, Pantuck CB, et al: Bupivacaine 0.01% and/or epinephrine 0.5 microg/ml improve epidural fentanyl analgesia after cesarean section. Anesthesiology 1998;89:1354–1361.

51. Vercauteren M, Vereecken K, La Malfa M, et al: Cost-effectiveness of analgesia after Caesarean section: A comparison of intrathecal morphine and epidural PCA. Acta Anaesthesiol Scand 2002;46:85–89.

52. Alahuhta S, Kangas-Saarela T, Hollmen AI, Edstrom HH: Visceral pain during caesarean section under spinal and epidural anaesthesia with bupivacaine. Acta Anaesthesiol Scand 1990;34:95–98.

53. Abouleish E, Rawal N, Rashad MN: The addition of 0.2 mg subarachnoid morphine to hyperbaric bupivacaine for cesarean delivery: A prospective study of 856 cases. Reg Anesth 1991;16:137–140.

54. Abboud TK, Dror A, Mosaad P, et al: Mini-dose intrathecal morphine for the relief of post-cesarean section pain: Safety, efficacy, and ventilatory responses to carbon dioxide. Anesth Analg 1988;67:137–143.

55. Dahl JB, Jeppesen IS, Jorgensen H, et al: Intraoperative and postoperative analgesic efficacy and adverse effects of intrathecal opioids in patients undergoing cesarean section with spinal anesthesia: A qualitative and quantitative systematic review of randomized controlled trials. Anesthesiology 1999;91:1919–1927.

56. Palmer CM, Emerson S, Volgoropolous D, Alves D: Dose-response relationship of intrathecal morphine for postcesarean analgesia. Anesthesiology 1999;90:437–444.

57. Milner AR, Bogod DG, Harwood RJ: Intrathecal administration of morphine for elective Caesarean section: A comparison between 0.1 mg and 0.2 mg. Anaesthesia 1996;51:871–873.

58. Uchiyama A, Nakano S, Ueyama H, et al: Low dose intrathecal morphine and pain relief following caesarean section. Int J Obstet Anesth 1994;3:87–91.

59. Jiang CJ, Liu CC, Wu TJ, et al: Mini-dose intrathecal morphine for post-cesarean section analgesia. Ma Zui Xue Za Zhi 1991;29:683–689.

60. Husaini SW, Russell IF: Intrathecal diamorphine compared with morphine for postoperative analgesia after caesarean section under spinal anaesthesia. Br J Anaesth 1998;81:135–139.

61. Kelly MC, Carabine UA, Mirakhur RK: Intrathecal diamorphine for analgesia after caesarean section: A dose finding study and assessment of side-effects. Anaesthesia 1998;53:231–237.

62. Stacey R, Jones R, Kar G, Poon A: High-dose intrathecal diamorphine for analgesia after Caesarean section. Anaesthesia 2001;56:54–60.

63. Sibilla C, Albertazz P, Zatelli R, Martinello R: Perioperative analgesia for caesarean section: Comparison of intrathecal morphine and fentanyl alone or in combination. Int J Obstet Anesth 1997;6:43–48.

64. Belzarena SD: Clinical effects of intrathecally administered fentanyl in patients undergoing cesarean section. Anesth Analg 1992;74:653–657.

65. Dahlgren G, Hultstrand C, Jakobsson J, et al: Intrathecal sufentanil, fentanyl, or placebo added to bupivacaine for cesarean section. Anesth Analg 1997;85:1288–1293.

66. Chung JH, Sinatra RS, Sevarino FB, Fermo L: Subarachnoid meperidine-morphine combination: An effective perioperative analgesic adjunct for cesarean delivery. Reg Anesth 1997;22:119–124.
67. Feldman JM, Griffin F, Fermo L, Raessler K: Intrathecal meperidine for pain after cesarean delivery: Efficacy and dose-response. Anesthesiology 1992;77:A1011.
68. Rawal N, Nuutinen L, Raj PP, et al: Behavioral and histopathologic effects following intrathecal administration of butorphanol, sufentanil, and nalbuphine in sheep. Anesthesiology 1991;75:1025–1034.
69. Connelly NR, Dunn SM, Ingold V, Villa EA: The use of fentanyl added to morphine-lidocaine-epinephrine spinal solution in patients undergoing cesarean section. Anesth Analg 1994;78:918–920.
70. Krukowski JA, Hood DD, Eisenach JC, et al: Intrathecal neostigmine for post-cesarean section analgesia: Dose response. Anesth Analg 1997;84:1269–1275.
71. Chung CJ, Kim JS, Park HS, Chin YJ: The efficacy of intrathecal neostigmine, intrathecal morphine, and their combination for post-cesarean section analgesia. Anesth Analg 1998;87:341–346.
72. Klamt JG, Garcia LV, Prado WA: Analgesic and adverse effects of a low dose of intrathecally administered hyperbaric neostigmine alone or combined with morphine in patients submitted to spinal anaesthesia: Pilot studies. Anaesthesia 1999;54:27–31.
73. Abouleish E, Rawal N, Tobon-Randall B, et al: A clinical and laboratory study to compare the addition of 0.2 mg of morphine, 0.2 mg of epinephrine, or their combination to hyperbaric bupivacaine for spinal anesthesia in cesarean section. Anesth Analg 1993;77:457–462.
74. Filos KS, Goudas LC, Patroni O, Polyzou V: Intrathecal clonidine as a sole analgesic for pain relief after cesarean section. Anesthesiology 1992;77:267–274.
75. Paech MJ, Pavy TJ, Orlikowski CE, et al: Postcesarean analgesia with spinal morphine, clonidine, or their combination. Anesth Analg 2004;98:1460–1466.
76. Pan PM, Huang CT, Wei TT, Mok MS: Enhancement of analgesic effect of intrathecal neostigmine and clonidine on bupivacaine spinal anesthesia. Reg Anesth Pain Med 1998;23:49–56.
77. Benhamou D, Thorin D, Brichant JF, et al: Intrathecal clonidine and fentanyl with hyperbaric bupivacaine improves analgesia during cesarean section. Anesth Analg 1998;87:609–613.
78. Baraka A, Noueihid R, Hajj S: Intrathecal injection of morphine for obstetric analgesia. Anesthesiology 1981;54:136–140.
79. Perez-Woods R, Grohar JC, Skaredoff M, et al: Pain control after cesarean birth: Efficacy of patient-controlled analgesia vs traditional therapy (IM morphine). J Perinatol 1991;11:174–181.
80. Cade L, Ashley J, Ross AW: Comparison of epidural and intravenous opioid analgesia after elective caesarean section. Anaesth Intensive Care 1992;20:41–45.
81. Eisenach JC, Grice SC, Dewan DM: Patient-controlled analgesia following cesarean section: A comparison with epidural and intramuscular narcotics. Anesthesiology 1988;68:444–448.
82. Harrison DM, Sinatra RS, Morgese L, Chung JH: Epidural narcotic and patient-controlled analgesia for post-cesarean section pain relief. Anesthesiology 1988;68:454–457.
83. Cade L, Ashley J: Towards optimal analgesia after caesarean section: Comparison of epidural and intravenous patient-controlled opioid analgesia. Anaesth Intensive Care 1993;21:696–699.
84. Stoddart PA, Cooper A, Russell R, Reynolds F: A comparison of epidural diamorphine with intravenous patient-controlled analgesia using the Baxter infusor following caesarean section. Anaesthesia 1993;48:1086–1090.
85. Anwari JS, Butt A, Alkhunein S: PCA after subarachnoid block for cesarean section. Middle East J Anesthesiol 2004;17:913–926.
86. Yost NP, Bloom SL, Sibley MK, et al: A hospital-sponsored quality improvement study of pain management after cesarean delivery. Am J Obstet Gynecol 2004;190:1341–1346.
87. Sinatra RS, Lodge K, Sibert K, et al: A comparison of morphine, meperidine, and oxymorphone as utilized in patient-controlled analgesia following cesarean delivery. Anesthesiology 1989;70:585–590.
88. Howell PR, Gambling DR, Pavy T, et al: Patient-controlled analgesia following caesarean section under general anaesthesia: A comparison of fentanyl with morphine. Can J Anaesth 1995;42:41–45.
89. Capogna G, Celleno D, Sebastiani M, et al: [Continuous intravenous infusion with patient-controlled anesthesia for postoperative analgesia in cesarean section: morphine versus buprenorphine.] Minerva Anestesiol 1989;55:33–38.
90. Sinatra R, Chung KS, Silverman DG, et al: An evaluation of morphine and oxymorphone administered via patient-controlled analgesia (PCA) or PCA plus basal infusion in postcesarean-delivery patients. Anesthesiology 1989;71:502–507.
91. Wittels B, Glosten B, Faure EA, et al: Postcesarean analgesia with both epidural morphine and intravenous patient-controlled analgesia: Neurobehavioral outcomes among nursing neonates. Anesth Analg 1997;85:600–606.
92. Brose WG, Cohen SE: Oxyhemoglobin saturation following cesarean section in patients receiving epidural morphine, PCA, or IM meperidine analgesia. Anesthesiology 1989;70:948–953.
93. Wittels B, Scott DT, Sinatra RS: Exogenous opioids in human breast milk and acute neonatal neurobehavior: A preliminary study. Anesthesiology 1990;73:864–869.
94. Baka NE, Bayoumeu F, Boutroy MJ, Laxenaire MC: Colostrum morphine concentrations during postcesarean intravenous patient-controlled analgesia. Anesth Analg 2002;94:184–187.
95. Sia AT, Thomas E, Chong JL, Loo CC: Combination of suppository diclofenac and intravenous morphine infusion in post-caesarean section pain relief—a step towards balanced analgesia? Singapore Med J 1997;38:68–70.
96. Siddik SM, Aouad MT, Jalbout MI, et al: Diclofenac and/or propacetamol for postoperative pain management after cesarean delivery in patients receiving patient controlled analgesia morphine. Reg Anesth Pain Med 2001;26:310–315.
97. Rashid M, Jaruidi HM: The use of rectal diclofenac for post-cesarean analgesia. Saudi Med J 2000;21:145–149.
98. Olofsson CI, Legeby MH, Nygards EB, Ostman KM: Diclofenac in the treatment of pain after caesarean delivery: An opioid-saving strategy. Eur J Obstet Gynecol Reprod Biol 2000;88:143–146.
99. Lim NL, Lo WK, Chong JL, Pan AX: Single dose diclofenac suppository reduces post-Cesarean PCEA requirements. Can J Anaesth 2001;48:383–386.
100. Dennis AR, Leeson-Payne CG, Hobbs GJ: Analgesia after caesarean section: The use of rectal diclofenac as an adjunct to spinal morphine. Anaesthesia 1995;50:297–299.
101. Bush DJ, Lyons G, MacDonald R: Diclofenac for analgesia after caesarean section. Anaesthesia 1992;47:1075–1077.
102. Wilder-Smith CH, Hill L, Dyer RA, et al: Postoperative sensitization and pain after cesarean delivery and the effects of single IM doses of tramadol and diclofenac alone and in combination. Anesth Analg 2003;97:526–533.
103. Lowder JL, Shackelford DP, Holbert D, Beste TM: A randomized, controlled trial to compare ketorolac tromethamine versus placebo after cesarean section to reduce pain and narcotic usage. Am J Obstet Gynecol 2003;189:1559–1562.
104. Pavy TJ, Paech MJ, Evans SF: The effect of intravenous ketorolac on opioid requirement and pain after cesarean delivery. Anesth Analg 2001;92:1010–1014.
105. Gin T, Kan AF, Lam KK, O'Meara ME: Analgesia after caesarean section with intramuscular ketorolac or pethidine. Anaesth Intensive Care 1993;21:420–423.
106. Cohen SE, Desai JB, Ratner EF, et al: Ketorolac and spinal morphine for postcesarean analgesia. Int J Obstet Anesth 1996;5:14–18.
107. Pavy TJ, Gambling DR, Merrick PM, Douglas MJ: Rectal indomethacin potentiates spinal morphine analgesia after caesarean delivery. Anaesth Intensive Care 1995;23:555–559.
108. Ambrose FP: A retrospective study of the effect of postoperative indomethacin rectal suppositories on the need for narcotic analgesia in patients who had a cesarean delivery while they were under regional anesthesia. Am J Obstet Gynecol 2001;184:1544–1547.
109. Hsu HW, Cheng YJ, Chen LK, et al: Differential analgesic effect of tenoxicam on the wound pain and uterine cramping pain after cesarean section. Clin J Pain 2003;19:55–58.
110. Elhakim M, Nafie M: I.V. tenoxicam for analgesia during caesarean section. Br J Anaesth 1995;74:643–646.
111. Sunshine A, Olson NZ, Zighelboim I, De Castro A: Ketoprofen, acetaminophen plus oxycodone, and acetaminophen in the relief of postoperative pain. Clin Pharmacol Ther 1993;54:546–555.
112. Sunshine A, Zighelboim I, Laska E, et al: A double-blind, parallel comparison of ketoprofen, aspirin, and placebo in patients with postpartum pain. J Clin Pharmacol 1986;26:706–711.

113. Rorarius MG, Suominen P, Baer GA, et al: Diclofenac and ketoprofen for pain treatment after elective caesarean section. Br J Anaesth 1993;70:293–297.

114. Sunshine A, Zighelboim I, Olson NZ, et al: A comparative oral analgesic study of indoprofen, aspirin, and placebo in postpartum pain. J Clin Pharmacol 1985;25:374–380.

115. Angle PJ, Halpern SH, Leighton BL, et al: A randomized controlled trial examining the effect of naproxen on analgesia during the second day after cesarean delivery. Anesth Analg 2002;95:741–745.

116. Diemunsch P, Alt M, Diemunsch AM, Treisser A: Post cesarean analgesia with ketorolac tromethamine and uterine atonia. Eur J Obstet Gynecol Reprod Biol 1997;72:205–206.

117. Moore A, Collins S, Carroll D, McQuay H: Paracetamol with and without codeine in acute pain: A quantitative systematic review. Pain 1997;70:193–201.

118. Montgomery JE, Sutherland CJ, Kestin IG, Sneyd JR: Morphine consumption in patients receiving rectal paracetamol and diclofenac alone and in combination. Br J Anaesth 1996;77:445–447.

24 Postoperative Pain Management for Patients with Drug Dependence

SRDJAN S. NEDELJKOVIĆ • AJAY D. WASAN

It is paradoxical to many practitioners that some of the patients most difficult to treat for postoperative pain are those who take the highest quantities of opioids. However, long-term opioid use has been associated with increased pain sensitivity,[1] and hyperalgesia has been found to occur in patients who take methadone and heroin long term.[2,3] Therefore, it is not surprising that patients who take opioids chronically will have a greater response to surgical pain. As the use of prescription opioids to manage chronic pain has increased, the chances that a patient undergoing surgery will have been taking high doses of opioids preoperatively has grown over the past two decades.[4,5] Some patients who take prescription opioids for chronic pain present with a history of taking escalating doses in the period leading up to surgery. On occasion, patients who are engaged in the illicit use of drugs present for surgery. Management of postoperative pain in patients who are dependent on drugs presents a significant challenge.

Broadly, patients who are drug dependent can be mismanaged in terms of control of postoperative pain in the following two ways: (1) they can be overtreated with excessive doses of analgesics or (2) they can be undertreated, resulting in inadequate pain relief and suffering. In addition to relieving pain, goals of treatment in the postoperative setting include maximizing functional advances and achieving rapid recovery of bowel function while minimizing side effects of analgesic therapy. Overtreatment of the drug-dependent patient can lead to adverse effects such as excessive sedation and can impede recovery from surgery. Patients with chronic pain who are overtreated may be discharged from the hospital on higher doses of narcotics than they required before surgery, possibly making outpatient management of their chronic pain syndrome more difficult. More commonly, patients who are drug dependent are undertreated in the postoperative period, sometimes because of fears of addiction, and are therefore at risk of experiencing excessive pain and psychological suffering.

In order to optimize pain management for the drug-dependent patient, it is important to know the concepts and definitions of dependence, tolerance, and addiction. The basis of substance abuse and the signs and symptoms of this disorder must be recognized. Pharmacological considerations, based on the substances that are administered, such as opioids, benzodiazepines, alcohol, cocaine, and other drugs, must be understood. Medical problems associated with substance abuse must be considered, including hepatitis, human immunodeficiency virus infection, and associated psychiatric disorders. Finally, the practitioner should develop a coordinated perioperative plan for how to manage postoperative pain, addressing the patient's physical and psychological needs. This plan should be discussed with the patient and other caregivers before surgery. Overall, an integrated approach should be taken by all members of the perioperative team in managing these challenging patients.

Concepts and Definitions of Drug Dependence and Substance Abuse

Patients undergoing surgery may be drug dependent because of legitimate medical needs, such as chronic pain, psychiatric conditions, or oncological syndromes. Common prescription drugs that cause dependence are the opioid analgesics and benzodiazepines. Other patients may be substance-abusing individuals who use prescription drugs illicitly or use illegal drugs such as heroin, cocaine, and marijuana. A key challenge in managing postoperative pain for patients who are drug dependent is to distinguish what form this dependence takes for the patient: Is the patient dependent on drugs only in the physiological sense, or is the patient drug addicted? Therefore, it is necessary to understand the different meaning of these two terms.

Physical dependence is a form of neurophysiological adaptation that occurs when a patient is exposed to various drugs, including opioids, benzodiazepines, certain antihypertensive medications, and tricyclic antidepressants. This is a physiological response that develops through pharmacodynamic substrate-receptor relationships. Patients who are dependent on such drugs exhibit an abstinence syndrome when these drugs are withdrawn. When opioids are abruptly discontinued, the abstinence syndrome involves signs and symptoms such as hypertension, tachycardia, diarrhea, insomnia, and other signs of psychomotor agitation. Studies have shown that there may be increased levels of norepinephrine available in the brain in patients who are experiencing opioid withdrawal.[6]

Many patients who take opioids or benzodiazepines chronically will become dependent on these drugs and exhibit withdrawal symptoms if the drugs are withheld. Reduced levels of dopamine receptors have been shown to persist for months after drug withdrawal,[7] a finding that may explain why some patients experience cravings for drugs long after the metabolism and elimination of the drug. Drugs with long half-lives, such as methadone, may be associated with a 6- to 8-week withdrawal period after discontinuation.[8]

Addiction describes the intermittent or constant craving for a drug to obtain pleasure or a sense of reward. It is marked by compulsive use of legal and/or illegal substances. Patients who are addicted often use a drug despite its harmful consequences and are preoccupied with efforts to obtain it. There is a loss of control in using the drug, and patients cannot regulate when or how much drug they consume. Addiction is considered a chronic, relapsing, and remitting psychiatric illness. Between episodes of addiction behaviors, patients can have years of "clean time" or sobriety in which the only consequence of their illness is a vulnerability to addiction if exposed to substances of abuse. Patients with a history of drug addiction are prone to recurrences that can overwhelm all their efforts to rigorously control their behavior. Despite long periods of

abstinence from drugs of abuse, alterations in neural mechanisms have been found that support the premise that an addiction disorder represents a lifelong susceptibility that can be reactivated even after a long time.[9,10]

There is substantial evidence that addiction is a brain disease, and it is now understood that addiction is primarily a neurobiological disorder. Exposure to a potential substance of abuse may cause a "switch" in the brain of a susceptible patient that changes the exposed patient's behavior from voluntary to compulsive.[11,12] After drug exposure and with repeated use, patients may lose the ability to regulate their drug-taking behaviors. In these patients, substances can "hijack" motivational priorities, perpetuating compulsive use (Fig. 24–1). Functional changes are seen in the dopamine-mediated reward system of the brain, such as in the left prefrontal cortex and the nucleus accumbens.[13] Feelings of euphoria and pleasure related to cocaine or methylphenidate use have been associated with increased dopamine levels in the brain.[7] Also, natural pleasure-inducing activities, such as eating, drinking, and having sex, have been found to stimulate the release of dopamine—similar to the release seen with euphoria caused by addictive drugs.[14] When opioids, stimulants, and ethanol are withdrawn, levels of dopamine in the nucleus

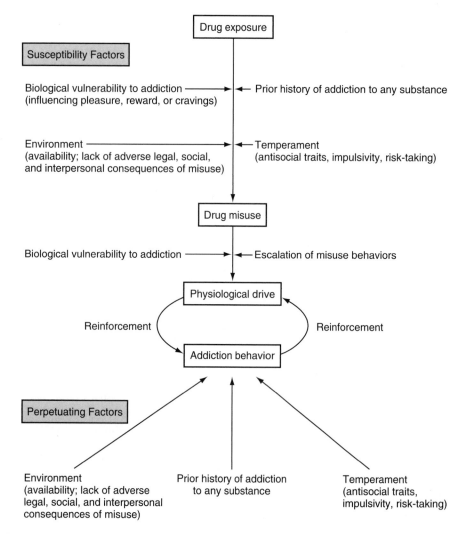

Figure 24–1 Pathway of addiction. (Adapted from Nedeljković SS, Wasan A, Jamison RN: Assessment of efficacy of long-term opioid therapy in pain patients with substance abuse potential. Clin J Pain 2002;18:S39–S51.)

accumbens drop.[15] Thus, the dopamine system is an important component of the reward-and-reinforcement mechanism that sustains an addiction.

Changes and neuroadaptations in the brain can result from repeated drug exposure. In most cases, repeated use is required to precipitate changes in brain function that are found in addiction. However, in some susceptible individuals, even brief exposure may be enough to instigate a permanent addictive disease. Addiction may be a heritable disorder, as genetic differences have been found in the endogenous opioid peptides and opioid receptors in the nervous system of animals prone to addictive behaviors.[12] The brain changes seen with opioid addiction have also been observed with amphetamines, cocaine, nicotine, and alcohol. This is termed *cross-addiction.* If a patient is dependent on one substance, there is a higher chance of addiction to other substances.[16] In addition, there is a high correlation between addictive drug use and other reward-seeking behaviors, such as smoking, gambling, impulsivity, and a history of experiencing multiple physical trauma.[12] Along with genetic and biological factors, social and environmental factors such as poor psychosocial support and drug availability play a role in the vulnerability to addiction.

Tolerance is a phenomenon by which patients require increasing amounts of a drug to achieve the same pharmacological effect. In a tolerant patient, a higher dose of an analgesic or psychoactive drug is necessary to produce the desired effect. Tolerance likely has a genetic basis and involves desensitization of the opioid receptors.[17] It is a normal physiological event, and its presence does not imply that a patient has lost control of the ability to regulate drug use. Tolerance occurs with most of the effects of opioids, with the exception of miosis and constipation. Tolerance to some of the side effects of opioid drugs can be advantageous, because tolerant patients are less likely to experience pruritus, sedation, or respiratory depression when given additional opioids. However, patients taking opioids over the long term may also become tolerant to their analgesic effects and to the effects of standard doses of opioids used for pain control in the postoperative period. Although the development of tolerance to the analgesic effects of opioids may be variable in its presentation and onset time, some studies have found that it occurs even after short exposure to these drugs.[18] Tolerance is more likely to develop in cases of prolonged duration of exposure and with higher doses of drugs. Drugs that are more potent (have a high intrinsic efficacy), like sufentanil, result in tolerance more slowly than those less-potent drugs (those with a low intrinsic efficacy), like morphine.[19] Dealing with issues of drug tolerance is an important aspect of postoperative pain management in drug-dependent patients, especially for those who are tolerant to the analgesic effects of opioids.

In the evaluation and management of postoperative pain in the drug-dependent patient, it is important to understand the differences and implications of dependence, addiction, and tolerance. Both tolerance and withdrawal responses can increase drug taking and support addiction behaviors. To avoid the abstinence syndrome in the perioperative period, drugs that can cause withdrawal reactions should be continued. Either the drug in question or an equivalent drug should be provided to all patients, regardless of whether they are abusing the drug or using it for legitimate needs. Patients who are tolerant to the effects of opioids may require higher doses of opioids to achieve analgesia. Because there is incomplete cross-tolerance between different opioids, some patients may benefit from the use of an opioid that is new to them. Patients should be asked about their history of drug addiction. Drug dosages should not be inappropriately escalated in patients who have had a history of substance abuse, and the goal should be to return to preoperative doses of drugs used for chronic pain or for addiction maintenance once the typical postoperative period has passed. More detailed recommendations on management of drug-dependent patients are given in "Perioperative Plan for the Drug-Dependent Patient."

Pharmacological Considerations for the Drug-Dependent Patient

The chances of encountering a drug-dependent patient undergoing surgery are substantial. Overall, the lifetime prevalence for alcohol abuse in the United States is estimated to be 14%, with more than 50% of these individuals in long-term abstinence.[20,21] For other drug addictions, the lifetime prevalence is 7%, with approximately 30% to 50% of these patients in long-term abstinence.[20,21] Patients who undergo surgery may be dependent on various types of drugs, including opioids, alcohol, sedatives (benzodiazepines and barbiturates), and stimulants, and they may also have developed a "habit" for marijuana. Each of these drug categories may manifest itself in different ways and presents challenges for the treating physician after surgery. Therefore, it is important to understand the symptoms and pharmacological considerations related to the use of each of these drugs.

ALCOHOL

Abuse and chronic use of alcohol constitute the most likely drug dependence problem to be encountered. It is estimated that more than 8 million persons in the United States are dependent on alcohol, compared with about 3.5 million who use illicit drugs (primarily heroin and stimulants).[22] Approximately 15% to 20% of patients who are hospitalized or who are in a primary care setting have a history of alcohol problems.[23] Low doses of alcohol may have a stimulant effect, suppressing central nervous system inhibitory systems. At higher doses, alcohol causes greater sedation and motor incoordination. Common signs and symptoms of alcohol withdrawal are nausea, tremulousness, insomnia, irritability, and a slight rise in body temperature. A rare consequence of alcohol withdrawal is delirium tremens, which can result in seizures, hallucinations, and dangerously high blood pressure. Patients who abuse alcohol may also have liver dysfunction, which may cause altered metabolism of analgesic drugs as well as anemia and thrombocytopenia.

Because alcohol administration enhances the function of N-methyl-D-aspartate (NMDA) receptors, NMDA antagonists may be useful in treating alcohol withdrawal.[24] Alcohol withdrawal has been found to enhance neurotransmission in excitatory glutamate pathways.[25] Benzodiazepines, which stimulate the gamma-aminobutyric acid (GABA) receptor, as well as carbamazepine and valproate, can reduce symptoms of alcohol withdrawal.[26] The risk of seizures and delirium is reduced when these drugs are used.[27] β-adrenergic drugs and clonidine may reduce some of the autonomic signs of withdrawal. After the withdrawal period, and as a component of addiction treatment, the use of opioid antagonists such as naltrexone can reduce ethanol consumption.[28] In patients who are untreated, withdrawal symptoms from alcohol peak at 72 hours, although patients may have symptoms such as insomnia for weeks.[29] Pharmacological treatment of alcohol withdrawal is rarely necessary for more than a week.

SEDATIVES (BENZODIAZEPINES AND BARBITURATES)

Benzodiazepines increase the effects of GABA, an inhibitory neurotransmitter, resulting in an anxiolytic and sedative effect. Withdrawal symptoms are more likely when benzodiazepines are discontinued in patients who have taken higher doses, who take drugs with a short half-life, or who are treated with these drugs for longer periods. Also, patients who have symptoms of anxiety, depression, personality psychopathology, and panic disorder may be more likely to have difficulty withdrawing from these drugs.[30] Prolonged use of benzodiazepines can result in seizures if these drugs are abruptly discontinued. Patients often experience insomnia, irritability, headaches, and tremors when withdrawing from benzodiazepines. Perceptual disturbances and severe anxiety may result. Severe manifestations of benzodiazepine withdrawal include convulsions, confusion, and psychosis.

It is recommended that withdrawal from benzodiazepines be done slowly. Although the first 50% of the dose can be tapered over 2 to 4 weeks, tapering of the final 50% may take much longer.[30] Signs of benzodiazepine withdrawal usually begin 2 to 10 days after the drug is stopped.[29] Some experts recommend converting patients to long-acting benzodiazepines, such as diazepam or clonazepam, so that there are fewer withdrawal symptoms between doses. The abuse potential of shorter-acting benzodiazepines is greater than that of longer-acting agents.[31] Withdrawal from benzodiazepines may take up to 1 year. The use of antidepressants, such as trazodone and imipramine, and anticonvulsants, such as carbamazepine and valproate, may be helpful in benzodiazepine withdrawal protocols.[30] Psychotherapeutic approaches for the management of anxiety without medications may also be beneficial.

OPIOIDS

In the United States, more than 15,780,000 prescriptions were written for long-acting opioids in 2003,[32] and it is estimated that approximately 750,000 persons are dependent on heroin.[22] Most commonly abused are rapid-acting drugs that produce pleasurable feelings (oxycodone, hydromorphone, methadone, fentanyl).[33] Drugs that can be crushed, inhaled, or injected (all methods for increasing the speed of onset and potency of action) are more likely to be abused. In some cases, it may be difficult to distinguish a patient who is escalating opioid use because of worsening chronic pain symptoms from an addict who is preoccupied with drug-seeking behavior.

Repeated administration of opioids causes both physical dependence and tolerance. Withdrawal from opioids often manifests as diffuse body aches, abdominal cramps, anorexia, diarrhea, and insomnia. Patients may yawn frequently. They may exhibit cravings for their opioid of abuse, may have

sympathetic and parasympathetic arousal, and may exhibit dilated pupils, rhinorrhea, goose bumps on the flesh, agitation, and tachycardia. In contrast to alcohol withdrawal, opioid withdrawal does not lead to seizures.

Withdrawal symptoms related to opioid dependence are treated with drugs such as diphenoxylate atropine (Lomotil) to control diarrhea, benzodiazepines to control anxiety and agitation, and α_2 agonists and beta-blockers to control sympathomimetic symptoms. The timing of withdrawal symptoms depends on the pharmacology of the drug that is used. Patients who take heroin may experience the greatest symptoms of withdrawal 36 to 72 hours after stopping the drug, and withdrawal may last for 7 to 10 days. For those who take methadone, the peak of withdrawal symptoms is at 72 to 96 hours, and withdrawal can last for more than 2 weeks[29] and even as long as 6 or 7 weeks.

Pharmacological methods of managing opioid addiction, such as using methadone, buprenorphine, and other drugs, are detailed in "Treatments for Drug Dependence and Addiction." α_2 Agonists (tizanidine and clonidine) and other drugs, such as beta-blockers, are administered to block the adrenergic response to withdrawal.

STIMULANTS (AMPHETAMINES AND COCAINE)

Amphetamines are often taken to produce euphoria, and some people take them to increase alertness and concentration. It is estimated that about 1 million persons in the United States are dependent on amphetamines.[22] These drugs can increase heart rate and blood pressure and release cortisol. Their prolonged use can lead to aggressive and paranoid behaviors. If stimulant drugs are withdrawn rapidly, patients may experience feelings of depression in addition to insomnia and anorexia. Depression usually lasts up to 48 hours but may persist in a milder form for approximately 2 weeks.[29]

Cocaine, also used as a stimulant, can lead to paranoid thoughts and a feeling of insects crawling under the skin. It blocks dopamine, norepinephrine, and serotonin uptake and can cause cardiac dysrhythmias, hypertension, and aggressive behavior. Another amphetamine-type drug is MDMA (3,4-methylenedioxymethamphetamine), commonly known as Ecstasy, which can cause euphoria, hallucinations, and a sense of well-being and empathy. Overdoses can lead to dehydration, heat stroke, cerebral hemorrhage, and the serotonin syndrome, which can cause death. Withdrawal from this drug can result in depression. It can be neurotoxic to serotonergic neurons,[34] and there is evidence that long-term cognitive impairments may occur after chronic use.[35]

In animal models, fluoxetine has been shown to block MDMA uptake into neurons, which may have a neuroprotective effect. However, no agents have been reliably efficacious for treating stimulant withdrawal. Beta-blockers may reduce hemodynamic symptoms of withdrawal.[36] Drugs that are indirect dopamine agonists, such as methylphenidate and amantadine, can reduce the incidence of recidivism for cocaine addiction.[37,38]

CANNABIS

Marijuana, which comes from the *Cannabis* plant, is an illegal drug that can be smoked or eaten. The use of this drug produces a sense of well-being, but higher doses can lead to depression, panic, and psychosis. Abstinence from marijuana is not known to cause a physical withdrawal syndrome. However, patients may experience psychological cravings for this drug. These patients may exhibit restlessness, anxiety, and insomnia when they stop using marijuana. Long-term use of this drug can cause memory problems.[39]

SUMMARY

Because addiction is considered a chronic and persistent disease, and because patients who have been addicted to substances are prone to recurrence of addictive behaviors, it is possible that exposure to drugs of abuse during the perioperative period may rekindle a latent addictive state. In individuals who previously abused substances, changes may have developed in the neural circuitry involving dopaminergic neurons located in the brain. Because of the possibility of cross-addiction, exposure to an opioid or benzodiazepine may stimulate cravings and other addictive behaviors, even in patients who had previously abused nonopioids such as alcohol and cocaine.

Maintaining abstinence from drugs of abuse is a complex process that depends not only on overcoming physical withdrawal from substances but also on developing social and coping mechanisms to avoid recrudescence.[10] Psychotherapy and behavioral modification programs may be helpful in this regard, including programs such as Alcoholics Anonymous and Narcotics Anonymous. Individuals who participate in these programs and who have pledged abstinence from drugs may understandably have anxiety about whether they will be exposed to substances of abuse during the perioperative period. In some cases, patients refuse anxiolytics or opioids, especially while awake before surgery, and prefer to use cognitive and behavioral strategies to relieve preoperative anxiety. Unfortunately, there have been reports of patients experiencing addiction relapse after being exposed to opioids given perioperatively.[10,40] Greater stress, anxiety, and poorly treated pain can all lead to requests for higher doses of opioids postoperatively,[41] even in patients whose addiction illness is in remission.

The perioperative management of patients who are prone to addiction must recognize that patients may be taking certain drugs to prevent relapse. These include disulfiram for alcoholics, acamprosate (reduces "reward" in alcoholics), naltrexone (opioid antagonist, also used for alcoholics), and methadone or buprenorphine (drug substitution for μ opioid receptor agonists). It is also important to understand that there is a higher incidence of psychiatric disorders in patients who have had substance abuse problems, including anxiety, depression, and psychosis, and that such patients may be taking a variety of pharmacological treatments with anesthetic and postoperative consequences.[10]

Treatments for Drug Dependence and Addiction

A number of pharmacological, psychological, and behavioral treatments have been proposed to manage patients with substance abuse disorders and drug addiction. Management of withdrawal depends on the drug of dependence. Because dopamine seems to play a role in the neurobiological reward system, efforts have been made to develop drugs that modify the dopaminergic system. For example, bupropion, which increases dopamine and noradrenaline levels in the synaptic cleft, has been found to be effective in treating nicotine addiction.[42]

ALCOHOL ABUSE

Alcoholics have been treated with disulfiram, which inhibits aldehyde dehydrogenase and causes acetaldehyde accumulation in patients who ingest alcohol. This accumulation causes a severely unpleasant reaction. Disulfiram also inhibits dopamine β-hydroxylase, possibly leading to an attenuated cardiovascular response during anesthesia.[10] Disulfiram can inhibit hepatic systems that are responsible for metabolism of drugs such as barbiturates, tricyclic antidepressants, and warfarin.[43]

Patients who have abused alcohol can be treated with μ opioid receptor antagonists such as naltrexone and nalmefene. These drugs reduce cravings for alcohol and, when an opioid is taken, increase the dose of opioid required to produce euphoria.[44] To simplify postoperative management, opioid antagonists should be stopped before surgery. If these drugs are continued during the perioperative period, patients will probably require higher doses of opioids to achieve analgesia. Other drugs that have been used to reduce cravings for alcohol are acamprosate and anticonvulsant medications, such as carbamazepine, valproate, and gabapentin.[45–47] In alcohol withdrawal, increased NMDA function occurs, and acamprosate, which antagonizes the NMDA receptor, has been shown to double abstinence rates.[35] Antidepressants in the selective serotonin reuptake inhibitor class, such as fluoxetine, and anxiolytics such as buspirone can reduce alcohol drinking in patients who are depressed or anxious.[48,49]

OPIOID ABUSE

The μ receptor subtype seems to play a key role in mediating cravings and reward in opioid abuse. Mice who lack this receptor exhibit no reinforcing behaviors for continuing to take morphine.[50] Drugs that are antagonists at the μ receptor, such as naltrexone, have been used to treat opiate addiction. The effects of drugs that inhibit the NMDA receptor, such as ketamine and memantine, may decrease opioid-induced tolerance.

Opiate withdrawal is accompanied by activation of the sympathetic nervous system. When opioids are discontinued, adrenergic activation of the locus ceruleus neurons in the brain is seen.[51] Manifestations of increased noradrenergic activity can be treated with α₂ agonists, such as clonidine, lofexidine, and tizanidine. These drugs have been shown to modulate withdrawal symptoms and decrease the sympathomimetic response to withdrawal. However, they may also cause hypotension, sedation, and bradycardia, although these side effects are less likely with tizanidine and lofexidine.

Because cravings for opiate drugs are greater when short-acting opiates are used, the use of methadone and buprenorphine, which have long half-lives, for the treatment of opioid addiction has been growing. Methadone is a full agonist at the μ receptor, but it may also have NMDA receptor antagonistic activity. Buprenorphine (Subutex) is a partial opioid agonist at the μ receptor and a κ receptor antagonist. Stimulation of κ receptors has been found to reduce dopamine levels and produce aversive responses.[13] Buprenorphine is also available in combination with naloxone, which is a μ receptor antagonist; this drug combination is called Suboxone. The peak effect of buprenorphine is at 100 minutes, and the effects return to baseline at 48 hours, with a half-life of 37 hours. It is usually prescribed as a single daily dose of 16 mg, given sublingually. Because buprenorphine is a partial agonist at the μ receptor, it gives a lower level of response at maximal receptor occupancy and it exhibits a "ceiling effect." However, because of its analgesic effects, some practitioners use it as an analgesic drug. Comparisons of the use of buprenorphine to methadone have shown similar results in the treatment of opiate addiction. Weaning programs for methadone often involve decreasing the dose by as little as 3% per week to as much as 5% per day. LAAM (L-acetyl-α methadol) is an alternative long-acting μ receptor agonist.

In patients who take any of these μ agonist-type drugs, the usual doses should be continued in the postoperative period. Otherwise, withdrawal may result, and increased pain is likely. Substituting these drugs for other opioids in the perioperative period only complicates management, in terms of both addiction control and analgesia. Similarly, using addiction-management drugs as analgesics and raising their doses makes it more difficult to return to their intended use after the patient has recovered from surgery. Management is simplified by maintaining agonist drugs used for addiction at their standard doses and using additional intravenous or short-term oral analgesics for acute pain after surgery.

OTHER ADDICTIONS

The endocannabinoid system, of which the CB-1 receptor is found in the brain, may play a role in the reward and cravings mechanism for various drugs, nicotine, and food. Long-term tobacco use has been found to stimulate the CB-1 receptor, and the reward response to morphine is reduced in mice lacking CB-1 receptors. Various cannabinoids have been found to increase the efflux of dopamine in the nucleus accumbens.[52] Rimonabant, which blocks the CB-1 receptor, has been shown to decrease cravings for food and nicotine, and drugs in this class may play a promising role in the management of opioid addiction.

From a psychological perspective, addictive drugs can produce euphoria, which acts as a positive reinforcer, stimulating further use. Similarly, taking addictive drugs can relieve symptoms of dysphoria or withdrawal, which are negative reinforcers and which also increase the motivational drive to obtain the drug. Cues in the environment can stimulate a conditioned response, such as cravings, which promotes further drug use.[13] Therefore, the reward system in the brain can become sensitized to environmental stimuli that are independent of physical withdrawal symptoms and that lead to increased drug use. Patients with risk-taking behaviors and psychiatric disorders are especially prone to abuse behaviors.[53,54] Therefore, cognitive-behavior therapies that focus on this type of aberrant behavior may play a role in the perioperative period in determining a treatment plan for the drug-dependent patient.

Perioperative Plan for the Drug-Dependent Patient

One of the most common challenges in the perioperative management of a drug-dependent patient is developing a treatment plan for a patient who is opioid tolerant. Patients who are opioid tolerant may be using prescription opioids for the management of chronic or cancer pain, or they may be abusing prescription opioids or other opioid-type drugs. Although there are similarities in managing patients who are tolerant to opioids regardless of their addiction status, there are additional considerations for the management of patients who both are dependent on opioids physiologically and have substance abuse problems. In either case, the issue of opioid tolerance in the perioperative period needs to be considered. A good treatment plan will address problems with acute pain after surgery, ongoing chronic pain, and psychological issues that may be affecting the patient.

PREPARING A TREATMENT PLAN

Whenever possible, it is important to prepare a plan for pain management for opioid-dependent surgical patients *before* surgery. Preoperatively, there should be an agreement on which service will be primarily responsible for managing pain, and all caregivers should achieve consensus on the treatment plan. This may necessitate that the surgical service consult with a pain management specialist prior to surgery. The care team should be aware that the patient's opioid dependence makes it more likely that the patient's pain will be undertreated postoperatively if precautions are not taken. Negative attitudes on the part of caregivers, educational deficiencies, and simple reluctance to prescribe drugs to a "recovering" addict may lead to poorly controlled pain. In addition, poorly treated pain can result in greater anxiety for the patient, along with low self-esteem and depression. Patients should be reassured that their history of substance abuse will not be a barrier to their receiving appropriate pain management after surgery.[10] For those patients in substance abuse treatment programs, it is prudent to confer with the mental health provider in order to optimize the perioperative plan.

Although less likely, it is possible that a patient will receive inappropriately high doses of opioids in the postoperative period and that he or she may engage in manipulative behavior to obtain excessive doses of opioids. The care team should keep in mind the planned surgical procedure and the anticipated levels of pain that may result. Continued use of an opioid postoperatively should be determined by the clinical picture of the patient after surgery. Preoperatively, an outline should be prepared specifying what interventions may be necessary for poorly controlled pain, and a strategy for tapering opioid doses postoperatively should be discussed with the patient.

PREOPERATIVE PERIOD

In the preoperative period, patients who take opioids regularly should be identified, and opioid-dependent or opioid-tolerant patients should be designated for special perioperative consideration. All patients should be questioned as to whether they have previous or current history of using alcohol, tobacco, opioids, benzodiazepines, and all other prescribed or illicit drugs that can cause dependence. Specifically, patients should be interviewed to determine what dose of opioids they are taking and over what period they have taken opioid drugs. In patients whose veracity is suspect, urine toxicology testing may play a role. Previous histories of surgical procedures and postoperative recovery should be obtained, with a focus on how the patient fared in terms of pain control. Intolerances to or experience of side effects to particular opioids should be identified. If the patient has a chronic pain syndrome, a description of the pain should be documented as well as how well the pain responds to the current opioid treatment.

Once the baseline pain management history is obtained, options for postoperative pain control should be delineated and discussed with the patient. It is important to understand the patient's expectations about postoperative pain control and to educate the patient about the expected course of surgery and recovery. The perioperative team should be aware of a patient's underlying chronic pain. Patients who report high levels of pain preoperatively will probably report higher levels of pain (visual analogue scale [VAS] scores) both before and after surgery. The treatment team may need to use alternative measurement scales to obtain an accurate picture of the severity of postoperative pain in these patients.

DAY OF SURGERY

On the day of surgery, patients who routinely take sustained-release opioids should take their usual dose of medication. Duration of action for most of these drugs is 8 to 24 hours, or even 72 hours for transdermal fentanyl. Therefore, having the patient take such a drug just prior to surgery enables baseline analgesic levels to be maintained during surgery and in the immediate postoperative period. Patients who neglect to take their usual opioids before surgery can be supplemented with intravenous formulations during surgery.

Because pain management may be more challenging for those who are tolerant to opioids, it is appropriate to counsel patients on the possibility that their pain levels may be more difficult to control. Correcting unreasonable expectations, such as being completely pain free after major surgery, may decrease postoperative levels of anxiety in some patients and reduce the dissatisfaction that may result from false hopes. Patients should be educated on the various methods to control pain postoperatively, including the use of patient-controlled analgesia (PCA), epidural and regional anesthetic techniques, and adjuvant medications such as anxiolytics, anti-inflammatories, and others. Depending on the type of surgery and expected recovery, patients may not be able to take their chronic pain medications orally, and alternative routes should be considered and prepared for. Patients should be allowed to take their usual analgesic drugs up to the time of surgery, along with other preoperative medications, often with a sip of water.

INTRAOPERATIVE ISSUES

Patients who are opioid dependent or opioid tolerant may require higher doses of analgesic drugs as part of their intraoperative anesthetic management.[16,55] Patient response may be measured in terms of cardiovascular responses to pain and, for those patients who are spontaneously breathing, changes in respiratory rates. Patients with increasing respiratory rates may require supplementation of intraoperative opioid. In addition, patients may benefit from the use of epidural or regional anesthesia to decrease nociceptive input from the area of surgery. They will be less likely to experience the adverse effects of high doses of opioids, such as respiratory depression. The anesthesia care team should communicate the patient's intraoperative opioid requirements and preoperative opioid use history to the postoperative care team, which may include staff in the post-anesthesia care unit as well as on the hospital floor or in the intensive care unit. This level of communication is important for all opioid-dependent patients and is especially vital if the patient is expected to remain intubated or pharmacologically paralyzed.

POSTOPERATIVE MANAGEMENT

In the postoperative period, patients who are opioid dependent may experience higher levels of pain. This may occur because preexisting analgesic use leads to increased postoperative requirements, tolerance to opioid drugs, and perhaps decreased efficacy of therapy. In some cases, caregivers underutilize analgesics.[56] In a review of 3058 postoperative patients, Rapp et al[55] found that 6.6% of patients had a history of long-term opioid use prior to surgery. Patients who used opioids before surgery were found to consume more opioid (24-hour usage = 135.8 mg morphine equivalent) via PCA postoperatively compared to opioid-naive patients (24 hour usage = 42.8 mg morphine equivalent). In spite of higher opioid usage, pain scores (VAS scores 0–10) were higher in the long-term opioid use group than in the opioid-naive group, both at rest (VAS 5 versus 3) and with movement (VAS 8 versus 6). Medications for anxiety were ordered postoperatively for 18.7% of the long-term opioid use group, compared with 0.6% of the opioid-naive group. The long-term opioid use group tended to use PCA longer (4 days versus 3) and had a lower incidence of nausea and pruritus related to opioid therapy. Patients with nonmalignant pain had higher opioid consumption and pain scores than those with a cancer diagnosis. Factors such as anxiety and depression, which are more prevalent in the chronic pain population, may also play a role in reports of higher postoperative pain in these patients. When patients attach a negative meaning to a surgical procedure, higher doses of analgesics may be used.[57] In addition to opioid tolerance and seeming loss of efficacy, it may be that patients with chronic pain who use opioids have negative perceptions of surgery that promote anxiety and fear and instigate higher opioid consumption.

One reason that a long-term opioid user is undertreated after surgery is that the patient's usual preoperative baseline dose of opioid is not continued. In some cases, patients are unable to take oral preparations immediately after surgery or the treatment team does not implement these prescriptions on a routine basis. Patients receiving long-term opioid therapy must resume their usual dose of opioid so that they continue to take baseline levels during their hospitalization. An exception to this rule would be the patient whose operation is expected to reduce his or her chronic pain. In most patients who are opioid dependent, a preexisting prescription for transdermal patches or oral opioids should be continued throughout the postoperative period; if they cannot take medications orally, their oral opioid regimen should be converted into a basal infusion of intravenous opioids, usually at about 50% of the dose equivalent, with supplemental doses provided as needed.

Another reason patients who are opioid dependent may experience additional pain after surgery is their tolerance to opioid drugs. Tolerance may necessitate that higher doses of opioid be given both intraoperatively and postoperatively to prevent pain. Therefore, it may take both a baseline dose of opioid and a higher intermittent dose of opioid to achieve analgesia in the opioid-dependent patient. Because tolerance to opioids can develop even after short-term use (days or weeks), even patients receiving brief courses of preoperative opioids should be monitored for signs and symptoms of opioid tolerance. Patients who are tolerant to opioids are more likely to experience increased pain and to require higher doses of opioids to relieve pain after surgery.[16] In some patients, long-term tolerance develops, so that patients are relatively insensitive to the effects of opioids even years after they have discontinued use. This phenomenon may be related to changes in neuronal plasticity, activation of NMDA receptors and glutamate, and greater production of spinal dynorphin, an endogenous opioid peptide.[16]

If a patient can resume oral intake within several hours after surgery, the baseline dose of orally administered chronic opioid therapy should be resumed. In addition, either an oral opioid or an intravenous PCA system should be implemented. For both oral and intravenous opioids, the intermittent dose may need to be higher to account for opioid tolerance, and this can be delivered via a PCA device. To reduce the effects of tolerance, it may be advantageous to use an opioid different from the one the patient is accustomed to. Because of interindividual variability in response to different opioids, changing from one opioid to another may provide better analgesia with fewer side effects in some patients.[58]

If a patient is unable to take opioids orally, the preoperative opioid dose should be converted into an equipotent intravenous dose, and 50% of it may be given as a baseline continuous intravenous infusion. If necessary, patients can use a PCA system to meet the remainder of their opioid requirement postoperatively. This technique allows optimal titration of analgesics to effect and reduces delays and anxiety related to potential withholding of analgesics. Although there is some concern that use of a PCA device may reinforce reward behaviors in addicts,[59] the use of PCA can reduce the risk of inadequate medication, and the probability that this modality would lead to an addiction problem is low. In case the predicted doses used in PCA are inadequate, an order for "rescue" doses should be implemented. These can be twice the level of "as-needed" patient-controlled doses. Repeated rescue doses should be permitted for the patient after evaluation by a nurse. In patients who use transdermal patches for analgesia, the patches should be continued in the postoperative period. Because hyperthermia can cause greater absorption of some transdermal medications, patients who demonstrate postoperative fevers may receive unexpectedly higher doses of opioids, and caregivers should be alerted to this possibility.

Patients who receive regional or epidural techniques for pain control may have lower needs for systemic opioids.

There may be improvements in functional activities when low-dose local anesthetic infusions are used. Also, spinal and epidural opiates have greater potency than opiates given via the oral or intravenous route. Therefore, reduced side effects of opioid therapy may be realized. However, it is unknown whether the use of regional techniques or spinal opiates in the perioperative period decreases drug cravings or relapse of addiction in opioid-dependent patients.[10] Even if a regional technique is used, continuation of preoperative opioids for such patients will probably be needed, at least at a portion of their long-term dose, to prevent withdrawal reactions or chronic pain that may exist outside of the area of regional analgesia. Pain relief will be optimized if patients who take opioids long term are permitted to continue at their usual doses. Complete discontinuation of opiates may result in significant pain complaints even in the setting of excellent regional anesthetic blockade. If there is a concern about excessive sedation, patients may be given approximately 50% of their baseline doses of opioid, at which level withdrawal reactions are unlikely. In any case, frequent reassessment of such patients and adjustment of doses may be necessary to achieve optimal pain control.

In addition to regional anesthetic techniques, the use of adjuvant drugs can decrease opioid requirements in the postoperative period. Nonsteroidal anti-inflammatory drugs (NSAIDs) can provide additional analgesia to that achieved using with morphine alone in the postoperative setting (although NSAID administration alone is usually inadequate). Such agents can be effective in reducing the amount of opioid consumed and therefore result in a lower incidence of opioid-related side effects after surgery. They can also provide additional analgesia to persons with particular types of pain, such as bony or musculoskeletal pain. However, the use of NSAIDs may be associated with gastrointestinal injury, renal problems, bleeding complications, cardiovascular complications, and delayed bone healing. For refractory pain in an opioid-resistant patient, ketamine has been used with some success.[60] An NMDA-antagonist, ketamine is known to enhance opioid analgesia, and its administration can reduce tolerance to opioid drugs. Finally, patients with excessive anxiety and fear related to surgery may benefit from the judicious use of benzodiazepines in the postoperative period, with care taken to avoid oversedation.

After surgery, once the patient's gastrointestinal function has recovered, an oral analgesic regimen can be recommenced. Again, if the patient had been taking a sustained-release preparation of an opioid for chronic pain, this should be continued at its preoperative dose if chronic pain is still an issue. For additional "as-needed" pain relief, patients may be given a standard short-acting opioid such as oxycodone, morphine, or hydromorphone. The patient who is tolerant to opioids may require higher doses of "as-needed" medications in the immediate postoperative period. A tapering schedule based on the level of pain and the type of surgery performed should be outlined for such a patient.

Dosages of postoperative pain medications in an opioid-dependent patient should be tapered over the same time span as opioids would be reduced in an opioid-naive patient after surgery. The treatment team must be alert for signs of abnormal drug-seeking behavior or loss of control over the reasonable use of postoperative analgesics. However, oral opioid doses may be higher in opioid-tolerant patients than in opiate-naive patients. Dosage tapering can be continued on an outpatient basis until the preoperative baseline dose of opioid used for chronic pain is reached. This process may take 1 to 2 months. Caregivers should avoid escalating the chronic pain medication dose to supplement acute postoperative opioid needs. Limited-quantity prescriptions should be dispensed, and a reasonable tapering schedule should be outlined. After discharge, the patient should be given an appointment with the pain management center to follow up on the course of drug tapering. More frequent follow-up and monitoring allow better evaluation of recovery and medication use as well as assessment of whether a transition to inappropriate use of analgesics is occurring. In some cases, dispensing of postoperative analgesics by a family member may reduce the chances of loss of control for the substance-abusing patient.

Postoperative Pain Management in the Addicted Patient

Use of addictive drugs can produce permanent alterations in the neurobiology of the brain. These changes can cause cravings for drugs and lead to relapse of addiction even years after a patient has stopped using the drug.[14] This process may make weaning from opioids after surgery particularly difficult for these patients. Exposure to psychological stress, environmental stimuli previously associated with drug use, or reexposure to the drug itself can cause a relapse of addictive behaviors. The likelihood of relapse may vary among patients and with the different drugs used. With opioid use, elevations of certain subtypes of glutamate receptors found in the brain may be responsible for relapse.[61] Long-term treatment with morphine may increase the expression of transcription factors and genes in mesolimbic structures, leading to a behavioral sensitization to addictive substances.[14,15] Finally, exposure to opioids can cause structural changes in brain neurons. Behavioral sensitization to opioids, along with neurobiological and structural factors, can be long lasting and persist for months or years. An individual with a history of substance abuse may therefore be prone to cravings and increased use of these drugs in the perioperative period and after surgery.

To stabilize a patient who is addicted to illicit drugs before elective surgery, one approach may involve substituting short-acting drugs with long-acting forms and then reducing the dose over a long period. Withdrawal from short-acting drugs may lead to adverse symptoms more frequently and may induce cravings, whereas drugs with a long half-life may induce lesser or more gradual symptoms of withdrawal. Detoxification from opiates is a long-term process; its successful accomplishment while the patient is recovering from surgery and having immediate postoperative pain is unlikely. Instead, detoxification and weaning measures can begin once the patient's postoperative pain has stabilized and the patient's recovery is well under way.

A special program must be developed for patients who are maintained on opioid antagonists such as naltrexone, mixed agonist-antagonist drugs such as nalbuphine and butorphanol (μ receptor antagonists and κ receptor agonists), or partial agonist-antagonist drugs such as buprenorphine (partial μ agonists and κ receptor antagonists). Patients who take pure μ antagonist drugs should discontinue use of such drugs at least 24 hours before surgery. Otherwise, it may be difficult to titrate opioids necessary for postoperative pain control; the antagonist drugs may impede the analgesic activity of μ agonists given for pain relief. For patients who take a mixed agonist-antagonist, there will be a ceiling effect to analgesia with these drugs. The drugs can competitively bind to μ receptors (because they are μ receptor antagonists) and block the action of μ agonists given postoperatively. Some practitioners have reported using supplemental μ agonist drugs as analgesics for patients who are taking partial-agonist regimens, such as buprenorphine (which is a partial μ agonist, having a ceiling effect for its μ agonism), with some improvement in pain control. Although this method of treatment may be adequate for patients after minor surgery, it is unlikely to be effective for patients who undergo surgery that is likely to produce more severe pain. A more prudent course would be to replace the mixed agonist-antagonist drug or the partial μ agonist drug with a full μ receptor agonist drug about 48 to 72 hours preoperatively and then resume the mixed drug after the acute phase of recovery has been completed. Usually, the original agent can be resumed within 5 to 7 days of major surgery. The goal should be to return the patient to the baseline drug regimen as soon as possible.

Conclusion

Managing drug-dependent patients in the perioperative period may be complicated by the physical and psychological nature of the substance use issue. Unfortunately, there are no prospective studies of suggested best practices. It is important to avoid undermedicating or overmedicating these challenging patients.

In addition to understanding the basic concepts of postoperative pain management, one must have knowledge of the neural and behavioral basis of addiction. Acquiring such knowledge may require consultations with specialists in addiction medicine as well as chronic pain. Knowledge of the pharmacology of drugs and frequent assessments of the patient are mandatory.

REFERENCES

1. Mao J: Opioid induced abnormal pain sensitivity: Implications in clinical opioid therapy. Pain 2002;100:213–217.
2. Compton P, Charavastra VC, Kintaudi K, et al: Pain responses in methadone-maintained opioid abusers. J Pain Symptom Manag 2000;20:237–245.
3. Laulin JP, Celerier E, Larcher A, et al: Opiate tolerance to daily heroin administration: An apparent phenomenon associated with enhanced pain sensitivity. Neuroscience 1999;89:631–636.
4. Collett B-J: Chronic opioid therapy for non-cancer pain. Br J Anaesth 2001;87:133–143.
5. Nissen LM, Tett SE, Cranoud T, et al: Opioid analgesic prescribing: Use of an audit of analgesic prescribing by general practitioners and the multidisciplinary pain center at Royal Brisbane Hospital. Br J Clin Pharmacol 2001;52:693–698.
6. Savage SR: Assessment for addiction in pain-treatment settings. Clin J Pain 2002;18(Suppl):S28–S38.
7. Volkow ND, Fowler JS, Wang GJ: Imaging studies on the role of dopamine in cocaine reinforcement and addiction in humans. J Psychopharmacol 1999;13:337–345.
8. Stoelting RK, Dierdorf SF: Anesthesia and Co-existing Disease, 2nd ed. New York, Churchill Livingstone, 1988, p 731.

9. McLellan AT, Lewis DC, O'Brien CP, Kleber HD: Drug dependence, a chronic medical illness: Implications for treatment, insurance, and outcomes evaluation. JAMA 2000;284:1689–1695.

10. May JA, White HC, Leonard-White A, et al: The patient recovering from alcohol or drug addiction: Special issues for the anesthesiologist. Anesth Analg 2001;92:160–161.

11. Nedeljkovic SS, Wasan A, Jamison RN: Assessment of efficacy of long-term opioid therapy in pain patients with substance abuse potential. Clin J Pain 2002;18:S39–S51.

12. McHugh P, Slavney P: Characteristics of motivated behaviors. In The Perspectives of Psychiatry. Baltimore, Johns Hopkins University Press, 1998, pp 165–177.

13. Koob GF, Le Moal M: Drug addiction, dysregulation of reward, and allostasis. Neuropsychopharmacology 2001;24:97–129.

14. Cami J, Farre M: Mechanisms of disease: Drug addiction. N Engl J Med 2003;329:975–986.

15. Nestler EJ: Molecular basis of long-term plasticity underlying addiction. Nat Rev Neurosci 2001;2:119–128.

16. Mitra S, Sinatra R: Perioperative management of acute pain in the opioid-dependent patient. Anesthesiology 2004;101:212–227.

17. Kieffer BL, Evans CJ: Opioid tolerance: In search of the Holy Grail. Cell 2002;108:587–590.

18. Jaffe JH, Martin WR: Opioid analgesics and antagonists. In Gilman AG, Nies AS, Rall TW, Taylor P (eds): Goodman and Gilman's The Pharmacological Basis of Therapeutics, 8th ed. New York, Pergamon, 1990, pp 485–521.

19. Sosnowski M, Yaksh TL: Differential cross-tolerance between intrathecal morphine and sufentanil in the rat. Anesthesiology 1990;73:1141–1147.

20. Kessler RC, McGonagle KA, Zhao S, et al: Lifetime and 12-month prevalence of DSM-III-R psychiatric disorders in the United States: Results from the National Comorbidity Survey. Arch Gen Psychiatry 1994;51:8–19.

21. O'Brien CP, McLellan AT: Myths about the treatment of addiction. Lancet 1996;347:237–240.

22. National Household Survey on Drug Abuse (NHSDA). Washington DC: Substance Abuse and Mental Health Services Administration (SAMHSA), 1999.

23. O'Connor PG, Schottenfeld RS: Patients with alcohol problems. N Engl J Med 1998;338:592–602.

24. Swift RML: Drug therapy for alcohol dependence. N Engl J Med 1999;340:1482–1490.

25. Davis KM, Wu JY: Role of glutaminergic and GABAergic systems in alcoholism. J Biomed Sci 2000;8:7–19.

26. Lejoyeaux M, Solomon J, Ades J: Benzodiazepine treatment for alcohol-dependent patients. Alcohol Alcohol 1998;33:563–575.

27. Adinoff B: Double-blind study of alprazolam, diazepam, clonidine, and placebo in the alcohol withdrawal syndrome: preliminary findings. Alcohol Clin Exp Res 1994;18:873–878.

28. Weiss F, Porrino LJ: Behavioral neurobiology of alcohol addiction: Recent advances and challenges. J Neurosci 2002;22:3332–3337.

29. Kosten TR, O'Connor PG: Management of drug and alcohol withdrawal. N Engl J Med 2003;348:1786–1795.

30. Rickels K, DeMartinis N, Rynn M, et al: Pharmacologic strategies for discontinuing benzodiazepine treatment. J Clin Psychopharm 1999;19(Suppl 2):12S–16S.

31. Griffiths RR, Wolf B: Relative abuse liability of different benzodiazepines in drug abusers. J Clin Psychopharmacol 1990;10:237–243.

32. Janssen Pharmaceutical Company: Memo, received November 14, 2004.

33. Fishbain DA, Rosomoff HL, Rosomoff RS: Drug abuse, dependence, and addiction in chronic pain patients. Clin J Pain 1992;8:77–85.

34. Boot BP, McGregor IS, Hall W: MDMA (Ecstasy) neurotoxicity: Assessing and communicating the risks. Lancet 2000;355:1818–1821.

35. Lingford-Hughes A, Nutt D: Neurobiology of addiction and implications for treatment. Br J Psychiatry 2003;182:97–100.

36. Kampman KM, Volpicelli JR, Mulvaney R, et al: Effectiveness of propranolol for cocaine dependence treatment may depend on cocaine withdrawal symptom severity. Drug Alcohol Depend 2001;63:69–78.

37. Grabowski J, Roache JD, Schmitz JM, et al: Replacement medication for cocaine dependence: Methylphenidate. J Clin Psychopharmacol 1997;17:485–488.

38. Alterman AI, Droba M, Antelo RE, et al: Amantadine may facilitate detoxification for cocaine addicts. Drug Alcohol Depend 1992;31:19–29.

39. Solowij N, Stephens RS, Roffman RA, et al: Cognitive functioning of long-term heavy cannabis users seeking treatment. JAMA 2002;287:1123–1131.

40. Wesson DR, Ling W, Smith DE: Prescription of opioids for treatment of pain in patients with addictive disease. J Pain Symptom Manag 1993;8:289–296.

41. Daley DC, Marlatt GA: Relapse prevention. In Lowinson JH, Ruiz P, Millman RB (eds): Substance Abuse: A Comprehensive Textbook, 3rd ed. Baltimore, Lippincott Williams & Wilkins, 1997, pp 458–467.

42. Ascher JA, Cole JO, Colin JN, et al: Bupropion: A review of its mechanism of antidepressant activity. J Clin Psychiatry 1995;56:395–401.

43. Hobbs WR, Rall TW, Verdoorn TA: Hypnotics and sedatives, alcohol. In Hardman JG, Limbird LE (eds): Goodman and Gilman's The Pharmacologic Basis of Therapeutics, 9th ed. New York, McGraw-Hill, 1996, pp 361–398.

44. Gonzalez JP, Brogden RN: Naltrexone: A review of its pharmacodynamic and pharmacokinetic properties and therapeutic efficacy in the treatment of opioid dependence. Drugs 1988;35:192–213.

45. Mueller TI, Stout RL, Rudden S, et al: A double-blind, placebo-controlled pilot study of carbamazepine for the treatment of alcohol dependence. Alcohol Clin Exp Res 1997;21:86–92.

46. Donovan SJ, Nunes EV: Treatment of comorbid affective and substance use disorders: Therapeutic potential of anticonvulsants. Am J Addict 1998;7:210–220.

47. Chatterjee CR, Ringold AL: A case report of reduction in alcohol craving and protection against alcohol withdrawal by gabapentin. J Clin Psychiatry 1999;60:617.

48. Cornelius JR, Salloum IM, Ehler JG, et al: Fluoxetine in depressed alcoholics: A double-blind, placebo-controlled trial. Arch Gen Psychiatry 1997;54:700–705.

49. Kranzler HR, Burleson JA, Del Boca FK, et al: Buspirone treatment of anxious alcoholics: A placebo-controlled trial. Arch Gen Psychiatry 1994;51:720–731.

50. Kieffer BL: Opioids: First lessons from knockout mice. Trends Pharmacol Sci 1999;20:19–26.

51. Rasmussen K, Beitner-Johnson DB, Krystal JH, et al: Opiate withdrawal and the rat locus coeruleus: Behavioral, electrophysiological, and biochemical correlates. J Neurosci 1990;10:2308–2317.

52. Robbe D, Alonso G, Duchamp F, et al: Localization and mechanisms of action of cannabinoid receptors at the glutamatergic synapses of the mouse nucleus accumbens. J Neurosci 2001;21:109–116.

53. Helmus TC, Downey KK, Arfken CL, et al: Novelty seeking as a predictor of treatment retention for heroin dependent cocaine users. Drug Alcohol Depend 2001;61:287–295.

54. Kavanaugh DJ, McGrath J, Saunders JB, et al: Substance misuse in patients with schizophrenia: Epidemiology and management. Drugs 2002;62:743–755.

55. Rapp S, Ready B, Nessly M: Acute pain management in patients with prior opioid consumption: A case-controlled retrospective review. Pain 1995;61:195–201.

56. Hamilton J, Edgar L: A survey examining nurses' knowledge of pain control. J Pain Symptom Manag 1992;7:18–26.

57. Chapman CR, Cox GB: Anxiety, pain and depression surrounding elective surgery: A multivariate comparison of abdominal surgery patients with kidney donors and recipients. J Psychosom Res 21;1977:7–15.

58. Woodhouse A, Ward EM, Mather LE: Intra-subject variability in post-operative patient-controlled analgesia (PCA): Is the patient equally satisfied with morphine, pethidine and fentanyl? Pain 1999;80:545–553.

59. Beattie C, Umbricht-Schneiter A, Mark L: Anesthesia and analgesia. In Graham AW, Schultz TK (eds): Principles of Addiction Medicine, 2nd ed. Chevy Chase, Md: American Society of Addiction Medicine, 1998, pp 877-890.

60. Weinbroum AA: A single small dose of postoperative ketamine provides rapid and sustained improvement in morphine analgesia in the presence of morphine-resistant pain. Anesth Analg 2003;96:789–795.

61. Carlezon WA Jr, Nestler EJ: Elevated levels of GluR1 in the midbrain: A trigger for sensitization to drugs of abuse? Trends Neurosci 2002;25:610–615.

25 Postoperative Pain Management in the Ambulatory Setting

NAVPARKASH SANDHU • SHYAMALA KARUVANNUR • DOMINIC HARMON

Owing to advances in anesthetic and surgical techniques and efforts to minimize costs, a growing number of surgical procedures are performed on an ambulatory (outpatient) basis.[1] As of 2003, 70% of surgical procedures in North America were performed on an ambulatory basis.[2] Though the majority of patients remain free of moderate to severe pain, 5% to 33% of patients may suffer considerable postoperative pain.[3,4] Pain is the most common cause of hospital admission or a visit to the emergency room after discharge.[1,5]

Ambulatory surgery is set to expand.[6] It has already expanded not only in terms of increasing complexity but also in terms of the selection of patients who are older and experiencing chronic illnesses such as diabetes and angina. Persistent pain after discharge following ambulatory surgery has numerous adverse effects. It is particularly harmful in older adults with underlying chronic conditions.[7] In this chapter, the evidence-based options for ambulatory pain management are reviewed to enable healthcare professionals to make appropriate analgesia choices for their patients.

Principles of Postoperative Pain Management in the Ambulatory Setting

PATIENT EDUCATION

Patient education has been shown to decrease anxiety and postoperative pain.[8,9] All instructions should be given both verbally and in written format. Patients should be informed about the likely duration of postoperative pain. This knowledge helps patients understand the limited duration of acute pain and prepares them psychologically to deal with it. It is important to note, however, that there is a disparity in reported pain levels after ambulatory surgery.[10] The literature is inconsistent, because measures of postoperative pain have not been systematically studied and reported in relation to specific operations.[10] A unified ambulatory surgery pain measurement strategy should be established so that patients can be informed about the intensity of pain they are likely to experience after specific procedures.

Patients should be familiar with the concept of pain assessment and the need to assess pain on a regular basis in order to modify analgesic treatment. They should be told about the choices for postoperative pain management, and they should discuss these options with their doctors. The stepladder pattern of choosing analgesics should be explained to patients (Fig. 25–1). Patients should be told to take oral analgesics "around the clock" rather than as needed. Patients should have information about how to troubleshoot problems with home-based analgesia[11]—for example, how to stop a home infusion device if they observe signs of toxicity or pump malfunction.

Patients should be given contact information for further advice after discharge. Physicians specializing in pain management should have access to a file, preferably computerized, with information on all ambulatory patients receiving home pump infusions, with special reference to flow rates of local anesthetic, other therapies prescribed, and any changes in therapy made by phone. This file will assure the patient that advice is available at all times in case of difficulty. Patients receiving continuous nerve blocks should be monitored by phone every day that the infusion is continued and for a day after removal of the catheter.

MULTIMODAL THERAPY

Kehlet et al[12] have proposed that "total or optimal pain relief allowing normal function cannot be achieved by a single drug or method without major strain on equipment or surveillance system or without significant side-effects." *Multimodal analgesia*, also known as "balanced analgesia," is a combination of acetaminophen, nonsteroidal anti-inflammatory drugs (NSAIDs), opioids, and local anesthetics. It is an attempt to maximize analgesia through additive or synergistic effects of drugs and to minimize side effects through reduction in dosage and the differences in side effect profiles. Multimodal analgesia is particularly relevant for ambulatory surgery.[12] Specific treatment combinations are chosen according to the type of surgery, patient medical and psychological characteristics, and the availability of home support. One of the goals

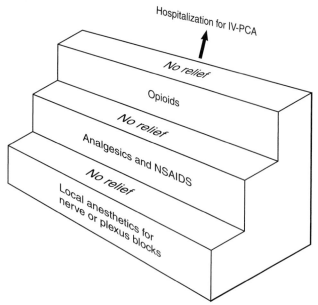

Figure 25-1 The successive steps in pharmacological choices for ambulatory patients. IV-PCA, intravenous patient-controlled analgesia.

of multimodal analgesia is to reduce the use of opioids during and after ambulatory surgery to prevent undesirable side effects such as sedation, confusion, nausea, and vomiting.

PREEMPTIVE ANALGESIA

Preemptive analgesia is an antinociceptive treatment that prevents establishment of altered processing of afferent input, which amplifies postoperative pain.[13] Overwhelming evidence from experimental studies shows the benefits of preemptive analgesia.[14] However, the results of clinical studies are controversial.[15] Difficulties in clinical studies have been associated with the different definitions of preemptive analgesia used.[13] Preemptive analgesia should prevent the establishment of central sensitization caused by incisional and inflammatory injuries during the period of surgery and the initial postoperative period.[13] Local anesthetics block pain impulses traveling to the central nervous system and decrease postoperative analgesic requirements.[16,17] To be effective in the immediate postoperative period, oral or rectal NSAIDs should be started before surgery.

PROTOCOL-BASED ANALGESIC MANAGEMENT

Protocol-based analgesic management can be a useful tool to standardize pain management strategies (Fig. 25–2). Use of protocols improves postoperative pain management.[18]

GENERAL AND REGIONAL ANESTHETIC TECHNIQUES

The choice of anesthetic techniques depends on patient and surgical factors. Major advances in ambulatory anesthetic techniques include the use of anesthetic agents of short duration and the growing use of regional anesthesia. The main disadvantage of general anesthesia is the high incidence of

postoperative nausea and vomiting (PONV) and moderate to severe pain, which may delay discharge.[19] New drugs and drug combinations, new needle and catheter designs, and introduction of imaging techniques have improved the quality and safety of regional anesthesia. Liposomal bupivacaine has been used in human volunteers in preliminary studies to prolong anesthesia up to 48 hours after intradermal injection.[20,21] Wider application of such agents will provide prolonged analgesia after single-shot injections and will revolutionize pain control in ambulatory patients.

A controversial issue in ambulatory surgery is whether regional anesthesia offers significant advantages over general anesthesia. Published data are conflicting.[22] All general and regional anesthetic techniques have advantages and disadvantages (Boxes 25–1 and 25–2). Acceptance of the technique by the surgeon and patient and the expertise of the anesthesiologist are paramount. It is essential that each unit audit its own complication rates, recovery room times, and patient opinions to determine outcome.

Regional anesthetic techniques include subcutaneous infiltration, intracavity and intra-articular instillation, field block, single peripheral nerve block, and plexus and neuraxial blocks. Regional anesthesia may be used as the sole anesthetic technique or in combination with general anesthesia to provide intraoperative and postoperative analgesia. Peripheral nerve blocks provide excellent analgesia with minimal adverse effects. The preoperative analgesia can be extended postoperatively through the use of peripheral nerve catheters. Neuraxial techniques are also an alternative to general anesthesia. Disadvantages include the time to perform and await onset of block and potential, though rare, neurological complications. Other regional anesthetic techniques appropriate for ambulatory surgery are peribulbar, retrobulbar, and topical anesthetics for ocular surgery, and intravenous regional anesthesia.

Continuous peripheral infusion techniques allow the rate of administration to be titrated and facilitate adjustment of drug concentrations and combinations. The use of patient-controlled regional anesthesia at home is a major advance in this field.

Several devices are used for ambulatory continuous nerve blocks. *Disposable pressure release devices* deliver local anesthetic at a preset rate. They are more expensive than programmable pumps but avoid the problem of retrieving programmable pumps sent home with patients. The Accufuser (McKinley Medical, Wheat Ridge, Colo) can deliver at fixed rates of 0.5, 1, 2, 4, 5, 8 and 10 mL/hr and give bolus doses of 0.5, 1 and 2 mL with lockout intervals of 15, 30 and 60 minutes. It is a simple mechanical device with a large reservoir that can last for 2 to 3 days (Fig. 25–3).

Programmable infusion pumps, such as the Gemstar Yellow (Hospira Inc., Lake Forrest, Ill) (Fig. 25–4), and PainPump2 (Stryker, Kalamazoo, Mich), are used with containers or larger bags containing local anesthetic for 2 to 3 days. These have the advantage of offering more choices for delivery rate and allow patient-controlled boluses as well.

ACETAMINOPHEN

Inexpensive and effective for mild pain, acetaminophen is well tolerated. It has multiple mechanisms of action.[23]

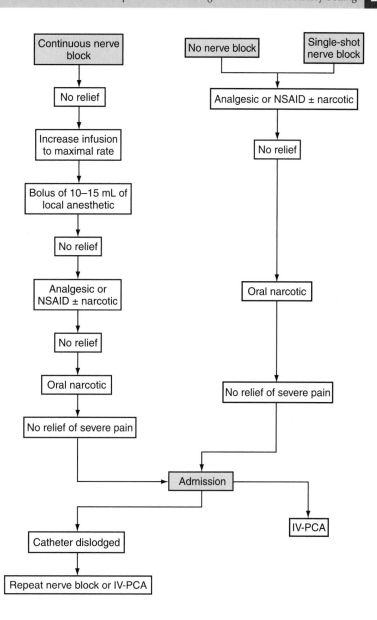

Figure 25–2 Flow chart depicting management of pain in ambulatory patients. IV-PCA, intravenous patient-controlled analgesia; NSAID, nonsteroidal anti-inflammatory drug.

BOX 25–1	ADVANTAGES OF REGIONAL ANESTHESIA TECHNIQUES

ADVANTAGES TO PATIENT

- Avoidance of general anesthesia
- Improved pain relief
- Decreased recovery time
- Decreased nausea and vomiting

ADVANTAGES TO SURGEON

- Rapid postoperative assessment possible

ADVANTAGES TO HOSPITAL

- Rapid recovery and earlier discharge
- Decreased postoperative nursing requirements
- Fewer unplanned admissions

BOX 25–2	DISADVANTAGES OF REGIONAL ANESTHESIA TECHNIQUES

- Onset is more time dependent
- Specific side effects
- Prolonged blockade may result in delayed discharge
- Surgeon cooperation required
- Expertise dependent
- Should be avoided postoperatively in patients with bony fractures complicated by large soft tissue swelling, owing to the risk of a compartment syndrome with such injuries. Pain, an early warning symptom of compartment syndrome, might be masked by regional anesthesia.

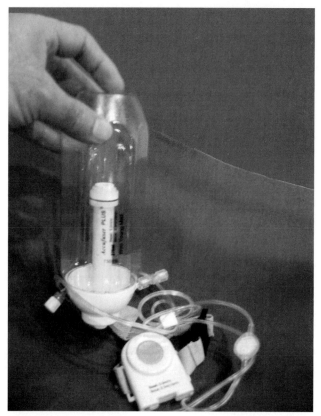

Figure 25–3 Accufuser (elastomeric pump) requires no batteries and has several choices of basal and bolus delivery through selection of tubes of varying diameter.

Unlike NSAIDs, it does not irritate the gastric mucosa, affect platelet function, or cause renal insufficiency. Acetaminophen has significant opioid-sparing effects.[24] The recommended rectal dose (up to 45 mg/kg) is higher than the oral dose (15 mg/kg) because of unreliable absorption from the rectal route. The maximum dose is 90 mg/kg in children and

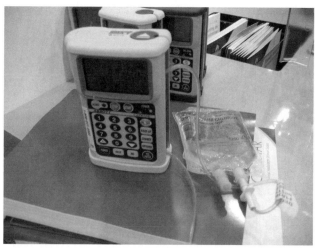

Figure 25–4 Gemstar Yellow (Hospira) is reusable, compact, and versatile—it can be programmed to deliver basal or bolus analgesia.

4 grams in adults in a 24-hour period. Acetaminophen is also used in combination with opioids for postoperative pain. The ceiling on the recommended dose of nonopioid limits the usefulness of combination drugs to the treatment of short-term mild to moderate pain (Table 25–1).

NONSTEROIDAL ANTI-INFLAMMATORY DRUGS

Unless contraindicated, all patients with postoperative pain should receive an NSAID.[25] The traditional NSAIDs, called *nonselective NSAIDs*, have significant gastrointestinal, hematological, and renal adverse effects, which are mediated through the inhibition of the isoenzyme cyclooxygenase-1 (Cox-1). These drugs help decrease opioid requirements. Examples are aspirin, ibuprofen, naproxen, and diclofenac (see Table 25–1). Aspirin should be avoided in patients with a history of peptic ulcer disease and in children (risk of Reye's syndrome). These drugs can be used alone or in combination

TABLE 25–1	Analgesics and NSAIDs		
Drug	**Dose and Route in Adults**	**Dose and Route in Children**	**Comments**
Acetaminophen	500–1000 mg every 3–4 hr PO Adult maximal dose 4000 mg/day	30–40 mg/kg loading dose; 10–15 mg/kg every 4–6 hr PO/PR Maximal dose in children 90 mg/kg/day	Toxic doses can cause hepatic toxicity
Aspirin	325–650 mg every 4–6 hr PO	12–20 mg/kg every 4–6 hr PO	Total 75 mg/kg/day in children Associated with Reye's syndrome Gastric irritation
Ibuprofen	200–800 mg every 6–8 hr PO	4–10 mg/kg every 6–8 hr PO	Gastric irritation, rarely thrombocytopenia, skin rashes, headache, dizziness, blurred vision, and toxic amblyopia
Ketorolac	Loading dose 30 mg IM/IV; 10 mg every 4–6 hr PO	0.5 mg/kg every 6–8 hr PO or IM	Use not to exceed 5 days Somnolence, dizziness, headache, gastrointestinal pain, dyspepsia
Naproxen	250–500 mg every 12 hr PO	5 mg/kg every 12 hr PO	Nausea, vomiting, gastric bleeding, drowsiness, dizziness, dermatological lesions, blood dyscrasias

IM, intramuscular; IV, intravenous; PO, orally; PR, per rectum.

TABLE 25–2	Dose Recommendations and Duration of Action of Cyclooxygenase (Cox-2) Inhibitors		
Drug	**Dose and Route in Adults**	**Duration (hr)**	**Cox-2/Cox-1 Activity**
Celecoxib	100–400 mg every 12 hr PO	4–8	8
Etoricoxib	60–240 mg PO	>24	106
Parecoxib	20 mg IM/IV	6–12	—
Rofecoxib	25–50 mg PO	12–24	35
Valdecoxib	20 mg PO	6–12	30

IM, intramuscular; IV, intravenous; PO, oral.

with opioids or nerve blocks. The choice of NSAID is based on the patient's medical condition.

Cox-2–selective NSAIDs appear to be as effective as nonselective NSAIDs in suppressing inflammation and providing analgesia for ambulatory surgery[26] with less risk of gastrointestinal toxicity. Another significant advantage of the Cox-2–selective NSAIDs is that they do not impair platelet function in the perioperative period.[27] Parecoxib is a long-acting injectable formulation that is effective in ambulatory surgery (Table 25–2).[28] Rofecoxib has been withdrawn by the manufacturer, and a warning has been added to the use of celecoxib and valdecoxib owing to the potential association of their long-term use with an increased incidence of myocardial infarction.

OPIOIDS

Usually a short-acting opioid, such as fentanyl, is started intraoperatively to supplement general anesthesia. In the postanesthesia recovery unit, intravenous fentanyl or morphine can be used for moderate to severe pain. After ambulatory surgery discharge, morphine is associated with more side effects than is fentanyl.[29] A long-acting oral opioid should be considered for surgery that is likely to result in moderate to severe postoperative pain after discharge.[30] Oral opioids commonly used in the postoperative period are listed in Table 25–3. Controlled-release oxycodone has a better side-effect profile than controlled-release morphine after ambulatory surgery discharge.[31] Adverse effects of opioids include constipation, nausea, vomiting, sedation, and respiratory depression. Patients should be given appropriate advice on how to manage these side effects.

NONPHARMACOLOGICAL TECHNIQUES

Nonpharmacological techniques can be used in the treatment of pain in the ambulatory setting.[32] The clinical efficacy of electroanalgesia techniques remains controversial owing to potential sources of bias and difficulty in quantifying the inherent placebo effect of the therapy. Other nonpharmacological techniques that have been used as analgesic adjuvants in the perioperative period are cryoanalgesia, ultrasound, and hypnosis.[33,34] Randomized clinical studies are required to establish effects of these modalities on analgesic outcome after ambulatory surgery.

Specific Procedures

ABDOMINAL SURGERY

Inguinal Hernia Repair

The ilioinguinal nerve can be blocked by a "double-pop" technique, in which 10 mL of local anesthetic is injected 2.5 cm superomedial to the anterior superior iliac spine. Even if neuraxial or general anesthesia is used, local anesthetic should be injected along the surgical incision. Alternatively, surgeons can inject 5 to 10 mL of 0.25% bupivacaine after exposure or at the end of surgery along the incision. NSAIDs and/or opioids should be given routinely before anesthesia ends. Pain can be decreased by having the patient press the wound with the palms during coughing or movement. Paravertebral block, which has been used for pain control, offers pain relief similar to that achieved

TABLE 25–3	Postoperative Oral Opioids		
Drug	**Dose and Route in Adults**	**Dose and Route in Children**	**Comments**
Morphine	10–20 mg every 2–3 hr	0.3 mg/kg every 3–4 hr	Cautious use in asthmatics Can cause respiratory depression in infants
Codeine	15–60 mg every 4–6 hr	1 mg/kg every 3–4 hr	Useful for moderate to severe pain Can be combined with acetaminophen
Morphine SR	15–30 mg every 6–8 hr	—	
Meperidine	50–150 mg every 3–4 hr	—	Contraindicated with monoamine oxidase inhibitors
Hydromorphone	2–4 mg every 4–6 hr	0.06 mg/kg every 3–4 hr	
Oxycodone	5–10 mg every 3–4 hr	0.2 mg/kg every 3–4 hr	
Oxycodone SR	10–20 mg every 12 hr	—	

SR, slow release.

by ilioinguinal nerve block and infiltration of the surgical incision.[35]

Appendectomy

Patients who undergo uncomplicated interval appendectomy can be sent home the day of surgery. The surgical wound should be injected with 5 to 10 mL of bupivacaine 0.25%. NSAIDs and opioids are used in the early postoperative period.

Laparoscopic Cholecystectomy

All incision sites used for laparoscopic cholecystectomy should be injected before incision with lidocaine 0.5% and after closure with 2 to 3 mL of bupivacaine 0.25%. An NSAID should also be given before discharge. Acetaminophen/codeine combinations are given as soon as the patient can take oral medications. Oral oxycodone may be used for patients with poorly controlled pain.

UROLOGICAL SURGERY

Circumcision can be performed with the use of penile block alone in adults. In children and infants, general anesthesia is also employed. Dorsal penile block can be performed with the use of 0.1 to 0.2 mL/kg of 0.25% bupivacaine in infants and children; it provides pain relief lasting 24 hours. Epinephrine should never be used because of risk of gangrene owing to vasospasm. Local application of EMLA (eutectic mixture of lidocaine 2.5% and prilocaine 2.5%) cream gives equivalent pain relief although its duration of action is shorter than that of dorsal penile block.[36] This measure can be easily repeated at home.[36] NSAIDs should be prescribed routinely, and opioids may be added.

Before orchidectomy, orchiopexy, or hydrocele repair, the spermatic cord can be grasped between index finger and thumb through the scrotal skin, and a 23-gauge needle passed into the cord. Bupivacaine 0.25% or ropivacaine 0.2% (3–4 mL) can be injected after intravascular placement of the needle has been ruled out. NSAIDs and opioids are also given. Scrotal skin should be injected with lidocaine prior to incision. Alternatively, the surgeon can inject 4 to 5 mL of 0.25% bupivacaine into the spermatic cord after exposing it. Supporting the testicles in a bandage or a scrotal support decreases postoperative pain. Alternatively, the ilioinguinal nerve is blocked near the anterior superior iliac spine.

PLASTIC SURGERY

Plastic surgery of the breast and abdomen can be followed by severe postoperative pain. Psychological overlay in patients undergoing these procedures may increase pain. They should receive NSAIDs, opioids, and anxiolytics. Paravertebral blocks using bupivacaine 0.5% (0.3 mL/kg) or ropivacaine can relieve postoperative breast pain for many hours.[37]

EAR, NOSE, AND THROAT PROCEDURES

In children undergoing tympanomastoid surgery, pain can be decreased on the day of surgery by a block of the great auricular nerve, a branch of the superficial cervical plexus.[38] Two milliliters of 0.25% bupivacaine with epinephrine 1:200,000 is injected subcutaneously at the midpoint of the posterior border of the sternocleidomastoid muscle. In addition, NSAIDs and opioids should be used.

GYNECOLOGICAL SURGERY

Surgical incisions can be infiltrated with 0.25% bupivacaine (maximum 2 mg/kg) at the end of gynecological surgery. NSAIDs and opioids should be prescribed. For uterine cramps, NSAIDs are especially helpful.[39]

UPPER EXTREMITY SURGERY

Shoulder Surgery

Shoulder and elbow operations are followed by a 25% incidence of severe pain.[4]

Interscalene Block. For operations around the shoulder, an interscalene block can be used as the primary anesthetic technique or as an adjunct to general anesthesia. Single-shot interscalene blocks provide excellent analgesia for the immediate perioperative period but may be insufficient after discharge from the hospital.[40] Shoulder arthroscopy or rotator cuff repair can be performed after interscalene block using nerve stimulation, paresthesias, or ultrasound guidance techniques. A catheter placed in the neck near roots/trunks through the interscalene groove[41] or through the paravertebral or posterior approach[42] facilitates postoperative pain control.

Patients can be discharged home with disposable infusion devices (e.g., Accufuser [McKinley Medical] or PainPump [Stryker]) or reusable programmable pumps like Gemstar Yellow (Hospira). Use of these devices should be coordinated with visiting home nurse services where feasible. These infusions, however, may not reliably control pain.[43] Patients may have to administer several boluses of local anesthetic to achieve control of pain.[43] Complications include incidental nerve blocks; phrenic nerve block, recurrent laryngeal nerve block, and stellate ganglion block should be explained to the patient.

Suprascapular Nerve Block. Suprascapular nerve blocks can be achieved by injection of 10 mL of a longer-acting agent such as bupivacaine or levobupivacaine 0.25% or ropivacaine 0.2% superior to the midpoint of the spine of the scapula. Although less effective than an interscalene block, suprascapular nerve block offers an alternative in patients with severe pulmonary disease, in whom phrenic nerve blockade may compromise respiration. The supraclavicular nerve block offers sufficient pain relief postoperatively.[44]

Surgery Distal to the Midpoint of the Arm

Infraclavicular Catheter. Infraclavicular brachial plexus catheter techniques avoid undesirable incidental blockade of the phrenic, recurrent laryngeal, or stellate ganglion nerves. Catheters here are more secure, and pericatheter leaks are uncommon. Pneumothorax is unlikely.

With the nerve stimulator technique, a vertical approach is commonly used. An 18-gauge insulated Touhy needle (Contiplex, B. Braun Medical, Bethlehem, Pa) is inserted beneath the coracoid process. After muscular twitches are obtained in the hand or forearm with a current of 0.3 to 0.4 mA, a 20-gauge catheter is threaded through the needle. A Stimulating catheter (Arrow International, Reading, Pa) allows stimulation of the plexus, and the position of its tip is confirmed before injection. If there is no response, the catheter may be manipulated to optimize the muscle twitch. Stimulating catheters have a limited role in the outpatient setting.

In the ultrasound-guided technique, the axillary vessels and brachial plexus are imaged below the clavicle in the area of the coracoid process of the scapula.[45] When the cords are best visualized, the transducer's position is labeled with a skin marker. The region is prepared with antiseptic solution and sterile drapes. A sterile cover containing conducting gel is put on the ultrasound transducer. A 17-gauge Touhy needle is introduced 1 to 2 cm cephalic to the transducer. The needle is directed between the axillary artery and vein, and local anesthetic is deposited around the medial brachial plexus cord. The needle is withdrawn into the pectoralis minor muscle and redirected between the axillary artery and lateral cord. After needle position is confirmed, local anesthetic is injected. The needle is then advanced a little deeper and, without release of pressure, the needle direction is changed to a more horizontal orientation and advanced between the posterior cord and the axillary artery. The third injection is delivered at this location, and a 20-gauge epidural catheter (Flextip [Arrow International]) is inserted.

The catheter position is now confirmed, and the catheter is withdrawn under imaging to bring the tip posterior to the axillary artery (Figs. 25–5 and 25–6). The catheter curls between the posterior and medial cords, and its position is better appreciated on withdrawal. Because the tip may be difficult to identify, 1 to 2 mL of air is injected through the catheter, and the point from which the air exits (usually hyperechoic or white) is seen. If the air spreads on both sides

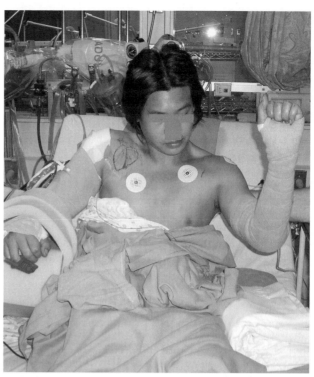

Figure 25–6 Open reduction and internal fixation of the radius fracture of the right arm and repair of multiple lacerations of the left arm were performed simultaneously with the use of bilateral infraclavicular blocks using ultrasound in this 14-year-old male patient. A right-side catheter was used for postoperative analgesia.

of the artery, the catheter position is satisfactory. If it moves toward the vein, the catheter should be withdrawn and the air test repeated. When in proper position, the catheter is fixed with a transparent dressing. With this technique, the catheter is unlikely to dislodge or leak because its path curves several times.

Axillary Catheter. An axillary catheter can be used for analgesia after operations of the hand, wrist, or elbow. The catheter entry site is through a moist area in the axilla, making these catheters more prone to infection. The needle can be introduced by a loss-of-resistance technique, or its location can be confirmed with electrical stimulation before the catheter is placed. Pericatheter leaks and dislodgments are more common with axillary than with infraclavicular catheters. Infusions at rates of 4 to 6 mL/hr of bupivacaine 0.25% or ropivacaine 0.2% are used; addition of patient-controlled boluses improves patient satisfaction.[46]

LOWER EXTREMITY OPERATIONS

Knee Arthroscopy

Knee arthroscopy is the most common ambulatory orthopedic procedure of the lower extremity. It can be performed with the use of femoral and sciatic blocks. When performed with central neuraxial block or general anesthesia, a continuous femoral nerve block is useful for control of postoperative pain. There are several other ways of supplying postoperative analgesia. A femoral nerve block (Figs. 25–7 and 25–8)

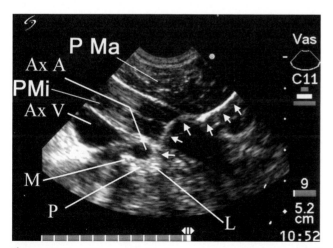

Figure 25–5 Ultrasonographic image of the cords of the brachial plexus and the catheter. L, M, and P label lateral, medial, and posterior cords, respectively. The catheter is marked by *white arrows.* AxA, axillary artery; AxV, axillary vein; PMa, pectoralis major muscle; PMi, pectoralis minor muscle.

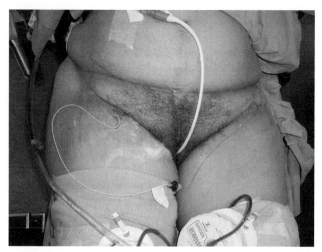

Figure 25–7 Bilateral femoral catheters provide postoperative analgesia for bilateral knee surgery.

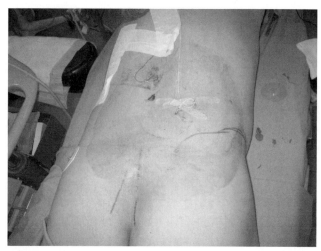

Figure 25–9 In a patient undergoing hip surgery, an epidural catheter was placed at the L2–L3 level, and a psoas compartment catheter was placed at the L4 level via the nerve stimulator technique.

or its variant, the fascia iliac block, gives better pain relief than intra-articular infusions.[47] A Contiplex or a Stimulating catheter may be placed via a nerve stimulator or ultrasound-guided technique (see earlier). NSAIDs in combination with an oral opioid may be added if the local anesthetic does not give adequate pain relief. The patient should be informed that there may be weakness of the quadriceps muscle and should use caution when trying to ambulate. The psoas compartment block and catheter techniques (Fig. 25–9) are alternatives that offer similar analgesia to that given by femoral catheters inserted below the inguinal ligament.[48] Bupivacaine solutions can be injected into the intra-articular space as a single injection or via a continuous catheter technique. Analgesia is less satisfactory than that provided by a femoral nerve block.[21]

Foot and Ankle Surgery

The sciatic nerve or its terminal branches can be blocked with either a single-injection or continuous-catheter technique. Use of this nerve block decreases the requirement for NSAIDs and opioids postoperatively.[49] The catheter should be inserted through the lateral hamstrings in order to secure it (Figs. 25–10 and 25–11).

▌ Summary

Successful ambulatory surgery depends on analgesia that is effective, has minimal adverse effects, and can be safely managed by the patient at home after discharge. A number of studies have established that the provision of effective postoperative analgesia is inadequate for a significant proportion of patients. Preemptive analgesia should be given to all patients unless there are specific contraindications.

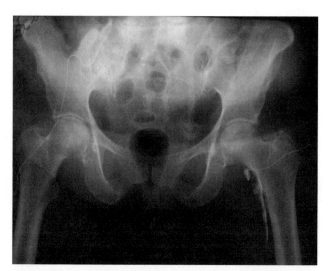

Figure 25–8 Radiograph of the patient shown in Fig. 25–7. The catheter on the right side was directed high up in the psoas compartment, and local anesthetic mixed with radiopaque contrast is spreading along the psoas muscle. The left catheter was placed posterior to the femoral nerve, below the inguinal ligament. The local anesthetic with radiopaque contrast is seen descending toward an unintended location. The two sides had equally satisfactory analgesia with continuous infusions.

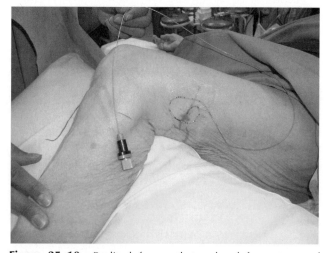

Figure 25–10 Popliteal fossa catheter placed for surgery and postoperative analgesia.

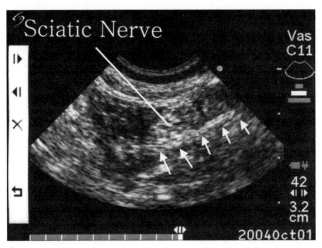

Figure 25–11 Ultrasonographic image of popliteal fossa catheter and sciatic nerve of the patient shown in Fig. 25–10, with approach using ultrasonography. *White arrows* mark the catheter lying anterior to the sciatic nerve.

A standardized multimodal postdischarge analgesic regimen tailored to each patient's expected postoperative pain levels should be prescribed. Patient follow-up by telephone questionnaire confirms whether surgical procedures result in mild or moderate to severe postoperative pain and determines the effectiveness of treatment regimens.

REFERENCES

1. Joshi GP: Postoperative pain management. Am J Orthop 2004; 33:128–135.
2. Pregler J, Kapur P: The development of ambulatory anesthesia and future challenges. Anesthesiol Clin North Am 2003;21:207–228.
3. Rawal N, Hylander J, Nydahl PA, et al: Survey of postoperative analgesia following ambulatory surgery. Acta Anaesthesiol Scand 1997;41:1017–1022.
4. Chung F, Ritchie E, Su J: Postoperative pain in ambulatory surgery. Anesth Analg 1997;85:808–816.
5. Mitchell M: Pain management in day-case surgery. Nurs Stand 2004; 18:33–38.
6. Coll AM, Ameen JR, Moseley LG: Reported pain after day surgery: a critical literature review. J Adv Nurs 2004;46:53–65.
7. McCaffery M, Pasero C: Pain: Clinical Manual, 2nd ed. St. Louis, Mosby, 1999.
8. Hekmat N, Burke M, Howell SJ: Preventive pain management in the postoperative hand surgery patient. Orthop Nurs 1994;13:3.
9. Goldsmith DM, Safran C: Using Web to reduce pain following ambulatory surgery. Proc AMIA Symp 1999;780–784.
10. Coll AM, Ameen JRM, Moseley LG: Reported pain after day surgery: A critical literature review. J Adv Nursing 2004;46:53–65.
11. Marquardt HM, Razia PA: Pre-packed take home analgesia for day case surgery. Br J Nurs 1996;5:1114–1118.
12. Kehlet H, Dahl J: The value of "multimodal" or "balanced analgesia" in postoperative pain treatment. Anesth Analg 1993;77:1048–1056.
13. Kissin I: Preemptive analgesia. Anesthesiology 2000;93:1138–1143.
14. Woolf CJ: Evidence of a central component of post-injury pain hypersensitivity. Nature 1983;308:686–688.
15. Moiniche S, Kehelet H, Dahl JB: A qualitative and quantitative systematic review of preemptive analgesia for postoperative relief: The role of timing of analgesia. Anesthesiology 2002;96:725–741.
16. Honama T, Imaizumi T, Chiba M, Niwa J: Preemptive analgesia for postoperative pain. Neurol Surg 2002;30:171–174.
17. Nguyn A, Girard F, Boudreault D, et al: Scalp nerve blocks decrease the severity of pain after craniotomy. Anesth Analg 2001;93: 1272–1276.
18. Chung F, McGrath B: Postoperative pain following discharge after ambulatory surgery. Can we do better? [abstract A20]. Can J Anaesth 2003;50:20A.
19. Rocchi A, Chung F, Forte L: Canadian survey of postsurgical pain and pain medication experiences. Can J Anaesth 2002;49:1053–1056.
20. Grant GJ, Barenholz Y, Bolotin E, et al: A novel liposomal bupivacaine formulation to produce ultralong-acting analgesia. Anesthesiology 2004;101:133–137.
21. Grant SA: Holy Grail of local anaesthetics and liposomes. Best Pract Res Clin Anaesthesiol 2002;16:345–352.
22. Rawal N: Analgesia for day-case surgery. Br J Anaesth 2001;87:73–87.
23. Smith HS: Acetaminophen (bench). In Smith HS (ed): Drugs for Pain. Philadelphia, Hanley & Belfus, 2003.
24. Korpela R, Korvenoja P, Meretoja OA: Morphine sparing effect of acetaminophen in pediatric day-case surgery. Anesthesiology 1999; 91:442–447.
25. Acute Pain Management Guideline Panel: Acute Pain Management: Operative or Medical Procedures and Trauma. (Clinical Practice Guideline AHCPR Publication No. 92-0032.) Rockville, Md, Agency for Health Care Policy and Research, 1992.
26. Karasch ED: Perioperative COX-2 inhibitors: Knowledge and challenges. Anesth Analg 2004;98:1–3.
27. Silverman D, Halaszynski T, Sinatra R, et al: Rofecoxib does not compromise platelet aggregation during anesthesia and surgery. Can J Anaesth 2003;50:1004–1008.
28. Barden J, Edwards J, McQuay H, et al: Oral valdecoxib and injected parecoxib for acute postoperative pain: A quantitative systematic review. BMC Anesthesiol 2003;3:1–8.
29. Claxton AR, McGuire G, Chung F, et al: Evaluation of morphine versus fentanyl for postoperative analgesia after ambulatory surgical procedures. Anesth Analg 1997;84:509–514.
30. Sunshine A, Olson NZ, Rivera J: Analgesic efficacy of controlled-release oxycodone in postoperative pain. J Clin Pharmacol 1996;26: 595–603.
31. Mucci-Lorusso P, Berman B, Silberstein P, et al: Controlled-release oxycodone compared with controlled-release morphine in the treatment of cancer pain: A randomized, double-blinded, parallel-group study. Eur J Pain 1998;2:239–249.
32. White PF: The role of non-opioid analgesic techniques in the management of pain after ambulatory surgery. Anesth Analg 2002;94: 577–585.
33. Hashish I, Hai HK, Harvey W, et al: Reduction of postoperative pain and swelling by ultrasound treatment: a placebo effect. Pain 1988;33: 303–311.
34. Gam AN, Thorsen H, Lonnberg F: The effect of low-level laser therapy on musculoskeletal pain: A meta-analysis. Pain 1993;52: 63–66.
35. Klein SM, Pietrobon R, Nielsen KC, et al: Paravertebral somatic nerve block compared with peripheral nerve blocks for outpatient inguinal herniorrhaphy. Reg Anesth Pain Med 2002;27:476–480.
36. Choi WY, Irwin MG, Hui TWC, et al: EMLA cream versus dorsal penile nerve block for post circumcision analgesia. Anesth Analg 2003; 96:396–399.
37. Kairaluoma PM, Bachmann MS, Korpinen AK, et al: Single-injection paravertebral block before general anesthesia enhances analgesia after breast cancer surgery with and without associated lymph node biopsy. Anesth Analg 2004;99:1837–1843.
38. Suresh S, Barcelona S, Young N, et al: Postoperative pain relief in children undergoing tympanomastoid surgery: Is regional block better than opioids? Anesth Analg 2002;94:859–862.
39. Huang YC, Tsai SK, Huang CH, et al: Intravenous tenoxicam reduces uterine cramps after Cesarean delivery. Can J Anaesth 2002;49: 384–387.
40. Wilson AT, Nicholson E, Burton L, Wild C: Analgesia for day-case shoulder surgery. Br J Anaesth 2004;92:414–415.
41. Klein SM, Grant SA, Greengrass RA, et al: Interscalene brachial plexus block with a continuous catheter insertion system and a disposable infusion pump. Anesth Analg 2000;91:1473–1478.
42. Borene SC, Rosenquist RW, Koorn R, et al: An indication for continuous cervical paravertebral block (posterior approach to the interscalene space). Anesth Analg 2003;97:898–900.
43. Singelyn FJ, Seguy S, Gouverneur JM: Interscalene brachial plexus block after open shoulder surgery: Continuous vs patient controlled infusion. Anesth Analg 1999;89:1216–1220.

44. Singlyn FJ, Lhotel L, Fabre B: Pain relief after arthroscopic shoulder surgery, a comparison of intraarticular analgesia, suprascapular nerve block and interscalene block. Anesth Analg 2004;99:589–592.

45. Sandhu NS, Capan LM: Ultrasound guided infraclavicular brachial plexus block. Br J Anaesth 2002;89:254–259.

46. Iskander H, Rakotondriamihary S, Dixmerias F, et al: Analgesia with continuous axillary block after severe hand trauma: Self-administration vs continuous infusion. Annales Francaises d'Anesthésie et de Réanimation. 1998;17:1099–1103.

47. Iskander H, Benard A, Ruel-raymond J, et al: Femoral blocks provide superior analgesia compared with intra-articular ropivacaine after anterior cruciate ligament repair. Reg Anesth Pain Med 2003;28:29–32.

48. Kaloul I, Guay J, Cote C, Fallaha M: The posterior lumbar plexus (psoas compartment) block provides similar postoperative analgesia after total knee replacement Can J Anaesth 2004;51:45–51.

49. Mendicino RW, Statler TK, Catanzariti AR: Popliteal sciatic nerve blocks after foot and ankle surgery: An adjunct to postoperative analgesia. J Foot Ankle Surg 2002;41:38–41.

26 Can We Prevent Chronic Pain after Surgery?

WILLIAM A. MACRAE

Epidemiological studies of patients attending pain clinics in the 1990s showed that surgery and trauma are major causes of chronic pain.[1,2] This finding led to publications on the general subject of chronic pain after surgery.[3-5] Until then, chronic pain after surgery had been a neglected topic, although pain after individual operations had been documented. The literature was fragmented and dispersed, so no overall picture was possible. This chapter does not go over this ground again, but discusses mechanisms, investigates what is known about risk factors, and points to possibilities for prevention. Those who wish to read about the general topic of chronic pain after surgery are referred to the references cited in this paragraph.

Chronic pain after surgery has many forms and presentations. Several different types of pain may occur after the same operation, and there are many mechanisms. In open thoracotomy, for example, in order to gain access to the chest, the surgeon has to either resect a piece of rib or spread the ribs. Either maneuver inevitably produces skeletal trauma to the ribs or to the joints at the posterior and anterior articulations. The intercostal nerves lie just deep to the inferior border of the ribs and are vulnerable to injury, which can cause neuropathic pain. The lungs or other viscera will also be affected by the operation and hence may contribute to the pain. Chest drains are often a source of pain.[6] After breast surgery, patients report many unpleasant symptoms, such as numbness, tingling, swelling, and sensitivity, which may cause as much distress as pain.[7,8] The pain may be phantom pain,[9] neuropathic pain caused by damage to the intercostobrachial nerve,[10] or scar pain.[11] It is clear, then, that even for a given operation, there is no one postsurgical pain syndrome, but rather a diverse group of problems.

It should also be obvious that these pain syndromes are not unique to postoperative states, but are similar to problems seen with other etiologies. The treatments are therefore not unique either; a neuropathic pain syndrome after surgery should be treated in the same way as any other neuropathic pain, be it diabetic neuropathy, traumatic, or post-herpetic neuralgia.[12] A postoperative mechanical musculoskeletal pain should be treated in the same way as other musculoskeletal problems.[13]

Mechanisms of Chronic Pain after Surgery

Any operation has the potential to cause chronic pain. There are many different mechanisms, but changes in the nervous system are the most important factor.

Neuropathic pain is complex, with many etiologies and mechanisms.[14] Obviously, nerve injury such as transection, stretching, or constriction causes changes. However, it is important to appreciate that the pain system responds to injury to other tissues as well.[15] One example that has been investigated extensively is thermal injury to the skin, such as sunburn. In the past, the pain after sunburn was explained as being caused by "damage to the skin." This is an inadequate explanation, as one would not expect injury to increase sensitivity in a sensory system; for example, an eye injury would not improve visual acuity. Thermal injury to the skin causes a cascade of changes; for example, inflammatory mediators are released from the damaged cells, which bathe the nerve endings of the C and Aδ fibers. This changes the nociceptors by reducing their thresholds and increasing excitability. The hyperexcitability occurs both at the periphery and in the spinal cord. The result is that previously innocuous stimuli are painful (allodynia), and more pain than usual is experienced from painful stimuli (hyperalgesia). It is this sensitization of the sensory nerves to the skin (caused by the damage) that causes the pain. In the same way that thermal injury causes sensitization, the inevitable injuries involved in surgery can also cause changes, resulting in sensitization and hyperalgesia.

Injury changes the nervous system not only at the periphery and the spinal cord but also at the brain. Remapping of the sensory cortex after deafferentation was first described in 1991.[16] This phenomenon has been widely described in humans after limb amputation.[17] It can occur soon after injury[18] and has been shown to change with time.[19] Plasticity also occurs in the thalamus.[20] Paradoxically, injury to the brain can cause misperceptions at the periphery, such as the case described by Halligan et al,[21] in which a patient experienced the sensation of having a third arm after a stroke.

Many different sorts of injury cause sensitization of the nervous system, both peripheral and central. This hypersensitivity may confer an evolutionary benefit by preventing an injured animal from further damaging itself, encouraging rest, and allowing healing. The sensitivity should return to normal after the injury has healed, but it does not always do so. Failure to return to normal from this injury-induced hyperalgesic state is probably one of the main causes of chronic pain after surgery. Why the system fails to adjust in this way is unknown. Animal work suggests that there is a genetic component to the development of neuropathic pain.[22,23]

Understanding the scale of the changes to the nervous system and the mechanisms that predispose to chronic pain after surgery is important for many reasons. Such an understanding can change the climate of blame that develops when patients have pain after an operation. It is not possible to perform surgery without some damage to tissues; a hyperalgesic state is induced after any operation, regardless of how it is done. Normally this state reverts to normal as healing occurs, but not always. Whether a patient experiences chronic pain after surgery is therefore more likely to depend on the "set" of the patient's nervous system than on precisely what the surgeon did. When patients have chronic pain after surgery it is inappropriate to assume that the surgeon has necessarily done anything wrong or to lay blame. It should also be clear that acting on simplistic notions about treatment, such as by performing simple nerve blocks or further surgery, is unlikely to help and may well do harm by causing further damage. The extent of the changes in the nervous system suggests that pharmacological, psychological, and behavioral therapies may be more beneficial to patients than invasive treatments.

Risk Factors

Most surgery is performed because the patient has a disease or injury that is amenable to improvement by surgery. In other cases, patients have cosmetic plastic surgery and surgery for social reasons, such as female sterilization and vasectomy. Also, some patients have inappropriate surgery. Many patients continue to have surgery for back pain despite evidence that in many cases it is unhelpful and may in fact make the problem worse.[24] Many patients with abdominal pain have visceral hyperalgesic syndromes, and these problems, too, may be made worse by surgery. Such patients can enter a vicious circle of repeated operations in the vain hope of cure or because of complications from previous operations.

Risk factors for chronic pain after surgery must therefore start with risk factors for diseases that lead to surgery. To prevent phantom pain and stump pain after limb amputation, the single most important strategy would be to eliminate smoking and obesity, because peripheral vascular disease and diabetes are the two most common reasons for amputation.[25] The risk factors for diseases such as breast cancer are complex, involving genetic, demographic, and lifestyle factors.[26] Screening and early detection will influence outcome in such diseases. These factors cannot be ignored if we are to take a realistic and broad view of risk factors for chronic pain after surgery.

DEMOGRAPHIC AND PSYCHOSOCIAL FACTORS

The influence of age has been reported in two studies of pain after breast surgery. Tasmuth et al[27] reported that younger patients have more pain postoperatively and over the long term as well as bigger tumors. Smith et al[28] found the incidence of chronic pain after mastectomy to be 26% in patients older than 70 years, 40% in those 50 to 69 years, and 65% in those 30 to 49 years. This study also showed that several other demographic factors related to age may be influential, such as marital status, housing, and employment.

Age does not seem to be a risk factor for phantom pain after upper or lower limb amputation.[29-31] Demographic factors do not seem to be important in pain after thoracotomy.[6,32]

Many studies have shown that pain is an important cause of disability.[33] Those who attribute their pain to a specific trauma (for example, an operation) report significantly higher levels of emotional distress, life interference, and pain severity than those whose pain had an insidious or spontaneous onset, regardless of the extent of objective physical findings.[34] This finding raises the possibility that by preparing patients better—for example, giving information about chronic pain before obtaining consent to surgery—we can change patients' perceptions, leading to better outcomes.[35]

PREOPERATIVE PAIN

In a careful study of the influence of preamputation pain on postamputation stump and phantom pain, Nikolajsen et al[36] showed that preamputation pain significantly raised the incidence of stump and phantom pain postoperatively and of phantom pain at 3 months. However, patients overestimated the severity of their preamputation pain 6 months after undergoing amputation (compared with their preamputation scores), and although patients stated that their phantom pain had been similar to their preamputation pain, these statements were not borne out by the patients' actual descriptions before and after amputation.

In a study of women undergoing mastectomy for breast cancer, Kroner et al[9] found a correlation between premastectomy breast pain and both phantom breast pain and nonpainful phantom breast sensations.

In patients undergoing thoracotomy for cancer, 48% of those who had been taking narcotics before thoracotomy went on to experience chronic post-thoracotomy pain, whereas only 5% of those who had not been taking narcotics did so.[37] Whether the postoperative pain was a continuation of the preoperative pain or a true postsurgical pain syndrome is impossible to say.

TYPE OF SURGERY

The incidence of chronic pain after surgery varies according to the type of operation and how it is performed. For example, Table 26–1 shows the incidences of chronic pain after various types of breast surgery.

In a study from Finland,[8] women undergoing surgery for breast cancer in high-volume surgical units suffered less chronic pain than those having operations in hospitals that had less experience in breast surgery.

TABLE 26–1	Incidence of Chronic Pain After Breast Surgery
Procedure	**Incidence (%)**
Breast reduction	22
Mastectomy	31
Breast augmentation	
Silicone	22
Saline	33
Submuscular	50
Subglandular	21
Mastectomy and reconstruction	
No implant	30
Implant	53

Modified from Wallace MS, Wallace AM, Lee J, Dobke MK: Pain after breast surgery: A survey of 282 women. Pain 1996;66:195–205.

Whether the cause of breast surgery influences the incidence of chronic pain is difficult to establish, because different operations are performed for malignant and benign conditions, and the type of surgery does influence the incidence of pain.[38]

The evidence for the effect of surgical technique on pain after thoracotomy is contradictory, with some papers showing a difference[6] but others showing no long-term difference.[39] The level and type of amputation does not appear to influence the incidence of phantom pain.[31]

In a review of pain after hernia repair, Callesen and Kehlet[40] reported that there was no difference between the various open techniques but that laparoscopic herniorrhaphy resulted in less pain and shorter convalescence than open repair. For cholecystectomy, the incidence of long-term right upper quadrant pain was reported as 3.4% after laparoscopic cholecystectomy but 9.7% after open cholecystectomy.[41]

Two studies from Finland have shown that chronic pain is equally common after thoracotomy for malignant disease and for benign disease.[32,42] Another study, however, found that chronic pain was more common after surgery for benign esophageal disease than for lung cancer.[6]

Cause of amputation does not influence the incidence of phantom pain.[31] Houghton et al[43] showed no difference in the incidence of phantom pain between traumatic and vascular amputees. This finding was confirmed in a study finding no difference between amputees whose amputations were of civilian or military origin.[44]

CONCOMITANT TREATMENTS

The data on the influence of other treatments is contradictory. Some studies have shown that radiotherapy and chemotherapy do not influence the incidence of chronic pain.[9] However, other studies have shown a higher incidence of chronic pain in patients who received chemotherapy and/or radiotherapy.[8,27] Smith et al[28] point out that it is difficult to unravel the relationship between the different treatments and pain because of confounding factors such as age.

In a study from the Mayo Clinic of children having limb amputations for either trauma or cancer, Smith and Thompson[45] showed that chemotherapy increased the risk of phantom pain considerably (Table 26–2).

GENETIC FACTORS

Why only some people have chronic pain after surgery is an interesting question. Clearly there are many factors determining individual susceptibility, and it seems likely that part of the reason will be genetic. Research in mice shows that there is a genetic influence in whether the animal suffers chronic pain after nerve injury.[22,23] Diatchenko et al[46] published the first paper demonstrating an association among a genetic polymorphism, pain sensitivity, and the risk of development of a chronic pain syndrome in humans. Some human pain syndromes have been shown to have a genetic component, and the clinical suspicion of many researchers in this field is that some of these conditions may be markers for a greater likelihood of development of chronic pain after injury. These conditions include migrainous headaches, fibromyalgia syndrome, irritable bowel syndrome, bladder frequency and urgency, and Raynaud's phenomenon (particularly bipolar, with both excessively cold extremities in cold weather and erythromelalgia ["burning-hot" feet], usually at night).

Against this possibility it must be said that many patients have several operations but experience chronic pain only after a particular one. Some patients who undergo bilateral operations have chronic postsurgical pain syndrome on one side but not the other. This is clearly a complex but fascinating area that will probably provide as many interesting questions as answers in the next few years.

PERIOPERATIVE PAIN

The question of whether perioperative pain is a risk factor for chronic pain has been the subject of many studies. It is of great importance, because perioperative pain is a factor over which we have some control. Early studies were confounded by the problem of patients' memory of past pain, a notoriously tricky subject. Studies have shown that patients are not good at accurately rating past pain. The past pain report is influenced by many factors, including the amount of pain suffered subsequently, especially at the time

TABLE 26–2	Phantom Pain in Pediatric Amputees	
Patients and Settings		**Incidence of Pain (%)**
Trauma-related amputees		12
Cancer patients		48
Chemotherapy before or at the time of amputation		74
Chemotherapy after amputation		44
No chemotherapy		12

Modified from Smith J, Thompson JM: Phantom limb pain and chemotherapy in pediatric amputees. Mayo Clin Proc 1995;70:357–364.

of remembering. Several studies comparing pain reports recorded in the perioperative period with reports of patients' memories of their pain several months later show poor correlation. It is therefore important that studies be prospective and that valid pain assessments be made in the perioperative period. Unfortunately, few studies fulfill these criteria, but when they have been met, the incidence of chronic postsurgical pain does correlate with postoperative pain intensity.[47]

Adequate treatment of pain around the time of the operation is correlated with a lower incidence of chronic pain after surgery. Whether there is a causal relationship is not yet clear. It is reasonable, however, to assume with our current level of knowledge that we should take all possible steps to minimize perioperative pain to try to prevent long-term problems.

Choice of Anesthesia and Analgesia in Reducing Chronic Pain

Many studies have looked at the influence of anesthetic technique on short-term postoperative pain. Two studies have examined pain for 10 days after surgery for which patients were randomly allocated to receive either local anesthesia or general anesthesia. In a study on patients undergoing hernia repair, Tverskoy et al[48] showed that patients who received either local anesthetic block and general anesthesia or spinal anesthesia had significantly less pain at 2 days than those who received only general anesthesia. At 10 days after operation, the group that had general anesthesia with local anesthetic still had significantly less pain than the general anesthesia alone group.

In an elegant study of pain after tonsillectomy and adenoidectomy in children, Jebeles et al[49] showed not only a decrease in pain scores but functional improvement in swallowing up to 10 days postoperatively in the children who received a preoperative local anesthetic infiltration. It is reasonable to assume that the local anesthetic given at the time of surgery protected the nervous system from the afferent nociceptive barrage during and immediately after the operation. This protection may prevent the sensitization that leads to chronic pain. Not all studies comparing regional anesthesia with general anesthesia show such benefit, however.[50]

In a study of chronic pain after cesarean section, patients who had chronic pain were more likely to have had general anesthesia rather than epidural anesthesia and had a higher recall of severe postoperative pain.[51]

Chronic pain after vasectomy is common, but the results of comparisons of local anesthesia with general anesthesia are contradictory.[52,53]

Prevention in the Preoperative Period

PREOPERATIVE ANALGESIA

The finding that preoperative pain and perioperative pain are associated with a higher incidence of chronic postsurgical pain led researchers to try delivering analgesia to patients prior to surgery. Animal work suggesting that pretreating with analgesics reduced changes in the nervous system formed a theoretical basis for this approach.[54] In a much-quoted study

by Bach et al,[55] patients who were to undergo lower limb amputation were given analgesia by epidural local anesthetic and opioid for 72 hours preoperatively. This study reported that the procedure reduced the incidence of phantom pain at 1 year, but there were methodological problems. Nikolajsen et al[56] subsequently conducted a randomized, double-blind, controlled trial to investigate the matter further. They showed no benefit in reduction of phantom pain and no change in hyperalgesia, allodynia, or wind-up–like pain.[57] Subsequent studies have also failed to show any convincing evidence that treating pain prior to amputation or other forms of surgery prevents long-term pain.

Many studies have shown that pain before amputation is a risk factor for chronic phantom pain. We must not abandon this important line of research, because phantom pain is usually resistant to treatment, so prevention is vital. The fact that no clinical effect for preemptive analgesia has been demonstrated should not blind us, however, to the possibility that it might be possible to reduce long-term problems by treating pain adequately perioperatively. It may be that the methods used in previous studies were inadequate to reduce afferent input sufficiently. Perhaps using combinations of drugs may make it possible to reduce chronic pain after surgery.

Several studies have investigated giving drugs preoperatively with the aim of reducing pain in the postoperative period, including gabapentin,[58-61] NSAIDs,[62] fentanyl and ketamine,[63] local anesthetic blocks,[64-66] and anesthetic blocks in combination with NSAIDs,[67] and clonidine and ketamine.[68] The results are contradictory, and there is a need for large randomized controlled trials, although the methodological problems should not be underestimated.

Pain after injury is mainly a hyperalgesic phenomenon. There is evidence that lidocaine infusion reduces secondary but not primary hyperalgesia caused by thermal injury, presumably through a spinal effect.[69] There is also evidence that ketamine given perioperatively reduces postoperative hyperalgesia.[68] These are both promising lines for further research.

PREOPERATIVE SCREENING OF HIGH-RISK PATIENTS

The presence of genetic risk factors opens up the possibility of screening. Patients who are deemed to be at particular risk could be prioritized to receive the best possible management to minimize that risk. There may be linked genetic factors, and many people working in this field believe that patients with other medical problems are more likely to experience chronic pain after surgery. Kalkman et al,[70] studying the factors predisposing to severe postoperative pain, showed that younger age, female sex, higher level of preoperative pain, larger incision size, and type of surgery (for example, abdominal or orthopedic) were independent predictors. Another approach to preoperative screening might be to assess the response to heat stimulation.[71]

As mentioned earlier, patients' beliefs about the cause and onset of their pain can influence the severity of pain and its impact on their lives. Education therefore has an important role to play in minimizing the problem of pain after surgery, especially because it seems increasingly obvious that the pain is not usually the surgeon's fault.

Complex regional pain syndrome develops in a surprisingly high number of patients after orthopedic surgery. It is a notoriously difficult problem to treat, so prevention is of great importance. Readers are recommended to read the review of this topic by Reuben.[72]

Conclusion

Because the treatment of chronic pain after surgery is often ineffective, prevention is paramount. Considering the amount of resources spent in most developed countries on surgical treatments, it is surprising that more resources are not devoted to improving long-term outcomes. There is a great need for well-designed, properly conducted studies to provide valid data on how to minimize chronic postsurgical pain. Perhaps the easiest way to reduce the amount of chronic postsurgical pain is to reduce the number of unnecessary operations.

REFERENCES

1. Davies HTO, Crombie IK, Macrae WA, Rogers KM: Pain clinic patients in northern Britain. Pain Clinic 1992;5:129–135.
2. Crombie IK, Davies HTO, Macrae WA: Cut and thrust: Antecedent surgery and trauma among patients attending a chronic pain clinic. Pain 1998;76:167–171.
3. Macrae WA, Davies HTO: Chronic postsurgical pain. In Crombie IK, Linton S, Croft P, et al (eds): Epidemiology of Pain. Seattle, International Association for the Study of Pain 1999, pp 125–142.
4. Perkins FM, Kehlet H: Chronic pain as an outcome of surgery. Anesthesiology 2000;93:1123–1133.
5. Macrae WA: Chronic pain after surgery. Br J Anaesth 2001;87:88–98.
6. Richardson J, Sabanathan S, Mearns AJ, et al: Post-thoracotomy neuralgia. Pain Clinic 1994;7:87–97.
7. Polinsky ML: Functional status of long-term breast cancer survivors. Health Social Work 1994;19:165–173.
8. Tasmuth T, Blomqvist C, Kalso E: Chronic post-treatment symptoms in patients with breast cancer operated in different surgical units. Eur J Surg Oncol 1999;25:38–43.
9. Kroner K, Knudsen UB, Lundby L, Hvid H: Long term phantom breast syndrome after mastectomy. Clin J Pain 1992;8:346–350.
10. Vecht CJ, Van der Brand HJ, Wajer OJM: Post-axillary dissection pain in breast cancer due to a lesion of the intercostobrachial nerve. Pain 1989;38:171–176.
11. Jung BF, Ahrendt GM, Oaklander AL, Dworkin RH: Neuropathic pain following breast cancer surgery: Proposed classification and research update. Pain 2003;104:1–13.
12. Sindrup SH, Jensen TS: Efficacy of pharmacological treatments of neuropathic pain: An update and effect related to mechanism of drug action. Pain 1999;83:389–400.
13. Main CJ, Williams AC: Musculoskeletal pain. Br Med J 2002;325:534–537.
14. Woolf CJ, Mannion RJ: Neuropathic pain: Aetiology, symptoms, mechanisms, and management. Lancet 1999;353:1959–1964.
15. Villanueva L, Dickenson AH, Ollat H: The Pain System in Normal and Pathological States. Seattle, IASP Press, 2004.
16. Pons TP, Preston E, Garraghty AK: Massive cortical reorganisation after sensory deafferentation in adult macaques. Science 1991;252:1857–1860.
17. Ramachandran VS, Hirstein W: The perception of phantom limbs. Brain 1998;121:1603–1630.
18. Borsook D, Becerra L, Fishman S, et al: Acute plasticity in the human somatosensory cortex following amputation. NeuroReport 1998;9:1013–1017.
19. Knecht S, Henningsen H, Hohling C, et al: Plasticity of plasticity? Changes in the pattern of perceptual correlates of reorganisation after amputation. Brain 1998;121:717–724.
20. Dostrovsky JO: Immediate and long-term plasticity in human somatosensory thalamus and its involvement in phantom limbs. Pain Suppl 1999;6:S37–S43.
21. Halligan PW, Marshall JC, Wade DT: Three arms: A case study of supernumerary phantom limb after right hemisphere stroke. J Neurol Neurosurg Psychiatry 1993;56:159–166.
22. Devor M, Raber P: Heritability of symptoms in an experimental model of neuropathic pain, Pain 1990;42:51–67.
23. Seltzer Z, Wu T, Max MB, Diehl SR: Mapping a gene for neuropathic pain-related behaviour following peripheral neurectomy in the mouse. Pain 2001;93:101–106.
24. Turner JA, Ersek M, Herron L, et al: Patient outcomes after lumbar spinal fusions. JAMA 1992;268:907–911.
25. Chaturvedi N, Abbott CA, Whalley A, et al: Risk of diabetes related amputation in South Asians vs Europeans in the UK. Diabet Med 2002;19:99–104.
26. American Cancer Society: What are the risk factors for breast cancer? Available at www.cancer.org/docroot/CRI/content/CRI_2_4_2X_What_are_the_risk_factors_for_breast_cancer_5.asp?sitearea=/
27. Tasmuth T, von Smitten K, Hietanen P, et al: Pain and other symptoms after different treatment modalities of breast cancer. Ann Oncol 1995;6:453–459.
28. Smith WCS, Bourne D, Squair J, et al: A retrospective cohort study of post mastectomy pain syndrome. Pain 1999;83:91–95.
29. Kooijman CM, Dijkstra PU, Geertzen JH, et al: Phantom pain and phantom sensations in upper limb amputees: An epidemiological study. Pain 2000;87:33–41.
30. Wartan SW, Hamann W, Wedley JR, McColl I: Phantom pain and sensation among British veteran amputees. Br J Anaesth 1997;78:652–659.
31. Jensen TS, Krebs B, Nielsen J, Rasmussen P: Immediate and long-term phantom limb pain in amputees: Incidence, clinical characteristics and relationship to pre-amputation limb pain. Pain 1985;21:267–278.
32. Kalso E, Perttunen K, Kaasinen S: Pain after thoracic surgery. Acta Anaesthesiol Scand 1992;36:96–100.
33. Larsson TJ, Bjornstig U: Persistent medical problems and permanent impairment five years after occupational injury. Scand J Soc Med 1995;23:121–128.
34. Turk DC, Okifuji A: Perception of traumatic onset, compensation status, and physical findings: Impact on pain severity, emotional distress, and disability in chronic pain patients. J Behav Med 1996;19:435–453.
35. Johnston M, Vogele C: Benefits of psychological preparation for surgery: A meta-analysis. Ann Behav Med 1993;15:245–256.
36. Nikolajsen L, Ilkjaer S, Kroner K, et al: The influence of preamputation pain on postamputation stump and phantom pain. Pain 1997;72:393–405.
37. Keller SM, Carp NZ, Levy MN, Rosen SM: Chronic post thoracotomy pain. J Cardiovasc Surg 1994;35:161–164.
38. Wallace MS, Wallace AM, Lee J, Dobke MK: Pain after breast surgery: A survey of 282 women. Pain 1996;66:195–205.
39. Landreneau RJ, Mack MJ, Hazelrigg SR, et al: Prevalence of chronic pain after pulmonary resection by thoracotomy or video-assisted thoracic surgery. J Thorac Cardiovasc Surg 1994;107:1079–1086.
40. Callesen T, Kehlet H: Postherniorrhaphy pain. Anesthesiology 1997;87:1219–1230.
41. Stiff G, Rhodes M, Kelly A, et al: Long-term pain: Less common after laparoscopic than open cholecystectomy. Br J Surg 1994;81:1368–1370.
42. Perttunen K, Tasmuth T, Kalso E: Chronic pain after thoracic surgery: A follow-up study. Acta Anaesthesiol Scand 1999;43:563–567.
43. Houghton AD, Saadah E, Nicholls G, et al: Phantom pain: Natural history and association with rehabilitation. Ann Roy Coll Surg Engl 1994;76:22–25.
44. Sherman RA, Sherman CJ: A comparison of phantom sensations among amputees whose amputations were of civilian or military origins. Pain 1985;21:91–97.
45. Smith J, Thompson JM: Phantom limb pain and chemotherapy in pediatric amputees. Mayo Clin Proc 1995;70:357–364.
46. Diatchenko L, Slade GD, Nackley AG, et al: Genetic basis for individual variations in pain perception and the development of a chronic pain condition. Hum Mol Genet 2005;14:135–143.
47. Katz J, Jackson M, Kavanagh BP, Sandler AN: Acute pain after thoracic surgery predicts long-term post-thoracotomy pain. Clin J Pain 1996;12:50–55.
48. Tverskoy M, Cozacov C, Ayache M, et al: Postoperative pain after inguinal herniorrhaphy with different types of anaesthesia. Anesth Analg 1990;70:29–35.

49. Jebeles JA, Reilly JS, Gutierrez JF, et al: Tonsillectomy and adenoidectomy pain reduction by local bupivacaine infiltration in children. Int J Pediatr Otorhinolaryngol 1993;25:149–154.

50. McCartney CJL, Brull R, Chan VWS, et al: Early but not long-term benefit of regional compared with general anesthesia for ambulatory hand surgery. Anesthesiology 2004;101:461–467.

51. Nikolajsen L, Sorensen HC, Jensen TS, Kehlet H: Chronic pain after Caesarean section. Acta Anaesthesiol Scand 2004;48:111–116.

52. McMahon AJ, Buckley J, Taylor A, et al: Chronic testicular pain following vasectomy. Brit J Urol 1992;69:188–191.

53. Paxton LD, Huss BK, Loughlin V, Mirakhur RK: Intra-vas deferens bupivacaine for prevention of acute pain and chronic discomfort after vasectomy. Brit J Anaesth 1995;74:612–613.

54. Woolf CJ, Chong M: Preemptive analgesia—treating postoperative pain by preventing the establishment of central sensitisation. Anesth Analg 1993;77:362–379.

55. Bach S, Noreng MF, Tjellden NU: Phantom limb pain in amputees during the first 12 months following limb amputation, after preoperative lumbar epidural blockade. Pain 1988;33:297–301.

56. Nikolajsen L, Ilkjaer S, Christensen JH, et al: Randomised trial of epidural bupivacaine and morphine in prevention of stump and phantom pain in lower limb amputation. Lancet 1997;350:1353–1357.

57. Nikolajsen L, Ilkjaer S, Jensen TS: Effect of preoperative extradural bupivacaine and morphine on stump sensation in lower limb amputees. Brit J Anaesth 1998;81:348–354.

58. Fassoulaki A, Patris K, Sarantopoulos C, Hogan Q: The analgesic effect of gabapentin and mexiletine after breast surgery for cancer. Anesth Analg 2002;95:985–991.

59. Dirks J, Fredensborg BB, Christensen D, et al: A randomised study of the effects of single-dose gabapentin versus placebo on postoperative pain and morphine consumption after mastectomy. Anesthesiology 2002;97:560–564.

60. Rorarius MGF, Mennader S, Suominen P, et al: Gabapentin for the prevention of postoperative pain after vaginal hysterectomy. Pain 2004;110:175–181.

61. Dierking G, Duedahl TH, Rasmussen ML, et al: Effects of gabapentin on postoperative morphine consumption and pain after abdominal hysterectomy: A randomised, double blind study. Acta Anaesthesiol Scand 2004;48:322–327.

62. Priya V, Divatia JV, Sareen R, Upadhye S: Efficacy of intravenous ketoprofen for pre-emptive analgesia. J Postgrad Med 2002;48:109–112.

63. Katz J, Scmid R, Snijdelaar DG, Coderre TJ, et al: Pre-emptive analgesia using intravenous fentanyl plus low-dose ketamine for radical prostatectomy under general anesthesia does not produce short-term or long-term reductions in pain or analgesic use. Pain 2004;110:707–718.

64. Katz J, Clairoux M, Kavanagh BP, et al: Pre-emptive lumbar epidural anaesthesia reduces postoperative pain and patient-controlled morphine consumption after lower abdominal surgery. Pain 1994;59:395–403.

65. Aguilar JL, Rincon R, Domingo V, et al: Absence of an early preemptive effect after thoracic extradural bupivacaine in thoracic surgery. Br J Anaesth 1996;76:72–76.

66. Gill P, Kiani S, Victoria BA, Atcheson R: Pre-emptive analgesia with local anaesthetic for herniorrhaphy. Anaesthesia 2001;56:414–417.

67. Espinet A, Henderson DJ, Faccenda KA, Morrison LMM: Does preincisional thoracic extradural block combined with diclofenac reduce postoperative pain after abdominal hysterectomy? Br J Anaesth 1996;76:209–213.

68. De Kock M, Lavand'homme P, Waterloos H: Balanced analgesia in the perioperative period: Is there a place for ketamine? Pain 2001;92:373–380.

69. Holthusen H, Irsfeld S, Lipfert P: Effect of pre- or post-traumatically applied lidocaine on primary and secondary hyperalgesia after experimental heat trauma in humans. Pain 2000;88:295–302.

70. Kalkman CJ, Visser K, Moen J, et al: Preoperative prediction of severe postoperative pain. Pain 2003;105:415–423.

71. Werner MU, Duun P, Kehlet H: Prediction of postoperative pain by preoperative nociceptive responses to heat stimulation. Anesthesiology 2004;100:115–119.

72. Reuben S: Preventing the development of complex regional pain syndrome after surgery. Anesthesiology 2004;101:1215–1224.

INDEX

Note: Page numbers followed by f, t, and b indicate figures, tables, and boxes, respectively.

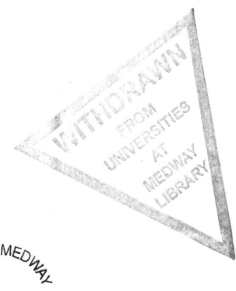